Pharmacology Review
SECOND EDITION

for MEDICAL STUDENTS

Clear ▪ Concepts
Student ▪ Centered
Memory ▪ Coded
Coherent and ▪ Concise
Coverage ▪ Complete
Simply ▪ Comprehensive

Pharmacology Review
Second Edition

Author: Dr S R Saif MBBS, MD, DCP, Registrar
Editor in chief: Dr M. Haider MD, JNMCH, AMU
Assistant Editors: Dr Zafar Niyaz MBBS, JNMCH, AMU, AIIMS and PGI Topper in PG Entrance
Dr Abrar MD (Cardiology), Grenada School of Medicine, New York
Dr Farrukh Siddique MD, Howard School of Medicine, Boston
Project Editor: Dr Mohd. Suhail MD, Chief Consultant, Muh. Medical Complex, Bahren
Art Editors: Dr Asim Suhail MBBS, USA
Dr Shahbaz Suhail
Dr Mehtab
Managing Editor: Dr Jahangir Warsi Ph.D, Lecturer, Michigan University
Compilation Editors: Dr Saif MBBS, JNMCH, AMU
Dr Zia Hashim MD (Medicine), PGI
Y N Arjuna Senior Vice President—Publishing, Editorial and Publicity, CBSP&D
Dr Zainab Z Rahman BDS, Rajiv Gandhi University of Health Science

Pharmacology Review

SECOND EDITION

for MEDICAL STUDENTS

S R Saif MBBS, MD, DCP

JN Medical College and Hospital
Aligarh Muslim University
Aligarh, UP (India)

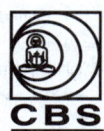

CBS Publishers & Distributors Pvt Ltd

New Delhi • Bengaluru • Chennai • Kochi • Mumbai • Pune
Hyderabad • Kolkata • Nagpur • Patna • Vijayawada

> *Disclaimer*
> Science and technology are constantly changing fields. New research and experience broaden the scope of information and knowledge. The author has tried his best in giving information available to him while preparing the material for this book. Although, all efforts have been made to ensure optimum accuracy of the material, yet it is quite possible some errors might have been left uncorrected. The publisher, the printer and the author will not be held responsible for any inadvertent errors, or inaccuracies.

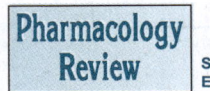

ISBN: 978-81-239-2473-1

Copyright © Author and Publisher

Second Edition: 2015
First Edition: 2005
Reprint: 2006, 2007, 2008, 2010, 2014

All rights reserved. No part of this book may be reproduced or transmitted in any form or by any means, electronic or mechanical, including photocopying, recording, or any information storage and retrieval system without permission, in writing, from the author and the publisher.

Published by Satish Kumar Jain and produced by Varun Jain for
CBS Publishers & Distributors Pvt Ltd
4819/XI Prahlad Street, 24 Ansari Road, Daryaganj, New Delhi 110 002, India.
Ph: 23289259, 23266861, 23266867   Website: www.cbspd.com
Fax: 011-23243014   e-mail: delhi@cbspd.com; cbspubs@airtelmail.in.
Corporate Office: 204 FIE, Industrial Area, Patparganj, Delhi 110 092
Ph: 4934 4934   Fax: 4934 4935   e-mail: publishing@cbspd.com; publicity@cbspd.com

Branches

- **Bengaluru:** Seema House 2975, 17th Cross, K.R. Road, Banasankari 2nd Stage, Bengaluru 560 070, Karnataka
  Ph: +91-80-26771678/79   Fax: +91-80-26771680   e-mail: bangalore@cbspd.com

- **Chennai:** 7, Subbaraya Street, Shenoy Nagar, Chennai 600 030, Tamil Nadu
  Ph: +91-44-26260666, 26208620   Fax: +91-44-42032115   e-mail: chennai@cbspd.com

- **Kochi:** Ashana House, No. 39/1904, A.M. Thomas Road, Valanjambalam, Ernakulam 682016, Kochi, Kerala
  Ph: +91-484-4059061-65, 67   Fax: +91-484-4059065   e-mail: kochi@cbspd.com

- **Mumbai:** 83-C, Dr E Moses Road, Worli, Mumbai-400018, Maharashtra
  Ph: +91-22-24902340/41   Fax: +91-22-24902342   e-mail: mumbai@cbspd.com

- **Pune:** Bhuruk Prestige, Sr. No. 52/12/2+1+3/2 Narhe, Haveli (Near Katraj-Dehu Road Bypass), Pune 411 041, Maharashtra
  Ph: +91-20-64704058, 64704059, 32392277   Fax: +91-20-24300160   e-mail: pune@cbspd.com

Representatives

- **Hyderabad** 0-9885175004
- **Nagpur** 0-9021734563
- **Vijayawada** 0-9000660880
- **Kolkata** 0-9831437309, 0-9051152362
- **Patna** 0-9334159540

Printed at: Shree Maitrey Printech Pvt. Ltd., Noida

*to help
all the doctors in providing
the best service in the world,*

*to make
India the best country on Earth*

and

*to make
Earth the best place under the sky*

This noble work is dedicated to the real service in alleviation of pain of the world by:

All the honest and dedicated scientists/ministers/secretaries/academicians/administrators/entrepreneurs/bureaucrats of India/world of past and present equally.

Azad Hind Fauj, All Freedom Fighters (known/unknown), Qurbaan Ali (exiled for life to Kalapani punishment by C.G. Atkin), Dr BR Ambedkar, Maulana Abul Kalam Azad, MK Gandhi, Namak Satya Gareh of Garhpura, Babur/Akbar/Ashoka/Chanakya/Aryabhat; President of India (Dr Rajendra Prasad, Fakhruddin A Ahmed, RV Raman, Dr Zakir Husain, APJ Abdul Kalam); Maulana Wali Rahmani, Dr M Rahman (Ex-VC AMU, IAS), Mother Teressa, Sarojini Naidu, A B Vajpayee, Rabindranath Tagore, Sir Allama Iqbal, BC Chaterji, Maharana Pratap, Kaader Khan, CV Raman, AR Rahman, Javed Akhtar, Barack Obama, Azim Premji, MGR, Jamshedji Tata, Mohd Yunus (Gramin Bank), the first CM of Bihar Mohammad Yunus; Ali Vardi Khan, Sir Syed Ahmed Khan, Prof Noorul Hasan (Education Minister), A A Fatmi (Ex-MoS, MHRD), Md Hanif Uddin (Madrasa Hanifia), Abdul Hameed, Bill Gates, Thomas Babington Macaulay (Jumrati & Sanichra for salary of teachers in Indian System of Education evolved), the first patriotic leader against British imperialism, Bahadur Shah Zafar, caretaker of Akbar in Mithila—Darbhanga Raj of MP.

Teachings and guidance of Guru Nanak, Gautam Budh, Bhavishya Puran (Verse 5) & Sama Veda (II, 6, 8), Moses, Jesus Christ, Ibrahim, Arabian Culture & Civilization, Hazrat Deewan Mohd Saadiq Ashraf (Rah), Shah Nasrullah (Reh), Khwaja Moinuddin Chisti (Reh), Khwaja Salim Chisti (Reh), Maulana Husain A Madni (Reh), Hazrat Nizamuddin (Reh), K Bandanawaz (Reh) and the great contribution of Royal Charter/Farman-E-Shahi of Akbar (Az-Gung-Ta-Sang-Az-Kosi-Ta-Dhosi) for Choudhry Hafiz Ali (Royal Teacher) and Choudhry Farid (Commander) of Jounpur now in Pehlam.

Founder of Internationally Acclaimed Ancient Universities of India (Vikramshila of Bhagalpur, Takhshila of Pakistan, Nalanda of Gaya, Madrasa of Bider & Culcutta), Shabarmati Ashram, Darul Oloom (Deoband), Jamiat Ulema Hind, Jamia Al-Azhar, Imaarat Shariah, Shibli College/Ghalib College/Maulana Azad College/Islamia Higher Secondary, Jamia Millia Islamia/Jamia Hamdard/MANUU/Osmania University/Alia University/Integral University/Al-Amin, Madrsatuloloom (Delhi), State's Madrasa Tuloloom (JUH, Bihar), All Jamia/Madaris, All Mobile Madaris (Tabligh); All true followers of fantastic hero Prophet Mohammed Saw, All noble works and beautiful minds of India/world in science/technology, literature and other education arena for the vertical progress of the nation/world so as to convert developing India into developed India, to make India the best country in the world and to make this world the best place under the sky, after all to complete the mission of the global brotherhood within global family as politics is the greatest global threat in making of the finest painless world and the only reason to destroy mankind but the solution of all issues rests in honesty.

Jai Bharat, Jai Hind: Jamia Urdu Hind.

Jo abr yahan se uthega
Sare jahaan par barsega
Ye abr hamesha barsa hai
Ye abr hamesha barsega

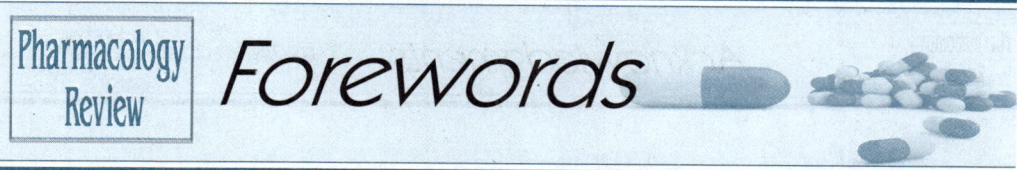

Forewords

The material presented in this book has been collected from valuable sources, compiled in a systematic arrangement, and is of value for easy revision for various examinations and as a basic need to prepare for class tests or professional examinations.

Chairman
Department of Pharmacology
JNMC, AMU
Aligarh

Writing the Foreword to a book conceived by an MBBS is a matter of my pleasure who felt the need for a book on pharmacology which is comprehensive and concise with state-of-the-art information on drugs to fulfil basic needs of all students preparing for various competitive examinations or for quick revision of the subject before the professional examination.

Targeted readers will derive the maximum benefit from this publication and help the author with comments and suggestions which will be well appreciated and suitably acknowledged.

Dr Md M Hyder
Aligarh

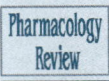 

Acknowledgments

When emotions are profound, words may not be sufficient to express thanks and gratitude. The wisdom, commitment and effort of many people made me transform this idea of my dream into a book.

Many people provided me valuable contributions and gave helpful comments. People worldover enjoy growing flowers, but only a few realize that one can grow a garden that will tell the time of the day.

My special thanks go to Mr SK Jain, Chairman and Managing Director, and Mr YN Arjuna, Senior Vice President—Publishing, Editorial and Publicity, CBSP&D, for their cooperation and direction at each and every step of publication.

I am thankful to Mr Karzan Lal Parashar for pagination, Mr Neeraj Prasad for cover design and Mr Anand Mohanty for proofreading the text.

I am sincerely indebted to Dr KC Singhal, Dr Shadab, Dr Shakeel, Dr Shah Farhan, Dr Suhail, Dr Shharyar, Dr Sarfraz, Dr Imteyaz, Dr Irshad, Dr Ekram, Dr Yasrab, Dr Yusuf, Dr Fazal, Dr Faraz, Dr Naseem Nizami, Dr Feroz, Dr Asif, Dr Javed, Dr Jubair and Dr Jamshed (Begusarai), Dr Anis, Dr Faiz, Dr Pervez, Dr Hifzur, Dr Mojahid, Dr Tauheed, Dr Tufail, Dr Arif and Dr Tazeen, Mohd Mustafa, MA, AMU; Prof Mohibul Haque, F/o Arts, AMU; Masoom Ali Sarwar, IAS; Gulam Ali, IAS; Syed Sabahat Husain, IAS; SL Dhani, IAS; Gudrun Nehar, IAS; teaching staff of Islamia Higher Secondary, Kasturba Vidyalaya, Siddiqa Girls High School and Middle School, Jamia Urdu Hind, Madrasa Hanifia for their help and guidance.

We are also thankful to the institutions, colleges, societies, trusts, etc. which have promoted our books and study materials (JUH) honestly:

Tamil Nadu Office: LR Sekar (B. TECH), MD, Ram Open School; JB Singaravel, Edisons Institute of Higher Studies, Britannia, Padi; TR Kavitha, JJSK Open School, Masthan Palli Street, Mannargudi; P Suresh KP, Suresh Open School, Dharmapuri; C. Vanitha, Annamalai Open School, Trichy Main Road, Dadagapatti Gate, Salem; Agniprava Open School, Madipakkam; Vesta Open School, Vesta Educational & Charitable Trust, Pallivasal Street, Puddukotti; Modern Open School, No: 1-A, Royal Nagar, Karunbu Kadai, Coimbatore; Stella Rani Open School, 16/9, 4th Cross, 5th Street, Kodungaiyur.

Punjab Office: Harkrishna Institute, Pakho Kalan, Barnala, Punjab.

Kashmir Office: Children and Women Welfare Society, Budgam, JK.

Bangalore Office: AI of Management and Technology Science, Bangalore.

Jewargi Office: S Poojari, Kanakashri Vidyapeeth, New Jewargi Road, Gulbarga.

Moulana Abul Kalam Azad Education and Charitable Welfare Society (R), Shahabaz Colony;

JN Education & Welfare Trust, Sharan, Nagar, Aland.

Hyderabad Office: NCI Academy, Nalgonda X Road, Malakpet, Hyderabad.

Mungeli Office: CG Council of School and Professional Education, Lormi, Mungeli, Chattisgarh.

Thiruvallur Office: Annai Saraswathi Educational and Research Trust, GNT Road, Thiruvallur.

West Bengal Office: Rabindra Education Centre, Bansdroni Rabindra Educational & Welfare Trust.

Dindigul Office: AA Jegan, AVNM Trust, Anna Nagar, Batiagundu, Dindigul.

Pondicherry Office: W R T Suresh, SRCC, Pondicherry.

Kharagpur Office: EIHS Educational Consultant Pvt Ltd, Jafala Road, Inda.

Avalur Office: Hafsa Open College, 7/82 Mosque Street, Avalur Pet; Annai Saraswathi Educational and Research Trust; Jayam Open School, Market Road; SRI Arunai Educational Trust; V. Murugan, Pooja Ashri Correspondence College, Mathalankulam Street, Tiruvannamalai.

Madras Office: Agniprava Open School, Madipakkam, Madras.

Secunderabad Office: MAA Tabrez, T.S. College of Tahera Sttar Educational Society, Ramnagar.

Kerala Office: S.R. Community College, Court Road, Alathur, Palakkad, Kerala; Ramesh K, Calicut, Kerala; Satheesh R, MIMS Marhaba Building, Ottapalam, Palakkad; Vinod TK, KIMS, Pollachi; Aiswaria KG, SRC College, Archana Business Centre, SRE Trust, Palakkad; Suresh BK, SR Community College, Mangalore; Unnikrishnan V, Sree Vinayaka Education, Sulur, Coimbatore; Vinod V, Sree Institute of Technology, Ernakulam; Abdul Nasar AA, Baron College IT, Thrissur, Kerala.

Assam Office: SSEC, Jana Kalyan High School, Tumni, Dhubri.

Karnataka Office: RJ Noble Educational Academy.

Chittor Office: Sai Yogesh Study Circle, John Complex, Opp ICICI Bank, Readspet.

Pondichery Office: Parthasarthi, AIMS Academy.

Shantiniketan Office: BIHM, Shantiniketan, Pravat Sarani, Bolpur, Birbhum, WB.

Madurai Office: Kings Academy, Park Road, Agarwal Eye Hospital, Arapalayam, Madurai.

Madras Office: MIOS, Radha Nagar, Main Road, Chrompet, Chennai.

Rajarajan Academy: Karuneegar Street, Adambakkam, Chennai.

Board of Madrasa Educational Society: Dr KM Ansar Ali, BMES, Karuneegar Street, Adambakkam.

Pune Office: R Kalsekar (Journalist), Mahad, Raigarh, Maharashtra.

Dr S R Saif

Pharmacology Review — *Preface*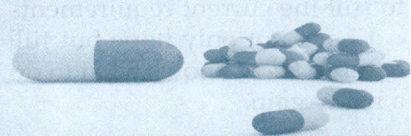

Though the deepest feelings are expressed by the sound of silence itself, it is my heart which is beating through these lines. The deepest truth is the simplest and the commonest. The most important thing in this world is not so much where we stand but in which direction are we going? If you think you can, you definitely can! Hence, try to achieve what you like, otherwise you have to like what you have achieved. What is it after all that turned an average person into a marvelous performer? If you do not, you have achieved half your failure. Therefore be firm with your goal but remain flexible with your approach. Destiny is not a matter of chance, it is a matter of choice. It is not a thing to be waited for, it is a thing to be achieved. Toppers do not do different things but they do the things differently.

What is your aim? Gaining command on the prescribed syllabus of the entrance/professional examinations or getting success in various examinations. Though both the aims look similar, it is not so. Success is achieved mainly due to *intelligence* and *technique of study*. This book is *technique of study*-oriented providing state-of-the-art information on drugs. I have focussed to make things better not bigger, thinking that if a little knowledge is dangerous, where is the man who has so much as to be out of danger. This review aims at providing state-of-the-art information on drugs and useful guidance to people concerned with various tests. Specialities of the review are that it is simple, precise, concise, complete, comprehensive, coherent, examination-oriented, coded and student-centered with the most recent information on drugs, including clinical pharmacology made amazingly simple with high-yield subject materials.

Flow charts and diagrams have been given to depict very important summary of the topics. The boxes have memory codes and important information of the text, which indeed is a very interesting part of the book.

Codes are relevant and serve as mnemonics (very easy to remember), e.g. code for side effects of METHYLDOPA.

M	Mental retardation,
E	Electrolyte imbalance,
T	Tolerance,
H	Hepatotoxicity and headache,
Y	'Yesness'—nodding due to parkinsonism,
L	Lactation in females,
D	Dry mouth,
O	Oedema,
P	Psychological upset, and
A	Anaemia (haemolytic).

The second edition of the book has been thoroughly revised, updated and enlarged to suit the current requirements of the students.

I have not only hope but full confidence that you will enjoy reading this book because *talent* knows what to do, *tact* knows how to do. Talent grows to gain, tact is a ready gain.

S R Saif MBBS, MD, DCP

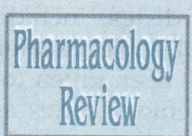

Pharmacology Review

FOR MEDICAL STUDENTS

presents simple, precise, coherent, concise, complete, comprehensive, coded, examination-oriented, student-centered with the state-of-the-art information on drugs and clinical pharmacology made amazingly simple with high-yield subject materials.

Pharmacology Review
Contents

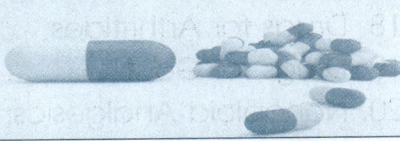

Forewords — vii
Preface — ix

Unit 1 — Introduction to Pharmacology

1. Definitions and Routes — 1
2. Pharmacokinetics — 6
3. Pharmacodynamics — 21
4. Adverse Effects — 33

Unit 2 — Drugs Acting on Nervous System

5. An Overview of Nervous System — 38
6. Cholinergic and Anticholinergic Drugs — 49
7. Adrenergic Drugs — 64
8. Antiadrenergic Drugs — 75
9. Drugs for Somatic Nervous System: Skeletal Muscle Relaxants — 87
10. Anaesthesias—General and Local — 94
11. Sedative-Hypnotics — 156
12. Anti-Seizure Drugs — 171
13. Alcohol — 179
14. Drugs for Mental Illness: Psychotropic Drugs, Psychopharmacological Agents — 185
15. CNS Stimulants, Cognition Enhancers, Hallucinogens and Psychostimulants — 201
16. Analgesics (Opioid) — 233

17. Antiparkinsonian Drugs — *243*
18. Drugs for Arthritides — *251*
19. Drugs for Gout — *255*
20. Nonopioid Analgesics: NSAIDs — *259*

Unit 3 — Hormones

21. An Overview of Hormones — *276*
22. Growth Hormone, Prolactin and Somatostatin — *282*
23. Gonadal Hormones — *286*
24. Hormonal Contraceptives — *303*
25. Drugs for Uterus — *308*
26. Drugs Acting on Thyroid Gland — *311*
27. Drugs Affecting Calcium Metabolism — *324*
28. Corticoids or Corticosteroids — *329*
29. Drugs for Glucose Metabolism — *338*

Unit 4 — Drugs Acting on CVS

30. An Overview of CVS — *354*
31. Cardiac Glycosides/Digitalis — *365*
32. Antiarrhythmic, Antianginal and Antihypertensive Drugs — *374*

Unit 5 — Drugs for Kidney

33. An Overview of Kidney — *412*
34. Diuretics — *416*
35. Antidiuretics — *432*

Unit 6 — Autacoids and Related Drugs

36. ACE Inhibitors — *436*
37. Antihistaminics — *448*
38. Drugs Related to 5-Hydroxytryptamine System — *457*
39. Platelet Activating Factor, Prostaglandins and Leukotrienes — *467*

Unit 7 — Drugs Affecting Blood

40. Drugs Affecting Coagulation, Bleeding and Thrombosis — 474
41. Fibrinolytic/Thrombolytic, Antifibrinolytic, Antithrombolytic, Antiplatelet Drugs — 488
42. Drugs for Hyperlipidemia — 498
43. Plasma Expanders — 509

Unit 8 — GIT Related Drugs

44. Drugs for Peptic Ulcer — 513
45. Emetics, Antiemetics, Digestants, Carminatives and Gallstone Dissolving Drugs — 525
46. Drugs for Constipation and Diarrhoea — 533

Unit 9 — Respiratory System

47. Drugs for Respiratory System — 543

Unit 10 — Antimicrobial Agents

48. Principles of Chemotherapy — 553
49. β-Lactam Antibiotics — 564
50. Tetracycline — 575
51. Chloramphenicol — 579
52. Aminoglycosides — 582
53. Macrolide and Other Antibiotics — 586
54. Sulfonamides and Cotrimoxazole (Bactrim) — 593
55. Quinolones and Fluoroquinolones — 598
56. Antitubercular and Antileprotic Drugs — 604
57. Antimalarial Drugs — 614
58. Antiprotozoal Agents — 623
59. Antifungal Agents — 629
60. Anthelmintics — 637
61. Antiviral Drugs — 647

Unit 11 — Chemotherapy

62. Anticancer Drugs, Immunosuppressants and Gene Therapy — 663

Unit 12 — Drugs for Community Medicine

63. Anaemia — 687
64. Poisoning and Antidotes — 694
65. Vaccines, Serum, Immunoglobulins, Immunopharmacology — 701
66. Dermatologic Pharmacology — 709
67. Vitamins — 717

Unit 13 — Classification of Drugs and Adverse Drug Reactions

68. Classification of Drugs (COD) — 737
69. Adverse Drug Reactions (ADR) — 770

Unit 14 — Newer Drugs and Drugs of Choice

70. Newer Drugs and their Uses — 784
71. Drugs of Choice (DOC) — 790

Index — 821

Pharmacology Review

for MEDICAL STUDENTS

In addition to MBBS and BDS students, this edition of the book also targets

candidates appearing in examinations like USMLE, PLAB, MD, MS, MLT, BPT, First-Aid (MMHW, Community Health of NIOS and IGNOU)

students pursuing courses in nursing, AIDS and human rights, sports and exercise medicine

all those aspiring to be medical representatives

all practising doctors/clinicians

and all students of allied and alternative systems of medicine.

*Whenever the history of all discoveries,
events and inventions of all times will be written,
the serendipity of penicillin and
the first demonstration of anaesthetic property of ether
for the painless surgery will be placed at the top
along with the other great discoveries, events and inventions.*

Unit 1
Introduction to Pharmacology

1
Definitions and Routes

Pharmacology is the branch of science that deals with drugs and their effective and safe use (most important purpose).

Drug is the "substance used to modify physiological or pathological states for the benefit of recipient." It is the single chemical substance that forms active ingredient of medicine (WHO 1966).

Poisons in small doses are the best medicines and useful medicines in too large doses are poisonous (**W**illiam **W**ithering, **d**iscoverer of **d**igitalis, 1789).

Medicine is an art founded on conjecture and improved by murder. Medicine in the hands of a fool is poison just as poison becomes medicine in the hands of the wise. (However, where safety and cure are concerned, expense and risk are no object.)

Homeopathy is a system of medicine founded by Christian Friedrich Samuel Hahnemann, a German physician (1755–1843).

> **Hippocrates**, the greatest physician in Greek medicine, is called "father of medicine".
> The early leader of Greek medicine was **Aesculapius** who bore two daughters:
>   A. **Panacea**, and
>   B. **Hygiea** (the goddess of health in Greek mythology).
> Discoverer of **yoga** method of treatment was **Patanjali**. The medical systems of truly Indian origin and development are **Ayurveda** and **Siddha**. **Dhanvantari** is the Hindu god of medicine. **Atreya** (about 800 BC) is acknowledged as the first great Indian physician and teacher. **Susruta** is called "father of Indian surgery".

Pharmacodynamics: What the drug does to the body.

For example, Adrenaline → Adrenoceptors
↓
Activates adenylcyclase
↓
↑ Intracellular cyclic 3'5-AMP
↓
Cardiac stimulation

> **Pharmacodynamics** is a description of the properties of drug receptor interaction, i.e. mechanism of drug actions.

Pharmacology Review

Pharmacokinetics: What the body does to the drug. It includes movement and alteration of drugs (absorption, binding, storage, distribution, biotransformation and excretion).

Pharmaceutics: It is the large scale manufacture of the drugs.

Pharmacotherapeutics: Application of pharmacodynamic information and knowledge of diseases for their prevention and cure.

Clinical Pharmacology: The scientific study of drugs in man. Its aim is to generate data for optimum use of drugs.

Drugs are of two types
1. **Chemotherapeutic agents** inhibit/kill parasite or cancer cells with minimum adverse drug reaction (ADR).
2. **Pharmacodynamic agents** have pharmacodynamic effects.

Pharmacy is the art and science of compounding and dispensing a drug for its administration. It includes identification, collection, purification, isolation, synthesis, standardization and quality control.

Toxicology is the study of poisonous effects of drugs and other chemicals to detect, prevent and treat.

Drug nomenclature has three categories of names:

Approved name
Brand name
Chemical and code name

ABC

1. **Proprietary/brand/trade name** is the name assigned by its manufacturer.
2. **Non-proprietary/generic/approved name** is the name accepted by a competent scientific body by international agreement through WHO. It is called **official name** after its appearance in the official publication.
3. **Chemical and code name.**

Drug Development and Testing

In vitro study	Animal testing	Clinical testing (phase 1, 2, 3)	Marketing (phase 4)	Availability
Biological product ↓ Lead compound ↑ Chemical synthesis	Efficacy Selectivity and mechanism	Drug metabolism and safety assessment	Post-marketing surveillance	Generics become available
→	→	→	→	
0 yr	2 yr	4 yr (investigational new drug)	8 yr (new drug application)	20 yr

Drug Names

Ending with	Category	Example
– ane	GA	Halothane
– azepam	BZD	Diazepam
– azine	Phenothaizine	CPZ
– azole	Antifungal	KTZ
– barbital	Barbiturate	Phenobarbital
– caine	LA	Lidocaine
– cainide	Antiarrhythmic	Flecainide
– cillin	Penicillin	Methicillin
– cycline	Antibiotic	Tetracycline
– ipramine	TCA	Imipramine
– ol	Beta-agonist	Isoproterenol
– olol	Beta-blocker	Propranolol
– operidol	Butyrophenone	Haloperidol
– oxin	Cardiac glycoside	Digoxin
– phylline	Methylxanthine	Theophylline
– pril	ACE inhibitor	Captopril
– relin	GnRH	Buserelin
– rinone	Antiarrhythmic	Amrinone
– terol	Beta-2 agonist	Albuterol
– tidine	H_2 blocker	Cimetidine
– triptyline	TCA	Amitriptyline
– tropin	Pituitary hormone	Somatotropin
– zosin	Alpha-blocker	Prazosin

Essential drugs are drugs satisfying the health care needs of majority of population available in adequate amounts and appropriate dosage forms at all times.

National drug list of India (1996) includes **279 drugs.**

Orphan drugs are the drugs which are not developed into usable medicine because the **cost** will not be recovered by the developer. These drugs are for diagnosis, prevention, treatment of rare diseases, without the expectation of cost of developing and marketing from the sales.

For example
- **B**aclofen
- **A**cetyl cysteine   BAD Drug
- **D**esmopressin, **D**igoxin **A**b **F**ab

Methazolamide, Ethoxzolamide and Dichlorphenamide MEDicine are obsolete diuretics. Thiazide is the most widely used diuretic. Bumetanide is Bigger in potency than furosemide.

Factors Governing Choice of Routes

1. Site of desired action.
2. Chemical and physical properties (solubility, stability, pH, irritancy, solid/liquid/gas).

Pharmacology Review

3. Route and extent of absorption.
4. Effect of digestive juices and first pass metabolism.
5. Patient's condition.
6. Dosage accuracy.
7. Rapidity.

Routes are of 2 types:
1. Local.
2. Systemic.

Local routes:
1. Topical (skin, mucous membrane).
2. Deeper tissues (intrathecal injection of AMB, lidocaine).
3. Arterial supply (anticancer drug infused in femoral and brachial artery for limb malignancies).

Systemic routes: Drugs are absorbed into the blood to be distributed all over the body through circulation.

1. **Oral** (oldest and commonest)
   Limitations:
   - Slower action.
   - Emetive (nausea and vomiting).
   - Some drugs are not absorbed (streptomycin).

Graphs of Various Routes

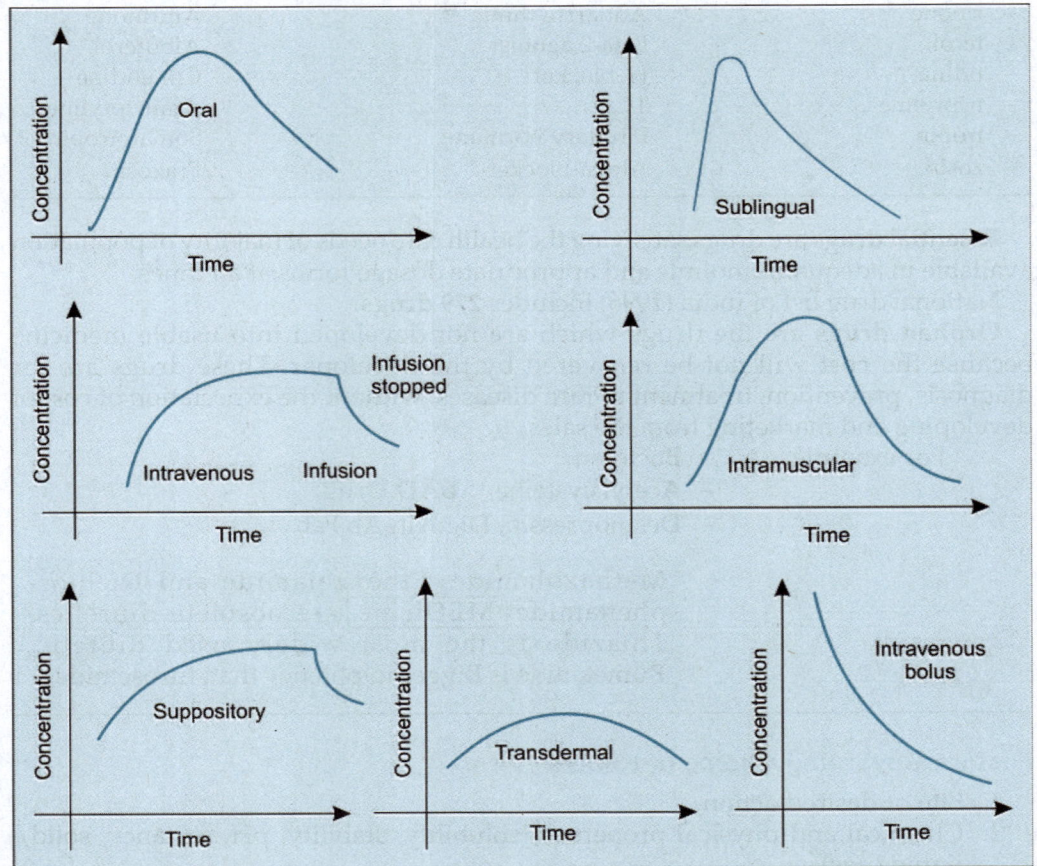

- Not used in uncooperative, unconscious, or vomiting patients.
- Destroyed by digestive juices (penicillin G, insulin) or liver (GTN, lidocaine, testosterone).

2. **Cutaneous** (highly lipid soluble drugs).

Transdermal therapeutic system (TTS): "This is a device to deliver drug into circulation at a constant rate via stratum corneum". The micropore membrane of TTS controls drug delivery rate which is less than **the slowest rate** of absorption from skin. TTS of GTN and estradiol is lasting **1–7 days** (available in India). Thickness of adhesive patches (TTS) is **0.2–0.4 mm.**

Advantage: Smooth plasma concentration of drug. Less ADR and first pass metabolism.

3. **Buccal/sublingual** and rectal routes bypass first pass metabolism and do not go through liver.
   - For lipid soluble and nonirritating drugs.
   - Taken under the tongue or crushed in the mouth, e.g. GTN.
4. **Rectal:** Irritant and unpleasant drugs in recurrent vomiting, etc.
5. **Inhalational:** GA, etc. → alveoli → rapid action.
6. **Nasal**
7. **Parenteral** (par = beyond, enteral = intestinal).

Use: In emergencies.

Disadvantages:
- Costlier.
- Painful/necrosis.
- Assistance needed (but self-injection is given in DM).

(a) **SC** (subcutaneous):
- More nerve involved.
- Less vessel involved.

(b) **IM** (intramuscular):
- Less nerve involved.
- More vessel involved.

(c) **Intradermal:**

(Drugs of **MW 100–1000** are **best** suited for absorption and distribution in the body)

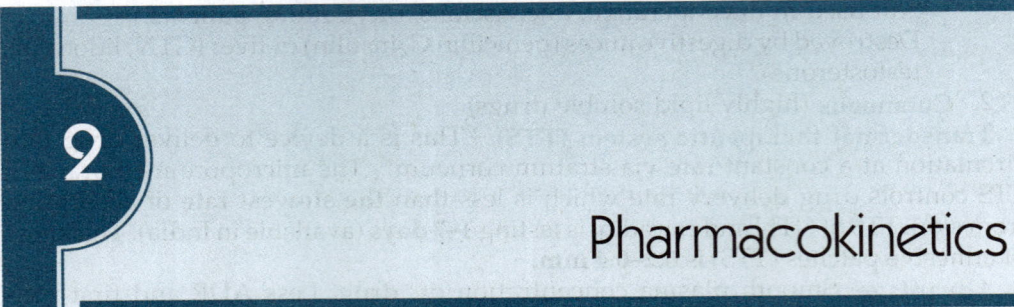

2. Pharmacokinetics

Pharmacokinetics (*pharmakon* = drug, *kinetics* = movement) is the quantitative study of the movement of drugs into and out of the body and includes uptake, distribution, biotransformation and elimination.

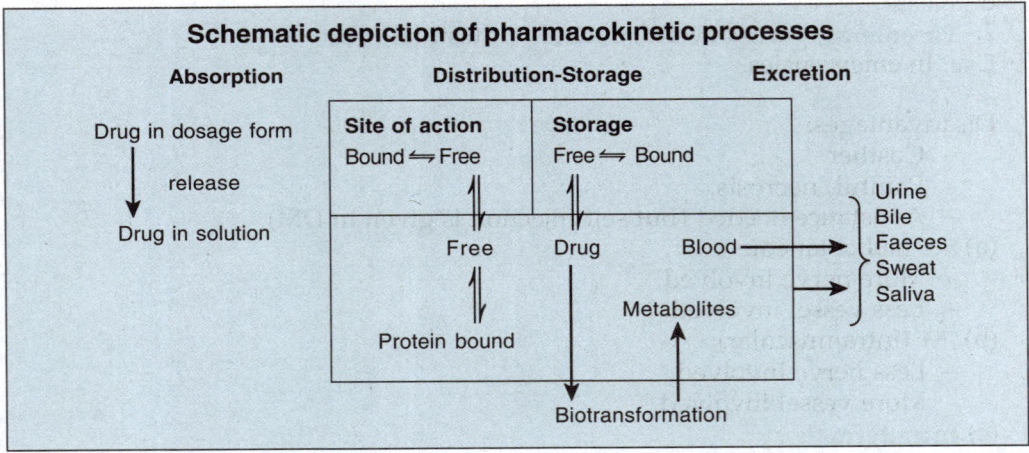

- It includes 4 processes: **M**etabolism, **A**bsorption, **D**istribution, **E**xcretion.

      MADE

- It entails clearance, distribution, volume, bioavailability.
- It determines dose, latency of onset, duration of action, time of peak action.
- All pharmacokinetic processes involve drug transport across biological membrane (thickness **100Å** bilayer).

Drug transports take place in the following ways:
1. **Passive diffusion.**
2. **Filtration.**
3. **Specialized transport.**

Passive diffusion: Most important and active role of the membrane is absent. **Strong electrolytes** are completely ionised at acidic and alkaline pH. But **most drugs** are weak electrolytes and their ionisation are **pH-dependent. Acidic drugs** are mainly unionised at pH of gastric acid, hence absorbed from the stomach and converted to ionised form within cell (pH 7) and slowly passed to ECF (ion trapping).

Basic drugs are mainly ionised at gastric pH and hence absorbed only from intestine on reaching, and attain higher concentration, intracellularly. Diffusion of non-ionised form of weak acid and weak base occurs through lipid membrane. Ionised drug → lipid insoluble → nondiffusible.

Lipid soluble unionised drug is reabsorbed and ionised lipid insoluble drug is excreted in urine. The former is pH independent and transport rate is directly proportional to lipid water partition coefficient of drug.

Biggest changes in the amount of ionised and nonionised form of drugs occur near pKa, with pH changes. At low pH in stomach, most weak acids are unionised and hence absorbed but weak bases are poorly absorbed due to ionisation. Ion trapping occurs with weak acids and weak bases due to pH difference on both sides of membrane. Ionised form is trapped on one side of the membrane (weak base on the side with lower pH and weak acid on the side with higher pH). At equilibrium, unionised concentration on both sides of membrane is equal.

Most drugs are unionised having high lipid solubility (related to O-W partition coefficient) and cross the membrane. Ionised drugs have low lipid solubility.

For weak acid, $pKa = pH + \log \frac{[\text{unionised}]}{[\text{ionised}]}$

Henderson-Hasselbalch equation for weak base,

$pKa = pH + \log \frac{[\text{ionised}]}{[\text{unionised}]}$

If pH = pKa, 50% is ionised and 50% is unionised.

Intestinal mucosa and RBC have small pores (4Å) and drugs with MW 100–200 are unable to penetrate. Capillaries (except those in brain which have tight junction) have large pore (40Å) and most drugs filter through it. Substances transferring ions across membrane are called ionophores.

Filtration: It is the passage of drugs through aqueous pores in the membrane. Capillaries with pores (40Å) filter most drugs, and depend on blood flow rate.

Specialized transports: They are: (1) Carrier mediated (active transport with energy needs, facilitated with no energy need). In active transport, excretion occurs in PCT. (2) Pinocytosis (process of transport across cell membrane by vesicles formation).

Absorption: (movement of drugs from its administration site into circulation). It is fast hence ignored in kinetic calculation.

- Most drugs are absorbed better when taken in empty stomach.
- Drugs have to cross membrane except when given IV.
- It depends on solubility, concentration, blood flow, routes, etc.
- It is increased by heat and exercise.
- Order of speed of absorption among different routes IM > SC > oral.

- Basic drugs are **best** absorbed from small intestine.
- **A**nticholinergic, **T**CA, **O**pioid, **M**etoclopramide alter gut wall motility. Methotrexate, neomycin, vinblastine damage mucosa.   **ATOM**
- Topical absorption depends on lipid solubility.
- **Penicillin** is destroyed by **acid** and **insulin** is destroyed by **peptidase** (orally ineffective).
- **Hyaluronidase** promotes spread and facilitates **subcutaneous absorption**.
- GTN, Clonidine, estradiol, and Hyoscine penetrate intact skin.   **HCG**
- **Corticosteroid** applied extensively on skin may produce pituitary-adrenal suppression.
- **Organophosphorus** compound coming in contact with skin produces systemic toxicity.
- Estrogen used locally in vagina can cause **gynaecomastia** in male partner.
- **Cornea** is permeable to **lipophilic** drug, e.g. physostigmine but not neostigmine.

Bioavailability (F): It is the rate and extent of drug absorption from dosage form/ unchanged form. It is **increased** in hepatic disease when drug is taken orally.

- Oral formulation of drug has same amount **(chemical equivalence)** but does not produce same blood level **(biological inequivalence)**. Small particle size increases absorption. Tablets and capsules may have diluents, binders, lubricants, stabilizing agents, etc.

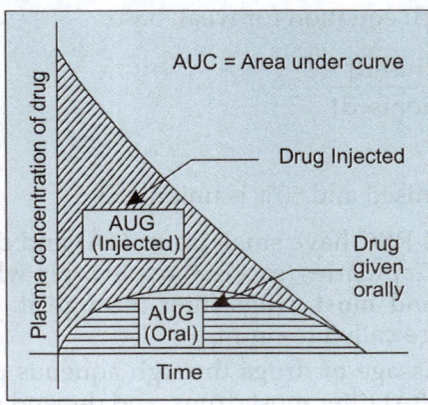

F = fraction of administered drug that reaches the systemic circulation.

$$F = \frac{AUC\ oral}{AUC\ injection} \times 100$$

It depends on:
1. Disintegration of a tablet.
2. Dissolution in the intestine.
3. First pass metabolism.
   - **Bioequivalence** occurs when drugs with equal F have same drug concentration versus time relationship.

Pharmacokinetics

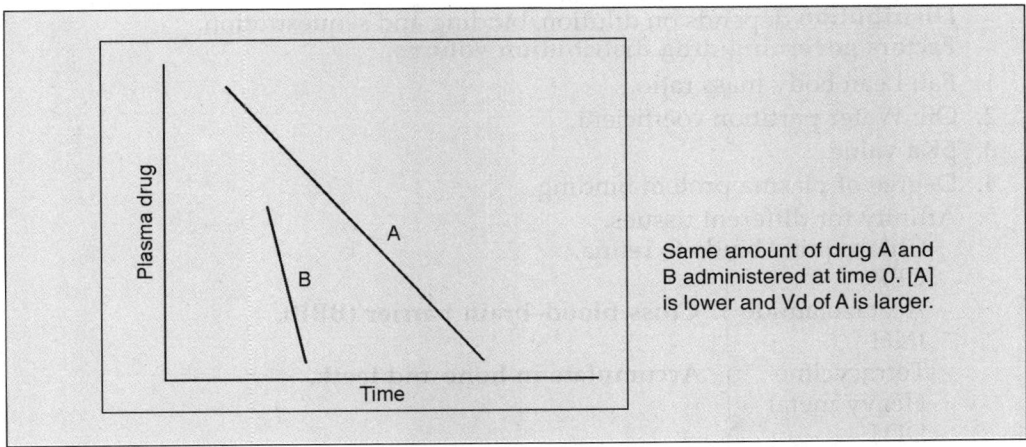

Same amount of drug A and B administered at time 0. [A] is lower and Vd of A is larger.

Distribution: Initial distribution of drugs depends on blood flow.

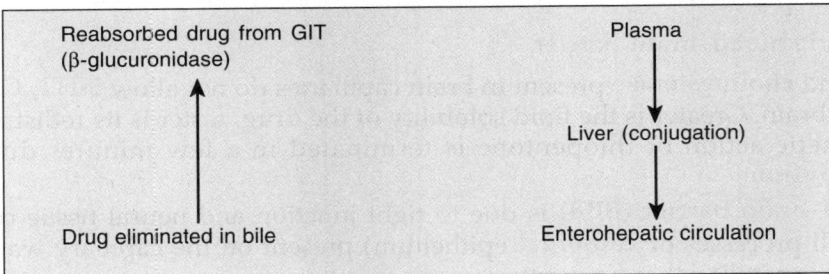

Apparent volume of distribution/final distribution (Vd) depends on lipid solubility, plasma protein binding and tissue binding. Drug metabolites have smaller Vd.

$$Vd = \frac{\text{Dose administration IV}}{\text{Plasma concentration}}$$

i.e. volume accommodating all drugs in the body with **same concentration throughout as in plasma**. Its Vd is larger →serum concentration is lower.

Distribution of drugs acts as a **reservoir** and only unbound drugs activate receptors. Bindings **slow** the onset of action and **prolong** the duration of action if eliminated in urine.

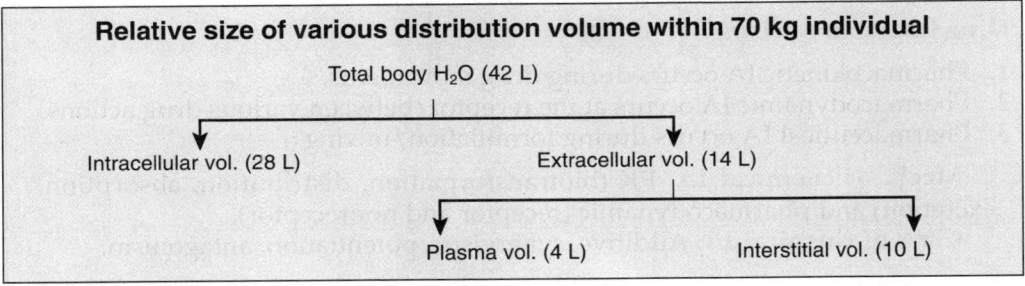

- Distribution depends on dilution, binding and sequestration.
- Factors governing drug distribution volume:
1. Fat: Lean body mass ratio.
2. Oil: Water partition coefficient.
3. pKa value.
4. Degree of plasma protein binding.
5. Affinity for different tissues.
   Chloroquine binds to retina.
   CPZ
   Acetazolamide $\Big\}$ Cross blood–brain barrier (BBB).
   INH
   Tetracycline $\Big\}$ Accumulate in bone and teeth.
   Heavy metal
   DDT
   Ether $\Big\}$ Accumulate in adipose tissue.
   Thiopentone

Enzymatic blood–brain barrier

MAO and **cholinesterase** present in brain capillaries do not allow **5-HT, CA, ACh** to enter brain. Greater is the lipid solubility of the drug, faster is its redistribution. Anaesthetic action of thiopentone is terminated in a few minutes due to its **redistribution**.

Blood–brain barrier (BBB) is due to tight junction and neural tissue covering (**glial** cell processes or **choroidal** epithelium) present on the capillary wall of the brain (here capillary has no pore).

A similar barrier called **CSF-barrier** is also present in **choroidal plexus**. Both prevent entry of **nonlipid soluble** drugs (streptomycin, neostigmine, hexamethonium). Inflammation increases permeability of these drugs.

BBB is **absent** at periventricular site of ant. hypothalamus and CTZ of medulla oblongata. Bulk CSF and drug flow occur through **arachnoid villi**.

Exit from CSF is independent of lipid solubility. **Placental membrane** is lipoidal passing lipophilic drugs only and some non-lipid soluble drugs also **(incomplete barrier)**. High degree of plasma protein bound drugs are restricted to **vascular compartment** and have **lower vol. of distribution plus prolonged action** and displace drugs bound with lower affinity.

Vitamin K and sulfonamide displace bilirubin, hence used in kernicterus in neonates.

Drug interactions (IA): 3P

1. Pharmacokinetic IA occurs during drug movements.
2. Pharmacodynamic IA occurs at the receptor/between various drug actions.
3. Pharmaceutical IA occurs during formulation/mixing.

Mech. of chemical IA: PK (biotransformation, distribution, absorption, excretion) and pharmacodynamic (receptor and nonreceptor).

Class of chemical IA: Additive, synergistic, potentiation, antagonism.

Pharmacokinetics

Serum bilirubin is increased by Sulfonamide, Vit. K, Diazepam, Oxytocin, Novobiocin, Salicylates
SK DONS

Serum bilirubin is decreased by Barbiturates, Phenytoin, Reserpine, Aspirin, Narcotics.
BP RAN

- Breast milk has lower pH (7) than plasma, hence Basic drugs are more concentrated in it.
- Ampicillin, Tetracycline, Phenolphthalein, OC, Refampin, Erythromycin participate in **enterohepatic circulation** and are excreted in urine.

AT PORE

Plasma protein binding: Most drugs bind to plasma protein.

(Acidic drugs →Albumin and basic drugs →α_1 acid glycoprotein)

Highly bound drugs do not displace each other. Acidic and basic drugs do not displace each other.

Biotransformation means chemical alteration of the drug in the body.

Nonpolar/lipid soluble is biotransformed into polar/lipid insoluble for excretion.

Most hydrophilic drugs are not biotransformed, hence excreted unchanged.

Hepatic metabolism is the **commonest one for drugs** (other organs are kidney, intestine, lungs and plasma).

Most drugs and their active metabolites get inactivated, e.g. propranolol. Inactive form **(prodrugs)** gets converted to active form in the body.

e.g. Levodopa (prodrug) ⟶ DA (active form).

CYP450/Cytochrome P450/Mono-oxygenase/MFO: It is the **most** versatile biocatalyst known. P450 means CO complex of its reduced form absorbs light strongly at **450 nm,** hence the name P450. CYP 3A4 means CYP (cytochrome P450), 3 (family 3), A (subfamily A) and 4 (4th member of the subfamily A). Out of 17 CYP450 gene families, only CYP1, 2, and 3 (total 8–10 isoforms) metabolise **most** drugs mostly in liver. CYP3A4 and 3A5 metabolise 50% of drugs in gut and kidney. **Highest** amount of CYP450 is found in gut and liver (but present in all tissues). MFO (Mixed Function Oxidase) means one oxygen of its molecule goes to water and the other to **ROH (drug-OH):**

RH + O_2 + $NADPH_2^+$ + CYP450 (reduced) →ROH + Water + NADP + CYP450 (oxidised)

Drug metabolism undergoes 2 phases

1. **Phase I:** Occurs in **SER** catalysed by CYP450 oxidase and causes polarity by hydroxylation (mainly) and oxidation. CYP450 involved here are **3A4/5, 2D6, 2C8/9, 1A1/2.** Phenobarbital causes hypertrophy of SER and **4**-fold production of CYP450 in **4** days (hence warfarin dose should be increased due to its metabolism by CYP450). **NICO** tine is changed into **CONI** tine by CYP2A6. Genetic polymorphism is **best** seen in CYP2D6 that leads to altered drug metabolising ability and metabolises more than 65 common drugs. Induction of CYP450 is biochemical mechanism of drug interaction. Induction means increase in CYP450 (phase I).

2. **Phase II:** Occurs in cytosol catalysed by cytoplasmic enzymes to conjugate the functional group of phase I with glucuronic acid/sulfate **(mostly)**, glutathione and acetate. Methylation also occurs.

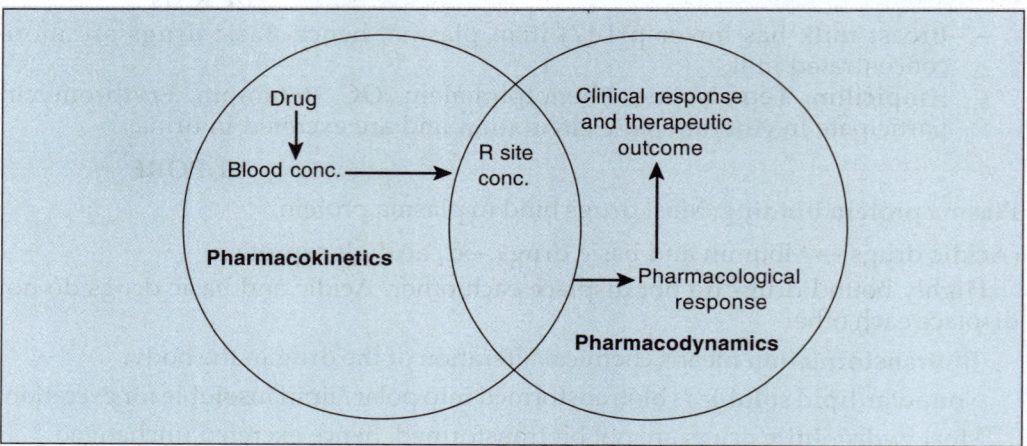

Biotransformation reactions (rxn):
1. **Nonsynthetic/phase I rxn (active/inactive).**
2. **Synthetic/conjugation/phase II rxn (mostly inactive metabolite).**

Phase I yields slightly polar, water-soluble, often active metabolites, involves cytochrome P450 (CYP450) and is lost first, by geriatric patient. Phase II yields very polar, inactive metabolites (renally excreted) and involves conjugation.

Nonsynthetic rxn

1. **Oxidation** is **mostly** carried by a group of **mono-oxygenase** in the liver which finally involves:
   CYP450 haemoprotein, CYP450 reductase, NADPH and O_2.
   CYP450 (MFO = mixed functional oxidase) is 30–100 in number.
   (oxidation = addition of O_2/negatively charged radical and removal of H_2/postively charged radical.) It is the **most important rxn.**
   In human being, **CYP3A4 and CYP2D6** biotransform the **largest** number of drugs. Highly lipid soluble drugs are metabolised by **MFO**.
2. **Reduction** also involves **CYP450** and occurs in **ER/cytosol**.
3. **Cyclization** involves ring formation from straight chain, e.g. proguanil.
4. **Decyclization** involves opening of **ring structure** of drugs.
5. **Hydrolysis:** Drug (ester) + H_2O $\xrightarrow{\text{esterase}}$ Drug (Acid + Alcohol).

Synthetic reaction involves **conjugation** of drugs and substrates from carbohydrates/amino acid **(energy dependent)** → Polar organic acid formation → Excretion in **urine/bile**.
1. **Acetylation** (drugs with amino/hydrazine residues + acetyl CoA), e.g. PAS, isoniazid.

2. **Glucuronide conjugation** occurs in ER (**most** important synthetic rxn). Drugs with hydroxyl/carboxylic acid group + glucuronic acid (UDPGA). Glucuronic acid is derived from **glucose** in the presence of **glucuronyl transferase**.
   For example, metronidazole, aspirin, chloramphenicol.
   SO_4^{2-}, acetyl, methyl, glycine, glutathione are also conjugated by **transferases**.
3. **Glycine conjugation:** (drugs with carboxylic group + glycine).
4. **Glutathione conjugation:** Drug + glutathione, e.g. paracetamol.
5. **Methylation:** Phenols and amines are methylated, e.g. adrenaline.
6. **Ribonucleoside/nucleotide synthesis:** activates purine and pyramidine antimetabolites.

Enzymes for drug metabolism

Enzymes also metabolize some drugs, e.g.

Drug	Enzyme
Adrenaline	MAO
Allopurinol	Xanthine oxidase
Procaine and succinylcholine	Plasma cholinesterase
Alcohol	Dehydrogenase

Two types of drug metabolising enzymes are:
1. **Microsomal** enzymes (present on SER in liver, kidney, GIT, lung) catalyse **most** of the glucuronide, hydrolysis, oxidation, reduction.
2. **Non-microsomal** enzymes (present in cytoplasm and mitochondria of liver cells and plasma) are flavoprotein oxidase, esterases, amidase, conjugases catalysing **all conjugation reaction except** glucuronidation, some oxidation, reduction and hydrolysis.

These enzymes are not inducible but show **genetic polymorphism.**

Microsomal and non-microsomal enzymes are deficient in newborn hence making more susceptible to many drugs, e.g. opioids.

Hofmann elimination: Drug inactivation in the body fluid by **spontaneous rearrangement** without the agency of any enzyme, e.g. atracurium.

A drug (quinidine) is metabolized by one isoenzyme (CYP3A4) and inhibits others (CYP2D6). For the same enzyme/cofactor, a drug competitively inhibits the metabolism of another.

Most drugs are metabolized by **nonsaturation kinetics** at therapeutic concentration (enzyme in excess).

If metabolism is dependent on blood flow as in liver, it is called **"blood flow limited metabolism".**

Carcinogenes, insecticides and drugs interact with DNA and increase microsomal enzyme protein synthesis **(CYP450 and glucuronyl transferase).**

A B C D
1 2 3 4
3A = 3 +1 = 4
(CYP3A4)
2D = 2 + 4 = 6
CYP2D6

Enzyme inducers are of 2 types:
1. Phenobarbitone type:
   - Induces CYP450 synthesis.
   - Increases liver weight and drug metabolism.

2. **3-methylcholanthrene type:**
   Does not increase CYP450 synthesis and liver weight.

When inducing agent is stopped, enzymes react with their original values over 1–3 weeks. As a result inducing drug metabolic rate is increased.

Rifampin, Glucocorticoids, Anticonvulsant, Macrolide induce **CYP3A** isoenzymes. **GRAM**

Barbiturates, Smoking, Phenytoin, Warfarin, Alcohol, Rifampin induce **MFO** and are metabolized by it. **BSF WAR and F = Phenytoin**

Phenobarbitone also induce	– CYP 2B1.
Rifampin also induce	– CYP 2D6.
Alcohol and 1NH also induce	– CYP 2E1.

Polycyclic hydrocarbons (benzopyrene and 3-methylcholanthrene of cigarette) induce **CYP1A**

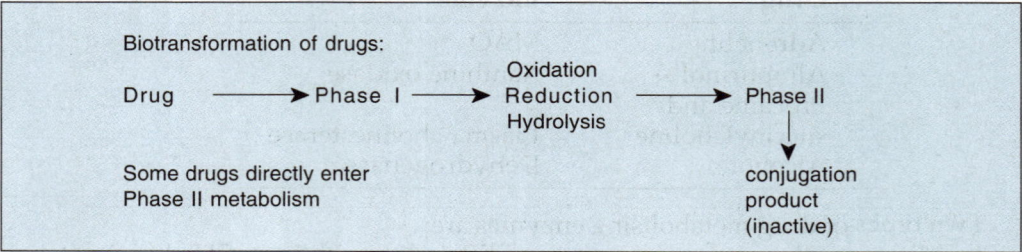

Consequences of microsomal enzyme induction
1. Decreased intensity/duration of action on inactivation by metabolism, e.g. OC failure.
2. Increased intensity of action on activation by metabolism and hence toxicity, e.g. paracetamol toxicity at low doses with enzyme inducers.
3. Faster metabolism of bilirubin and steroids (endogenous substrates).
4. Increased porphyrin due to depressed δ-**aminolevulinic acid synthetase** leads to acute intermittent porphyria.

Warfarin, phenytoin, OC, imipramine, doxycycline, theophylline, griseofulvin, phenylbutazone, tolbutamide, chloramphenicol are metabolically effected by enzyme induction.

Intermittent use of inducer drug may need adjustment of dose of another drug prescribed on regular basis, e.g. oral hypoglycemic, antiepileptic, antihypertensive, oral anticoagulants.

Inducing agents are Barbiturates, Phenytoin, Phenylbutazone, Griseofulvin, Glutethimide, Rifampin, Ethanol, Tobacco smoking, DDT, 3-methylcholanthrene, 3, 4-benzpyrene.

Tolerance occurs if the drug induces its own metabolism.

Uses of enzyme induction
- Liver disease.
- Chronic poisoning.
- Cushing's syndrome (phenytoin decreases it).
- Congenital nonhaemolytic jaundice (phenobarbitone clears it).

Pharmacokinetics

First pass (presystemic) metabolism

It occurs with orally administered drug. It is the drug metabolism from the site of absorption into systemic circulation during its passage.

Orally, it takes place in liver and intestinal wall. It also occurs in skin and lungs.

Drugs of high first pass metabolism

- **L**idocaine
- **I**soprenaline
- **M**orphine   } not given orally — **LiMIT**
- **H**ydrocor**t**isone
- **T**estosterone

- **P**ropranolol
- **S**albutamol
- **V**erapamil   } given orally — **PSVT**
- Pe**T**hidine

Increased oral bioavailability occurs in

1. Hepatic disease
2. If two drugs competing with each other are given concurrently, e.g. propranolol and CPZ.

Drug excretion

Elimination = Metabolism and excretion

1. **Urine:** Kidney is the **commonest** channel for the excretion of **most** of the drugs →excretes all water-soluble substances.
   Hydrophilic/lipophobic substances are **most** efficiently eliminated by kidney due to no reabsorption from tubule.
   Most drugs are ultimately eliminated by kidney. Glomerular capillaries have pores larger than usual hence all non-protein bound drugs, irrespective of their lipid solubility, are filtrated.
   Only nonlipid soluble and highly ionised drugs are excreted from tubules. Weak bases in acidic urine and weak acid in basic urine are **ionised** and hence excreted more. Drugs using some active transport compete with each other. Tubular transport mechanism is under-developed at birth, hence duration of action of drugs is increased in neonates. Effect of urinary pH change on drug excretion is **greatest with pKa between 5 and 8.** Organic acid and base transports are from blood to tubular fluid and vice versa **(bidirectional).**
2. **Faeces:** Unabsorbed drugs and drugs derived from bile are excreted in faeces. Liver transports organic acids, bases and steroid into **bile. Large polar compounds are actively excreted into the bile**.
3. **Exhaled air.**
4. **Milk:** Lipid soluble and less protein bound drugs enter breast milk by **passive diffusion**.
5. **Saliva and sweat:** For example, rifampin, Li, etc.

Most hydrophilic drugs are excreted unchanged, e.g. streptomycin, neostigmine.

Kinetics of elimination: Elimination usually follows **first** order kinetic. Drug elimination means sum total of metabolic inactivation and excretion. For drug that is not metabolised, is only excreted.

Clearance (CL) is the theoretical volume of plasma from which drug is completely removed in a unit time.

Pharmacology Review

CL = Elimination rate/C   Unit of CL = vol./time, C = plasma concentration

1. **First order (exponential) kinetics (most common)**

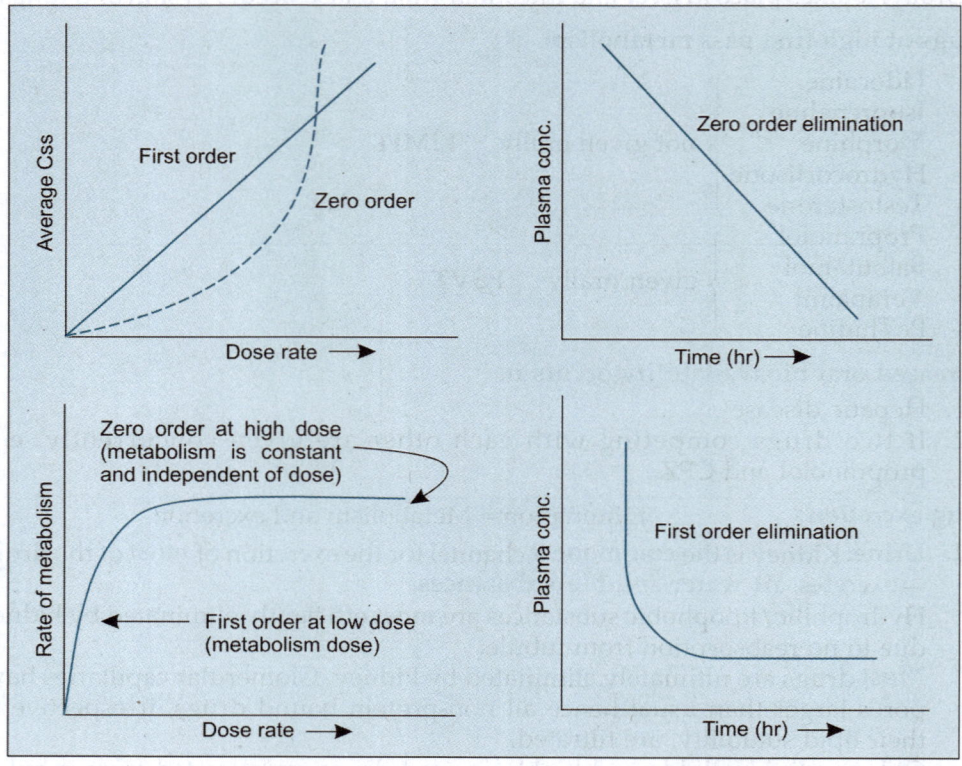

Elimination rate is directly proportional to drug concentration (CL = constant). Doubling the dose will double Css if drugs follow first order kinetic.
(Css = drug concentration at steady state).
Drug dose effect on metabolic rate (see box above)

$$\left(\text{in first order } V = \frac{V_{max}[C]}{K_m}, \text{ in zero order } V = \frac{V_{max}[C]}{[C]}\right)$$

2. **Zero order (Linear) Kinetics:** Elimination rate is constant **(Michaelis Menten Kinetics)** and independent of drug concentration. Constant amount of drug is eliminated per unit time. CL decreases with increase in concentration. It is capacity limited metabolism. **H**eparin, **E**thambutol, **P**henytoin, **A**spirin (at high doses) follow zero order kinetic.   **HEPArin**
(**W**arfarin, **A**lcohol and **A**ntiepileptic (phenytoin), **T**olbutamide and **T**heophylline also   **zero WATT**).

3. **Half-life (t½):** Time taken for plasma concentration of drug to be reduced to **half of its original value.**

Measures (effect/concentration) declines by half.

t½ = 0.7 V/CL

In 1 t½ →**50%** elimination. In 2 t½ →50 + 25 = **75%** elimination. In 3 t½ →50 + 25 + 12.5 = **87.5%** elimination. In 4 t½ →87.5 + 6.25 = **94%** elimination. Nearly complete drug elimination takes place in **4–5 t½**.

Value of t½ is measured in 3 ways: (1) **plasma t½**—P concentration decreased to ½, (2) **biological effect t½**—effect/active metabolites decreased to ½, (3) **biological/elimination t½**—total amount in the body decreased to ½.

In **first order kinetic, t½ remains constant** because volume and CL do not change with dose. In **zero order kinetic,** t½ increases with dose because clearance progressively decreases.

Drugs with short t½ are digoxin, choloroquine, long-acting sulfonamide and need **loading + maintenance** dose for rapid therapeutic effect with long-term safety.

Loading dose is the single/repeated doses given in the beginning to attain target concentration rapidly.

$$\text{Loading dose} = \frac{\text{Target concentration} \times V}{F}$$

If t½ is 3 hrs, administration should be 6–12 hrly.
Drug action is increased by:
- Prolonging absorption from the site of administration.
- Increasing plasma protein binding.
- Retarding metabolic rate and renal excretion.

Plasma concentration monitoring is significant in **H**ypoglycemic, **G**A, **G**uanethidine, **R**eserpine, **A**ntihypertensive, **M**AO inhibitor, **L**evodopa, **O**meparazole, oral **A**nticoagulant, **D**iuretics. **Half GRAM LOAD**.

Drugs with low safety margin are anticonvulsant, antidepressant, Li, antiarrhythmic.

Ethinyl group addition of estradiol makes it longer acting and suitable for OC. Doses per day of a drug is determined by t½ and the difference between minimum therapeutic and toxic concentration.

t½ of some important drugs:

Important drugs	t½
Digitoxin	200 hrs
Digoxin	48 hrs
Verapamil	4 hrs
Propranolol	4 hrs
Insulin	< 1 hr
Heparin	1 hr (t½ increases up to 5 hrs at >100 U/kg)
Doxycycline	18 hrs
Penicillin G	½ hr
Cotrimoxazole	11/9 hrs

(Contd.)

(Contd.)

Important drugs	t½
Ciprofloxacin	4 hrs
Metronidazole	6 hrs
Ofloxacin	6 hrs
Vancomycin	6 hrs
Ceftriazone	8 hrs
Tetracycline	8 hrs

MOVe = 6 hrs

Most of the antimicrobials, other than mentioned here have t½ → 1–2 hrs.

Safety margin/therapeutic index/therapeutic range (TI)
Range between dose for minimum therapeutic effect and dose for maximum acceptable ADR.

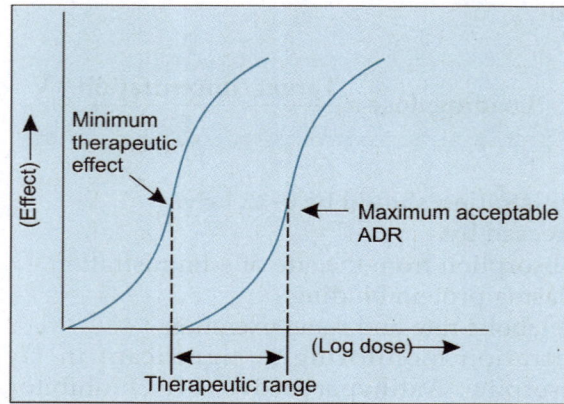

Maintenance dose is the dose to be repeated at specified interval of time to attain target concentration so as to maintain the *same* by balancing elimination.

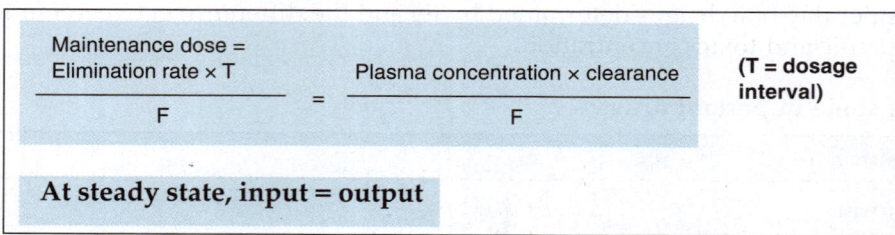

$$\text{Maintenance dose} = \frac{\text{Elimination rate} \times T}{F} = \frac{\text{Plasma concentration} \times \text{clearance}}{F} \quad (T = \text{dosage interval})$$

At steady state, input = output

Faster infusion rate does not change the time to achieve steady state. Only Css changes.

Inhibition of drug metabolism
Ethanol inhibits methanol. Phenytoin, phenylbutazone, warfarin, and chloramphenicol inhibit tolbutamide. Chloramphenicol inhibits cyclophosphamide.

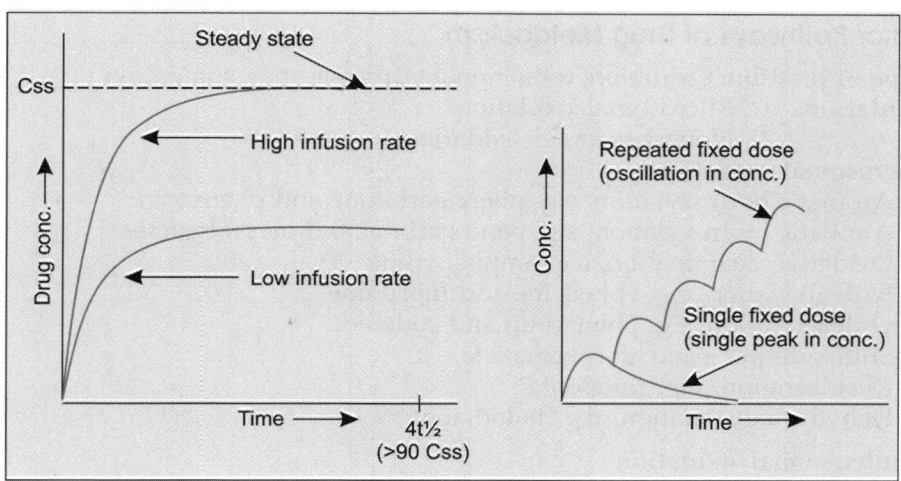

Cimetidine inhibits propranolol, lidocaine and theophylline. Allopurinol inhibits 6-mercaptopurine and azathioprine. Propranolol inhibits lidocaine metabolism by decreasing hepatic blood flow. Salicylates inhibit probenecid.

Active metabolites of some drugs

Drugs		Active metabolites
Amitriptyline	–	Nortriptyline
Codeine	–	Morphine
Chloral hydrate	–	Trichloroethanol
Diazepam	–	Desmethyl diazepam
Digitoxin	–	Digoxin
Imipramine	–	Desipramine
Phenacetin	–	Paracetamol
Phenylbutazone	–	Oxyphenbutazone
Primidone	–	Phenobarbitone and phenylethylmalonamide
Spironolactone	–	Canrenone
Trimethadone	–	Dimethadione
Prodrug		**Active form**
Benorylate	–	Aspirin + paracetamol
Becampicillin	–	Ampicillin
Cyclophosphamide	–	Aldophosphamide
	–	Phosphoramide mustard
	–	Acrolein
Enalapril	–	Enalaprilat
Levodopa	–	DA
Prednisone	–	Prednisolone
Sulfasalazine	–	5-aminosalicylic acid

Major Pathways of Drug Metabolism

Type of reaction: Oxidation, reduction, hydrolysis and conjugation.
Oxidation: 1. Microsomal oxidation
2. Nonmicrosomal oxidation

Microsomal oxidation
- A. Aromatic hydroxylation, e.g. phenobarbitone and phenytoin.
- B. Aliphatic hydroxylation, e.g. pentobarbital and meprobamate.
- C. Oxidative deamination, e.g. amphetamine.
- D. N-dealkylation, e.g. ephedrine and morphine.
- E. O-dealkylation, e.g. phenacetin and codeine.
- F. Sulfoxidation, e.g. chlorpromazine.
- G. Desulfuration, e.g. thiopental.
- H. Dehydrohalogenation, e.g. halothane.

Nonmicrosomal oxidation
- A. Alcoholic oxidation, e.g. ethanol.
- B. Aldehydic oxidation, e.g. acetaldehyde.

Reduction
- A. Azoreduction, e.g. sulfasalazine.
- B. Nitroreduction, e.g. chloramphenicol.

Hydrolysis
- A. De-esterification, e.g. procaine and meperidine.
- B. Deamidation, e.g. lidocaine.

Conjugation
- A. Glucuronidation
    - a. Phenolic OH, e.g. salicylates.
    - b. Alcholic OH, e.g. oxazepam
    - c. Carboxyl, e.g. salicylates.
    - d. Amine, e.g. sulfamethoxazole.
    - e. Sulfhydryl, e.g. disulfiram.
- B. Glysine conjugation, e.g. salicylic acid and fenfluramine.
- C. Glutathione conjugation, e.g. acetaminophen.
- D. Sulfate conjugation, e.g. steroids and terbutaline.
- E. Methylation:
    - a. Aromatic amines, e.g. oxprenolol.
    - b. Catechols, e.g. levodopa.
- F. Acetylation:
    - a. Aromatic amines, e.g. sulfisoxazole and procainamide.
    - b. Hydrazides, e.g. isoniazid.

3. Pharmacodynamics

PharmacodynaMics means Mechanism of action.

Principles of drug action

Drugs based on gene impart new function but drugs alter the pace of ongoing activity. Drugs bind with receptor by ionic, covalent, hydrogen bonds and van der Waals forces.

1. **Stimulation:** Adrenaline stimulates heart. Pilocarpine stimulates salivary gland. Excessive stimulation leads to depression of that function.
   For example, CNS stimulation by picrotoxin
   ↓
   Convulsion
   ↓
   Coma
   ↓
   Respiratory depression

   > Targets for drug actions are Receptors, Ion channels, Carrier molecules, Enzymes
   > **RICE**

2. **Depression:** Barbiturates inhibit CNS. Quinidine inhibits heart. Most drugs are not classified as stimulant/depressant.
   For example, ACh
   — Inhibits SA node in heart
   — Stimulates intestinal smooth muscle.

3. **Replacement:** Use of substances in deficiency state.
   For example, insulin in DM.

4. **Irritation:**
   Mild →stimulation (bitters increase secretion).
   Strong →inflammation, necrosis.
   Counter-irritant increases blood flow.

5. **Cytotoxic action:** For parasites/cancer cells without effecting host cells.

Mechanism of drug action

A. Physical action: May be

- Radioactivity (^{131}I).
- Osmotic (mannitol).
- Adsorptive (charcoal).
- Radioopacity (contrast media such as $BaSO_4$, urogram).

ROAR

B. **Chemical action:** Drugs act extracellularly, e.g. Al (OH)$_3$ neutralises gastric acid (antacids).
   NaHCO$_3$ (acidifying agent) and NH$_4$Cl (alkalinising agent) react with buffers in plasma to alter pH of urine. Oxidising agents inactivate alkaloids. Chelating agents sequester toxic metals.
C. **Enzymatic action:** Enzymatic stimulation increases affinity for substrate (km decreases).
   Enzyme protein synthesis occurs by induction but not by stimulation (km constant).
   Enzymatic inhibition

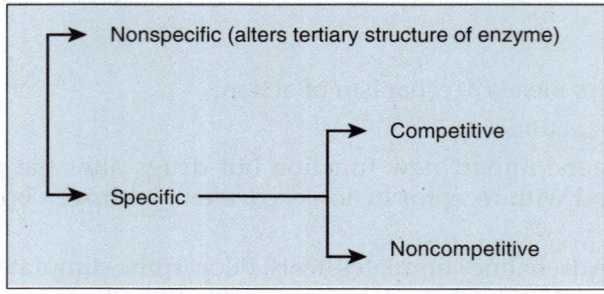

Competitive inhibition
1. K_m **increased,** V_{max} **constant, equilibrium type:** Physostigmine competes with ACh for cholinesterase. Allopurinol competes with hypoxanthene for xanthene oxidase.
   Carbidopa and methyldopa compete with levodopa for dopa decarboxylase. Warfarin competes with vitamin K for enzyme synthesising clotting factor in the liver.
2. K_m **increased,** V_{max} **decreased, non-equilibrium type:** Organophosphate reacts with cholinesterase (covalently). Methotrexate has 50,000 times higher affinity for DHF reductase than DHFA.

   Noncompetitive inhibition (reaction with adjacent site, not with catalytic site): K_m constant, V_{max} decreased.

Drugs react with enzymes

Acetazolamide	C. anhydrase
NSAID	COX
Nialamide	MAO
Tranylcypromine	MAO
Digoxin	**Na$^+$K$^+$ ATPase**
Theophylline	Phosphodiesterase
Enzyme induction	No change in
Noncompetitive inhibition	affinity (K_m constant)

Enzyme stimulation decreases K_m. Competitive inhibition increases K_m.

D. **Through receptors:** Receptors are macromolecules to bind and interact with drugs. They are regulatory molecules **mostly** protein. They are also called **binding sites** capable of generating response. They are **heteropolymeric** (many nonidentical subunits). On stimulation, quaternary structure changes opening central cation channel.

Receptors exist in **dynamic state** and are regulated by ongoing activity. Prolonged deprivation of agonist in tonically active system leads to supersensitivity of receptor. Unmasking/proliferation of receptor is called **up-regulation** (prolonged contact with antagonist leads to formation of new receptors called up-regulation). Decreased synthesis/increased destruction of receptor is called **down-regulation** (number of receptor decreases on continuous exposure to agonist). Receptors exist in 2 **interchangeable** states. $R_1 \rightleftharpoons R_2$

Agonist binds to R_1, antagonist binds to R_2. Partial agonist binds to R_1 and R_2. They may be on the surface/inside the cell and specific agonist combines with them to initiate the response.

Agonist: Stimulates the receptor to produce response and has **IA=1 (maximum)** and affinity, e.g. Adrenaline (IA=Instrinsic activity).

Antagonist: Inhibits action of agonist on receptor and has affinity but **no IA (IA=0)**, e.g. atropine.

Inverse agonist: Stimulates receptor to produce response in the **opposite direction** to that of agonist. It has affinity but **IA=0 to –1**, e.g. DMCM.

Partial agonist: Stimulates receptor to produce **submaximal effect**.
– Antagonises the action of full agonist.
– Has affinity but submaximal IA (IA = 0 to 1), e.g. nalorphine.

Ligand: It is the molecule attached selectively to a particular receptor/sites. **Spare R** means maximum response at less than maximum R occupation.

Silent receptor: It is the site for binding drugs without pharmacological response called **drug acceptor or site of loss**.

Receptor occupation theory

1. Intensity of response is directly proportional to fraction of receptor occupied by drug, and **maximum response** occurs when all receptors are occupied.
2. Drugs exert **all-or-none action** (no partial activation).
3. Drug and receptor stand in rigid **"Lock and Key"** relationship.

Affinity is the ability of drug to combine with receptors.

Efficacy/intrinsic activity (IA) is the ability of a drug to activate receptors after receptor occupation (**maximum** response elicited by drug).

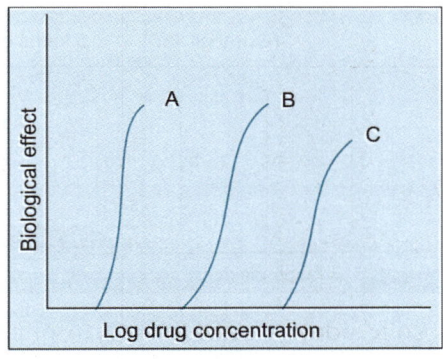

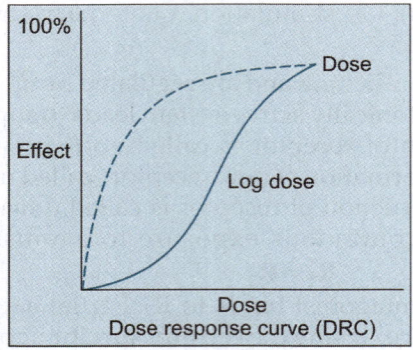

Dose response curve (DRC)

Drug potency is the amount of drug needed to produce certain response.

Dextropraopranol is **100 times** less potent in beta receptor blockade than **levoisomers**.

Potency A > B but same efficacy.

A/B > C in potency and efficacy.

In IA and potency as analgesic, **morphine > aspirin.**

As CNS depressant, diazepam > phenobarbitone in **potency** and less than cyclopentolate in **IA**.

Drug action: Drug combination with receptor resulting in **conformational** changes in receptor (for agonist) and inhibition of conformational changes in receptor (for antagonist).

Drug effect is the ultimate change in biological function as a result of drug action, through a series of **intermediate steps (transducer)**.

Drug receptor interaction obeys **law of mass action**. So, DRC is a **rectangular hyperbola**. DRC is **sigmoid** on logarithmic scale. Response is **directly proportional** to exponential (log) function of dose. **Drug efficacy** is directly proportional to height of DRC. Steep slope indicates that a moderate increase in dose will markedly increase the response.

Function of receptors

(i) Recognition of specific ligand molecule.
(ii) Transduction of signal into response. Receptor has effector domain and ligand binding domain.

Transducer mechanism: Mechanism of translation of receptor stimulation into functional response; there are **4 categories of the mechanism:**

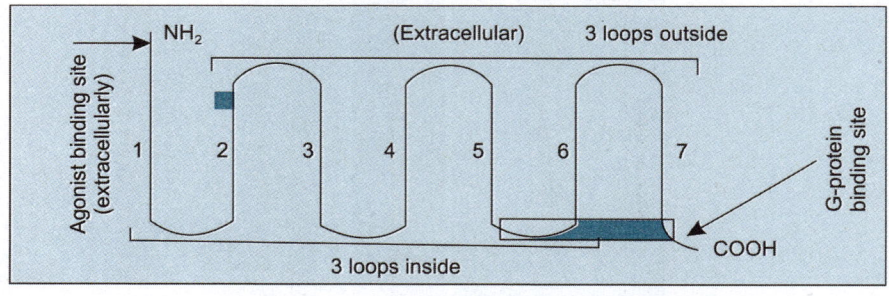

(Cytosolic side)   **COOH = C**ytosolic side

1. G-protein coupled receptor.
2. Receptor with intrinsic ion channel.
3. Enzymatic receptor.
4. Transcription factors.

1. **G-Protein coupled receptor** (see box above): G-protein coupled receptor molecule has **7α-helical membrane spanning hydrophobic amino acid segments** which run into **3 extracellular and 3 intracellular loops**. G-proteins float in membrane with exposed domain lying **cytosolic side** and are **heterotrimeric (α, β, γ, subunits)**. **On activation**, GTP displaces GDP which is bound to exposed domain. Active α-subunit carrying GTP gets detached from β, γ-subunits to react and acts as GTPase to hydrolyse GTP into GDP. Ca^{++} release occurs in waves. G-protein coupled receptor functions through **3 pathways**:

   A. Adenylcyclase (AC)
   AC activation → ↑ cAMP intracellularly (2nd messenger)
   ↓
   Activates cAMP dependent protein kinase (PKA)
   α
   Effect (channel, carrier, protein, enzyme)

   B. Phospholipase C (PLC)
   PLC activation
   ↓
   PIP_2 hydrolysis
   ↓
   IP_3 and DAG (2nd messenger)
   ↓
   IP_3 ⇒ ↑Ca^{2+} from intracellular organelles depots.
   DAG ⇒ PKC activation by Ca^{++}.
   ↓
   ↑ cytosolic Ca^{++} (3rd messenger)
   ↓
   CAM and PKC activation.

Inhibitory G-protein (Gi) inhibits both AC and PLC activation.

PIP_2 = Phosphatidyl inositol 4,5-bisphosphate
IP_3 = Inositol 1,4,5-triphosphate
DAG = Diacylglycerol
CAM = Calmodulin

   C. Channel regulation: Activated G-proteins open/close ion channels to cause hyperpolarisation/depolarisation/intracellular Ca^{++} concentration change, e.g. Gs → opens Ca^{++} channel in cardiac and skeletal muscles; Gi and G_0 → open K^+ channel in cardiac and smooth muscles and close Ca^{++} channels in neurons.

1. **G-protein-linked second messengers**
Except D_1, all receptors of type **ON**e causes c**ON**tractility.

Receptor	G-protein class	Major functions
α_1	q	Increases vascular smooth muscle contraction
α_2	i	Decreases sympathetic outflow, decreases insulin release
β_1	s	Increases heart rate, increases contractility, increases renin release, increases lipolysis, increases aqueous humor formation
β_2	s	Vasodilation, bronchodilation, increases glucagon release
M_1	q	CNS
M_2	i	Decreases heart rate
M_3	q	Increases exocrine gland secretions
D_1	s	Relaxes renal vascular smooth muscle
D_2	i	Modulates transmitter release, especially in brain
H_1	q	Increases nasal and bronchial mucus production, contraction of bronchioles, pruritus and pain
H_2	s	Increases gastric acid secretions
V_1	q	Increases vascular smooth muscle contraction
V_2	s	Increases H_2O permeability and reabsorption in the collecting tubules of the kidney

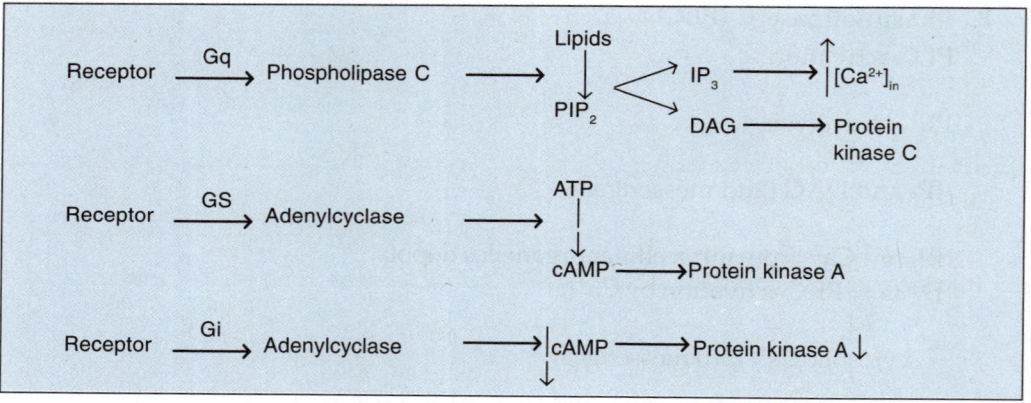

2. **Receptors with intrinsic ion channel**
   Receptors have channel for (Na^+, K^+, Ca^{2+}, Cl^-).
   Agonist binding opens the channel causing hyperpolarization/depolarization or change in cytosolic ion composition, e.g.:
   - Nicotinic cholinergic R
   - GABA–A R
   - Glycine (inhibitory) R
   - $5\text{-}HT_3$ R
   - Excitatory amino acid R (NMDA, etc.). Receptor (R) is **pentameric protein**, has **fastest** onset and offset response.
3. **Enzymatic receptors** are enzymatic proteins. Agonist binding sites lie on **outer** face of plasma membrane. Catalytic sites lie on **inner** face of plasma membrane. Both domains are interconnected by **single peptide chain**. In **most** cases, enzyme

Pharmacodynamics

is **tyrosine protein kinase**. Other enzyme is **guanylyl cyclase**, acts through cAMP as 2nd messenger in the cytosol and activates cAMP-dependent protein kinase.

4. **Tanscription factors** are cytoplasmic/nuclear soluble proteins (responding to lipid soluble chemical messenger) which penetrate the cell specific genes, attach receptor protein to express themselves and synthesise mRNA hence protein. All steroidal hormones, TH, vitamins A and D function in this way (**slowest** action).

Combined effect of drugs

A. **Synergism** (↑ed action taking place in the same direction).
   1. **Additive:** Effect of drug A + B = effect of drug A + effect of drug B.
   2. **Supradditive (potentiation):** For example, effect of drug A + B > effect of drug A + effect of drug B.
   One component is always inactive here, e.g.
   Sulfonamide + Trimethoprim (sequential blockade). Tyramine + MAO inhibitors (increasing releasable CA store).

B. **Antagonism** (when one drug inhibits the action of another drug).
   For example, effect of drug A + B < effect of drug A + effect of drug B.
   May be 1. **Physical**.
           2. **Chemical** (direct binding of drug by another drug without involving receptor, e.g. heavy metal chelator).
           3. **Functional:** (i) insulin and glucagon (physiological) on blood sugar level; (ii) Histamine and adrenaline on BP and bronchial muscle.
   Opposite action of 2 agonists at different receptors occurs in physiological antagonism, e.g. ACh and NE on heart rate.

Competitive	Noncompetitive
1. Maximum response is attained by increasing agonist dose (surmountable/reversible antagonism). Parallel shift of DRC occurs to right (IA = 0)	Maximum response is suppressed (unsurmountable antagonism).
2. Antagonist decreases agonist **potency**, e.g. ACh-atropine.	Antagonist decreases agonist **efficacy**, e.g. Bicuculline–diazepam.
3. Parallel rightward shift of agonist DRC:	Flattening of agonist DRC:
(graph: Response vs dose; Agonist curve and Agonist and antagonist curve shifted parallel to right, both reaching 100)	(graph: Response vs dose; Agonist curve reaching 100, Agonist and antagonist curve flattened, lower maximum)
(Competitive surmountable antagonist)	(Competitive unsurmountable antagonist/noncompetitive antagonist)

4. Receptor: Anticholinergics decrease intestinal spasm induced by cholinergic agonists but not by histamine /5-HT because they act through different set of receptors.

Antagonism may be competitive and noncompetitive (due to **covalent** bond formation).

Competitive inhibition = K_m increases, no change in V_{max}.
NOncompetitive inhibition = NO change in K_m, V_{max} decreases
UNcompetitive inhibition = K_m and V_{max} decrease (Under Normal)

Dosage (appropriate amount of drug for the **response of choice** in a patient) is:
- **Standard dose** (dose appropriate for **most patient**).
- **Target level dose** (empirical dose given in the beginning and adjusted for target level).
- **Regulated dose** (modifies regulated body function).
- **Titrated dose** (optimal dose obtained by titrating it with acceptable ADR).
- **Toxic dose.**
- **Therapeutic dose.**
- **Prophylactic dose.**

Fixed dose combination
Advantages
- Better patient compliance.
- Convenient.
- Synergistic.
- Counteraction of ADR.

Disadvantages
- Additional ADR and expense.
- Dose unadjusted of most drug.
- Contraindication of one component.
- Contraindication of whole preparation.

RECEPTORS
Receptor with intrinsic ion channel ⎤
Enzymatic receptor   ⎥
Coupled with G-protein   ⎬ Types
Expression through gene regulation   ⎦
Proteins usually
Transduction into response on substance combination
On the membrane/inside cytoplasm or nucleus
Radiological studies for their identification
Specifically bind with ligand

Factors modifying drug action
1. Genetics
2. Route, time of administration and environmental factor
3. Age
4. Sex
5. Psychological factor
6. Tolerance
7. Body size
8. Pathological state
9. Species and race
10. Cumulation

GRASP The BPSC

Body size
Individual dose = $\dfrac{BSA (m^2)}{1.7}$ × average adult dose.

Pharmacodynamics

$$= \frac{BW(kg)}{70} \times \text{average adult dose}.$$

BSA = Body surface area = $BW(kg)^{0.42} \times H(m)^{0.72} \times 0.0072$.

Age

1. **Pediatric pharmacology**

   Child dose $= \dfrac{Age}{Age + 12} \times$ adult dose (Young's formula).

   $= \dfrac{Age}{20} \times$ adult dose (Dilling's formula).

   $= \dfrac{Age}{24} \times$ adult dose (Cowling's formula).

   Newborn has low GFR and immature tubular transport which reach to maturity after **5th month and 7th month respectively**.
   After 1 year, drug metabolism is faster than adult.

   1. Gray baby syndrome
   – Chloramphenicol (ADR)
   2. Kernicterus due to unconjugated bilirubin accumulation in CNS.

   – Corticosteroid causes growth suppression.
   – Androgen causes early fusion of epiphysis (stunting stature).
   – Newborn has more body water and less body fat than adult. Hence, water soluble drug will have higher volume and lipid soluble drug will have lower volume.
   – Plasma protein binding is reduced in (approximately) first year.
   – Metabolism is decreased (oxidation, glucuronidation).
   – GFR and tubular function are decreased.
   – t½ of **D**iagoxin, **P**henytoin, **T**heophylline, carbamazepine is shorter in children (>1 year).   **DPT**

   Dose of digoxin = 8–12 mg/kg/d whereas it is 3–5 mg/kg/d in adults.

2. **Geriatric pharmacology**
   – In elderly, renal function declines, hence dose is decreased.
   – Elder has smaller body mass, less body water and more body fat, hence water soluble drug has lower Vd and lipid soluble drug has higher Vd.
   – Reduced plasma albumin reduces bound drug in plasma.
   – Reduced renal excretion and reduced hepatic metabolism occur.
     CNS drugs cause more confusion and CVS drugs cause more effect.
   – Overall, elderly patients need smaller dose of most drugs.

   Sex: Females have smaller body size hence lower dose. Antihypertensive drugs effect the sexual function of male only. Gynaecomastia occurs in male only.
   In pregnancy, GIT motility is decreased, fluid expands, albumin decreases, acid glycoprotein increases, renal blood flow increases. Hepatic microsomal enzymes undergo induction.

   Species and race: Indians have better tolerance of thiacetazone than whites.

Genetics: G6PD deficiency causes <u>haemolysis</u> with primaquine (oxidizing drug) showing different metabolic rate.

Route, e.g. $MgSO_4$ — Oral (purgation)
— Topical (decreases swelling)
— IV (decreases BP)

Psychological factor: Efficacy depends on beliefs, attitudes and expectation.

Placebo is inert substance (lactose, distilled water) but few person responds to a placebo (placebo reactor).

Uses of placebo
1. Clinical trial (dummy medication).
2. To patient without need.

It may release endorphins in brain (analgesic). Analgesic action is checked by naloxone.

Pathological state
1. In GIT disease: Amoxycillin absorption is decreased but that of cephalexin and cotrimoxazole are increased.
2. In cirrhosis: Bioavailability is increased.
   Albumin is decreased.
   Metabolism is decreased.
   Elimination is decreased.
3. In renal disease: Albumin is decreased.
   BBB permeability is increased, e.g. BZD, barbiturates, etc.

Contraindication in renal disease
  – Tetracycline causes uremia.
  – Sulfonamide causes crystalluria.
  – NSAID and carbenoxolone cause fluid retention.
    – Cephaloridine.
    – Cephalothine.
    – Aminoglycoside.
    – Cyclosporine.
    – Penicillin.
    – Phenformin induces lactic acidosis.
    – Vancomycin.
    – K^+ sparing diuretic.
    – Thiazide decreases GFR, worsens uremia.

4. **In CHF:** Decreased absorption occurs from GIT due to edema and vasoconstriction, e.g. procainamide and hydrochlorothiazide.

5. **In thyroid disease:** Hypothyroid patient is more sensitive to digoxin and CNS depressant. **Hyperthyroid** patient is more sensitive to arrhythmic action but resistant to inotropic action of digoxin.
   Digoxin elimination is directly proportional to thyroid function.

6. **Other modified drug response:** Thiazide causes more decrease in edematous patient. Adrenaline and digitalis cause arrhythmia in MI. Phenothiazines cause tolerance in schizophrenia. Morphine causes respiratory failure in head injury.

Imipramine
Atropine   } Cause urinary retention in prostatic hypertrophy.
Furosemide

Hypnotics cause confusion and delirium in severe pain. Cotrimoxazole causes ADR in AIDS.

Cumulation occurs when administration is more than elimination, e.g. chloroquine causes retinal damage.

Tolerance (means higher drug dose needed for a given response) may be:
- Cross-tolerance.
- Tachyphylaxis.
- Drug resistance in antibiotics.
- Natural (black races tolerate mydriatics).
- Acquired.

Acquired tolerance In most drugs specially CNS depressant, tolerance develops to only sedative action of chlorpromazine, phenobarbitone and analgesic euphoric action of morphine.

Cross-tolerance is directly proportional to closeness of drugs, e.g. alcohol tolerates GA and barbiturates.

Complete tolerance occurs between morphine and pethidine. Partial tolerance occurs between morphine and barbiturates.

Tachyphylaxis (tachy = fast, phylaxis = protection) means rapid tolerance development, e.g. ephedrine and tyramine release CA in the body more than synthesis.

Pathway	Rate limiting enzyme
1. Melatonin synthesis	Serotonin N-acetylase
2. Cholesterol synthesis	HMG-CoA reductase
3. Melanin synthesis	Tyrosinase
4. Fatty acid synthesis	Acetyl CoA carboxylase
5. Lactose synthesis	Synthetase
6. Purine synthesis	Glutamine-PRPP-amidotransferase
7. CA synthesis	Tyrosine hydroxylase
8. Urea formation	Carbamoyl phosphate synthetase
9. Adipose tissue lipolysis	Hormone sensitive lipase
10. Citric acid cycle	α-Ketoglutarate dehydrogenase
11. Gluconeogenesis	FDPase, pepcarboxykinase
12. Glycogenesis	Glycogen synthetase
13. Glycogenolysis	Glycogen phosphorylase
14. Glycolysis	Phosphofructokinase
15. Haembiosynthesis	δ-Alasynthetase

Pharmacology Review

Some important drugs	Mechanism of action
Dantrolene	Direct skeletal muscle depressant
Spironolactone	Aldosterone receptor antagonist
Pirenzepine	M_1 cholinergic receptor blocker
Acetazolamide	Carbonic anhydrase inhibitor
Succinyl choline	Depolarising neuromuscular blocker
d-tubocurarine	Competitive NM junction blocker
Prazosin	Selective α_1 blocker
Metoprolol	β_1 blocker
Labetalol	$\alpha + \beta$ blocker
Clonidine	α_2 blocker
Dobutamine	β_1 and α_1 agonist
Mannitol	Osmotic diuresis
Guanethidine	Nonadrenergic uptake blocker
Naloxone	Competitive antagonist of morphine
Aminophylline	Phosphodiesterase inhibitor
Digoxin	Inhibits $Na^+ K^+$ ATPase
Captopril	ACE inhibitor
Acetylcholine	Activation of cholinoceptors
Phenylephrine	Release of intracellular Ca^{++} ion
Amiodarone	Blocks $Na^+ K^+ Ca^{++}$ channels, blocks α and β receptors
Isoprenaline	AC activation
Ouabain	$Na^+ K^+$ ATPase inhibitor
Procaine	Na^+ channel blocker

Adverse Effects

Adverse Drug Reaction (ADR): It is the undesirable and unavoidable consequence of a drug at therapeutic dose and includes **all kinds of noxious effects**.

All drugs have ADR (whenever drug is given, risk is taken).

Effective therapy depends not only on the correct choice but also on the correct use of drugs. Incorrect use of drugs may lead to ADR called **negative ADR** (Adverse Drug Reaction).

- **Commonest diseases** of sufferers are CVS/respiratory system diseases and DM.
- **Commonest drugs** are diuretics, digoxin, antimicrobials, K^+, analgesic, tranquilizers, insulin, aspirin, steroid, antihypertensive, warfarin.
- **Commonest ADR** is related to GIT, skin, mental alertness, plasma K^+ concentration.

Severity of ADR
1. Minor
2. Moderate
3. Severe (permanent damage)
4. Lethal (contributes to death)

Causes of ADR
1. **Non-drug factors**
   - Extrinsic (environment, prescriber).
   - Intrinsic (age, sex, genetics, disease, habit, allergy, personality).
2. **Drug factor:** Intrinsic (use of drugs and drug interaction).

Classification of ADR **ABCDE**

1. **Type A (80%)/Augmented:** Occurs in every case, is predictable and dose-related, e.g. ↓BP.
2. **Type B (20%)/Bizarre** occurs in some people and is not dose-related, it is unpredictable and is due to hereditary. It has **most** drug fatalities, e.g. allergy. Types A and B are main types of ADR.
3. **Type C/Continuous:** It is due to long-term use.

4. **Type D/D**elayed, e.g. carcinogenesis.
5. **Type E/E**nding of use, e.g. rebound adrenocortical insufficiency.

Selected topics from classification and causes

1. Intolerance
2. Toxic effect
3. Idiosyncrasy
4. Side effect
5. Iatrogenic (physician induced) disease
6. Teratogenicity
7. Secondary effect
8. Mutagenicity and Carcinogenicity
9. Photosensitivity
10. Allergy
11. Drug dependence
12. Drug withdrawal Reaction

ADR: IT IS ITS MCP (Most common problem)

1. **Side effect** is unwanted and unavoidable effect at therapeutic dose, e.g. dryness of mouth due to atropine.
2. **Secondary effect** is indirect consequence of primary action of drug, e.g. corticosteroids weaken host defence mechanism leading to activation of latent TB.
3. **Toxic effect** is the consequence of excessive pharmacological action of drug due to prolonged use or overdose, e.g. hepatic necrosis from paracetamol overdose. Respiratory failure from morphine overdose.
   Commonest involved organs are CNS, CVS, kidney, bone marrow, liver, lungs, skin.
   > Poison is a substance endangering vital function.
   – Emesis is not attempted in comatose patient and in kerosene poisoning for fear of aspiration into lungs.
   – Universal antidote:
   Charcoal : Strong tea : Milk of magnesia (most important)
       2   :   1   :   1
4. **Intolerance** is appearance of characteristic toxic effect at therapeutic doses, e.g. triflupromazine induces muscular dystonia.
5. **Idiosyncrasy** is genetically determined abnormal reactivity to a chemical, e.g. barbiturates cause excitement and mental confusion.
6. **Teratogenicity** is drug capacity to cause foetal defect on administration to pregnant mother, e.g. thalidomide disaster (1958–61) caused phocomelia (seal like limbs) and multiple defects in babies.

Drugs effect at 3 stages

a. Fertilization and implantation (conception to 17 days): Pregnancy failure is often unnoticed.
b. Organogenesis (18 to 55 days of gestation): *Most vulnerable* period.
c. Development (56 days onward).

Human Teratogenic Drugs

Drugs	Defect
Anticancer	Death and multiple defect
Androgen	Virilization, limbs and cardiac defect
Antithyroid	Hypothyroidism, foetal goiter
Thalidomide	Phocomelia, multiple defects
Progestin	Virilization of female foetus
Stilboesterol	Vaginal CA
Corticosteroid	Cleft palate and lip, cardiac defect
Tetracycline	Teeth, bone defect, etc.
Phenytoin	Cleft lip/palate, microcephaly
Phenobarbitone	Multiple defect
Warfarin	Nose, eye, hand defect, growth retardation
Carbamazepine	Neural tube defect
Lithium	Foetal goiter, cardiac defect
Sodium valproate	Neural tube defect (spina bifida)
Indomethacin/aspirin	Premature ductus arteriosus closure
Isotretinoin	Craniofacial heart, CNS defect

7. **Carcinogenicity and mutagenicity:** Drugs cause cancer and genetic defect usually by drug oxidation, e.g. anticancer drugs, radioisotopes, estrogens, tobacco.

8. **Drug induced/iatrogenic/physician induced diseases** are functional diseases caused by drugs, e.g.

INH	Hepatitis
Hydralazine	DLE
Antipsychotic	Parkinsonism
Salicylates and corticosteroid	Peptic ulcer.

9. **Drug allergy/drug hypersensitivity** is an immunologically mediated reaction independent of drug dosage.
   In supersensitivity, response is highly increased. Hypersensitivity reaction is of 6 types:

   i. Type I/**A**naphylactic
   ii. Type II/**C**ytolytic reaction } Humoral   **ACID**
   iii. Type III/**I**mmune complex
   iv. Type IV/**D**elayed reaction (cell mediated).
   v. Type V/LATS (long acting thyroid stimulator).
   vi. Type VI/GUHD.

   i. **Type I/anaphylactic/immediate reaction:** IgE fixed to mast cell → Ag-Ab reaction on exposure to drug on mast cell surface, releasing mediators (5-HT, histamine, LTC_4 and D_4, PG, PAF)
   ↓
   angioedema, itching, asthma, anaphylactic shock.

ii. **Type II/cytolytic reaction**
   (IgG/IgM) + (Drug/Tissue component)
   ↓
   Ag – Ab reaction on re-exposure on cell surface
   ↓
   Complement activation and cytolysis
   ↓
   SLE, organ damage, hemolysis, agranulocytosis, thrombocytopenia.

iii. **Type III/retarded/Arthus reaction** (duration 1–2 weeks)
   IgG + drug →Ag – Ab complex
   ↓
   Binding complement and precipitating on vascular endothelium
   ↓
   Destructive inflammatory response
   ↓
   Rashes, serum sickness (fever, LAP, arthralgia), polyarthritis nodosa, S.J. syndrome (erythema multiforme), arthritis, nephritis, myocarditis, CNS symptoms.

iv. **Type IV:** Ag + ereceptor of T cell
   ↓
   T cell sensitization
   ↓
   Lymphokines (attract granulocytes)
   ↓
   Contact dermatitis, photosensitization
   ↓
   Reactions develop in >12 hrs.

Treatment of allergy

Anaphylactic shock, or angioedema of larynx } 0.5 mg adrenaline SC then antihistaminics and IV glucocorticoids may be given.

Bronchospasm (adrenaline followed by glucocorticoid).
Type II, III, IV: Glucocorticoids.

Drugs causing allergic reactions
- Antibiotics
- ACE inhibitor
- Methyldopa
- Hydralazine
- Phenothiazine
- Carbamazepine
- Phenylbutazone
- Salicylates
- Allopurinol

10. **Drug dependence:** Drugs altering mood and feelings leading to withdrawal from reality (euphoria) and taken for self-satisfaction which is more important than basic needs. It is self-medication for non-therapeutic purposes. Stimulant drugs produce no/little dependence.

    Dependence is
1. Physical
2. Psychological
3. Drug abuse
4. Drug addiction
5. Drug habituation

Physical dependence: Altered physiological state due to repeated use of drug necessitating its use to maintain physiological equilibrium. Drug withdrawal causes **withdrawal syndrome (abstinence syndrome).**

Nervous system acts normally in the presence of drug called neuroadaptation, e.g. BZD, opioid, etc.

Reinforcement is the ability of the drug to reinforce the user for repeated use, e.g. cocaine, etc. Faster the drugs act, more reinforcing these are, e.g. weak reinforcers are BZD.

Drug abuse is the social disapproval of the manner and purpose of drug use.

Drug addiction is the compulsion for drug use. Most addicts relapse after withdrawal, e.g. LSD.

Drug habituation is less compulsive drug use. Withdrawal causes only mild discomfort, e.g. Tea, tobacco.

11. **Drug withdrawal reactions:**

Corticosteroid withdrawal	Acute adrenal insufficiency
Clonidine withdrawal	Severe HTN and sympathetic over activity
β-blocker withdrawal	Worsening of MI and angina pectoris
Antiepileptic drug withdrawal	Seizures

12. **Photosensitization** (cutaneous reactions due to drug and radiation).

    1. Photoallergic: Drug →CMI response $\xrightarrow{\text{light (320–400 nm)}}$ dermatitis.

    2. Phototoxic: Drug in skin

$$\downarrow \text{light (290–320 nm)}$$
$$\text{Photochemical reactions}$$
$$\downarrow$$
$$\text{Photobiological reactions}$$
$$\downarrow$$
$$\text{Local tissue damage (sunburn like)}$$
$$\downarrow$$

Desquamation, edema, hyperpigmentation, e.g. demeclocycline

Drugs causing photoallergy
- CPZ
- Chloroquine
- Sulfonamide
- Sulfonylurea
- Griseofulvin

Unit 2
Drugs Acting on Nervous System

5. An Overview of Nervous System

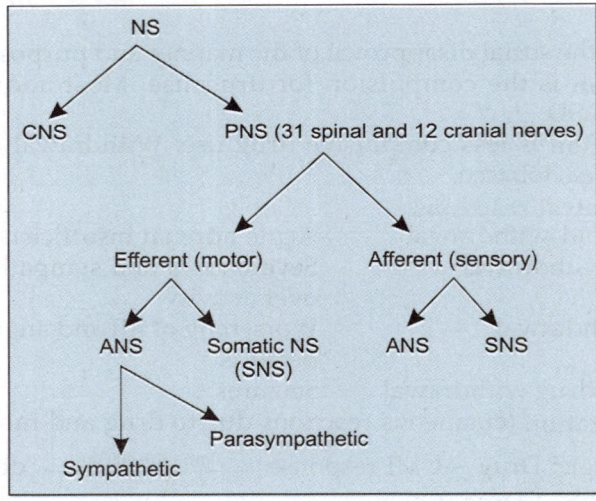

- ANS functions **below conscious level and** controls **visceral functions (cardiac and smooth muscles and exocrine gland)**.
- SNS is **single myelinated** nerve for voluntary control, e.g. skeletal muscle control.
- Sympathetic (thoracolumbar) NS has **2 chains of ganglia** on each side of the spinal cord.

Afferents of ANS
Most visceral nerves are mixed with nonmyelinated visceral afferent nerve fibres having cell bodies in the dorsal root ganglion of spinal nerve and sensory ganglion of CN.
- All organs have ANS **except** skeletal muscle.
- Preganglionic and somatic nerve fibres are **myelinated** but postganglionic nerve fibres are **nonmyelinated**.
- Level of activity of innervated organ is algebraic sum of sympathetic and parasympathetic tone.

An Overview of Nervous System   39

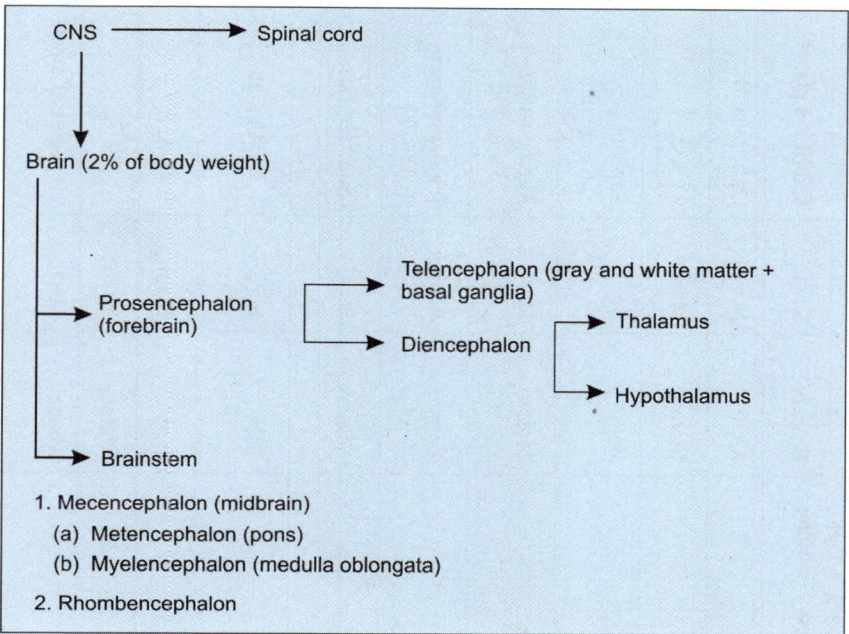

- **Refractory period** of atrial fibre is decreased by sympathetic and parasympathetic fibres.
- **Central autonomic connections** are: (1) **midbrain and medulla** (for respiratory, pupillary, vagal control, etc).

(2) **Hypothalamus (highest)**

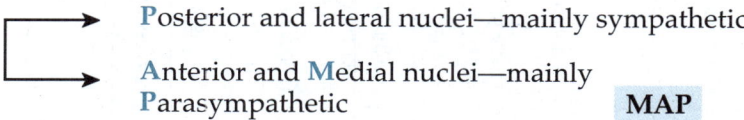

- Lateral column in the thoracic spinal cord contains cells for sympathetic outflow.
- **Autonomic efferent /motor limb**
  → Sympathetic (vessels, gland, hair follicle).
  → Parasympathetic (gastric and pancreatic gland).

But most organs receive both sympathetic (predominate in stress) and parasympathetic (predominate in satiation and rest) nerves.

Sweet gland, piloerector muscle and some vessels have postganglionic sympathetic cholinergic supply.

Neurohumoral transmission: It occurs through synapses and neuro-effector junctions by the release of humoral (chemical) transmitters (DA, 5-HT, GABA, Peptides, Purines) which are present in the prejunctional neurone and released on stimulation.

CNS has >10 and ANS has mainly 2 neurotransmitters (ACh, NE).

Table 5.1

Lieing	L	CN				128 = Sensory 10,975 = Both Rest = Motor	Some	Passage ways of CN
		CN	I	(oLfactory) smell	Sensory		Some	Cribriform plate I
People	dicaPrio	CN	II	(oPtic) sight	Sensory		Say	Optic canal II
Cause	Conditioned	CN	III	(oCulomotor) accommodation	Motor		Marry	CO_2
Trouble	Titanic	CN	IV	(Trochlear) accommodation	Motor		Money	
To	To	CN	V	(Trigeminal) mastication	Both		But	Superior orbital fissure III to VI
All	Award	CN	VI	(Abducens) eye movement	Motor		My	Middle meatus VII to VIII
Featuring	Featuring	CN	VII	(Facial) facial movement (anterior 2/3 taste)	Both		Brother	Jugular foramen IX to XI
Very	Very	CN	VIII	(Vestibulocochlear) hearing and balance	Sensory		Says	Sun Meri Jaan
Good	Good	CN	IX	(Glossopharyngeal) posterior 1/3 taste	Both		Big	F. RoTUndum V_2
Villain	Villain	CN	X	(Vagus) talking	Both		Brain	F. OvAl E V_3
And	And	CN	XI	(Accessory) head turning	Motor		Matters	
Hero	Hero	CN	XII	(Hypoglossal) tongue movement	Motor		Most	Hypoglossal canal

Table 5.2: Difference between somatic and autonomic nervous systems

Somatic	Autonomic
1. **Supply**—skeletal muscles	All others
2. **Distal most synapse**—within CNS	Outside CNS
3. **Nerve fibres**—myelinated	Presynaptic—myelinated Postsynaptic—non-myelinated
4. **Peripheral plexus**—absent	Present
5. **Neurotransmitter**	All presynaptic—ACh Postsynaptic parasympathetic—ACh Postsynaptic sympathetic—ACh/NA
6. **Effect of nerve section on organ** paralysis and atrophy	No paralysis No atrophy

Table 5.3: Difference between sympathetic and parasympathetic nerves

Sympathetic	Parasympathetic
1. Origin: T_1 to L_3 Thoracolumbar (thoracic and lumbar region)	1. CN III, VII, IX, X, S_{2-4}: (Craniosacral—brainstem and sacral region)
2. Ganglion away from organ	2. Close to organ
3. Pre- and postganlionic 1:20 to 1:100	3. 1:1 to 1:2 (exception-enteric plexus)
4. Function: Stress and emergency control, fight or flight reaction	4. Food assimilation and energy conservation
5. Transmitter: NA (major) and ACh (minor)	5. ACh

Steps in neurohumoral transmission
- Impulse conduction
- Transmitter release
- Action on postjunctional membrane
- Postjunctional activity
- Termination of transmitter action

1. **Impulse conduction:** Resting transmembrane potential (-80 mV inside) by high K^+ efflux and low Na^+ influx.

    ↓

    On stimulation, ↑ Na^+ conductance (influx)

    ↓

    $+20$ mV inside (reverse polarisation—depolarisation), K^+ efflux for repolarisation

    ↓

    Action potential (AP) generation

    ↓

    Ion channel activation by the generation of local circuit of the next excitable part of the membrane.

    ↓

    AP propagation.

Na⁺ K⁺ pump is electrogenic pump, pumping 3Na⁺ ion outside for each 2K⁺ ion inside the cell. This creates about –4 mV on the inside, beyond that, diffusion alone creates negativity.

Na⁺ K⁺ leak channel has 100 times more permeability for K⁺ than Na⁺. Na channel is 5000 times more permeable than K⁺ channel.

Change in potential from –80 mV to +20 mV takes 2 msec. Na channels open and close within 2 msec but K⁺ channels open slower than Na⁺ channels.

Voltage gated Na⁺ K⁺ channel

Both activation and inactivation of Na⁺ channel (Na⁺ influx) but only activation of K⁺ channel (K⁺ efflux) occur during potential change from – ve to + ve.

1. Resting
2. Na⁺ activation
3. Na⁺ inactivation
4. K⁺ activation

Hydrated K⁺ is smaller than hydrated Na⁺, hence only K⁺ can move out and Cl⁻ move in (hyperpolarisation).

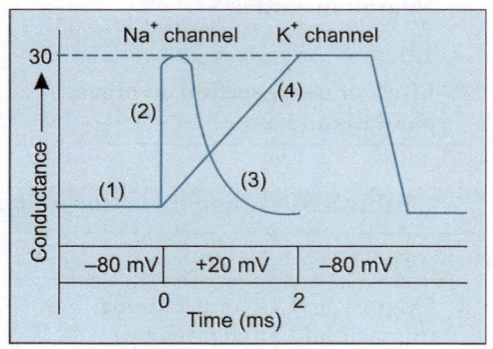

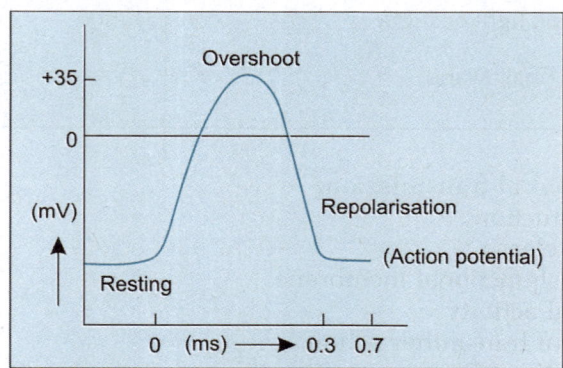

Tetrodotoxin (from puffer fish) ⎤ Selectively abolish increased

Saxitoxin (from shell fish)   Na⁺ conductance in nerve fibre.

2. **Transmitter release:** Neurotransmitter is stored in synaptic vesicles of prejunctional nerve ending. It occurs by vesicle fusion with axonal membrane after Ca⁺⁺ entry due to impulse.
3. **Action on postjunctional membrane**: Released transmitter combines with receptor on postjunctional membrane and causes excitatory/inhibitory postsynaptic potential (EPSP/IPSP).

EPSP is caused due to ↑ permeability for all ions. This leads to depolarisation by Na^+/Ca^+ influx and K^+ efflux.

IPSP is caused due to ↑ permeability for smaller ions. Since hydrated K^+ is smaller than hydrated Na^+, it leads to hyperpolarisation by K^+ efflux and Cl^- influx (permeable for smaller ions →hydrated K^+ is smaller than hydrated Na^+).

4. **Postjunctional activity:** Suprathreshold EPSP generates a propagated postjunctional AP which is stabilised by IPSP.
5. **Termination of transmitter action:** After combination with receptor, transmitters either are degraded (e.g. ACh) or actively uptaken into prejunctional membrane.

Co-transmission: In ANS, co-transmitter is also present in the same neurone but in the different vesicles, e.g. purine (ATP, adenosine), peptides (VIP, NPY, substance P, enkephalin, somatostatin) and PG. In most cases, combination is:
– VIP with ACh.
– ATP with ACh and NA.

NPY causes vasoconstriction which is found in vascular adrenergic nerves.

Exception: ATP is stored with NA in the same vesicles.

Ion channels are: (i) **voltage** sensitive (electrically gated), e.g. Na channel on axon and K and Ca channel on cell body and dandrites, (ii) **transmitter sensitive** (ligand gated/R operated) found on cell body and synapses. **R channel coupling** occurs through: (i) **R-acting** directly on **channel proteins,** (ii) R-coupled to ion channel through **G-protein,** (iii) R-coupled to G-proteins to modulate **2nd messengers** which secondarily modulate channels. Ion current of a channel is **EPSP** (Na or Ca channel opening and K channel closing) or **IPSP** (K or Cl^- channel opening). Fast IPSP is blocked by $GABA_A$ R antagonist and slow IPSP by $GABA_B$ R antagonist. Receptors may be ionotropic (directly gated cation selective channel such as NMDA R) and metabotropic (G-protein coupled 2nd messenger system such as glutamate R). **Most** nerves of CNS are excited by glutamate and aspartate.

Inhibitory presynaptic auto-R occurs on cholinergic and noradrenergic nerves causing each transmitter to inhibit its own release (autoinhibitory feedback). Presynaptic $\alpha_2 R$ inhibits NA release and β_2 stimulates NA release (presynaptic R of DA, PG, AT II, 5-HT and enkephalin of adrenergic nerves modulates NA release). Release of transmitter stores from vesicles requires Ca^{2+} entry through its channel and triggers interaction between vesicular proteins **(synaptobrevin, synaptogramin)** and nerve ending membrane proteins **(syntaxin, SNAP)**→ fusion of vesicular and nerve ending membranes → pore opening to extracellular space and neurotransmitter release. NE of chromaffin granule is converted to E in cytoplasm by phenylethanolanine-N-methyl transferase and taken up into granule.

---

cAMP activates pKa and **DAG** activates **pKc**.
cAMP and IP_3 are related to Ca^{2+}.

DAG = 3 letters = PKC.
4 letters = cAMP = IP_3 = Ca^{2+}.

Pharmacology Review

Outlay of ANS

CNS	Peripheral
Somatic (motor nerve)	ACh, Nm → skeletal muscle
ANS Parasympathetic (ciliary muscle, gastric and pancreatic gland)	ACh → N_N → ACh → M
Sympathetic (vessel, spleen, sweat gland, hair follicle)	ACh → N_N → NA (Major) → α, β; ACh (Minor) → M; DA → D
	ACh (adrenal medulla) → Adrenaline in blood

Autonomic innervation of male sexual response:
Erection is mediated by **Parasympathetic** NS. | Point and Shoot |
Emission is mediated by **Sympathetic** NS.
Ejaculation is mediated by somatic and visceral nerves.

Molecular mechanisms of action (also see pages 26 to 28)

Cholinergic ⟶ Muscarinic (M_1–M_5)
⟶ Nicotinic (N_M, N_N)

Adrenergic ⟶ α ($α_1$, $α_2$)
⟶ β ($β_1$–$β_3$)

Dopaminergic: D_1–D_5.

3 major effector pathways of G-protein coupled receptors (GPCR)

A. Adenyl cyclase pathway:

- β-adrenoceptors
- $α_2$-adrenoceptors

A = AC
T = Two   ATB
B = Beta

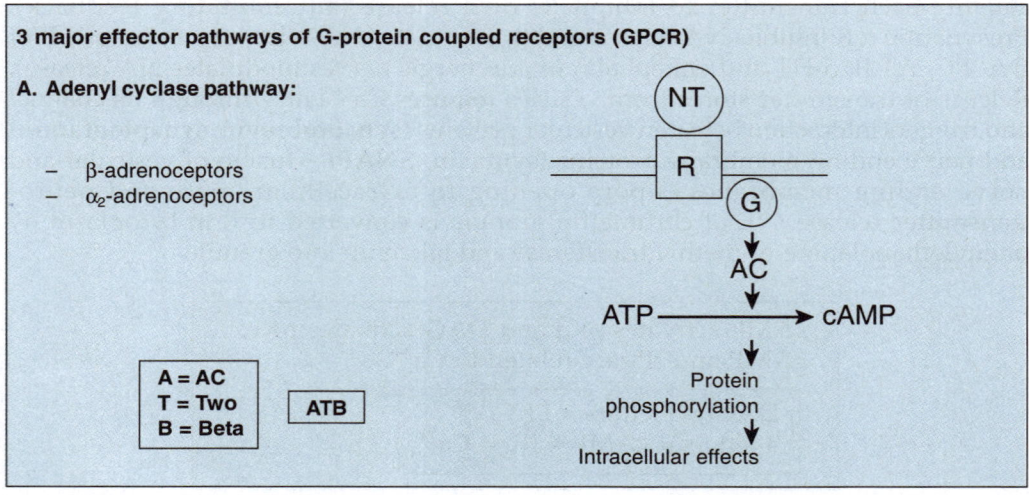

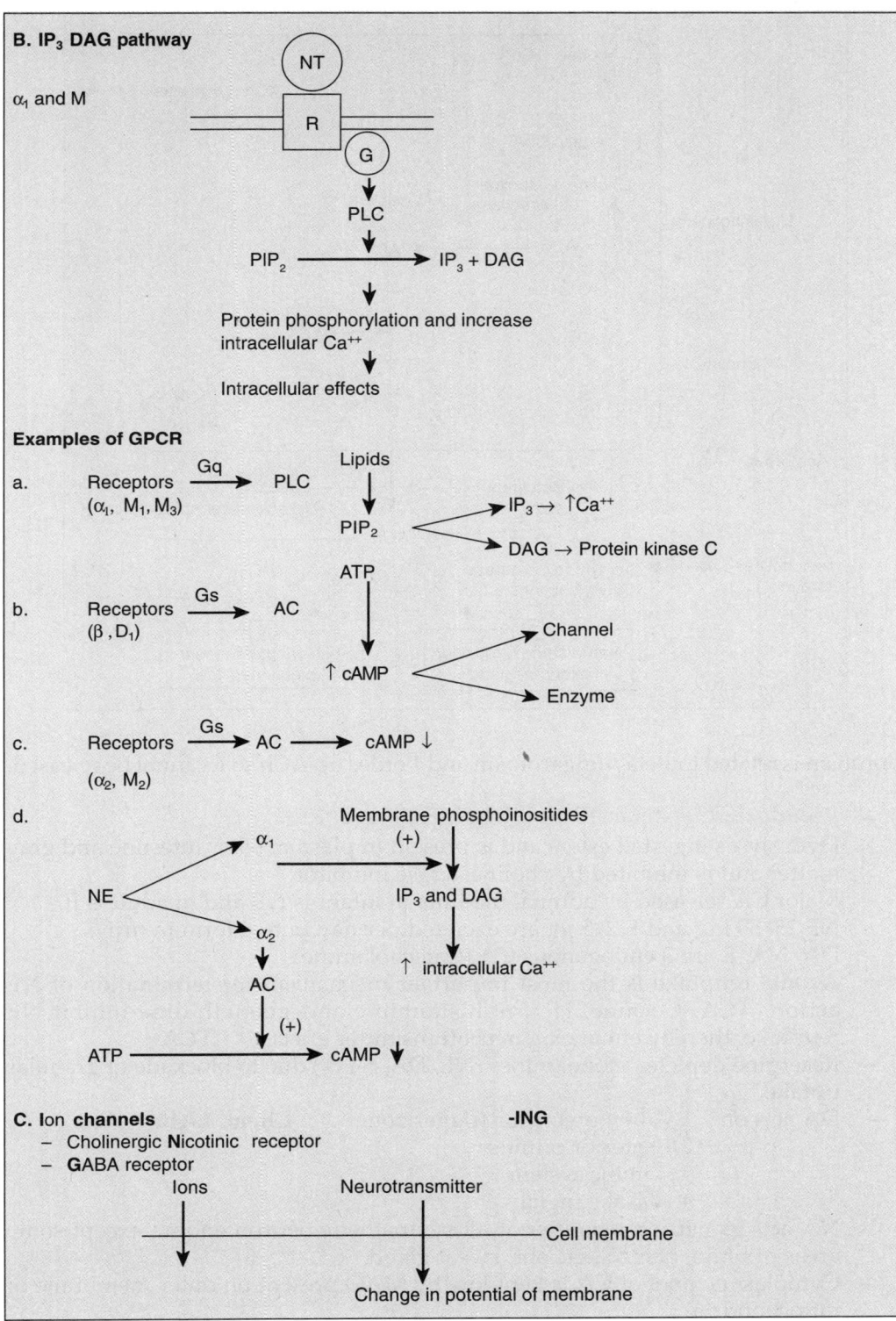

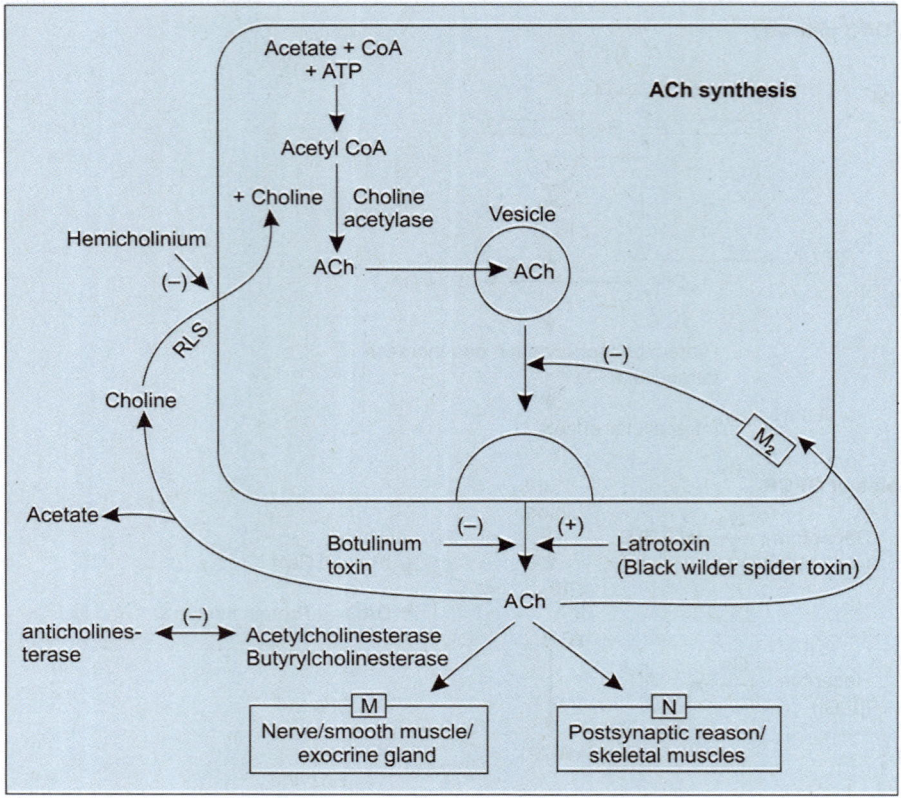

Botulism is related to **B**eta **B**ungarotoxin and **B**ottles up ACh so it cannot be released.

- **Pseudocholinesterase/Butyrylcholinesterase**
  Hydrolyses ingested esters and is present in plasma, liver, intestine and gray matter and is inhibited by cholinesterase inhibitor.
- Major CA released by adrenal medulla in infant is NE and in adult is E.
- NE 25–50 mg and E 2–5 µg are excreted per day in free form in urine.
- DA, NA, E are 3 endogenous CA (Catecholamine)
- Axonal reuptake is the most important mechanism for termination of NE action. **T**CA, **C**ocaine, H_1 **A**ntihistaiminic and guanethidine inhibit NE reuptake, thereby enhancing neurotransmitter effects.   **TCA**
- Reserpine depletes monoamines (NE, DA, 5-HT) due to blockade of granular uptake.
- DA acts on   1. **Chem**oreceptor trigger zone   **Chem. LAB.**
  2. **A**nterior pituitary
  3. **L**imbic system
  4. **B**asal ganglia
- NA acts as neurotransmitter at all sympathetic neuron ending except some areas of brain, hair follicle and sweat gland.
- Cytoplasmic pool of CA is kept low by MAO present on outer membrane of mitochondria.

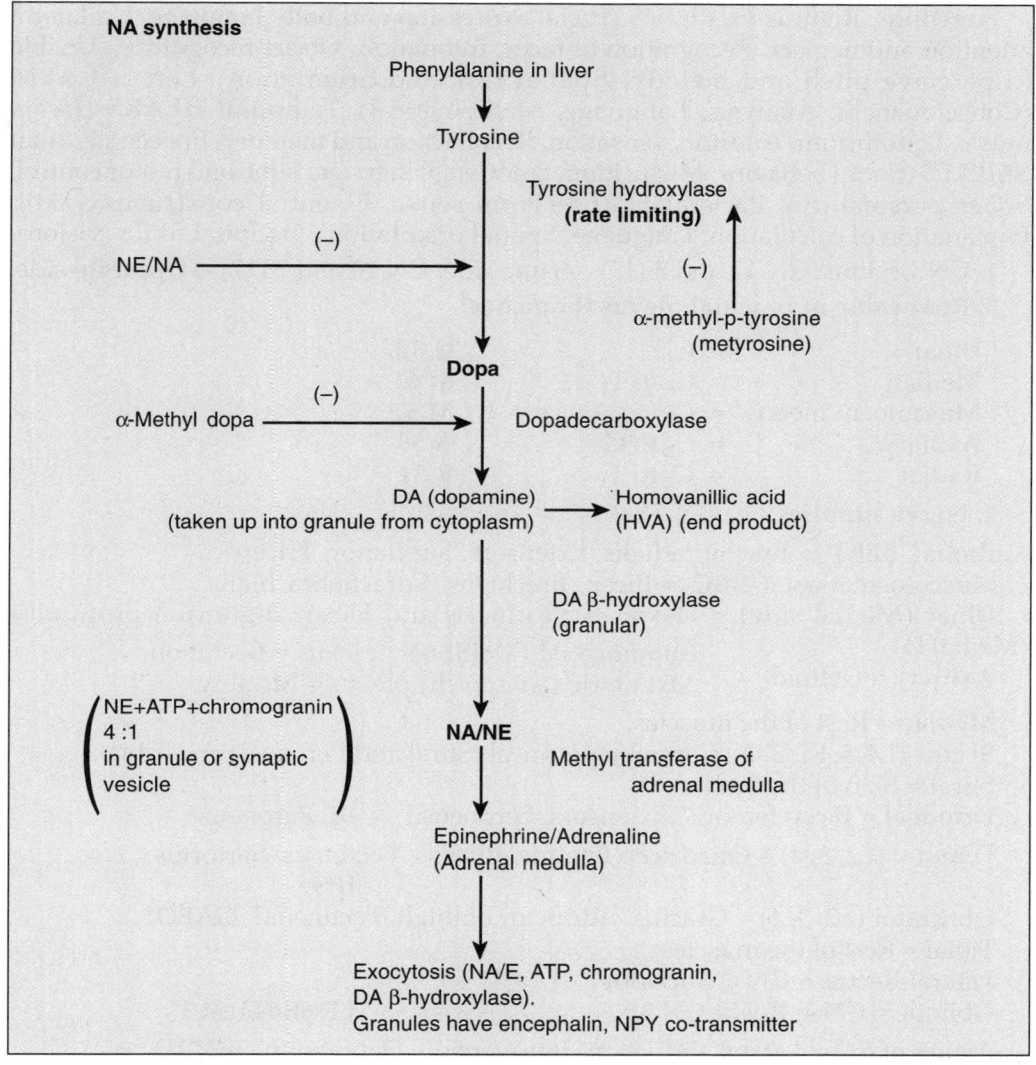

Methoxy hydroxymandelic acid in urine (vanillyl mandelic acid/VMA) (90% of NE metabolite).

1. **Cerebral hemisphere:** Normally, one out of two hemispheres is dominant (for analytical process) or nondominant (for visuospatial relation). But in mania, schizophrenia, and other psychiatric disorder, the right ½ has nothing left in it and the left ½ has nothing right in it.

Functions: Right is **FURIOUS** (**F**acial expression and body language, **U**nilateral attention and neglect, **R**ecognition of faces, **I**ntonation, **O**bject recognition, **U**nable to percieve pitch and melody, **S**patial task and orientation). Left is **CALM** (**C**onsciousness, **A**nalysis, **L**anguage, **M**athematical), Temporal **HEARS** (**H**ears music, **E**quilibrium, **A**uditory sensation, **R**ecollection and memory, **S**peech), Frontal **SMELLS** (**S**ocial behavior, **M**icturition, **E**motion, **L**anguage, **L**imb and motor control, **S**ober personality), Parietal **FEELS** (**F**orm sense, **E**ssential constructive skill, **E**xplanation of calculation, **L**anguage, **S**patial orientation), Occipital **SEES** (vision).

2. **CN Lesions:** CN 12 and 5 (17)→Same side. CN 10 and 7 (17)→Opposite side.

3. **Root value of brachial plexus (branches)**

Ulnar	= C_8T_1	U 81
Median	= C_6 to T_1	M 61
Musculocutaneous	= C_5 to C_7	M 57
Axillary	= C_5 to C_6	A 56
Radial	= C_5 to T_1	R 51

4. **Nerve supplies**

Radial BEST = **B**rachioradialis, **E**xtensors, **S**upinator, **T**riceps.
Musculocutaneous BBC = **B**icep, **B**rachialis, **C**orachobrachialis.
Ulnar (**M**edial side) = **F**lexor carpi ulnaris and **F**lexor digitorum profundus (**M**edial ½)
Axillary = **D**eltoid

Submuco**S**al (Mei**SS**ner) plexus = **S**ecretion.
Myenteric (Auerbach) plexus = **M**otility.

Median = Rest of the muscles.
Sciatic (L4, 5, S1, 2, 3): Common peroneal (**S**ural and **P**eroneal) and **T**ibial.
Sural = **S**kin of the limb.
Peroneal = **B**icep femoris, **E**xtensors, **P**eroneus. **BE Peroneus**
Femoral (L2, 3, 4) = Quadricep femoris, **I**lliacus, **P**ectineus, **S**artorius
IPS
Obturator (L2, 3, 4) = **G**racilis, **A**dductor of thigh, **P**ectineus? **GAPO**
Tibial = Rest of the muscles.
Lateral Rectus = CN 6, **S**uperior
Oblique = CN 4, **Rest** = CN 3. **LR 6S04 rest 3**

Action of **SO** = **L**ateral abduction, **I**ntroversion, **D**epression. **SOLID**

5. **Erb's palsy: D**amage to **C**5 and 6 of **B**rachial plexus leading to **A**bsent Moro and bicep reflex. **ABCDE**

Cholinergic and Anticholinergic Drugs

Cholinergic Drugs
(Cholinomimetic, Parasympathomimetic)

Cholinergic agonist: Classification

1. **Directly acting**
   (a) **Est**ers — **Me**thacholine, **Ac**etylcholine (ACh), **B**ethanechol and **Ca**rbachol   `My ABC LMNOP`
   (b) **Alkaloids** — **A**recoline, **L**obeline, **M**uscarine, **N**icotine, **O**xotermorine, **P**ilocarpine
2. **Indirectly acting/anticholinesterase**
   Reversible and irreversible

Reversible   `sin (PAP) END`
- **P**hysostigmine (Eserine)
- **A**mbenonium, **R**ivastigmine
- **P**yridostigmine
- **E**drophonium
- **N**eostigmine
- **D**emecarium

Tacrine, Rivastigmine, Galantamine, Donepezil } Used for Alzheimer's disease

Irreversible
- **T**abun, Sarin, Soman (nerve gas for chemical warfare)
- **D**i **I**sopropylfluorophosphate (dyflos/DFP)
- **M**alathion   `TIME Please`
- **E**chothiophate
- **P**arathion

Acetylcholine (as prototype): Analogues of ACh are quarternary compounds.
Action: Nicotinic and muscarinic.
Two binding sites are for ACh, one binds the quarternary nitrogen and the second binds carboxyl oxygen.

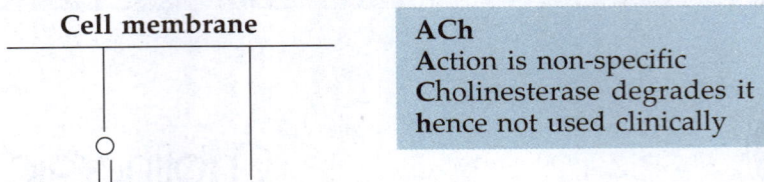

Mechanism: Directly acting cholinergic agonists **mimic** the effect of ACh by binding directly to cholinoceptors.

Disadvantage of ACh: It has short duration of action, activates all cholinoceptors present in most internal organs.

Cholinoceptors
(1) **Muscarinic receptor** is present in cardiac and smooth muscle, eye, vessel, respiratory tract, glands of GIT, sweat gland and CNS (all subtypes).
Types: M_1, M_2, M_3, M_4, M_5
      └─────┘
       Well defined

Muscarinic receptors are stimulated by muscarine and inhibited by atropine. CNS (cortex, basal ganglia, spinal cord) has both N_N and muscarinic receptor (mainly M_1). Muscarinic agonist and α_2 agonist inhibit ACh release at autonomic neuro-effector due to autoreceptor site but not in ganglia and skeletal muscles. Endothelial cells of all vessels have muscarinic receptor for smooth muscle relaxation. ACh stimulates and atropine blocks all 3 subtypes of muscarinic receptor.

	M_1	M_2	M_3
1. Location and functions	Autonomic ganglia and gastric gland	Depressant effect on heart	Smooth muscles for contraction and exocrine gland for secretion
2. Transducer mechanism	Increase cytosolic Ca^{++} through IP_3/DAG	Decrease cAMP, K^+ channel opening	Increase cytosolic Ca^{++} through IP_3/DAG

(2) **Nicotinic receptor** N_M/N_I Stimulated by nicotine and inhibited
    (2 types) $N_G/N_N/N_2$ by hexamethonium.

N_M is stimulated by PTMA (phenyltrimethyl ammonium) and nicotine, and inhibited by tubocurarine/α-Bungarotoxin/curare.
It is present on skeletal muscles. $N_{Muscle} \; N_{Nerve}$

N_N is present in autonomic ganglia, adrenal medulla and CNS. It is stimulated by nicotine/DMPP (dimethylphenyl piperazinium), and inhibited by hexamethonium/trimethaphan. It causes CA release in adrenal medulla.

Nicotinic cholinergic receptor
(a) 8 nm in diameter.
(b) 5 subunits $(2\alpha + \beta + \delta + \gamma)$/pentamer
(c) 2 molecules of ACh bind to 2α subunits, rest subunits moving apart opening central pore of 0.7 nm, to allow passage of partially hydrated ions (Na^+, K^+, Ca^{++}, Cl^-, etc.). Positive charges lining the channel block the passage of anions.

Muscarinic action
- M_1: Present in CNS → stimulatory
- M_2: Present in heart → inhibitory
- M_3: Present in smooth muscle → contraction
- Endothelium → Release NO → vasodilatation

Exocrine glands →↓ secretion
1. Hyperpolarisation of SA node causes ↓ impulse generation → bradycardia.
2. ↑ RP at AV node and His–Purkinje fibres → slow conduction, ↑ atrial contraction, flutter and fibrillation.
3. ACh → muscarinic receptor on endothelium → EDRF/NO (nitric oxide) → vasodilatation.
4. Smooth muscle contraction in most organs causes ↑ peristalsis and ↑ tone in GIT and relaxation of sphincter → bowel evacuation. Contraction of detrusor and relaxation of trigone and sphincter → bladder voiding.
   Bronchial muscle contraction → asthma precipitation.
5. ↑ed secretion of all parasympathetic innervated glands (salivation, lacrimation, sweating, gastric secretion, tracheobronchial secretion).
6. Contraction of circular muscle of iris → miosis →↓ IOP. Contraction of ciliary muscle. Eye accommodated for near vision

Nicotinic action (ACh acts only at high doses).
1. ACh stimulates both sympathetic and parasympathetic nerves (action at N_N receptors) present on postsynaptic neuron. It does not cross BBB but on direct injection to brain, it causes stimulation followed by depression.
2. It causes contraction of skeletal muscles (action at N_M receptors)
   - Intra-arterial injection → twitching and fasciculation.
   - IV injection → no effect due to rapid hydrolysis of ACh.

Interaction (IA)
1. AntiChE potentiates ACh mainly and to a lesser extent methacholine, bethanechol, carbachol also.
2. Atropine antagonises muscarinic action.
3. Adrenaline antagonises ACh.

Methacholine
- Hydrolysed by AChE.
- Stimulates both cholinoceptors (N and M).
- Acts selectively on CVS.

Carbachol
- Not hydrolysed by AChE or pseudocholinesterase.
- Stimulates both cholinoceptors (N and M).
- Acts selectively on GIT and bladder.

Bethanechol
- Stimulates only muscarinic receptor.
- Stimulates selectively smooth muscle of GIT and bladder.
- It is the only systemically effective cholinergic agonist.
- Used in paralytic ileus, non-obstructive urinary retention, bladder atony, congenital megacolon, gastroesophageal reflux.

Arecoline
- Found in betel nut *Areca catechu*.
- Has nicotinic and muscarinic actions.
- Responsible for watering of mouth during chewing of pan.

Muscarine
- Found in mushroom (*Amanita muscaira and inocybe*)
- Causes mushroom poisoning.

Types of mushroom poisoning
1. Early/muscarinic, treated by atropine.
2. Late/phalloidin type → inhibits RNA and protein synthesis → damages GIT mucosa, liver and kidney.
3. Hallucinogenic/anticholinergic action is due to isoxazole of *A. muscaria*.

Pilocarpine is obtained from *Pilocarpus microphyllus*. It is tertiary amine acting on **M-receptor**. The only cholinomimetic alkaloid used clinically.

Mechanism
1. It stimulates muscarinic receptor.
2. It causes sweating and salivation, miosis and ciliary muscle contraction.
3. Small dose → ↓ BP

   Large dose → ↑ BP due to ganglionic stimulation.

PK: Lipid soluble. Hence
- Penetrates cornea used in eye.
- Easily absorbed
- Crosses BBB

U: Used as miotic
1. Open angle glaucoma.
2. To counter the effect of mydriatics.
3. To break adhesion of iris (miotic is alternated with mydriatic).

Anticholinesterase (AntiChE)

Mechanism: This inhibits cholinesterase → ↑ ACh in synaptic space.

AntiChE and ACh are same in action
Action is reversible/irreversible (due to covalent bond formation).

Action
1. Lipid soluble agents (organophosphate and physostigmine) cross BBB and thus have CNS effects. They have more marked muscarinic effects.
   Lipid insoluble agents (neostigmine) do not cross BBB and do not have CNS effects. They have more marked nicotinic effects (skeletal muscles and ganglia)
2. AntiChE in skeletal muscle → ACh release → no immediate hydrolysis → repetitive receptor binding → twitching and fasciculation.
   In curarised and myasthenic muscle, it causes ↑ force of contraction.
   High doses → persistent depolarization → inhibition of neuromuscular transmission → weakness and paralysis.
3. It stimulates muscarinic receptor of ganglia.
   At high doses → inhibition of transmission due to persistent depolarization of ganglionic nicotinic receptor.
4. Over all effects on CVS depend on agents and doses.
   Muscarinic action →↓ HR and ↓ BP.
   Ganglionic stimulation → ↑ HR and ↑ BP.
   Ganglionic blockade with high doses and action on medullary centre cause stimulation followed by inhibition.

PK: (a) **Physostigmine:** Rapidly absorbed orally, penetrates cornea, crosses BBB. Excreted after hydrolysis by ChE. **L**ipid soluble, **M**iotic in glaucoma, **N**atural and **O**rally absorbable **(LMNO)**.
(b) **Others:** Poorly absorbed. Not cross BBB. Neostigmine (water soluble, used in myasthenia gravis, synthetic and poor orally absorbable). Edrophonium (shortest acting) causes respiratory failure. Excreted unchanged in urine (poor hydrolysis).
(c) **Organophosphates:** Absorbed from all sites even from intact skin and lungs. Hydrolysed (parathion most toxic).

Contraindication of ChE inhibitor (AntiChE)
1. Asthma, respiratory failure (most important)
2. Peptic ulcer (increase gastric secretion).

U: 1. **Alzheimer's disease** (degeneration of cholinergic neurones → dementia), treated by cerebroselective AntiChE **Tacrine,** Gallentamine, Rivastigmine, Donepezil.
2. **Belladonna poisoning** (Anticholinergic): Physostigmine IV crosses BBB.
3. **Cobra bite:** Neostigmine + Atropine inhibit respiratory paralysis.
4. **Drug overdose:** TCA, phenothiazine and antihistaminics have additional anticholinergic property. Treated by physostigmine. With GA and diazepam, physostigmine causes arousal effect.
5. **Postoperative decurarisation:** Neostigmine preceded by atropine.
6. **PSVT.**
7. **Urinary retention/postoperative paralytic ileus:** Bethanechol used.
8. **Myasthenia gravis (1 in 10000 population)**
   Auto Abs against $N_M R$ at skeletal muscle end plate.
   ↓
   Decrease in N_M to 1/3 of normal.
   ↓
   Weakness and fatigue of muscle with recovery after rest.
   AntiChE inhibits AChE → ↑ ACh to act on $N_M R$ over large area.

Treatment

- Neostigmine (DOC) 15 mg oral QID is used because it is water soluble, does not cross BBB; no CNS side effects. Has more marked nicotinic effects).
- In case of intolerance → atropine to counter muscarinic side effects.
- Corticosteroid → ↓N_MR-Ab synthesis. Prednisolone 30–60 mg/d → remission in **80%** in advance cases.
- Azathioprine and cyclosporine inhibit N_MR-Ab synthesis.
- Plasmapheresis to remove Ab.
- **Thymectomy** (complete remission) because thymus has modified muscle cells with N_MR on their surface (a source of **Ag** for N_MR-Ab in myasthenic patient).
- **Cholinergic weakness** occurs due to over-treatment with AntiChE which causes persistent depolarization of muscle end plate. Late cases with high doses requirements of AntiChE alternatively experience cholinergic and myasthenic weakness, which require opposite treatment, and are differentiated by:

a. Tensilon edrophonium test

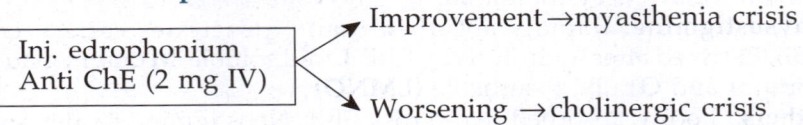

b. Provocative test

0.5 mg IV
d-tubocurarine (N_M receptor antagonist)
↓
Weakness in myasthenia.

9. **As miotic:** Only lipid soluble drugs used, e.g. physostigmine, pyridostigmine.
   - To encounter the effect of mydriatics.
   - To break adhesion of iris (miotics are alternated with mydriatics).
   - **In glaucoma:** Optic nerve damage due to raised (>21 mm Hg) IOP.

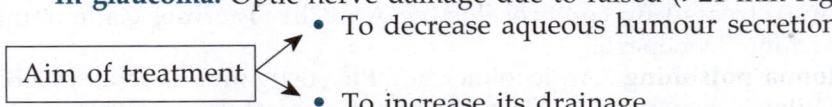

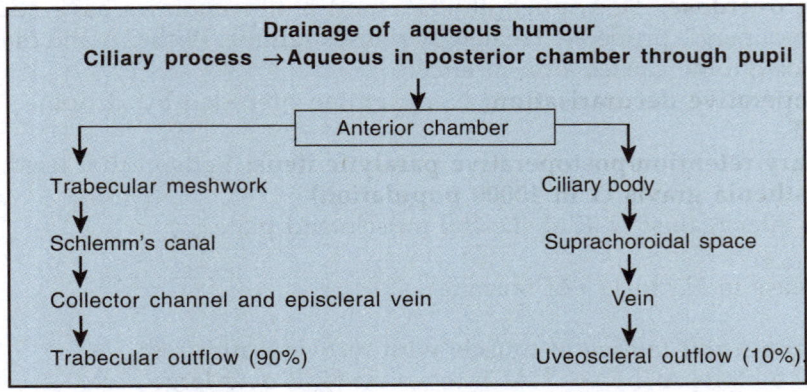

Cholinergic and Anticholinergic Drugs

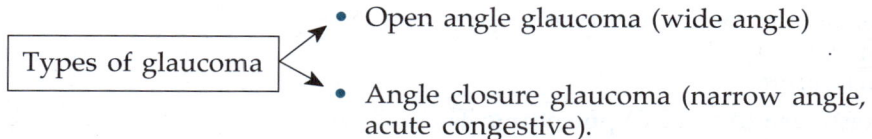

Types of glaucoma
- Open angle glaucoma (wide angle)
- Angle closure glaucoma (narrow angle, acute congestive).

Open angle glaucoma is due to degenerative disease effecting patency of trabecular meshwork.

Treatment of open angle glaucoma (ocular hypotensive drugs)

A. β blockers (DOC)
   Advantages over miotic are:
   (a) No effect on pupil size, ciliary tone, outflow facility.
   (b) Reduce aqueous formation.
   (c) Ocular β blockers are lipophilic.

   Ocular ADR

   Blepharoconjunctivitis, **A**llergy, **D**ryness and **B**urning

   For example, Timolol and Betaxolol.   **BAD Burning**

B. Miotics: Increase tone of ciliary muscle and sphincter pupillae → ↑ outflow leading to ↓ IOP. Therapy is started with the lowest effective concentration and increased later, e.g. **pilocarpine** (constricts pupil and decreases IOP). If not effective, **Pilocarpine + Physostigmine** combination is given.

C. α agonist: Adjuvant to miotics/β blocker.

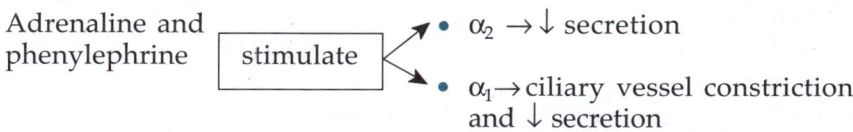

Adrenaline and phenylephrine — stimulate
- $\alpha_2 \to$ ↓ secretion
- $\alpha_1 \to$ ciliary vessel constriction and ↓ secretion

Adrenaline stimulates $\beta_2 \to$ ↑ outflow through trabecular meshwork.

Dipivefrine (prodrug of Adr.) —esterase of cornea→ Adrenaline.

Apreclonidine ⎫
Brimonidine ⎭ → ↓ aqueous production via α_2 action

D. Acetazolamide: It decreases aqueous formation by limiting the generation of HCO_3^- ion in ciliary epithelium.

E. $PGF_{2\alpha}$: Increases uveoscleral outflow, e.g. latanoprost.

Treatment of narrow angle glaucoma
- Loss of vision is due to **40–60 mm Hg IOP** (aqueous outflow blockade).
- Antimuscarinic (pupillary dilator) induces this glaucoma (iris dilates and drainage of intraocular fluid is obstructed).

Drugs are
   a. β blocker.
   b. Pilocarpine → sphincter pupillae contraction
         ↓
      spreads iris mass centrally (less contact with lens)
         ↓
      pupillary block removed and free iridocorneal angle.
      But if IOP is high → iris muscle fails to respond.

c. Hypertonic mannitol/glycerol
   d. Acetazolamide.
   e. Apraclonidine.

Anticholinesterase (AntiChE) poisoning: There is excess of acetylcholine leading to symptoms similar to parasympathetic nervous system stimulation.

Local muscarinic manifestations at the site of exposure induce **DUMBELS** syndrome:

Defecation
Urination
Miosis
Bronchoconstriction and ↑ Bronchial secretion
Emesis
Lacrimation
Salivation

Vascular collapse and coma (↓ BP→baroreceptor → stimulation of efferent sympathetic tone to heart)

Respiratory failure → death

Treatment: It must be given within 24 hrs because enzymes undergo aging and become resistant to hydrolysis.

Termination of further exposure.
Airway maintenance
Breathing maintenance
Circulation maintenance   **A B C D**
Drug therapy with antidote

1. **Atropine:** The single most important agent to counteract muscarinic symptoms. Dose—**2 mg IV/10 min** till pupil dilates (up to 200 mg/d). Atropine is for all cases of antiChE (carbamates/organophosphate) poisoning.
2. **Cholinesterase reactivator:** Pralidoxime and obidoxime.

Obidoxime is more potent than pralidoxime. Pralidoxime (2-PAM) is ChE regenerator and chemical antagonist (not R blocker).

Mechanism: It has quarternary nitrogen and attaches to anionic site of enzyme (unoccupied site), and oxime end reacts with phosphorus atom attached to esteratic site → oxime phosphonate formation
→ ChE reactivation.

It is chemical antagonist and regenerates active ChE. It acts more at ChE of skeletal muscle but does not cross BBB.

Phosphorated ChE is reactivated a million times faster if –OH group in the form of oxime is present instead of water.

U: Organophosphate AntiChE poisoning.
CI: Carbonate poisoning because anionic site of enzyme is not free.

Chronic organophosphate poisoning

Leads to polyneuritis, demyelination.
Sensory disturbances occur first.
Unknown mechanism
No specific treatment.

Rivastigmine: Cerebroselective AntiChE for AD. Carbamate derivative of physostigmine.
Mech: Inhibits both AChE (mainly G1 isoform) and BuChE. Enhanced cholinergic transmission in brain.
PK: Lipid soluble (enters brain). Carbamyl residue introduced by the drug into enzyme dissociates slowly →10 hours inhibition of cerebral AChE despite 2 hours plasma half-life of the drug. ADR = mild.
U: AD

Donepezil
Mech: Cerebroselective and reversible AntiAChE.
PK: Half-life = 70 hours, hence given OD. ADR = mild.
U: AD (the most effective cholinergic agent).

Galantamine: Natural alkaloid. Derived from daffodil.
Mech: Nicotine agonist and AntiAChE.
U: AD.

Anticholinergic Drugs
(Parasympatholytic)

All of them are competitive antagonists and act on **2 types of receptors: Muscarinic receptor** (autonomic effector, CNS blocker) and **Nicotinic receptor** (neuromuscular and ganglionic blocker).

Drugs having antimuscarinic actions are: **ATP, ADP**

Anticholinergic, TCA, Phenothiazine, Antihistaminic, Disopyramide, Pethidine.
Natural alkaloids are obtained from solanaceae family. Atropine is obtained from **Atropa belladonna** and **Datura stramonium** having alkaloid **ester of tropic acid** with **tropine base**. Atropine is **racemic. Levoisomers** are more active than dextroisomers. Hyoscine is obtained from *Hyoscyamus niger* with **scopine base** in place of tropine base acting on **eye and glands.**

Classification
1. **Natural alkaloids:** Atropine, hyoscine (scopolamine).
2. **Semisynthetic derivatives:** Homatropine, homatropine methylbromide, hyoscine butylbromide, ipratropium bromide, Tiotropium bromide.
3. **Synthetic compound**
   a. **Mydriatics:** Cyclopentolate, tropicamide.
   b. **Antisecretory–antispasmodics**
      1. **Quarternary compounds:** Propantheline, oxyphenonium, clidinium, penthienate, pipenzolate methyl bromide, mepenzolate methyl bromide, isopropamide, glycopyrrolate.
      2. **Tertiary amines:** Dicyclomine, pirenzepine, telenzepine. oxybutymin, flavoxate, talterodine.
4. **Antiparkinsonian:** Trihexyphenidyl (benzhexol), procyclidine, biperiden, benztropine, cycrimine, ethopropazine.

Atropine (as prototype)
Action

1. It blocks **all MR**.
2. It decreases **salivary (maximum), sweat, lacrimal,** and **tracheobronchial secretion** (M_3 blockade). Sensitivity of atropine is **minimum** on gastric gland and smooth muscle.
3. It stimulates **CNS** such as **medullary centre** (motor, respiratory) and inhibits **vestibular excitation + motion sickness.** High doses cause hallucination, delirium, respiratory depression and coma. But hyoscine produces central depressant effects at low doses and excitation at high doses.
4. It causes **tachycardia (most prominant)** due to blockade of M_2 **R on SA node** →**vagal tone decreases** HR **(max. in young adult)** since parasympathetic (as well as sympathetic) tone is maximum. Increased HR and vasomotor centre stimulation raise BP. **Histamine release** and direct vasodilation (at high doses) lower BP. Vessel has no parasympathetic tone hence no raised BP.
5. **Body temperature** is increased at high doses due to inhibition of sweating and stimulation of temperature regulating centre of hypothalamus (children more sensitive for atropinic fever).
6. It causes mydriasis and light reflex loss, due to parlysis of dilator pupillae (M_3 R blocked) leading to photophobia, ↑ IOP due to obliteration of iridocorneal angle. Cycloplegia due to paralysis of ciliary muscles (M_3 R blocked) leads to blurring of vision. My**D**riasis → contraction of **D**ilator pupillae (α_1 agonist) and relaxation of sphincter pupillae (antimuscarinic and ganglionic blocker). **Miosis**→contraction of sphincter pupillae (AntiChE, Muscarinic agonist) and relaxation of dilator pupillae (α_1 blocker, adrenergic blocker).
7. **All visceral smooth muscle** innervated by parasympathetic motor are relaxed by M_3 blockade →tone and amptitude of contraction decrease → constipation.
8. It causes **bronchodilatation** and reduces airway resistance in COPD and asthma. Histamine, PG and kinin increase vagal activity but atropine partially blocks vagal reflex. Atropine has **relaxant** action on urinary and biliary tract.
9. It has mild LA action.
10. Sensitivity to atropine: Saliva, sweat and bronchial secretion > eye, bronchial muscle and heart > smooth muscle and gastric gland.
11. **Hyoscine** inhibits impulse conduction across cholinergic link in pathway leading from vestibular apparatus to VC.
12. **Scopolamine** is similar to atropine except it is more effective in **CNS**.

PK: Atropine and hyoscine absorbed form GIT. 50% atropine—hepatic metabolism. Rest atropine—excreted unchanged in urine. $t\frac{1}{2}$ = 3–4 hrs. Hyoscine more completely metabolised and crossed BBB.

IA of atropine: It delays gastric emptying hence absorption of **most drugs** are slowed such as levodopa is more degraded peripherally and less reached to brain requiring increased dose. But digoxin and tetracycline absorption is increased due to longer transit time in GIT.

Cholinergic and Anticholinergic Drugs

CI of atropine: Narrow iridocorneal angle (may lead to precipitation of glaucoma due to obliteration of angle). **Elderly patient** with prostatic hypertrophy (may lead to urinary retention).

ADR and toxicity of atropine and its congeners (poisoning of datura/belladonna/beautiful lady/pupil dilator plant):

Manifestations:	
— **D**ilated Pupil.	Dum
— **D**ysphagia.	Dum
— **D**elirium.	Diga
— **D**ifficulty in talking.	Diga
— **M**outh dry.	Mousam
— **B**lurred vision.	Bhiga
— **B**P decreased leading to CVS collapse.	Bhiga
— **B**reathing paralysis.	Bin
— **P**hotophobia.	Piye
— **M**icturition difficulty and constipation.	Mein
— **T**emperature raised.	To
— **G**ait drunken.	Gira
— **H**allucination (visual).	Hai
— **A**taxia.	Allah
— **S**carlet rash.	Surat
— **A**bnormal behavior (psychosis).	Aapki
— **S**kin dry and hot.	Subhan
— **A**uditory hallucination.	Allah

Atropine (a) Muscarinic antagonist: **D**ilates pupil and **D**ecreases acid secretion in acid-peptic disease, urgency in mild cystitis, and respiratory secretion. It causes increased body temprature, rapid pulse, dry mouth, flushed skin, disorientation and mydriasis with cycloplegia. Atropinic fever is more dangerous.
(b) Parasympathetic block effects: Red as beet, Mad as hatter, Hot as hare, Dry as bone, Bloated as bladder.
(c) Blocks: **S**alivation, **L**acrimation, **U**rination, **D**efecation. `SLUD`

Diagnosis: Methacholine 5 mg/neostigmine 1 mg SC fails to induce typical muscarinic effects.

Treatment: Termination of source of exposure.
      Airway maintenance.   `A B C D E F G`
      Breathing maintenance.
      Circulation maintenance.
      Drugs   – Physostigmine (2 mg SC/IV) Neostigmine is not given since it does not cross BBB
          – Darkroom for rest.
          – Use of ice bag due to **f**ever.
          – Diazepam in convulsion.
      ECG monitoring

Fluid (IV/oral).
Gastric lavage with **tannic acid**.
($KMnO_4$ is used in all types of alkaloidal poisoning except atropine and cocaine).

U of anticholinergic agents

1. As *mydriatic and cycloplegic* in corneal ulcer, keratitis, choroiditis, iritis, iridocyclitis **(Mydricain = atropine + adrenaline+procaine)**. For breaking adhesions between iris and lens, fundoscopy, refraction testing, a shorter acting mydriatic is used, e.g. tropicamide, cyclopentolate, homatropine. (For breaking adhesions of iris, midriatic alternated with miotic.)
2. **A**sthma, Bronchitis and COPD: Drugs →bronchodilation →may lead to infection and alveolar collapse due to drying up of secretion. **Reflex vagal activity** →bronchoconstriction and increased secretion leading to **A**sthma, Bronchitis and COPD.
   Inhaled anticholinergic produces slower response than inhaled sympathomimetic. Adrenaline (α action) causes mucosal decongestion. Theophylline also causes mucosal decongestion. Acute exacerbation of COPD and asthma not responding to $β_2$ agonist alone is treated with—$β_2$ agonist + ipratropium.
3. As **C**ardiac vagolytic to encounter bradycardia.
4. **M**otion sickness: Hyoscine **(most effective)**. Prophylaxis = 0.2–0.4 mg oral/IM transdermal patch containing 1.5 mg hyoscine for 3 days applied behind pinna. Scopolamine (DOC).
5. **P**arkinsonism as adjuvant to levodopa and in drug induecd **extrapyramidal syndrome.**
6. Sedation and **A**mnesia during labour **(Twilight sleep)** and was also used as lie detector in World War II.
7. **P**oisoning (to antagonise muscarinic effect) due to AntiChE, mushroom, neostigmine (used for myasthenia gravis, decurarisation and cobra envenomation).
8. As anti**S**pasmodic in **GIT** (pylorospasm, gastritis, nervous dyspepsia). Renal and biliary colic. Drug induced and functional diarrhoea. Spastic constipation. Enuresis (urination) in chidren (imipramine preferred). Dysmenorrhoea.
9. As antisecretory in:
   — Peptic ulcer by checking gastric secretion, pirinzepine/telenzepine preferred.
   — Parkinsonism by checking excessive sweating and salivation.
   — Pulmonary embolism by checking reflex secretion.
   — Preanesthetic medication by checking respiratory secretion and laryngospasm.

USES OF ATROPINE:	MAMC PASS
Motion sickness	Parkinsonism and poisoning
Amnesia and sedation	Aasthma, bronchitis, COPD
Mydriasis and cycloplegic	antiSecretory
Cardiac vagolytic	antiSpasmodic

10. Atropine should not be used as mydriatic because:
    - Pupil dilates in 30–40 min.
    - Cycloplegia takes place in 1–3 hrs.
    - Subject is incapable to see for about a week.

In children, atropine is used as mydriatic since tone of their eye muscles is more.

Central anticholinergics/antiparkinsonian drugs: Cheap, lesser ADR but lower efficacy than levodopa.

Mech: Have **higher central: Peripheral anticholinergic action ratio** than atropine, along with **H_1 antihistaminic property,** but is **better tolerated** by older patients. **Anticholinergics** are the only drugs effective in drug induced (phenothiazine) parkinsonism. Reduce the **unbalanced cholinergic action in striatum** of parkinsonism, **all producing 25% improvement in clinical features** lasting **6 hrs** after single dose. **Hypokinesia** is effected **least** and **tremor** is benefited more than rigidity. **Peripheral action** controls **sialorrhoea**. Symptoms of parkinsonism **best relieved** by anticholinergics (benztropine) are **tremors.**

ADR: **Same** as atropine because pharmacological profile is **similar** to atropine. **Confusion and loss of memory** common in elderly.

CI: Obstructive GI disorder. Angle closure glaucoma, BPH.

U: In **mild case** and **levodopa contraindicated patient**. They are **the only drugs** effective in drug induced parkinsonism (benztropine—**DOC**). Trihexyphenidyl is **the commonest** used drug (start with the **lowest** doses).

Quarternary compound
Common features
  – Incomplete oral absorption.
  – Not penetrate brain and eye.
  – Slow elimination.
  – Higher nicotinic blocking property.
  – Neuromuscular blockade at high doses.

Uses
1. **Hyoscine butyl bromide (quarternary compound):** Esophageal spasm, gastrointestinal spasm.
2. **Atropine methonitrate:** Abdominal colic, hyperacidity, asthma.
3. **Homatropine methyl bromide** (ganglionic blocker): Antispasmodic.
4. **Hyoscine methyl bromide** (bronchodilator): Antispasmodic, antisecretory.
5. **Ipratropium bromide:** COPD, Asthma.
6. **Propantheline (most popular anticholinergic):** Gastritis, peptic ulcer.
7. **Oxyphenonium:** Peptic ulcer, GI hypermotility.
8. **Penthienate:** Hypermotility, hyperacidity.
9. **Clidinium + BZD:** Nervous dyspepsia, gastritis, peptic ulcer.
10. **Pipenzolate methyl bromide/mepenzolate methyl bromide:** Flatulent dyspepsia, infantile colic.
11. **Isopropamide:** Nervous dyspepsia, hyperacidity.
12. **Glycopyrrolate:** Preanesthetic medication.
13. **Oxybutynin:** Overactive bladder, flavoxate also.

Dicyclomine
Mech.: Smooth muscle relaxant, antiemetic action, antispasmodic action.
Uses: Motion sickness, morning sickness.

Pirenzepine
Mech.: It blocks M_1R. Blockade causes inhibition of gastric secretion.
PK: t½ —11 hrs. Excreted unchanged in urine.
Uses: Peptic ulcer.

Mydriatics
Homatropine: Pupil dilates in 45–60 min. **Mydriasis** lasts 1–3 days. **Accommodation** recovers in 1–2 days.

Cyclopentolate: Mydriasis and cycloplegia occur in 30–60 min and last about a day.
Uses: Iritis, uveitis, refraction, fundoscopy.

Tropicamide: It is the **quickest** (20–40 min) and **briefest** (3–6 hrs) mydriatic.
Uses: Refraction, fundoscopy.

DRUGS ACTING ON AUTONOMIC GANGLIA

Ganglia has adrenergic R, dopaminergic R, peptidergic R, cholinergic (N_N and M_1) R.

Classification
Ganglionic stimulants
1. **Nicotinic agonist (selective):** Nicotine **(small dose)**, lobeline, DMPP, TMA (tetramethyl ammonium).
2. **Muscarinic agonist (nonselective):**　　　　　**A-CAP**
   ACh, Pilocarpine, Carbachol, AntiChE.

Ganglion blocking agents
1. **Persistent depolarising blockers:** Nicotine (large dose), AntiChE (large dose).
2. **Competitive blockers:** Hexamethonium, Pentolinium, Mecamylamine, Pempidine, Trimethaphan.　　**PMT HP**

Mech: Ganglionic blockers block **entire output** of ANS at nicotinic R (N_N/N_G R) by blocking ion channel of ANS. They inhibit both sympathetic and parasympathetic ganglia (**major limitation**). Since most of the organs are supplied by both sympathetic and parasympathetic nerves and one of the supplies is dominant, the effect of ganglion blocker will be opposite to the effect of the dominant nerve supply.

ADR of ganglionic blockers
(a) **Vasodilatation** (inhibition of sympathetic)
(b) **Inhibition of parasympathetic:** Tachycardia, Mydriasis, Cycloplegia, Constipation, Micturition difficulty, Inhibition of salivation, Impotence　**MIT, MIC**
(c) **Anhydrosis** (sweat gland inhibition by sympathetic nerve).

Hemodialysis is useless in the following poisonings: **ABCD**
Anticholinergic (organophosphates).
BZD
Compound like kerosene oil
Digitalis

Atropine does not block vagally mediated gastrin secretion because mediator of vagal effect is GRP, not ACh.

Adrenergic Drugs

β_1 is mainly in heart and β_2 smooth muscles including lungs.

In the body heart is 1 and lungs 2

Except D_1, all receptors of type ONe cause cONtraction

Sympathomimetic = Actions similar to adrenaline.

Odd numbered receptors are stimulatory (M_1, M_3, α_1, β_1, β_3)

Even numbered receptors are inhibitory (M_2, α_2, β_2)

Adrenergic R
1. α R: (a) α_1 (α_1A, α_1B, α_1C).   (b) α_2 (α_2A, α_2B, α_2C).
2. β R: β_1, β_2, β_3.

Dopaminergic R: (a) stimulatory: D_1, D_5.   (b) inhibitory: D_2, D_3, D_4.

R.	Pathway	Functions
α_1	↑ IP_3/DAG, ↑ PLA_2	Contraction of smooth muscle (vessel, GU, pilomotor, bronchi, radial, ciliary, and sphincters of gut), Arrhythmia, Gut-Relaxation (nonsphincter), Enhanced glucose (glycogenolysis and gluconeogenesis, K^+ release from liver), gland-Secretion. $\boxed{CARES}$
α_2	↓cAMP, ↑ K^+ Ch., ↑↓Ca^{++}, ↑ IP_3/DAG	↓central Sympathetic flow, ↓ Insulin release, ↓Transmitter release (NA and ACh), vasoconstriction and platelet aggregation. ↓ renin secretion $\boxed{SIT}$
β_1		Cardiac stimulation, ADH and salivary amylase secretion, Renin release, and relaxation of gut (no hyperpolarisation). $\boxed{CAR}$
β_2	↑cAMP	Smooth muscle (vessel, bronchi, gut, GU, visceral, ciliary, splenic vessel) relaxation, Kontraction of sKeletal muscle. (K^+ uptake, glycogenolysis), insulin and glucagon secretion, glycogenolysis and gluconeogenesis in liver, histamine release inhibition.
		B_2 = DI/DIlute/Relax: Functions of B_2 are generally, either dilation or relaxation wherever it is found.
β_3	↑ Ca^{++} Ch.	Lipolysis and thermogenesis in adipose tissue. α_2 = inhibition of lipolysis. Other receptors involved in lipolysis and thermogenesis are α_2, β_1, β_2.

Effects of Autonomic Nerve Activity on Organ Function

Organ	Sympathetic	Parasympathetic (M₃ mainly)
Eye	α_1 = radial muscle C (mydriasis). β_2 = ciliary muscle R (far vision). Ciliary epithelium = secretion ↑ β_2 and ↓ α_2.	C of circular muscle (miosis) and ciliary muscle (near vision). Lacrimal secretion M_3
Heart	β_1 = stimulate all parameters (P)	M_2 = depresses all P.
Arterioles (α C and β D)	Coronary systemic vein C α_1, α_2 and D β_2; mucosa, skin and salivary glands C α_1, α_2; sk. ms. C α_1, and D β_2; cerebral C α_1; lung and abd. viscera C α_1, and D β_2; renal C α_1, α_2 and D β_1, β_2, D_1; splanchnic C α_1 and D β_2, D_1; ciliary C α_1; D_1 in coronary and cerebral D.	Coronary C; all D except renal, abdominal viscera, splanchnic and vein (systemic).
Tracheo-bronchial ms.	β_2 = dilates bronchioles (smooth ms) α_1 = ↓ secretion β_2 = ↑ secretion	C of bronchioles. ↑ secretion (secretion)
GIT	α_1, α_2, β_2 = R of stomach. α_1 = sphincters C. α_1, α_2, β_1, β_2 = R of intestine. α_2 = inhibits gut secretion	↑ gut C and secretion R of sphincters. ↑ peristalsis (M_3 only)
Genitourinary tract	β_2 = R of detrusor (bladder) and uterus. α_1 = ejaculation/trigone, sphincters and uterus C, ↑ tone and motility of ureter. Renin release ↑ (β_1) and ↓ (α_1).	Trigone and sphincter R. Penile erection. Detrusor (bladder) C. Uterus (variable).
Skin	α_1 = C of pilomotor smooth muscle and sweating on palms.	Generalised sweating.
Metabolic functions Glands	α_1, β_2 = ↑ gluconeogenesis/glycogenolysis in liver. β cell secretion = ↑ (β_2) and ↓ (α_2). α_1 = **thick** salivary (K^+ and H_2O) secretions	**Thin** salivary secretion
Gallbladder and duct	β_2 = R (Relaxation)	C (contraction)
Adrenal and spleen	Spleen capsule = C α_1 and R β_2.	N = secretes E and NE (M also)

Most vessels have uninnervated M_3 → EDRF (No) → Vasodilation. C = Contraction, R = Relaxation, sec. = Secretion, D = Dilatation, ms. = Muscle.

Mechanism of adrenergic receptors (R)

1. β actions → ↑ cAMP → cAMP dependent PK phosphorylation:
   a. **Liver and muscle** → stimulate glycogen phosphorylase and inhibit glycogen synthetase → ↑ glucose, hyperlactacidemia.
   b. **Liver** → K^+ release → hyperkalemia → hypokalemia due to K^+ uptake in muscle α_1 and β_2 = glycogenolysis and gluconeogenesis.
   c. **Adipose tissue** → stimulates lypolysis → ↑FFA and ↑ O_2 use.
   d. **Heart** → phosphorylation of **Troponin** → ↑ interaction with Ca^{++} → ↑ force of contraction.

Heart →phosphorylation of **Phospholamban** →sequestration of Ca^{++} from sarcoplasmic reticulum →**relaxation**.
   e. Pancreas →α cell → ↑glucagon and β cell → ↑ insulin.
2. **α Action** →Stimulates G protein in smooth muscle →↑IP_3/DAG →↑ Ca^{++} from intracellular organelles →stimulation of calmodulin dependent MLCK → myosin phosphorylation →**contraction** ($α_1$).
3. **Prejunctional $α_2$ R** →↓ cAMP →blocks neural Ca^{++} channel →↓ NA release → stimulate Ca^{++} channel →**hyperpolarisation**.
4. **Stimulation of $α_2$ of gut** →hyperpolarisation of cholinergic neurone →↓release of ACh →↓ tone.
   Stimulation of $α_1$ R of smooth muscle →↑ K^+ efflux →hyperpolarisation → **gut relaxation**.
5. **In β cell**: Stimulation of $α_2$ R. →↓cAMP →↓ **insulin release**.

Classification   IAM PM'S BRAND
1. **Direct sympathomimetics (bind and activate R):**
   Adrenaline, **NA**, **I**soprenaline, **P**henylephrine, **M**ethoxamine, **S**albutamol, **R**itodrine, **M**idodrine, **A**praclonidine, **B**rimonidine.
2. **Indirect sympathomimetics:** Tyramine (releases NA to act on R).
3. **Mixed action sympathomimetics:**   **MAME**
   Amphetamine, **E**phedrine, **M**etaraminol, **M**ephentermine.

Sympathomimetics
1. Catecholamines (CA) have **catechol** in structrue (**L-form** more active— parenterally/inhalationally).
2. Phenylethylamine—**no catechol** (more active orally).

NA with **$NaHCO_3$** causes rapid oxidation, hence never mix both of them together. Order of agonist potency for α = **Adr > NA > Iso** and for β = **Iso > Adr > NA**   **ANI = Alfa**
Adrenaline acts at all R. NA acts at all R except $β_2$.
Isoprenaline acts at all R except α.

Adrenaline	= All
NA	= 2 Letters →Not Act on 2 ($β_2$).
Iso	= 3 Letters →Acts on $β_1, β_2, β_3$ = 3.

Actions of adrenaline: Actions similar to sympathetic stimulation (fight or flight reactions).
1. Adrenaline is physiological antagonist of histamine.
2. It increases HR by stimulating **SA** node. It stimulates **AV** node and Purkinje fibres → ↑BP →SA node depression by reflex bradycardia (stimulation of vagus nerve mainly with NA) →↑ force of contraction → tension and relaxation accelerated →↓RP.

Reflex effects are more important than direct effects on heart [**Reflex effects** on heart (blocked by atropine) **predominate** over direct beta effects if NA is agonist]:

It causes **vasoconstriction (α)** in skin, mucosa and kidney and **vasodilatation ($β_2$)** in skeletal muscle, liver and coronaries (arterioles most effected).

Vasodilation predominates in organs where ↑ blood supply is required during fight/flight.

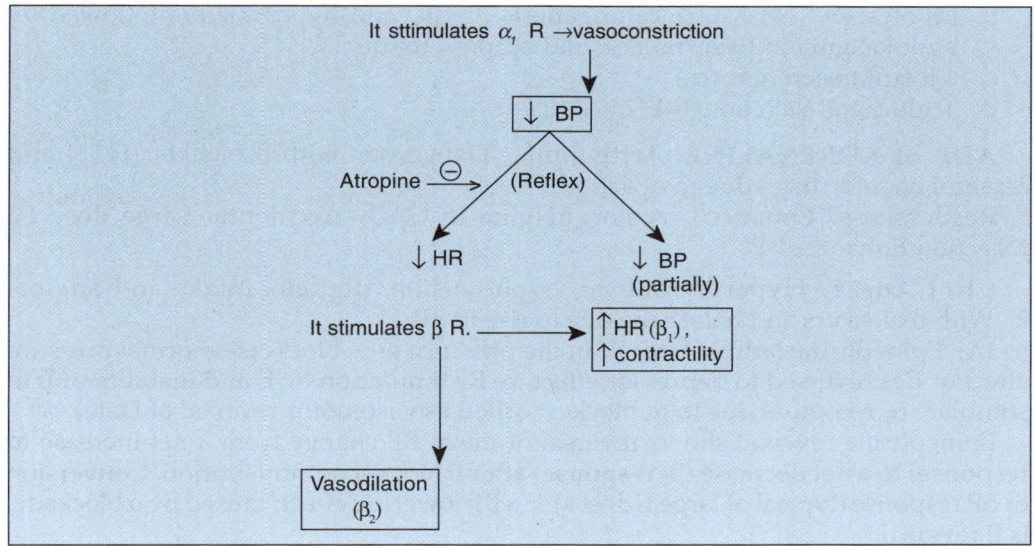

It causes ↑ **BP (systolic and mean)** and ↓BP (diastolic) and ↑ **pulse** pressure. (Sensitivity $β_2 > α$ hence peripheral resistance decreases). NA causes ↑ BP (systolic, mean, diastolic) and ↑ **cutaneous vasoconstriction** due to $α$ action.

Isoprenaline causes ↑ systolic BP and ↓ diastolic BP ($β_1$— cardiac stimulation and $β_2$—vasodilatation) but mean BP falls.

3. Adrenaline and isoprenaline cause bronchodilation ($β_2$). Adr.→$β$ R stimulation →↑ cAMP in mast cell→↓Ag:Ab relaxation induced mediator release. **Adr. →$β$ R** stimulation →↑cAMP in bronchial muscle cell → relaxation → bronchodilation. At high doses of Adr.→pulmonary edema due to blood shifting from systemic to pulmonary circuit.
4. Actions on eye:
   (i) It causes contraction of radial muscle of iris ($α_1$)→mydriasis.
   (ii) $α_1$ → ciliary vasoconstriction →↓ aqueous formation →↓ IOP
   $α_2$ → ↓ secretory activity of ciliary epithelium →↓ IOP
   $β_2$ → ↑ secretory activity of ciliary epithelium → ↑ IOP
   Facilitation of trabecular outflow →↓ IOP
   Net effect is ↓IOP.
5. It causes gut relaxation ($α$ and $β_2$ stimulation).
6. It causes **contraction of uterus** in non-pregnant ($α$) and its relaxation at term in pregnant ($β_2$).
7. It causes relaxation of detrusor ($β_2$) and constriction of trigone and sphincter ($α_1$) finally leading to **inhibition of micturition.**
8. It contracts splenic capsule ($α_1$) to pour more RBC in circulation.
9. It stimulates $α$ R. in motor nerve ending of **skeletal muscle** → ↑ACh → neuromuscular transmission.

10. Poor penetration into CNS; it causes **excitation** followed by **depression** on direct inj. It stimulates α_2 R. in brainstem→↓sympathetic outflow → ↓BP and ↓HR.
11. It causes:
    a. glycogenolysis → hyperglycemia and hyperlactacidemia (β_2).
    b. Lipolysis→↑ FFA (β_3), calorigenesis ($\beta_2+\beta_3$) and hyperkalemia followed by hypokalemia in liver, muscle and adipose tissue.
    c. ↓ insulin secretion (α_2).
    d. ↑ glucagon secretion (β_2).

ADR of ADRENALINE: **A**rrhythmia, **D**angerous with β blocker (HTN and cerebral haemorrhage due to α_1 action).
Restlessness, **E**nhanced tremor, a**N**gina in CAD, **A**ccidental **L**arge dose **IV** i**N**jection **E**nhances BP.

CI of Adr: 1. Hyperthyroidism, hypertension, digitalis intake and angina. 2. With β blockers and halothane due to rise in BP.

IA: Epinephrine (adrenaline) IV in the presence of α_1 blockers→normal pressure effect of E is reversed to depressor effect, β_2 R stimulation by E and inability of E to stimulate α_1 receptors due to α blocker (called as vasomotor reversal of Dale).

Epinephrine reversal shows reversal of mean BP change from a net increase (**α response**) to a net decrease (**β_2 response**) after α blocker administration. Conversion of BP response (typical of large E doses) to a BP lowering effect; caused by α blockade, is E reversal.

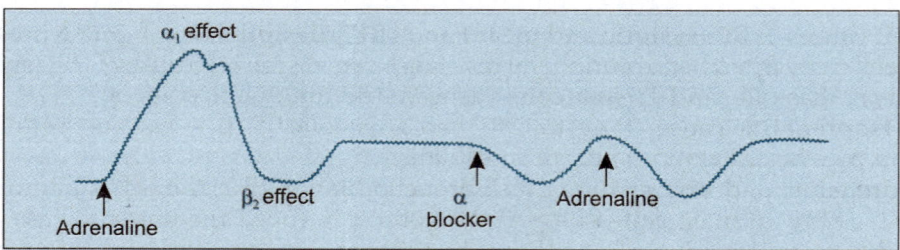

Uses of adrenaline

1. **Allergic disorders:** Urticaria, angioedema, anaphylaxis, laryngeal edema. **DOC** in anaphylaxis (0.5 mg IM).
2. **Cardiac arrest** →Adrenaline stimulates the heart. CPR (designed by **Kouwenhoven**) is also done.
3. **Stokes-Adams syndrome** (transition of partial to complete heart block = cardiac arrest). Adrenaline/isoprenaline.
4. **Hypotension:** Anaphylactic shock →adrenaline (DOC) 0.5 mg SC/IM. It raises BP, counteracts bronchospasm and laryngeal edema.
5. **Local bleeding control** (skin, bleeding gums, mucous membrane, epistaxis). Adrenaline (1:10,000 concentration)/ephedrine/phenylephrine. In gastric erosion and stress ulcer →NA.
6. **Insulin hypoglycaemia** →Adrenaline, but glucose is given as soon as possible.
7. **Reversible airway obstruction (DOC–Adr)** (Adr →The **fastest** acting bronchodilator when inhaled). β_2-mediated relaxation.
8. Mixed with local anaesthetic to increase duration of action.

Therapeutic Classification of Adrenergic Drugs

I. **Pressure agents**
   Noradrenaline
   Ephedrine
   Dopamine
   Phenylephrine
   Methoxamine
   Metaraminol
   Mephentermine

II. **Cardiac stimulants**
   Adrenaline
   Isoprenaline
   Ephedrine
   Dobutamine
   IDEA

III. **Bronchodilators**
   Isoprenaline   **I AM FAST**
   Salbutamol (Albuterol)
   Orciprenaline (Metaproterenol)
   Formeterol
   Adrenaline
   Salmeterol, Terbutaline.

IV. **Nasal decongestants**
   Ephedrine
   Pseudoephedrine
   Phenyl Propanolamine
   Phenylephrine
   Naphazoline
   Oxymetazoline   **NOX**
   Xylometazoline

V. **CNS stimulants**
   Ephedrine   **MADE**
   Amphetamine
   Dexamphetamine
   Methamphetamine

VI. **Anorectics**
   Fenfluramine
   Dexfenfluramine
   Mazindol, **SIBU**tramine
   For My Darling SIBU

VII. **Uterine relaxant and vasodilators**
   Isoxsuprine   **SIT**
   Salbutamol
   Terbutaline, Ritodrine

Dopamine (DA)
Mechanism
1. Acts peripherally on D_1, α and β, receptors. Sensitivity: $D_1 > \beta_1 > \alpha$.
2. D_1 in renal and mesenteric vessels →**most sensitive** →**IV infusion of low doses** →**increase intracellular cAMP**→**vasodilatation**→**increase GFR and sodium excretion.** 15 times more sensitive on D_1 than D_2.
3. — D_1 agonist at **low doses.**
   — β_1 agonist at **intermediate doses.** Stimulates heart →↑ BP
   — α agonist at **high doses** →vasoconstriction.
4. DA depletion in basal ganglia →**parkinsonism.**
   DA excess in CNS →**Schizophrenia.** D_2 depresses CNS.
5. At **normal dose** of DA → ↑ cardiac output and ↑ BP (systolic).

PK: Not cross BBB. Dose = 3–10 µg/kg/min (IV) in cardiogenic shock.
U: — **Shock** (septic/cardiogenic) — **DOC and CHF** (↑ BP and ↑ urine outflow. It dilates renal and mesenteric vessels by D_1 action).
— **MI and Cardiac Surgery.** Doses (µg/kg/min): Renal = 1 to 5, cardiac = 5 to 10, vasopressor = 10 to 20, NE = >20.

ADR of DOPAMINE: DA must be administered after hypovolemia correction. **O**verdose (↑ sympathomimetic action), **P**ain (angina, headache), **A**rrhythmia, **M**AO + DA = dangerous, **I**schaemic **N**ecrosis and **E**mesis.

Amphetamine: It is **synthetic** compound which crosses BBB and has CNS effects and has **same** pharmacological profile as **ephedrine**. **D-isomer > L-isomer** in potency on CNS. D-isomer shows **maximum** selectivity.

Mechanism: It is **indirect sympathomimetic** (i.e. causes NE release and stimulates α and β). Absence of catechol in structure allows for good penetration into CNS. Actions in CNS are more prominent with dextroamphetamine and with amphetamine. It has **weak analgesic, antiemetic and anticonvulsant** actions, hence potentiates analgesic, anti-epileptics and antimotion sickness drugs.

CNS effects (due to endogeneous CA release) are
— ↑ Concentration
— ↓Appetite and ↓Fatigue (↑ work capacity)
— Respiratory centre of stimulation
— Euphoria
— Improved athelitic performance (drug has been included in **DOPE test**) followed by deterioration.
— wakefulness due to stimulation of Reticular activating system.
— ↑ Span of attention
— ↑ Talkativeness
— ↑ **Alertness**
— Improved mood
— ↑ Motor activity.
— ↓appetite due to inhibition of hypothalamic feeding centre.

CARE
FIRST AIM

ADR:
— **Irritability and insomnia**
— **High dose IV:**
  • Hallucination
  • Abdominal cramp
  • Vascular collapse
  • Excitement
  • Psychosis
  • Arrhythmia
  • Convulsion and Coma →death
  • Euphoria

HAVE PACE

— ↓ appetite → starvation → acidic urine → ↑ ionisation of amphetamine at acidic pH→rapid excretion of drug.

Treatment of toxicity: Urine acidification and CPZ to control α effects.

Uses:
— Narcolepsy
— Obesity
— Hyperkinesis in children (mildest grade of mental retardation)
— Attention deficit disorders
— Drug of abuse used by Teenagers seeking thrill/kick
— Epilepsy
— Parkinsonism
— Nocturnal enuresis in children (has central action and increases tone of vesical sphincter)

NO HATE Please

Ephedrine: Obtained from Ephedra vulgaris.
Mechanism: It acts on **α and β R** (direct action). It is indirect sympathomimetic, releases NA. It has $\alpha + \beta_1 + \beta_2$ actions (similar to NA).
PK: Crosses BBB and causes stimulation.
It is resistant to MAO, hence effective orally.
Uses:
— Mild chronic bronchial asthma
— Postural hypotension in neurological disorder.
— AV block (commonest cause of isolated heart block in adult → AV nodal sclerosis).
— Hypotension during spinal anaesthesia.

Dobutamine: Derivative of DA.
Mechanism:
— Acts on α and β R. At clinically employed doses, only B_1 action. Therefore, considered as selective β_1 agonist.
— increases force of cardiac contraction and CO.
Uses: As an inotropic agent in:
— CHF
— MI
— Cardiac surgery
— Cardiogenic shock (DOC)

Pseudoephedrine is **stereoisomer** of ephedrine (little β_2 agonist).
Uses:
— Decongestant of nose and eustachian tube
— Alternative to phenylpropanolamine

Phenylephrine
Mechanism: Selective α_1 agonist. It raises BP by vasoconstriction
Uses:
— Mydriatic (fundus examination)
— Decreases IOP by vasoconstriction of ciliary body
— As nasal decongestant

Methoxamine: α_1 agonist stimulant
Uses: — As pressor agent.

Metaraminol: α action
Uses: — As pressor agent.

Mephentermine
Mechanism:
— Stimulates α and β.
— Releases NA.
— Cardiac stimulation and vasoconstriction
↓
↑ CO, ↑ BP (systolic and diastolic)
↓
↑BP (mean)
+ve chronotropic effect is counterbalanced by **vagal stimulation** due to rise in mean BP.
PK: Crosses BBB
Uses:
— Hypotension due to spinal anesthesia and surgery.
— Shock in MI.

Selective β₂ stimulants
- **Orciprenaline** (β₂: β₁ least selective)
- **Salbutamol** (β₂: β₁ highest, 10 times)
- Terbutaline
- Salmeterol   **TOSS**
- Formoterol
- Ritodrine
- Bambuterol

Actions
- Bronchodilatation
- Vasodilatation
- Uterine relaxation

PK: Orciprenaline (metaproterenol) is not a substrate for COMT, hence **orally effective**.

Uses:
- Bronchial asthma
- As uterine relaxant to delay premature labour.
- In hyperkalemic familial periodic paralysis, due to ↑ K^+ uptake by muscle.
- AV block (orciprenaline)

ADR:
- Muscle tremor **(most important)**
- Tachycardia
- Arrhythmia

Isoproterenol: Smooth muscle relaxation (β₂)
ADR: — ↑ HR

Terbutaline and salbutamol (Albuterol): Efficacy **similar** to isoprenaline.
Mechanism: Selective β₂ agonist → bronchial smooth muscle relaxation

PK:
- Duration of action of terbutaline — 6 hr.
- Peak bronchodilation of terbutaline — 10 min.
- Presystemic metabolism in gut wall.
- Oral bioavailability—50%
- Slower metabolism, longer duration of action.
- Greater oral efficacy is due to non-catecholamine structure of both salbutamol and terbutaline.

ADR:
- Skeletal muscle tremor **(Commonest)**
- Arrhythmia on oral use.
- ↓BP → reflex induced tachycardia on oral use.
- Palpitation
- Restlessness
- Nervousness
- Ankle edema
- Throat irritation

CI:
- Heart disease
- Ruptured membrane, toxaemia of pregnancy and foetal distress

U:
- Bronchial asthma (both are currently **the most popular drugs**)
- As tocolytics (delivery postponed by 70%)

Complication: Cardiovascular (↓BP, ↑ HR, pulmonary edema).
Metabolic (↑ sugar and ↓K^+).

Isoprenaline

Mechanism: β_1 and β_2 agonist.
ADR:
— ↑ HR.
— Myocardial damage on IV administration.

Nasal decongestants

— α agonist
— Local vasoconstriction
— **Imidazole** (selective α_2 agonist)
— **N**aphazoline   **NOX**
— **O**xymetazoline
— **X**ylometazoline

ADR:
— Atrophic rhinitis and anosmia due to **persistent vasoconstriction** on long-term usage.
— Absorbed from nose to cause systemic ADR (↑ BP, CNS depression) Use cautiously in hypertensives and in those receiving MAO inhibitor.

Isoxsuprine: Orally effective long-acting, also beta stimulant acting directly as smooth muscle relaxant.
ADR: Tremor, dizziness, flushing and tachycardia.
Uses:
— As **uterine relaxant** for threatened abortion and dysmenorrhoea. (Terbutaline also used).
— **PVD** (Buerger's disease, Raynaud's phenomenon, gangrene, diabetic vascular insufficiency): **Directly acting vasodilator + Isoxsuprine.**
Ritodrine (β_2) to postpone labour.

Anorectic agents (weight reducing agents): **All are equally effective,** develop tolerance and are given 1 hour before each meal (TDS).
These inhibit feeding centre.

Fenfluramine: It has tranquillizing effect and is **most commonly** used anorectic agent in **India**

Mechanism: It increases serotonergic transmission in brain.
Amphetamine and Mazindol act on NA/DA pathways.

PK: t½—20 hr.
Dexfenfluramine is **dextroisomer** of fenfluramine and has **same** mechanism, efficacy and ADR.

ADR:
— **D**iarrhoea.
— **D**rowziness.
— **D**ry mouth.
— **D**epression.
— **L**oss of libido.
— **L**ethargy and **L**ight headedness.

(DDL = Dilwale Dulhania Lejainge)

Uses: — Obesity (**Commonest**—dexfenfluramine)
Sibutramine: Lost weight (3–9 kg) regained after discontinuation.

Mech: NA and 5-HT reuptake inhibitor without antidepressant action. Thermogenesis (β_3).
ADR: **M**ood swings, **A**nxiety, **D**ecreased sleep, **A**che in chest and gut due to constipation, **M**outh dry, **T**achycardia and BP raised even death.

MADAM Tensed

Newer α_2 agonists used in glaucoma are **apraclonidine** and **brimonidine**.
Newer α_1 agonist used in chronic orthostatic hypotension due to inadequate sympathetic tone is **midodrine**.
Excitatory drugs (**L**SD, **A**mphetamine and **C**ocaine) **LAC**k physical dependence.

Conditions = DOC (Drug of Choice)

1. Anaphylactic shock = Adr.
2. Sudden cardiac arrest = Adr and CPR
3. Shock with decreased renal output = DA
4. Cardiogenic Shock = Dobutamine
5. Complete heart block = Isoprenaline
6. Anorectic = Fenfluramine
7. Narcolepsy = Amphetamine
8. Hyperkinetic child syndrome also called as attention deficit hyperactivity disorder (ADHA) = Amphetamine
9. Diagnosis of pheochromocytoma = Phentolamine
10. Preoperative control of HTN in pheochromocytoma = Phenoxybenzamine
11. Intraoperative control of HTN in pheochromocytoma = Sod. nitroprusside.
12. Hypertrophic obstructive cardiomyopathy = Propranolol
13. Arrhythmia in thyrotoxicosis or Pheochromocytoma = Propranolol
14. Malignant HTN (HTN emergency) = Labetalol
15. Benign prostatic hypertrophy = Tamsulosin, finasteride
16. Prophylaxis of migraine after more than 4 attacks = propranolol
17. Treatment of acute attack of migraine = ergotamine, sumatriptan
18. Anxiety induced tremor = Propranolol
19. Glaucoma = Timolol preferred, Betaxolol, Levobunolol.

8. Antiadrenergic Drugs

Competitive Antagonists at α and β Adrenergic Receptors

α-Blockers

Antiadrenergic drugs act on adrenergic nerve always **reducing sympathetic functions**.

Classification: α blockers
1. **Equilibrium type (competitive/reversible)**
   A. **Selective:** (a) α_1: Doxazosin, Prazosin, Terazosin, Trimazosin. Tamsulosin (uroselective α_{1A} blocker).
   (b) α_2: Roumolscine, Yohimbine.
   B. **Nonselective:** Ergotamine, Ergotoxine, Dihydroergotoxine, Dihydroergotamine, Tolazoline, Phentolamine, Ketanserin, Chlorpromazine
2. **Nonequilibrium type (irreversible):** Phenoxybenzamine, Dibenamine.

Ergot alkaloid is adrenergic antagonist with which **Dale** demonstrated "Vasomotor reversal phenomena".

Actions of α blockers
1. ↓ vasoconstriction of α blocker → ↓ peripheral resistance → ↓BP → interference of postural reflex → syncope and dizziness on standing.
2. **α** blocker → blockade of pressor action of adrenaline → ↓BP due to vasodilatation (β action)/(vasomotor reversal of Dale). Orthostatic hypotension (most important).
3. ↓ mean arterial pressure → reflex tachycardia.
4. α_2 blockade → NA release.
5. α blockade of radial iris muscle → miosis.
6. α blockade of nasal blood vessels due to vasodilation → **nasal stuffiness**.
7. α blockade of intestine → inhibition of relaxant sympathetic effect → ↑ intestinal mobility.
8. α blockade ↓ BP → ↓ renal blood flow → ↓GFR → Na retention and ↑ blood volume → β_1 stimulation → **renin secretion**.

9. α blockade in vas deferens and related organs → inhibition of ejaculation → impotence.
10. Tone in smooth muscle of trigone and sphincter of bladder and prostate ↓ → ↓ urine flow.

Phenoxybenzamine is **alkylating** agent due to formation of reactive intermediate and forms strong covalent bond with a adrenoceptor.

Mechanism: It cyclizes spontaneously in the body giving rise to a reactive **ethyleniminium** reacting with α R by forming **covalent bond.** $α_2$ blockade causes ↑ **NA release** from sympathetic nerves and also **inhibits NA uptake** →↓ BP (postural hypotension). Covalent bond formation results in competitive insurmountable **(irreversible)** antagonism.

PK: Orally—eratic and incomplete. Penetrate brain. **Most** drugs excreted in urine. Dose—60 mg/d IV (in 1 hr)/oral.

ADR: IV→nausea, vomiting. **Oral** →tiredness, lethargy, depression. SC/IM→irritation.

Uses: Phenoxybenzamine/phentolamine controls HTN during **clonidine withdrawal** and **cheese reaction** in patients on MAO inhibitors. Phenoxybenzamine used in pheochromocytoma with β blocker.

Tolazoline
Mechanism: Vasodilatation and cardiac stimulation. 5-HT R inhibition. Has histamine like gastric secretogogue and ACh like motor action on intestine.

ADR: Salivation, lacrimation, sweating, nausea, vomiting, cramps, chills, peptic ulcer, tachycardia, nervousness.

Phentolamine (nonselective, reversible α blocker): It is quick and short-acting.
Mechanism: — Blocks $α_1$ and $α_2$ R →↑ **NA release**.
 — It is competitive surmountable antagonist.

Uses: HTN due to cheese reaction and clonidine withdrawal. Vosoconstriction due to extravasated NA IV infusion (**most** suitable α blocker).

Prazosin: It is moderately potent antihypertensive, selective competitive $α_1$ blocker. α blocker fails to manage essential HTN as vasodilatation is compensated by cardiac stimulation. **Exception** is prazosin.

Mechanism
1. It blocks sympathetically mediated vasoconstriction →↓BP.
2. It **dilates arteriole more than veins**—postural hypotension →dizziness and fainting as **first dose effect.**
3. It inhibits **phosphodiesterase**→↑ cAMP in smooth muscle →vasodilatation (dilates resistance > capacitance vessels).
4. It decreases **LDL and TG** and increases HDL.
5. It counteracts **insulin resistance**—suitable for DM (but not for **neuropathy** → postural hypotension).
6. Haemodynamic effect→↓TPR and mean BP with slight ↓in venous return and CO (**similar** to directly acting vasodilator).

ADR: — First dose syncope
 — **Postural hypotension,** headache, drowsiness, dry mouth.
 — Weakness, rash, nasal blockade, blurred vision.

Antiadrenergic Drugs

- Impaired ejaculation
- Palpitation (reflex tachycurdia)

PK:
- **Effective orally** (bioavailability 60%).
- Highly bound to plasma protein (**α acid glycoprotein**).
- Oral dose →peak fall in BP after 5 hr and effect lasts 12 hrs.
- Hepatic metabolism and excreted in **bile**.
- t½ →**2–3** hrs.
- **Terazosin** is similar to prazosin except bioavailability **90%** and t½ →12 hr.

Uses:
- **HTN** and coronary heart disease.
- **LVF** by decreasing preload and afterload.
- **Raynaud's** disease.
- **Prostatic hypertrophy** (BPH) ($α_1$ inhibition in prostate and bladder trigone).

Doses:
- starting →0.5 –10 mg BD
- maintenance →2 – 6 mg/d

(**Doxazosin** and **Trimazosin** are congeners of prazosin).

Yohimbine
Mechanism:
- Selective $α_2$ blocker.
- Blocks 5-HTR.
- ↑ HR, ↑ BP due to NA release and central sympathetic outflow.

Uses of α blockers

Surgery Parmanently (Medicine Partially) Cures BPH: Sock, Penile erection, Migraine, Peripheral vascular disease, CHF, BPH, Pheochromocytoma, Hypertension.

1. **Secondary shock:** α blocker (because it shifts blood from pulmonary to systemic circulation. Reflex vasoconstriction due to **blood/fluid loss** causes this shock.
2. **Migraine:** Ergotamine **(most effective)** in moderate to severe attack.
   For **A**cute **E**pisode: 5-HT agonist, e.g. Sumatriptan. **A**nalgesics.
   Ergot alkaloids, e.g. Ergotamine. For prevention: **A**ntiserotonergics, e.g. Pizotifen. **B**eta blockers, e.g. Propanonol. **C**CB, e.g Flunarizine. Anti-**D**epressants, e.g. Amitriptyline.   **ABCD**
3. **CHF:** Prazosin (but salt and water retention in **most patient** on chronic use). ACE inhibitor preferred.
4. **BPH:** Prazosin and Terazosin→$α_1$ inhibition in bladder trigone, prostate and urethra→↓smooth muscle tone→**complete** emptying of bladder. Tamsulosim (uroselective-$α_{1A}$ R antagonist) preferred.
5. **HTN:** α blockers **except** $α_1$ selective antagonists, e.g. prazosin have failed because vasodilatation is compensated by cardiac stimulation. **Phentolamine/phenoxybenzamine** used in HTN during **clonidine withdrawal and cheese reaction** in patient on MAO inhibitor.
6. **PVD:** Ischemia is **most potent vasodilator** in skeletal muscle. Tolazoline, prazosin and phenoxybenzamine are used in intermittent claudication, Raynaud's phenomenon and acrocyanosis.

7. **Pheochromocytoma** (called **10% tumour**) **is the commonest adrenal medulla cell tumour.** Its **commonest extrapyramidal site** is →**organ of Zuckerkandl** at bifurcation of aorta.

   Commonest symptom →headache.
   Method of choice for location →CT scan.
   Diagnosed by estimation of urinary CA metabolites **(VMA, normetanephrine).**
   Phentolamine Test: 5 mg phentolamine IV over 1 min in recumbent subject →>35 mm Hg systolic and >25 mmHg diastolic decrease in BP is indicative of pheochromocytoma.
   Tumour→↑ CA→↑ HTN→urinary CA metabolites (VMA, normetanephrine) are diagnostic.
   Treatment: Phenoxybenzamine followed by removal of tumour.

8. **Erectile dysfunction**
   a. **Papaverine** (3–20 mg) with/without 1 mg phentolamine in corpus cavernosum. Priapism (10%) produced is reversed by blood aspiration from corpus cavernosum or by phenylephrine.
   Complications: Penile fibrosis on repeated injection, Penile **D**eviation, Local **h**aematoma, **P**aresthesia   **PhD**
   Alternative to papaverine—alprostadil (PGE$_1$).
   b. **Sildenafil.**

Sildenafil/VIAGRA/Penegra/Cavetra

In March 1998, it was approved. It sets millions of bedroom on fire and was hailed as **medical miracle.** Viagra came to **India** by name Penegra/Cavetra (Sildenafil citrate) in **Jan. 2001.**

> SildenaFIL FILLS the PENis (PENegra)

Viagra for plant **(Nambi, 2000)** promises an **agricultural boom** both in terms of quality and quantity. This is a new herbal preparation having the potential to solve all the food scarcity problems and to wipe out poverty from the face of the earth.

Mechanism

NO released from nerve endings and endothelium during sexual stimulation causes formation of cGMP which is responsible for relaxation of smooth muscles of corpus cavernosus and blood vessels supplying it → cavernosal engorgement and penile erection. PDE-5 is the isoenzyme of phosphodiesterase which is responsible for degradation of cGMP in corpus cavernosus. Inhibition of this enzyme by sildenafil causes ↑ cGMP →↑ relaxation of smooth muscle →↑ penile erection.

PK: Orally active, oral absorption 40%, t½→4 hrs in men <65 yr, penile erection (degree and duration) increased 80%, dose: 50–100 mg 1 hr before intercourse (for men >65 yr—**25 mg**).

ADR (due to vasodilatation) of SILDENAFIL: Sex unsafe in CAD, **IA** with nitrate most dangerous due to **L**ow BP, **D**izziness, **H**eadache, **H**ypotension**,** MI. **D**yspepsia, **E**ye dysfunction, **N**otable change (perception of brightness), Nasal congestion, Visual disturbance. Impairment of colour discrimination due inhibition of retina (PDE 6). **A**ngina, **F**lushing, **I**nhibitor of PDE 5, **L**ess inhibition of PDE 6.

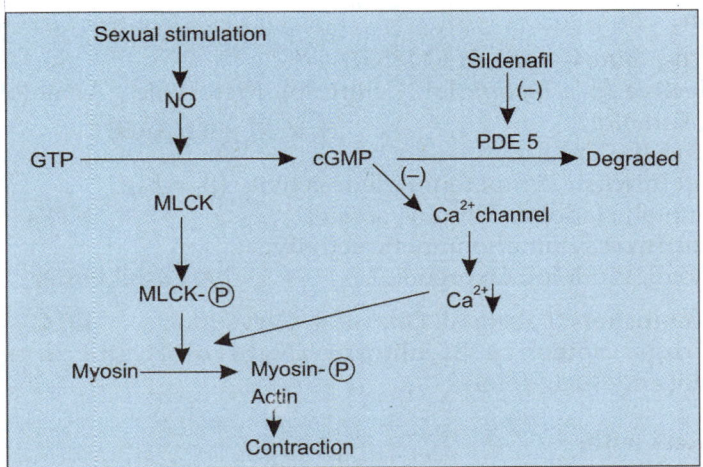

U: For penile errection. (Normally all drugs have **S**ide effects but **S**ildenafil has **front** effects also.)

CI: **K**idney and **L**iver dis., **P**eptic ulcer, **D**isorder of blood, CHD and those taking nitrates. **KLPD**

> Drugs to improve **P**enile tumescence: **P**hosphodiesterase inhibitor, e.g. sildenafil, **P**apaverine, **P**hentolamine, **P**rostaglandins, e.g. alprostadil
> **5P**

Male Erectile **D**ysfunction (**MED**):
MEDicine **STOP** (**S**SRI, **T**hioridazine, methyld**O**pa, **P**ropranolol).
Ethanol
DM

> Pure α agonist slows HR via baroreceptor reflex and pure β agonist enhances HR. α and $β_1$ stimulation→reflex ↑ in vagal outflow→reflex bradycardia.
> Pulse pressure is slightly increased by NA and is markedly increased by E and isoproterenol. ↓HR caused by NA is due to baroreceptor reflex activation of vagal outflow to heart. Typical dose-dependent effects of E on BP are β effects (isoproterenol-like) at small doses and α effects (NA-like) at large doses.

β-Blockers

They are structurally **similar** to CA, have **bulky alkyl substitution on N and oxymethylene bridge near aromatic ring**. All are **competitive blockers**. Propranolol blocks $β_1$ $β_2$ but has weak $β_3$ blockade action. **L-isomers** are active forms. Most **agonists and antagonists** have **isopropyl substitution**. Intrinsic sympathomimetic = partial agonistic.

Classification

1. **Selective** (β_2): Butoxamine, ICI 118551
2. **Cardioselective** (β_1): Bisoprolol, Celiprolol, Metoprolol, Atenolol, Acebutolol, Betaxolol, Esmolol.   **A to M = B CAME**
3. **Nonselective** (β_1 and β_2):
   a. **Without intrinsic** sympathomimetic activity ($\beta_1 = \beta_2$):
      Propranolol, Nadolol, Timolol, sotalol.   **NTPs**
   b. **With intrinsic** sympathomimetic activity:
      Alprenolol, Pindolol, Oxprenolol.   **A Postal Order**
   c. **α and β blockers:** Labetalol, Dilevalol, Carvedilol.   **DLC**
4. **Newer drugs:** Selective β_1 blocker (Nabivolol) and α_1 + β blockers (Medroxalol and Bucindolol).

> **β blockers with:**
> Shortest t½ — Esmolol (10 min)
> Longest t½ — Nadolol (14–24 hrs)
> Highest bioavailability — Pindolol (90%)
> Lowest bioavailability — Alprenolol (10%)
> Maximum LA property — Propranolol.

Propranolol (as prototype): It has β_1, β_2 and weak β_3 action. **L-isomer** is more active.

Actions

1. It suppresses anxiety in short-term stressful situation (suppresses tremors, palpitation).
2. LA action—as lidocaine.
3. It blocks β_2 R →↑ **bronchial resistance.**
4. It blocks adrenergically provoked tremor in skeletal muscle.
5. It decreases aqueous humour formation →↓ **IOP.**
6. It blocks **uterus relaxation** which occurs due to isoprenaline and selective β_2 agonist.
7. It blocks adrenergically induced lypolysis →↑ **Plasma TG,↓ FFA and ↑ LDL/HDL ratio.** It **prevents glycogenolysis** in heart, skeletal muscle and liver.
8. It decreases CO, HR, and force of contraction and **prolongs** systole by retarding conduction. Cardiac work and O_2 consumption are decreased along with total coronary blood flow reduction (inhibition of vasodilatation through β R). It **reduces** RP and automaticity. AV conduction is delayed. It **blocks** cardiac stimulation by adrenergic durgs but not that by digoxin, Ca^{++}, glucagon and methylxanthine. It blocks fall in BP and vasodilatation and increases BP rise caused by adrenaline (there is **re-reversal of vasomotor reversal** that is seen after **α blocker**). Subendocardial area (site of ischemia in angina patient) is unaffected. Hence, oxygen supply is improved in angina patient. **TPR** (total peripheral resistance) is increased due to inhibition of β vasodilatation but CO is decreased. With continued treatment, resistance vessels adapt reduced CO →↓ TPR →↓BP (systolic and diastolic) **(most likely explanation** of antihypertensive action). Propranolol→↓ renin release (β_1 action) from kidney→↓BP.

Antiadrenergic Drugs

> **Actions of propranolol:**
> ↓CO,
> ↓ renin secretion,
> ↓ NA release and ↓ CNS sympathetic output,
> ↓ AV conduction velocity,
> ↓ HR and ↓ contractility →↓O_2 demand.

9. **As antihypertensive:** Most β blockers maintain antihypertensive actions over **24 hrs** with **single daily** dose despite short and different plasma t½ and all exert **similar** antihypertensive effects. Nonselective β blockers increase **TG and LDL/HDL ratio. Most effective drugs** for preventing sudden cardiac death in post-MI are **ACE inhibitor and β blocker.** Drugs with sympathetic action decrease vascular resistance by $β_2$ agonism.

10. **As antianginal:** No vasodilatation. Flow to **ischaemic area** does not decrease due to favourable redistribution and decrease in endo-cardial wall tension. Acts by **decreasing cardiac work** and O_2 **consumption** marginally at rest and importantly during exercise/anxiety by limiting the increase in these modalities (HR↓, mean BP↓, inotropic action↓). All β blockers are equally effective in classical angina (decrease frequency and severity of attacks and increase ex-tolerance). **Non-selective** worsens variant angina due to vasoconstriction ($β_2$ blockade). **High doses** worsen classical angina due to ↑ O_2 demand (ventricular dilatation and systolic prolongation). β blockers worsen **coronary vasospasm** ($β_2$ blockade).

11. **Mechanism of antiarrhythmic action:** Propranolol reduces **slope of phase 4 depolarisation** leading to reduction of automaticity in SA node, AV node, PF and other ectopic foci (with ↑ refractoriness), prolongs ERP of AV node (antiadrenergic action) and impedes AV conduction **(most important action).** Reduced excitability. Suppression of slow channel responses and after depolarisation induced by CAs. Prolongation of PR interval **(most prominent)** due to sensitive AV node. Depression of contractility and BP < with Quinidine. ↓cAMP and ↓Ca^{++} **currents** suppress abnormal pacemakers.

PK:
- Absorbed orally
- Penetrates brain
- Hepatic metabolism depends on hepatic blood flow. **Chronic propranolol use** decreases hepatic blood flow. Oral bioavailability is increased (t½ is prolonged).
- Low bioavailability is due to first pass metabolism.
- **Higher doses** increase bioavailability and prolong t½.
- t½ 3 hr.
- **Meal** increases bioavailability due to decreased first pass metabolism.
- Plasma concentration = 0.1–0.3 µg/ml.
- Propranolol →**Hydroxypropranolol** (active) excreted in urine mostly as glucuronides.
- **90%** bound to plasma protein.
- IV dose is **1/3** of oral dose.
- Dose: 0.5–2 mg/kg/d only orally (BD, TDS or QID)

- **High dose**—Quinidine like direct membrane stabilising action.
  Clinical dose—antiarrhythmic due to adrenergic blockade.
- 1 mg/min. IV (maximum 5 mg)

IA:
- Additive depression of SA node and AV conduction with verapamil and digitalis but safe with dihydropyridines (e.g. nifedipine) since DHPs do not suppress AV node.
- Reduces lidocaine metabolism by decreasing hepatic blood flow.
- Increases CPZ bioavailability by decreasing first pass metabolism.
- α agonist causes ↑ BP due to inhibition of $β_2$ receptors on blood vessels.
- Cemetidine inhibits propranolol metabolism.
- NSAIDs attenuate antihypertensive action of β blocker.
- It delays recovery from hypoglycaemia due to insulin and oral antidiabetics. Warning signs of hypoglycaemia mediated through sympathetic stimulation (e.g. palpitations, tremors) are suppressed.

ADR:
- ↓CO →Na^+, water retention due to haemodynamic adjustment.
- Bradycardia
- Worsening of COPD
- Prinzmetal's angina due to coronary constriction (α mediated)
- ↑ TG and ↑ LDL and ↓HDL increase the risk of coronary disease.
- **Nightmares** and **insomnia (lipid soluble drugs).**
- **Hypoglycaemia.**
- **Rebound HTN, worsening of angina** and **sudden death** on withdrawal after chronic use due to **supersensitivity** of β R occurring as a result of reduction in agonist stimulation.

> **ADR of β blocker:** Asthma, and impotence, less with agents having intrinsic sympathomimetic activity.
> CVS effects (CHF, ↓HR, AV block).
> CNS effects (sedation, sleep alteration) not seen with lipid insoluble agents.

- Tiredness and decreased exercise capacity due to decreased glycogenolysis and lypolysis and **blunting** of $β_2$ mediated ↑ blood flow to exercising muscle.
- Inhibition of vasodilatation ($β_2$ R).
  ↓
  worsening of peripheral vascular disease (PVD).

CI of β blocker
- **A**sthma at rest (due to bronchoconstriction)
- Heart **B**lock
- **C**HF (due to depressant effect on heart).
- **D**M, PVD and pulmonary disease.   **ABCD**

Timolol is contraindicated in myasthenia gravis.

CI of propranolol: Prinzmetal angina, **P**VD, **P**artial/complete heart block, **P**ulmonary disease (bronchial asthma due to bronchoconstriction), **P**lasma lipid profile altered.   **5P**

Precaution in propranolol use in
- **Variant angina** (β blockade →increase coronary spasm).
- **CCB use** (both are cardiac depressant).
- **Withdrawal** from treatment (risk of anginal attack).

Uses of β blocker (summary)
- Angina pectoris
- BP raised
- Cardiac arrhythmia
- Dissecting aortic aneurism
- Essential tremor
- Failure (CHF)
- Glaucoma
- Hypertrophic cardiomyopathy
- Infarction (MI)
- Anxiety
- Migraine
- Thyrotoxicosis
- Pheochromocytoma

ABCDEFGHI And Medulla Tumour Pheochromocytoma

Non-Cardiac uses of β blocker:
Thyrotoxicosis
Migraine
Anxiety
Glaucoma
Essential tremor

TBM AGE
= Neonate-Child

Uses of β blocker
1. **HTN** (atenolol **DOC**).
   Effective in 35% when used alone.
   Young non-obese hypertensive (**DOC**)
   (specially with IHD, post-MI and psychological stress).
2. **Angina pectoris:** All β blockers
3. **Cardiac arrhythmia**
   - WPW syndrome.
   - Suppresses tachycardia, extrasystole (provoked by emotion and exercise), atrial flutter and fibrillation (slow AV conduction).
   - 2nd choice in PSVT (↓ re-entry at AV node).
   - Alternative to digitalis in controlling ventricular rate.
   - Digitalis induced arrhythmia by blocking sympathetic component.
4. **MI**
   - Prophylaxis (inhibits reinfarction, sudden death and fibrillation) after acute MI for 1.5–3 yrs to reduce ischaemic damage.
   - Limits infarct size by decreasing O_2 consumption.
   - Inhibits ventricular fibrillation.
5. **CHF:** β blockers contraindicated in compensated HF but **$β_1$ blockers** useful.
6. **Dissecting aortic aneurysm** decreases cardiac contractile force
7. **Glaucoma**
8. **Essential tremor:** Non-selective β blocker.
9. **Hypertrophic cardiomyopathy**
   β blocker increases CO during exercise only.
10. **Thyrotoxicosis**
    - Inhibits peripheral conversion from T_4 to T_3.

- During thyrotoxicosis (thyroid storm) →**most valuable** due to quick symptomatic relief.
- Also given in preoperative preparation.
- Combination propylthiouracil + glucocorticoid + β blocker.

11. **Pheochromocytoma**
    - Controls tachycardia and arrhythmia but β blocker is used after the use of α blocker otherwise dangerous rise in BP takes place due to unopposed α action.
    - Sympathetically mediated arrhythmia of halothane and pheochromocytoma.
12. Migraine (pulsatile vasodilatation in brain causes pain)
    - Chronic prophylaxis—**propranolol most effective.**
    - Ergotamine (amine alkaloid of lysergic acid) is **most effective** drug against migraine.
13. **Anxiety** (nervousness and panic, e.g. exam. etc):
    Anxiety symptoms (↑ BP, palpitation, tremor, GI hurrying) are due to sympathetic overactivity (hence β blocker is useful).

Cardio-selectivity (metoprolol, atenolol, acebutolol)
— More potent in blocking $β_1$ **(cardiac)** than $β_2$ **(bronchial)** R. But selectivity is **lost** at higher doses.
— Safer in DM, bronchospastic disease
— Lower incidence of cold hand and feet ($β_2$ is not blocked so vasoconstriction is prevented).

Membrane stabilising activity (propranolol, oxprenolol, alprenolol, acebutolol) has antiarrhythmic action.

Lipid insolubility (nadolol, sotalol, atenolol)
— Incompletely absorbed orally.
— Excreted unchanged in urine.
— t½ →6–20 hrs.
— Lipid soluble agents have hepatic metabolism and t½ →2–6 hrs.

Sotalol: Nonselective, lipid insoluble. Has antiarrhythmic property.

Mechanism

1. Prolongs **repolarisation** by blocking cardiac K^+ channel →widened AP and ↑ ERP **(the most characteristic function of class III antiarrhythmic).**
2. It is not Na^+ channel blocker (not depress conduction in fast response tissue but delays AV conduction).

Uses: — VT
— AF/AFl

Limitation: — APD prolongation and QT risk of torsade de pointes.

Nadolol: Nonselective, long-acting.

PK: — Water soluble
— Not metabolised
— t½ →15 hrs

U: — HTN

Atenolol: Water soluble
Mechanism: Selective $β_1$ blocker

Antiadrenergic Drugs

Uses: — HTN and angina (commonest used β blocker)

Timolol, Metipranolol, Cartiolol, Levobunolol, Betaxolol are used topically in eye. **A**tenolol, **N**adolol and **S**otalol **A**re **N**ot **S**oluble in lipid.

Timolol
Uses: — HTN, angina, MI prophylaxis (given orally)
Glaucoma (given topically)

Pindolol: Has intrinsic sympathomimetic activity ($\beta_1 = \beta_2$)
Uses: — HTN

Acebutolol: — β_1 cardioselective agent
— Partial agonist.
— Membrane stabilising.
PK: — t½—10 hrs.

Acebutolol →**diacetolol** (active metabolite) →excreted by kidney.

Metoprolol: Cardioselective β_1 blocker.
Mechanism: Blocks cardiac stimulation like propranolol. Less bronchoconstriction in asthma. Less masking of hypoglycaemia in DM than propranolol.
PK: >90% metabolised. Slow and fast hydroxylators of metoprolol.
ADR: Mild
CI and precaution same like propranolol.
Uses: Cold hands and feet. MI (IV) but generally given orally.

Esmolol: Ultrashort acting β_1 blocker.
PK: t½ <10 min. Inactivated by **esterases** in blood.
Uses: PSVT, AF/AFl, MI and HTN in surgery in emergency. Arrhythmia associated with anaesthesia.

Alprenolol: It is β_1 selective.

α + β blocker

Labetalol: First α + β blocker which has **4 stereoisomers,** each having distinct profile of action. Antihypertensive action is **similar to methyldopa** on chronic use (α_1 + β blockade).

Pharmacological properties
1. **Non-selective antagonist for β_1 and β_2** but selective antagonist for α_1.
2. **β blocking potency** →1/3 that of propranolol.
   α blocking potency →1/10 that of phentolamine.
3. Has **no** β_1 but weak β_2 agonistic activity. **5 times** more potent in blocking β than α R.
4. **At low doses** → acts like proranolol.
   At high doses → (acts like propranolol and phenoxybenzamine)
   → ↓CO and ↓TPR.
5. ↓BP is due to α_1 and β_1 antagonism and β_2 agonism. Initially ↓ CO (due to β_1 blockade) →↓CO and ↓TPR (β_1, α_1 blocked, β_2 agonism)
6. Labetalol increases limb blood flow and **inhibits NA uptake** by adrenergic nerve endings.
7. **Central β blockade** →↓ sympathetic outflow from CNS.
8. ↓ **renin release** from JG cells and **inhibition of CA uptake** from adrenergic nerve terminals.

Mechanism of action

At low doses β_1 blockade →↓ CO→BP ↓ and ↓ Renin release.

At high doses α_1 antagonism →vasodilation →↓ TPR →↓ BP
β_2 agonism

Uses

1. **IV**→ rapid BP↓ in cheese reaction and **clonidine withdrawal,** etc.
   Orally →in severe and resistant cases. Dose: 6 mg/kg/d, TDS.
   HTN especially when not controlled by β blocker only.
2. Pheochromocytoma.

ADR: — Postural hypotension **(most important)**
— Failure of ejaculation.
— Rashes and liver damages.

Dilevalol

1. **Is α + β blocker, selective β_2 agonist.**
2. **4 times** more potent in blocking β_1 and β_2 R but **6 times** less potent in blocking α_1 R than labetalol.
3. ↓BP due to β_2 mediated vasodilatation.
4. Dose: 200–800 mg OD.

Carvedilol

Mechanism

1. $\beta_1 + \beta_2 + \alpha$ blocker.
2. Vasodilatation due to α blockade.
3. Has **antioxidant** property.

Uses: CHF, HTN.

Tamsulosin

1. Is **selective α_1 A blocker.**
2. **Increases urine flow** and decreases residual urine in BPH without altering BP/HR.

9. Drugs for Somatic Nervous System: Skeletal Muscle Relaxants

The NM blockers are structurally related to ACh and are either antagonists (nondepolarising type) or agonists (depolarising type) on NR.

These act at neuromuscular **junction/muscle fibre** itself/centrally in **cerebrospinal axis** to cause paralysis/to decrease muscle tone.

Classification
1. **Peripherally acting**
   a. **Directly acting:** Quinine, Dantroline Sod.
   b. **Neuromuscular blocker**
      A. **Depolarising blocker:** Succinylcholine (SCh, Suxamethonium), Decamethonium (C-10)
      B. **Nondepolarising (competitive) blocker:**
   Short-acting: Mivacurium
   Intermediate acting: Vecuronium, Rocuronium, Atracurium.
   Long-acting: Pancuronium, Pipecuronium, Doxacurium, d-Tubocurarine, Gallamine triethiodide, Cisatracurium, Rapacuronium.
2. **Centrally acting**
   a. **BZD** and cyclobenzaprine.
   b. **GABA** derivative: Baclofen.
   c. **Mephenesin** group: Mephenesin, Methocarbamol, Carisoprodol, Chlorzoxazone, Chlormezanone.
   d. Central α_2 agonist: Tizanidine.

Muscle relaxation potentiating agents	
Aminoglycosides	ATP
Tetracycline	ABC
Polypeptide antibiotic	
Antiarrhythmic	
Beta blocker	
Calcium channel blocker	

Neuromuscular blockers (all are quarternary compound).

Competitive blocker: Curare **first** used in arrow poison, is obtained from *Strychnos toxifera* and **Chondrodendron**.

Curare →Tubocurarine and toxiferin (active principles).
(Muscle group **most** sensitive to muscle relaxant is neck muscle).

Mechanism: All blockers have **same** mechanism. They block N_M →EPP (End Plate Potential) decreased below threshold for muscle AP.

Safety factor is **5** at neuromuscular junction, EPP is decreased to **20%** of normal amplitude for muscle paralysis to occur. Decreased safety factor occurs in GA, myasthenia gravis, aminoglycoside (↓ ACh). Neostigmine group drugs increase safety factor. N_M has **5 subunits** (α_2, β, ε, γ, δ). **Cationic head of 2 ACh** binds negatively charged group of 2α subunits →Na^+ channel opening. Competitive blockers have > **one quaternary N^+ atom** for the attraction to the **same site** (these are thick bulky molecules, termed **Pachycurare** by Bovet). *Neuromuscular blockers block cholinergic transmission at neuromuscular junction acting either agonist (depolarising type) or antagonist (nondepolarising type).*

At low doses: They combine with N_M R and prevent binding of ACh →inhibition of muscle contraction.

At high doses: These block **ion channels** of end plate →flaccid.

Competitive muscle relaxant (MR) causes ganglionic block mostly by	
Galamine	Go
Trimethaphan	To
Pancuronium	Panki
D-Tubocurarine	Dukan

Mechanism of depolarising agents

Phase I: Drugs attach to N_M R and act like ACh to depolarise the junction without effecting acetylcholinesterase →Na channel opening, depolarising the R →transient twitching of muscle **(fasciculation)**.

Phase II: Repolarisation due to continuous depolarisation →Na^+ channel blocked →**Resistance to depolarisation and muscle flaccid.**

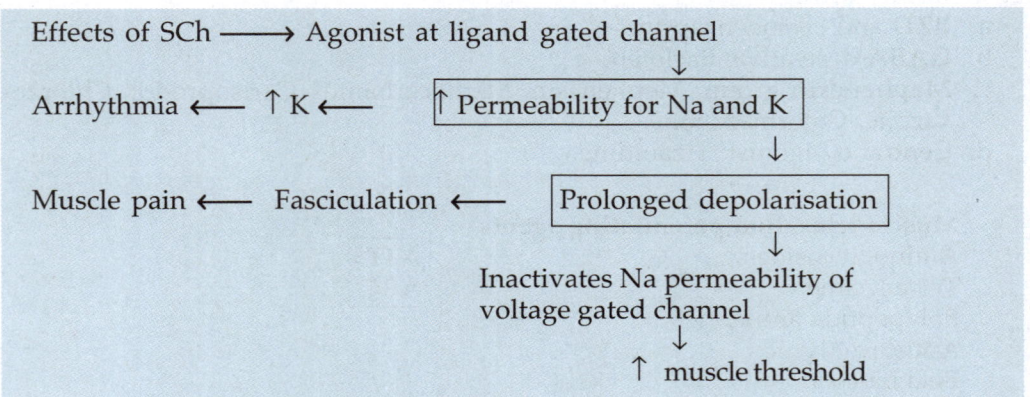

Actions of neuromuscular blockers
1. **In skeletal muscle,** competitive blockers produce paralysis:
   Order of paralysis: Finger and Eyes → Limbs → Face and neck → Trunk → Intercostal muscle→Diaphragm (effected lastly) →no respiration. **ELFTID**
   (Recovery takes place in **reverse order—diaphragm first**)

C-10 causes **flaccidity** and order of paralysis is: Neck and Limbs →Face, Jaw, Eye, Pharynx → Trunk → Respiratory muscle.   **LFTR**

Temperature lowering intensifies block. **Cathodal current** to end plate enhances block.

2. **Competitive blockers (d-TC maximum)** block and SCh stimulates N_N of autonomic ganglia.
3. **Mast cells**
↓d-TC due to bulky cationic nature of molecule.
Histamine release (heparin also)
↓
Hypotension, bronchospasm and increased respiratory secretion.
4. **d-TC** (naturally occurring skeletal muscle relaxant obtained from *C. tomentosum*) causes ↓BP due to: ↓venous return, histamine release and ganglionic blockade.
5. **Gallamine, pancuronium, vecuronium** → vagal ganglionic blockade → ↑ HR.
6. **Gallamine, pancuronium** →   inhibit muscarinic R.→↑ HR.
7. ↓HR ← muscarinic R ←   **SCh**   → initially stimulates
    stimulation   vagal ganglia
                                     ↓
                                    ↓HR

after vagal stimulation,
it stimulates symp. ganglia
↓
↑ HR

PK: All neuromuscular blockers are quarternary compound, hence **not abosrbed orally** (given IV), **not cross BBB and placenta.**

— SCh composed of 2 ACh molecules (completely metabolised)
↓ **pseudocholinesterase** present in liver and plasma.
Succinylmonocholine
↓
Succinic acid + choline.

If **pseudocholinesterase** is absent, phase II blockade takes place leading to muscle paralysis and apnoea. Abnormal enzyme is detected by determining **Dibucaine number** in the serum of the individual. Paralysis recovers in about **5 min.**

It is the **commonest** used muscle relexant with **shortest** action.
Ontset of action →1–2 min.
Duration of action →6 min.
Test for ability to metabolise SCh →**Dibucaine number**
(it identifies patient with abnormal pseudocholinesterase).

— **Gallamine (synthetic)** is not metabolised. Others are partly metabolised. All nondepolarising agents are given parenterally.
Unchaged drug is excreted in **urine and bile.**
Duration of action → 45 min
Dose: 1 mg/kg.

— **Pancuronium (synthetic steroidal** compound **5 times** more potent than d-TC).

— **Atracurium:** Not metabolised by enzyme. **4 times** less potent than pancuronium. Inactivated by spontaneous non-enzyme molecular rearrangement **(Hofmann elimination)** to form laudanosine in addition to that by **cholinesterase.**
Order of potency: Pancuronium > Atracurium > d-TC.
Mg^{2+}, AntiChE, Isoflurane and Li + potentiate phase I block

MAIL

d-TC
- **Not cross BBB and placenta**
- Duration of action →25–40 min.
- **First** synthesized by **curare king.**
- Neonates more sensitive.
- **Antagonists:** Edrophonium, neostigmine, pyridostigmine (antiCh E acts by increasing availability of ACh).
- Ether has synergistic action.
- Lowering temp. decreases blockade.
- Cathodal current to end plate lessens blockade.
- Dose: 0.3 mg/kg.

ADR: SCh
1. ↓BP, ↓HR **(histamine release).**
2. **Malignant hyperpyrexia** (treatment →dantrolene—DOC)
3. **Myalgia**
4. **Myoglobinuria and myoglobinemia.**
   It is **the only skeletal muscle relaxant** causing **bradycardia.**

Gallamine
Tachycardia and arrhythmia due to inhibition of parasympathetic ganglia and cardiac vagolytic effect.
d-TC: — Histamine release
— Ganglia blockade

Vecuronium
Lacks histamine release and ganglionic action. It is the only competitive muscle relaxant having no effect on CVS.

Toxicity
- Respiratory paralysis + apnoea **(most important).**
- Flusing common with d-TC.
- ↓BP and CVS collapse especially in hypovolemic patient with newer drug.
- Arrhythmia and cardiac arrest especially with SCh in digitalised patient.
- Asthma precipitation due to **histamine release.**
- Postoperative **muscle soreness** with SCh.

CI—Gallamine: **Nephrotoxicity and pregnancy** (crosses placenta).

Uses: SCh
- For passing tracheal tube and laryngoscopy (dose = 1 mg/kg).
- Convulsion and trauma **(SCh—commonest)**
- Adjuvant to GA **(most important)**

Atracurium
- Bronchial asthma.
- Liver and kidney failure.
- Ocular surgery (competitive blockers paralyse extraocular muscle).

Vecuronium: Bronchial asthma

d-TC: Myasthenia gravis (for provocative test = 0.5–2 mg).

IA
- **SCh + Thiopentone Sod.** in the **same syringe** react chemically.
- **CCB** potentiates neuromuscular blocker.
- **Sympathomimetic** enhances ACh release →↓ competitive block.
- **Diuretics** enhance competitive block due to hypokalemia.
- **Corticosteroid (high dose)** reduces competitive blockade while propranolol, diazepam and quinidine enhance it.
- **AntiChE** reverses competitive blockade. Hence, neostigmine (IV 0.5–2 mg) is used at the end of operation after long-acting blockers.
- **GA** potentiates competitive blockers. **Ketamine** also intensifies non-depolarising blockade.
  Fluorinated anaesthesia causes phase II blockade by SCh.
- **Aminoglycosides** compete with Ca^{++} and reduces ACh release (potentiate competitive blockers).
  Tetracycline (by chelating Ca^{++}), **clindamycin, polypeptide** and lincomycin potentiate competitive blockers.

Advantage of newer neuromuscular blockers
- **Minimal histamine release.**
- **Minimal** ganglionic and cardiovascular effects.
- **Easy reversal.**

Baclofen
Baclofen is **G-protein coupled selective $GABA_B$ R agonist**—a centrally acting skeletal muscle relaxant (inhibitory neurotransmitter in spinal cord is **GABA and Glycine**). Baclofen inhibits Both poly- and mono-synaptic activation of motor nerve.

Mechanism: GABA R   – $GABA_A$ R
              – $GABA_B$ R

$GABA_A$ R is intrinsic ion channel R →enhances Cl^- **conductance** (inhibited by **bi-cuculline** and facilitated by **BZD**).

Drug hyperpolarises neurons by enhancing K^+ **conductance** and altering Ca^{++} **flux**. It acts in spinal cord to depress both polysynaptic and monosynaptic reflex. Action is blocked by **SACLOFEN**.

PK: Abosrbed orally. t½→3–4 hrs. Excreted unchanged in urine (centrally acting muscle relaxant given orally/parenterally).

ADR: Ataxia, confusion, drowsiness, weakness, withdrawal syndrome (seizures, ↑ HR, hallucination).

U: Severe spasticity of spinal cord origin.

MephenesIN: Acts at **spinal INternuncial neuron** which modulates reflexes maintaining muscle tone and reducing muscle spasm due to inhibition of polysynaptic excitation of motor nerve.

Carisoprodol
- Relaxant and sedative.
- Analgesic, antipyretic, anticholinergic actions are weak.

Uses: Musculoskeletal disorder associated with muscle spasm.

Chlormezanone: Relaxant and sedative, antianxiety and hypnotic, no clinical use as relaxant.

ADR: Gastric irritation and sedation (most important).

ADR of centrally acting muscle relaxants
- All are sedative.
- Reduce muscle tone.
- Depress selectively spinal and supraspinal polysynaptic reflexes involved in the regulation of muscle tone.
- Polysynaptic pathways for wakefullness maintenance are depressed.

Uses of centrally acting muscle relaxant
- Acute muscle spasm.
- Anxiety and tension.
- Backache and neuralgia.
- Orthopaedic manipulation (BZD/methocarbamol).
- Tetanus: Diazepam (**commonest**) and methocarbamol (alternative).
- Electroconvulsive therapy (BZD/SCh).
- Spastic neurological disorder: Descending pathway impairment in the cerebrospinal axis→**spasticity,** cerebral palsy, spinal injury, multiple sclerosis.

Dantrolene: Directly acting muscle relaxant.

Mechansim: It uncouples contraction from muscle membrane depolarisation (Ca^{++} release from ER is reduced). Slow contracting **"antigravity muscle"** is effected less than fast contracting **"twitch" muscle.**

PK: Absorbed from GIT, penetrates brain and causes sedation, hepatic metabolism, renal excretion, t½—9 hrs.

ADR: Muscular weakness **(dose limiting)**, diarrhoea and liver toxicity.

Uses
1. **Oral (4 mg/kg/d QID)**
   - Reduces voluntary power.
   - Reduces spasticity in multiple sclerosis, **cerebral palsy, paraplegia, hemiplegia** and upper motor neuron (UMN) disorder.
2. **IV (1 mg/kg)**
   - **Malignant hyperthermia—DOC** (due to persistent release of Ca^{++} from SR induced by fluorinated (halothane) GA and SCh in genetically susceptible person).
3. **Neuroleptic malignant syndrome.**

Quinine: Enhances **RP** and reduces **excitability** of motor end plate leading to reduction of response to repeated neuron stimulation.

Progabide is $GABA_{A \& B}$ agonists.

Drugs impairing neuromuscular transmission
Antibiotic: Aminoglycoside, polymyxin, tetracycline, trimethoprim.
Antiarrhythmic: Quinidine, procainamide.
β blocker: Propranolol, timolol.
Quinine, Li, Mg, methoxyflurane, phenothiazine.
Drugs inactivated **by Pseudocholinesterase** of liver and plasma:
— SCh
— Ester type LA
— Propanidid

Cisatracurium: R-Cis enantiomer of, and 4 times more potent than atracurium with slower in onset but similar in duration of action.
Mech: Same as atracurium.
PK: Hofmann elimination, not hydrolysed by plasma cholinesterase. No histamine release (most important).
(Rapacuronium has withdrawn due to bronchospasm and death).
Tizanidine: TizaNIDINE is a congener of cloNIDINE.
Mech: Inhibits excitatory amino acid release in spinal interneurons, facilitates glycine, reduces muscle tone and spasm and blocks polysynaptic reflex.
PK: Absorbed orally. First pass metabolism. Renal excretion. Half-life 3 hours.
ADR: Dry mouth, insomnia, hallucinations, elevated LFT values.
CI: With clonidine.
U: Spasm (neurological and muscular).

Cyclobenzaprine
Mech: It interferes with polysynaptic reflexes in brainstem that maintains skeletal muscle tone. Has sedative and antimuscarinic actions.
ADR: Confusion and visual hallucination.
U: Acute muscle spasm but ineffective in muscle spasm due to cerebral palsy/spinal cord injury.

10 Anaesthesias—General and Local

An ideal anaesthetic drug induces anaesthesia smoothly and rapidly and permits rapid recovery as soon as administration ensues. No single anaesthetic drug achieves these desirable effects and is without some disadvantages when used alone. Modern practice of anaesthesia involves, most commonly, the use of combinations of drugs.

Anaesthesias: 2 types—Local (LA) and General (GA).

LA: Means **reversible** loss of sensory perception in a **restricted area** by blocking generation and conduction of impulse at **all parts of neuron.** It causes loss of sensation in a body part without the loss of consciousness or the impairment of central control of vital functions. Plasma levels of LA are highest with block and lowest with subcutaneous infiltration. It acts at **peripheral nerve** and **minor surgery** is done.

It uses Na channel as the primary means of AP generation.

GA: Reversible loss of all sensation and **consciousness** causing abolition of reflexes and relaxation of muscle. Acts at **CNS,** involves **whole body, major surgery** is done.

Earliest LA discovered serendipitously in the late 19th century, **cocaine by Neimann.**

Sigmund Freud studied cocaine's physiological actions and Corl Koller used it as LA in eye surgery in 1884.

Horace Wells (1844, a dentist) used **N$_2$O (nitrous oxide) first time** as **laughing** gas. Modern anaesthesia (thiopental) dates from 1930. In 1940, curare was used as muscle relaxant.

First inhalational anaesthesia was discovered in (1776) by **Priestley.**

Level of LA in spinal block does not change with change in posture after **10 min.**

LA can also be produced by **ice, CO$_2$ snow, ethyl chloride spray,** etc.

Diethylether was used for the **first time** by **William Morton** (1846).

LA is **weak base** with **amphiphilic property** (pKa = 8 to 9).

$$LAH^+ \rightleftharpoons LA \longrightarrow \quad LA \rightleftharpoons LAH^+ \text{ Nerve cell memb.}$$

Cationic form is the most active form at the receptor site.

Only uncharged form crosses the membrane →charged form interacts with binding site. All LAs carry at least one amine function.

Typical LA structure: Chemically, LA consists of a benzene ring separated from tertiary amide either by ester or amide linkage and this intermediate chain divides it as ester and amide linked LA.

> Hydrophilic secondary/tertiary amine charged by picking up hydrogen ion
> +
> Alkyl chain with ester/amide linkage
> +
> Aromatic residue (lipophilic) for penetration into membrane

- Ester linked LA is more prone to hydrolysis than amide linked LA and has shorter duration of action with half-life <1 hour. Ester-linked LA is hydrolysed by butyryl ChE (pseudo ChE). Amide linked LA is hydrolysed by CYP450 in the order of prilocaine (fastest) > etidocaine > lidocaine > mepivacaine > ropivacaine > bupivacaine (slowest).
- High incidence of allergic reactions of ester linked LA is due to PABA and its solution is unstable. In amide linked LA, incidence of allergic reactions is low and solution is stable (not destroyed even by autoclaving).

a. **Amide linked LA:**   AmiDe LA has "Double i" in name
   1. **Long-acting:** Etidocaine, bupivacaine, ropivacaine, dibucaine (**longest**-acting LA)
   2. **Intermediate-acting:** Lidocaine, mepivacaine, prilocaine

   These are more intense, longer-acting and bind to α_1 **acid glycoprotein** in plasma with **no cross-sensitivity and no hydrolysis** by **esterase**.

b. **Ester-linked LA:** Cocaine, Procaine, Tetracaine

   Benzocaine, chloroprocaine (**shortest**-acting LA).

   These are used on mucous membrane due to short duration of action, less intensity and hypersensitivity. **All** are short-acting **except** tetracaine (long-acting). The only naturally occurring LA—**cocaine.**

Classification: LA

INJECTABLE
a. **Low potency, short duration**
   — Procaine
   — Chloroprocaine (shortest duration)
b. **Intermediate potency and duration**
   — Lidocaine (lignocaine)
   — Prilocaine, cocaine, mepivacaine
c. **High potency and long duration**
   — **A**methocaine (tetracaine)
   — **R**opivacaine, etidocaine   **A Red Blood Cell**
   — **B**upivacaine
   — **C**inchocaine dibucaine (longest duration)

Pharmacology Review

SURFACE ANAESTHESIA
a. **Soluble:**   `TLC`
 — **T**etracaine
 — **L**idocaine
 — **C**ocaine

b. **Insoluble**   `BOB`
 — **B**enzocaine
 — **B**utamben (butylaminobenzoate)
 — **O**xethazaine

> Dyclonine, cyclomethycaine, and proparacaine are LA used in other countries.

GA
INHALATIONAL
a. **Gas**
 — N₂O (nitrous oxide)
b. **Volatile liquids**   `SIDE`
 — Ether
 — Halothane
 — **S**evoflurane
 — **I**soflurane
 — **D**esflurane
 — **E**nflurane
 — Methoxyflurane

INTRAVENOUS
a. **Inducing agents**   `TEMP`
 — **T**hiopentone sodium
 — **E**tomidate
 — **M**ethohexitone sodium
 — **P**ropofol
b. **Slower-acting durgs**
 BZD: Diazepam, lorazepam, midazolam.
 Dissociative anaesthesia: Ketamine.
 Neurolept analgesia: Fentanyl + Droperidol.
c. **Others**
 — Cyclopropane
 — Chloroform
 — Trielene
 — Dexmedetomidine
d. **Opioid analgesics**   `FARMS`
 — **F**entanyl
 — **A**lfentanil
 — **R**emifentanil
 — **M**orphine
 — **S**ufentanil

Mechanism of action of LA: (Acts by blocking voltage-gated Na⁺channel). Drug in undissociated (non ionized) form penetrates the axonal membrane and inside it gets dissociated (ionized). This ionized form binds to receptor situated in **sodium channel** in inactivated state from inner side, blocking the channel and thus preventing depolarization and hence action potential. LA enters at node of Ranvier. Ionised cationic LA **(active)** in open channel at inner face →R within voltage sensitive Na⁺ channel ─────────────────────┐
                                                    ↓

↑ Threshold of channel
↓
Na⁺ permeability fails
(reduced Na⁺ ion entry
during upstroke of AP)
↓
Depolarisation fails to
reach threshold potential
↓
Conduction block

— Ca^{++} reduces Na⁺ channel inactivation. High doses block K⁺ channel.
— Na⁺ channel has activation gate near extracellular mouth and Inactivation gate at Intracellular mouth. **At resting state,** activation gate is closed. LA crosses the membrane in its **lipophilic form** and re-ionises to bind **LA R** in intracellular mouth. LA R is present in S_6 **segment of domain IV** of voltage-gated Na⁺ channels which are formed of β_1 (36,000 daltons), β_2 (33,000 daltons) and α (2,60,000 daltons) subunits. α subunits are formed of 4 damains (I to IV) with each domain having 6 transmembrane sements ion α-helical conformation and a membrane reentrant pore loop.

Amino acid residues of short segments between SS_1 and SS_2 are the most critical determinants of ion conductance and selectivity of the channel. After it opens, the channel inactivates within a few microsecond due to closure of an inactivation gate. The frequency dependence of LA action depends critically on the rate of dissociation from the receptor site in the pore of Na channel. A high frequency is needed for LA so that drug binding during AP exceeds drug dissociation between AP. Dissociation of smaller and more hydrophilic drugs is more rapid, so a higher frequency of stimulation is needed to yield frequency dependent block. This block of ion channel is most important for the actions of antiarrhythmics. Resting membrane is less sensitive to LA. Most LA is voltage and time dependent. Resting state has lower affinity for LA than activated (open state) and inactivated channels. Recovery from LA induced block is 10–1000 times slower than the recovery of channels from normal inactivation.

Batrachotoxin, aconitin, veratridins and scorpion venom bind to receptors within the Na⁺ channel and prevent inactivation, act as agonists leading to longed inflex of Na. Tetrodotoxin and saxitoxin bind to receptors near extracellular surface and block them. High LA dose increases threshold for excitation, slows impulse conduction, declines the rate of rise of AP and its amplitude and abolishes the generation of AP. Tetrodotoxin and saxitoxin are two of the most potent known toxins.

Reduction in change of P_{Na} and P_k in **activated nerve** membrane leads to LA. Effect on **resting** membrane **absent**.

Effects on **nerve** are:
- ↓ amplitude
- ↓ rate of rise
- ↓ conduction velocity
- Axonal conduction blockade

Duration of action:
- Shortest — Chloroprocaine
- Longest — Dibucaine (600 min)

Delhi To Bombay
- — Tetracaine (480 min)
- — Bupivacaine (360 min)

Potency and duration of action are enhanced by alkalinization. In inflamed areas, LA is less effective due to high vascularity and rapid wash out.

- Na^+ channel is formed of **a large α and 2 small (β₁ and β₂) subunits**.
  α subunits → 4 domains (I–IV) → each domain has 6 segments (S_1 to S_6).
- **Resting nerve** is more resistant to blockade than conducting nerve. LA enters axon at **nodes of Ranvier only**.
- **Stock solution** of LA is **acidic (ionised)** which is neutralised before anaesthesia can occur.

Local action of LA

1. It blocks **nerve** (motor, sensory), **synapses, neuromuscular junction and R** and reduces **ACh release**. It causes voluntary muscle **paralysis**. Fixed number of nodes of Ranvier (at least 2/3 successive nodes) must be blocked to prevent conduction. Hence, smaller fibres are blocked more rapidly. Sensitivity to LA block decreases with increasing fibre size consistent with high sensitivity for pain sensation mediated by small fibers and low sensitivity for motor function mediated by large fibres. It is unlikely that fibre size determines sensitivity under steady state condition. The thicker the nerve, the farther apart the nodes tend to be hence the greater resistance to block them.
   In infiltration block of large nerves, LA first develps proximally and then spreads distally as the drug penetrates the core of the nerves (proximal sensory fibres are located in the mantle in the core of the trunk). Pregrancy enhances susceptibility of LA due to unknown cause.

    - **M**yelinated fibre is blocked more easily than nonmyelinated fibre of same diameter.
    - **P**reganglionic type B is blocked before smaller unmyelinated type fibre.
    - **S**maller diameter nerve fibre with closely spaced node of Ranvier is more sensitive than larger diameter nerve fibre.
    - **A**utonomic fibre is more sensitive than somatic fibre.
    - Sensory nerve is blocked before motor nerve due to its smaller size and less myelin (but both are inherently equally sensitive). Based on fibre diameter the nerve fibre are classified as type A, B being the thickest and C the thinnest.

Table 10.1: Size and susceptibility to block nerve fibres

Fibre type	Function	Myelination	Conduction velocity (m/s)	Sensitivity to block	Diameter (micron)
Type A α (Alpha)	Proprioception, Motor AMP	Heavy	70–120	+	6–22
β	Touch, pressure	"	30–70	++	6–22
γ	muscle spindle/ tone	"	15–30	++	3–6
δ (Delta)	Pain, Touch Temperature DPT	"	15–30	+++	1–4
Type B	Preganglionic sympathetic	Light	3–15	++++	<3
Type C	Dorsal root— pain, touch Sympathetic— postganglionic	Absent	0.5–2.3	++++	0.4–1.2

Two factors which determine the sensitivity of nerve fibres to local anaesthetics are fibre diameter and myelination therefore type B fibres (myelinated) are more readily blocked than type C (non-myelinated) inspite being of thinner diameter than B. So sequence of block is type B→type C→ Aδ and in functional terms it is autonomic (mediated by C and B fibres)→sensory (mediated by C and also Aδ fibres) → sensory →autonomic.

Among sensory fibres, sequence of blockade is temperature (cold before hot) → pain → touch → deep pressure → proprioception.

Frequency of nerve stimulation: A stimulated nerve will be blocked early.

— **At tongue: Order of taste sense:** Bitter lost first →sweet and sour → salty (last).

2. **LA with vasoconstrictor**
   — Reduces systemic toxicity of LA due to **reduced absorption.**
   — Causes **neurosis** of local tissue due to reduced O_2 supply.
   — **Prolongs duration of action** due to reduced passage to circulation.
3. Most LA is used in the form of acidic salt (HCl) which is stable and soluble and dissociation is delayed in abnormal acidic medium such as infection.

Petency
Correlates with lipid solubility.
Minimum concentration (Cm) of local anaesthetic that will block nerve impulse conduction.

Onset of action
Depends on number of factors like dose and concentration.
pKa: It is the pH at which a local anaesthetic is 50% ionized and 50% non-ionized. Since local anaesthetics are weak bases, agents with pKa

closer to physiologic pH will have more drug in non-ionized form which can diffuse through axonal membrane and so onset will be rapid. That is why lignocaine with pKa of 7.8 is fast acting than bupivacaine (pKa 8.1). This is the rationale of adding soda bicarbonate to local anaesthetic which increases the pH and so more drug available in non-ionized form.

Likewise in ischemic tissue, onset of block will be delayed (in acidic pH more drug will be in ionized form).

It is less effective in inflammatory area due to **low pH** and **ionised form**. **Mucous membrane** has low buffering capacity (does not neutralise acidity of LA) hence it is not anaesthetised. pKa must be **7– 9** so that both **charged and uncharged** form of LA should be available.

4. It causes cardiac depression, ↑ RP, antiarrhythmia and ↓ BP (due to sympathetic blockade but **cocaine** is sympathomimetic → ↑ BP).
5. **All LAs** cause neural inhibition, initially inhibiting **inhibitory neurons** causing stimulation and at high doses, inhibiting **all neurons** thus flattening of waves in ECG. Hence, **all LAs** cause stimulation followed by depression. Most serious ADR of LA is convulsion and the best prevention is small dose.

Differential Block

It depends on concentration. A drug at lower concentration will produce only sensory block while at higher concentration can produce motor block.

Systemic Effects and Toxicity

Toxicity is proportional to potency.

Cardiovascular system

- Except cocaine all local anaesthetics are vasodilators in clinically used concentrations.
- All local anaesthetics have negative inotropic action on myocardium.
- These agents depress the conduction system.
- At higher doses, local anaesthetics can produce ventricular arrhythmias. So combined action like bradycardia, decreased myocardial contractility, ventricular arrhythmias, hypotension can produce cardiac arrest.
- Cardiotoxic potential of bupivacaine is much higher than that of lignocaine.

Central nervous system: Central nervous system is the first system involved in local anaesthetic toxicity. Typical sequence is excitation followed by depression of cerebral tissue (*inhibitory neurons are more sensitive than excitatory neurons*). Signs and symptoms are circumoral numbness, dizziness, tongue paresthesia, visual and auditory disturbances, muscle twitching, tremors, convulsions followed by coma and death.

Treatment

- Convulsion can be controlled by diazepam or thiopentone.
- Maintain adequate ventilation and oxygenation. CNS toxicity is more with bupivacaine than lignocaine.

Respiratory system: Lignocaine depresses hypoxic drive. Direct depression of medullary respiratory centre can occur at high doses.

Immunologic: Allergic reactions are very common with esters but rare with amides. The reaction with amides is because of the preservative (methyl paraben) it contains. Cross sensitivity does not exist between agents of same class.

Local toxicity: When directly injected into nerve, local anaesthetics can damage the nerve. When directly injected into muscle, they are myotoxic.

Local anaesthetics with adrenaline can cause necrosis and gangrene if used in ring block because following structure have end arteries:
- Fingers
- Toes
- Penis
- Pinna

Methaemoglobinemia: Seen with prilocaine, benzocaine and very rarely with lignocaine.

Treatment: IV methylene blue 1% (1 to 2 mg/kg).

Malignant hyperthermia: Lignocaine can cause malignant hyperthermia in susceptible individuals.

Commercial Preparations

Although local anaesthetics are weak bases but their commercial preparations are made acidic (pH to around 6) to enhance their chemical stability so they are available as hydrochloride salts. Local anaesthetics containing adrenaline are made even more acidic (pH around 4) because adrenaline can become unstable at alkaline pH. Antimicrobial preservatives (methylparaben) is added to multidose vials or spinal and epidural anaesthesia preservative free preparations should be used.

PK of LA: Soluble surface anaesthesia →rapidly absorbed from mucous membrane. **Amide-linked** LAs are bound to plasma α_1 **glycoprotein,** are degraded by **dealkylation** and **hydrolysis** in microsomes. **Ester-linked** LAs are hydrolysed by **esterase** and **pseudocholinesterase** in the liver (except cocaine). Lungs can also excrete significant amount of LA (bupivacaine, lignocaine, prilocaine). Due to poor water solubility of LA, renal excretion of unchanged drug is only <5%.

Ester of intermediate chain is broken down by **butyrylcholinesterase** in blood. **Amide** is metabolised by **amidase** and CPY450 in liver.

Drugs metabolised by pseudocholinesterase (plasma cholinesterase) are:

CAMPS

- Chloroprocaine (ester LA)
- Amethocaine (ester LA)
- Mivacurium (non-depolarising muscle relaxant)
- Procaine (ester LA) and propanidid (IV anaesthesia)
- Succinylcholine (depolarising muscle relaxant)

Duration of Action

It depends on:
1. **Dose:** Increased dose increases the duration.
2. **Pharmacokinetic profile of drug:** It includes
   - **Plasma protein binding** (α_1 acid glycoprotein): Agents with high protein binding like bupivacaine has prolonged action.
   - **Metabolism:** Esters are metabolized by pseudocholinesterase and amides are metabolized in liver by microsomal enzymes. Esters have small duration of action than amides.

3. **Addition of vasoconstrictors:** Vasoconstrictors decrease the systemic absorption of local anaesthetics in blood, so increases the concentration thereby increasing the duration of action. Vasoconstrictors used are:
   - **Adrenaline:** In a concentration of 1 in 2 lakhs. Duration of both sensory and motor blockade is increased by addition of epinephrine to lignocaine but only sensory block is prolonged if epinephrine is added to bupivacaine with no effect on motor blockade.

   Xylocaine with adrenaline should not be used for
   - Ring block of fingers, toes, penis, pinna (absolute contraindication).
   - When an inhalational agent especially halothane which sensitizes myocardium to adrenaline is used.
   - Myocardial ischemia patients.
   - Severe hypertensives.
   - Intravenous regional anaesthesia (Beir's block).
   - **Phenylephrine:** In a concentration of 1 in 2 lakhs. Other vasoconstrictors which can be used are noradrenaline and felypressin (octopressin), a synthetic derivative of vasopressin.
4. **Sodium bicarbonate:** Addition of sodium bicarbonate increases both onset and duration of action. Sodium bicarbonate increases the onset by making the pH more alkaline so more drug is available in unionized form. Later carbon dioxide released from sodium bicarbonate metabolism enters intracellularly making the pH more acidic making more drug to be available in ionized form, thereby increasing the duration of action also.

   So addition of sodium bicarbonate:
   1. Enhances the onset of action.
   2. Increases the duration of action.
   3. Improves the quality of block.
   4. Decreases the pain of injection.

Systemic Absorption

It depends on:
1. **Site of injection:** It is proportionate to the vascularity of the site of injection. Systemic absorption is highest after intercostal nerve block.
2. **Addition of vasoconstrictors:** This is the most important factor. Addition of vasoconstrictor increases the margin of safety by decreasing the systemic absorption that is why **maximum dose of xylocaine (lignocaine) with adrenaline is 7 mg/kg (500 mg) while without adrenaline is 3 mg/kg (200 mg).**

Hydrophobicity enhances both the potency, toricity and duration of action of LA due to reduced metabolism by enzymes and more LA available at the site of action.

ADR of LA
— **Order of effects of cocaine on CNS**
   Euphoria → Excitement → Confusion → Restlessness → Tremor and muscle twitching → Convulsion → Unconsciousness → Respiratory depression and Death.   **ECRT-CURD**
— Local tissue **necrosis** due to reduced O_2 supply with LA + vasoconstriction.
— Bupivacaine → **highest local tissue necrosis.**
— Chloroprocaine → **neuropathy.**

- Hypersensitivity reaction especially with **ester type LA.**
- ↓BP, arrhythmia, vascular collapse.

Methods of Local Analgesia

A. **Topical (surface anaesthesia):** All local anaesthetics except mepivacaine, bupivacaine and ropivacaine can be used for surface (topical) analgesia (penetration of procaine and chlorprocaine is very poor after topical application).
B. **Infiltration anaesthesia:** Local anaesthetic is infiltrated at operation site.
C. **Nerve blocks:** Drug is injected around the nerve supplying the operation site.
D. **Intravenous regional anaesthesia (Beir's block).**
E. **Central neuraxial blocks:** Which includes spinal and epidural anaesthesia.
F. **Refrigeration analgesia:** It is topical analgesia produced by CO_2 snow, ice cooling, ethyl chloride spray. It blocks the nerve conduction at local site.

Cocaine

1. A **natural alkaloid** from leaves of *E. coca*. **The only naturally occurring LA.** The only LA having **sympathomimetic** properties and causing vasoconstriction.
2. **First** used by Karl Coller for **ocular anaesthesia** in 1884 (is **the earliest** used anaesthesia). First isolated by Nieman.
3. **Protoplasmic poison** → tissue necrosis.
4. **CNS stimulation** with marked effect on mood and behaviour.
   CNS excitement is manifested as enphoria, agitation, violence, hyperexcitability, convulsion, apnea and death.
5. Stimulates:
   Vagal centre → ↓BP
   Vasomotor centre → ↑BP
   Vomiting centre → Vomiting
   Temperature regulating centre → Pyrexia
6. **Blocks E/NE uptake** into nerve in the periphery → potentiates directly acting and suppresses indirectly acting sympathomimetic effects. It causes **mydriasis and vasoconstriction.** Not injected.
   Sympathetic stimulation causes tachycardia, hypertension and arrhythmia. It is potent vasoconstrictor.

PK: It is the only ester metabolised in the liver (not by pseudo ChE) and one metabolite ecgonine is CNS stimulant.

U: Surface LA.

CF: IV route.

Chloroprocaine: It is metabolised **most rapidly,** has **shortest** duration of action (150–20 minutes) and **lowest** systemic toxicity. It is more **neurotoxic** than others. Chloroprocaine is a chlorinated derivative of procaine and was introduced in 1952. Its plasma half-life is 25 seconds.

Muscular back pain is due to tetany in the supraspinus muscles which is a consequence of Ca^{2+} binding by EDTA included as preservative of 2-chloroprocaine of epidural LA. Most acidic (pH = 33).

U: Maximum safe dose for procaine and chloroprocaine is 1 g.

CI: It is contraindicated in spinal anaesthesia due to causing paraplegia and cauda equina syndrome.

Procaine: First synthetic LA synthesised by **Einhorn in 1905.**

1. Acts for 30–60 min. It is stored in cool place to prevent hydrolysis.
2. Hydrolysed in plasma and liver →PABA release →antagonises the action of sulfonamide.
3. Procaine + benzylpenicillin = **procaine penicillin** acts for 24 hrs due to **slow absorption**. Like amethocaine (tetracaine) it inhibits bacteriostatic action of sulfonamide and P-aminosalicylic acid.
4. Amide derivative of procaine is **procainamide** (classical antiarrhythmic). AOC and drug for malignant hyperthermia.

Lidocaine (Lignocaine): The **most popular and the most widely used LA**, first synthesised in 1943 by **Lofgren** and **first used by Gordh.** It also has antiarrhythmic action. On injection, it prevents conduction within **3 min.**

ADR: Drowsiness, **A**ltered taste, **M**ental clouding and blurred vision, **T**innitus. (Dose related neurological effect—**commonest**). **MDAT**

Overdose causes muscle twitch, arrhythmia, convulsion, ↓BP, coma, respiratory arrest, fits and paresthesia (decreased by urine acidification →↑ excretion). Amides (6 letters) have **2 "i"** in LA and t½ = **2 to 6 hrs.**

Mechanism of action of Lidocaine

1. **All cardiac effects** are direct action. **Suppression of automaticity** in ectopic foci is **the commonest cardiac action**. Rate of O phase depolarisation is reduced only in the presence of hyperkalemia. **Reduced conduction** specially in depolarised cell. **Reduced APD** in PF and ventricular muscle. Less marked reduction in ERP (hence **ERP/APD** is enhanced). Effect on APD and ERP of atrial fibres **absent. Suppression of re-entrant** ventricular arrhythmia either by abolishing one way block or by producing 2 ways block.
2. Blocks **inactivated Na⁺ channel** more than open state. **Depolarised/damaged fibres** effected more than normal ventricular and conducting fibres. **Lack of effect** on channel recovery leads to inefficacy in atrial arrhythmia. QT interval reduces.

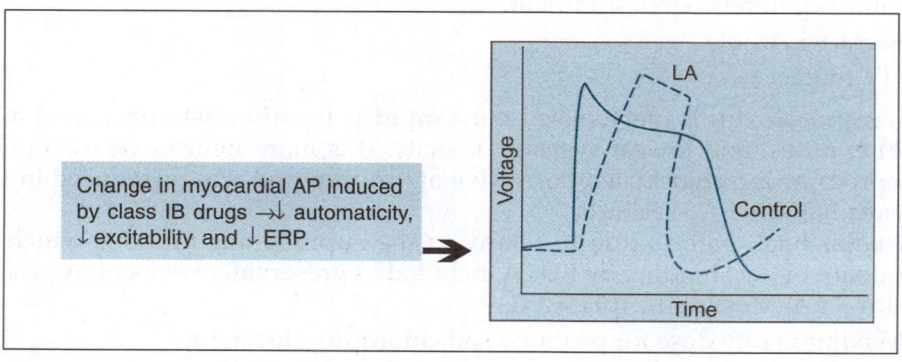

Change in myocardial AP induced by class IB drugs →↓ automaticity, ↓ excitability and ↓ ERP.

Action of LA on heart is **frequency dependent (state dependent)** with the **highest** activity at the higher frequency. Thus, it acts preferentially on arrhythmic muscle. Lidocaine is vasoineffective.

Lignocaine is the main drug used. Its features are:
Locally administered as local anaesthetic.
Inactive orally so...
Given IV. For antiarrhythmic action, which is due to...
Na^+ channel blockade which occurs in...
Only inactive state of Na^+ channels.
CNS side effects like convulsions occur on high doses.
Action lasts only 15 minutes due to rapid redistribution.
Inhibits Purkinje fibres and ventricles but...
No effect on AVN, SAN, so...
Effective in ventricular arrhythmias only (not supraventricular).
Emergency uses like to prevent arrhythmia following MI, cardiac surgery and digitalis toxicity.

3. No mydriasis and cycloplegia.

PK of lidocaine: Absorbed orally. **75%** plasma protein bound. Duration of action →10–12 min due to rapid redistribution. **Hydrolysed, conjugated** and **deethylated** in liver. Excreted in urine, pKa = 7.8

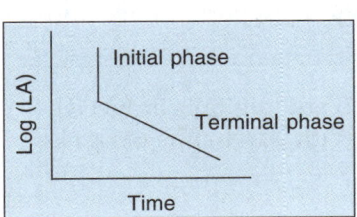

t½ = Early distribution phase—**8 min** and later elimination phase—**2 hrs.**
t½ is enhanced in **CHF** due to ↓ in volume of distribution and hepatic blood flow. Therapeutic plasma concentration—**2–5 µg/ml.**
Dose: 1–3 mg/min. IV or 1.5 mg bolus + 0.5 mg/20 min IV. Solution is stable containing preservative methylparaben.

(**Xylocard** and **Gesicard** injections are specially made for cardiac use and contain no preservative). Elimination of lidocaine follows 2 compartment kinetics, thus repeated dosing enhances duration of therapeutic effects (*see* Graph). Vasoconstrictors prolong LA action.

IA of lidocaine: Cimetidine enhances plasma level. **Propranolol** enhances t½ by reducing hepatic blood flow.

Drusg that effect LA

- Adrenal steroid and etomidate suppress hypothalamo-pituitary-adrenal axis.
- Aminoglycosides potentiate neuromuscular blocker drugs.
- AntiChE potentiates suxamethonium.
- Antiepileptic agents are essential to arrest status epilepticus.
- Antihypertensives of all kinds complicate LA due to hypotension.
- Beta blockers prevent homeostatic sympathetic cardiac response to cardiac depression.
- Diuretics cause hypokalemia which potentiate neuromuscular blockers and GA.

- Psychotropic drugs (neuroleptics) synergise or potentiate with opioids, hypnotics and GA.
- MAO inhibitor with pethidine/ephedrine causes hypertension.

U: Used as **both surface and injection** anaesthesia (DOC). As LA →**maximum** dose without adrenaline is **3 mg/kg** and with adrenaline is **7 mg/kg**.

Vasoconstrictor (adrenaline) reduces local blood flow, slows absorption rate of LA and prolongs its effect. The final concentration of adrenaline is 1 in 2,00,000. Vasoconstrictor is not used for nerve block of extremity due to reduced blood flow causing organ damage.

Alternative vasoconstrictor "felypressin" has no effect on HR and BP, hence it is preferred in EVS disease. Sympathetic nerve blood is used in vascular disease to induce vasodilation.

Duration of effect without adrenaline (3 mg/kg) is 454–60 minutes and with adrenaline (7mg/kg) is 2–3 hours. Sympathetic, sensory and motor blockade need the highest concentration of LA.

1. Ventricular **T**achycardia and arrhythmia **(DOC)** due to rapid developing and titrable action. Ventricular fibrillation and premature ventricular complex. Digitalis induced ventricular arrhythmia. Acute MI (prophylaxis).
2. **R**egional anaesthesia (0.5% LA) IV.
3. **E**pidural anaesthesia (1.5% LA).
4. **S**urface application (4% LA).
5. **I**nfiltration (1–2% LA).
6. **N**erve block (1–2% LA).
7. **S**pinal anaesthesia—5%. Injection is made **heavy** or hyperbaric by adding 7.5% **dextrose** and **light** by adding **saline**.

The **RESINS**

> DOC in ventricular tachycardia and VES (acute MI and digitalis induced)
> **Dose:** 1–1.5 mg/kg/min. Maximum safest dose: With adrenaline 6 mg/kg and without adrenaline 3 mg/kg.

CI: Malignant hyperthermia. Lidocaine releases Ca^{2+} from sarcoplasmic reticulum.

Prilocaine: Pharmacological profile similar to that of (more common in neonates due to less resistance of fetal Hb to oxidants and immaturity of enzymes) lidocaine but one of its metabolite (O-toluidine) causes **methaemoglobinemia.** Treatment: 1. **Ascorbic acid,** 2. **Methylene blue** 2 mg/kg (converts Met. Hb →Cynomet. Hb). Drugs causing methemogobinemia are compounds of introgen, chloroquine, primaquine, chlorobenzene, benzocaine, prilocaine, dapsone, sulfonamide, phenacetin, etc. **Lidocaine + prilocaine** cause lowering of melting point, that are mixed in **equal** proportion at 25°C. It is the **safest** LA. Other than liver, it is metabolised in kidneys, lungs and by amidase.

U: 1. **Alternate** to lidocaine infiltration.
2. Most suitable for Bier's IV block.
3. Dose: 5 mg/kg and with adrenaline 8 mg/kg. Dose over 600 mg causes Met. Hb, hence contraindicated in both cases.

Dibucaine: Most potent, most toxic and **longest**-acting LA. A quinoline derivative.
U: As surface anaesthesia in:
1. Anal canal.
2. Spinal anaesthesia.

Tetracaine (Amethocaine): is **PABA ester.** It inhibits the action of sulfonamide and paraminosalicylic acid. Duration of action is more than lidocaine. Both surface and conduction block anaesthesia. **10 times** as potent and toxic as procaine.

U: ENT (eye, nose, throat), tracheobronchial tree, spinal and caudal anaesthesia.

ADR: More toxic and potent due to slow action but blood concentration is the **same** even after IV and tracheobronchial spray.

Etidocaine

It was introduced in 1972. Its onset of action is similar or comparable to that of lidocaine and its duration of action and cardiotoxicity are similar to that of bupivacaine.

Bupivacaine: Lipid soluble and analgesic. Commonly used LA.

4 times more potent than lidocaine and the solution is stable available as 0.5%. Hepatic metabolism with half-life = 3½ hrs. Duration of effect without E is 2–3 hrs and with E is 3–5 hrs. Addition of E has no effect on motor blockade, it prolongs only duration of sensory block. Maximum safe dose in 2 mg/kg, with/without E. Most cardiotoxicity is due to high tissue and protein binding making resuscitation prolonged and difficult. Treatment is bretylium (DOC). Lidocaine is racemic mixture of S and R isomers and the R isomer is cardiotoxic. But bupivacaine has more sensory than motor blockade, has made it prolonged analgesic.

Order to cardiotoxicity and CNS toxicity: Bupivacaine > ropivacaine > lidocaine. But reversal of sodium channel and rapid clearance from circulation for cardiotoxicity is more frequent with ropivacaine than bupivacaine and causes more toxicity in bupivacaine including motor sensory blockade. Ropivacaine, alfentanil and midazolam are hydrolysed by CYP3A4, hence concomitant use of the two latter agents slow metabolism of rupivacaine.

ADR: Ventricular tachycardia, **maximum cardiotoxic,** cardiac depression hence not used for IV regional anaesthesia. Most common ECG finding of bupivacaine is slow rhythm with broad QRS complex. **Highest** local tissue irritancy. Levobupivacaine is the S-enantiomer of racemic bupivacaine and is less cardiotoxic than bupivacaine.

U: 1. **S**pinal (0.5–1%).
    2. **I**nfiltration.
    3. **N**erve block (0.5% LA).   **SINEO**
    4. **E**pidural (0.5% LA).
    5. **O**bstetrics (opioid+LA is given for pain relief).
    6. DOC in isobaric spinal anaesthesia as it is the **most potent.**

Ropivacaine: Bupivacaine congener. Blocks A_δ **and C > A_β fibres** in pain transmission. Duration of action similar to that of bupivacaine.

U: Postoperative and labour pain. More motor-sparing than bupivacaine.

Mepivacaine

It was introduced in 1957. Its pharmacological properties are similar to those of lidocaine but it is toxic in neonate due to lower pH of neonatal blood and duration of action is slightly longer than lidocaine.

Butamben and Benzocaine: Not absorbed from **mucous membrane.** Both are **PABA** derivatives, hence antagonise sulfonamide. Benzocaine has low aqueous solubility.

Table 10.2: Summary of properties of local anaesthetics

Drug	Potency	t 1/2	Duration of action		pKa	Maximum safe dose (mg/kg)	Comments
			Without adrenaline	With adrenaline			
Esters							
Procaine	+		15–30 minute	30–90 minutes	8.9	12 mg/kg	Shortest acting
Chloroprocaine	+		15–25 minute	30–90 minutes	9.0	12 mg/kg	
Cocaine	++		—	—	8.7	3 mg/kg	Used for topical anaesthesia. Potent vasoconstrictor
Tetracaine	++++		2–3 hours	3–5 hours	8.2	3 mg/kg	
Amides							
Lignocaine	++	1.6 hrs	45–60 minutes	2–3 hours	7.8	3 mg/kg (without adrenaline) 7 mg/kg (with adrenaline)	Most commonly used local anaesthetic
Prilocaine	++		45–60 minutes	2–3 hours	7.8	8 mg/kg	Can cause methaemoglobinemia
Mepivacaine	++		45–60 minutes	2–3 hours	7.6	4.5 mg/kg	
Etidocaine	++++		2–3 hours	3–5 hours	7.7	4 mg/kg	
Bupivacaine (sensoricaine, marcaine)	++++	3.5 hrs	2–3 hours	3–5 hours	8.1	2 mg/kg	Very commonly used local anaesthetic
Ropivacaine	++++		2–3 hours	3–5 hours	8.1	3 mg/kg	Less cardiotoxic than bupivacaine
Dibucaine	++++	4 hrs	2.5–3.5 hrs	3.5–5.5 hours	8.8	1 mg/kg	Longest acting, most potent, most toxic

U: Sore throat, stomatitis, wounds/ulcers.
Oxethazaine: Ionises even at **low pH**, hence anaesthetises **gastric mucosa.**
ADR: Drowsiness and dizziness when dose is **>100 mg/d.**
U: Gastritis and gastroesophageal reflux. Heart burn of pregnancy. Irritable bowel disease: reduces gastrocolic reflex so reduces **post-prandial surgery.**

Dyclonine HCI

It has a rapid onset of action and a duration of effect comparable to that of procaine.
U: Mucous membrane and skin.

Pramoxine HCI

It is a surface LA that is not a benzoate ester. It reduces cross-sensitivity reactions in patients allergic to other LA, but is too irritating to be used within nose or on the eye.

Lecithin coated microdroplets of methoxyflurane can produce local analgesia. All amide LAs can be autoclaved without undergoing any chemical change.

Site of Action of Drug

1. Anterior and posterior nerve roots (main site of action).
2. Mixed spinal nerves.
3. Drug diffuses through dura and arachnoid and inhibits descending pathways in spinal cord.

Table 10.3: *Local anaesthetics for epidural anaesthesia*

Drug	Concentration
Chloroprocaine	2–3%
Lignocaine	1–2%
Mepivacaine	1–2%
Prilocaine	2–3%
Bupivacaine	0.25–0.5%

Surface anaesthesia: Only **superficial layer** is anaesthetised by surface anaesthesia. **Dilute** solution of LA is infiltrated under the skin in the area of operation to block **sensory nerve endings** (used for minor operation). LA is injected around **nerve trunks** to anaesthetise area distal to injection. **All nerves** coming to a particular area are blocked after LA injection SC **nerve block** lasts longer than **field block** or **infiltration anaesthesia.** Dyclonine is surface anaesthesia.

Maximum dosages for topical use are 300 mg, lidocaine, 150 mg cocaine and 50 mg tetracaine.

Only LA which is
1. Naturally occurring, vasoconstrictor, **earliest** used → cocaine.
2. Intradural injection contraindicated, causes paraplegia → chloroprocaine.
3. LA of choice in malignant hyperpyrexia → procaine.
4. **Safest,** causes **maximum Met Hb** so contraindicated in the same → prilocaine.
5. Vision effective (neither dialator nor constrictor) → lignocaine.

6. Completely hydrolysed in body and not excreted → amethocaine.
7. Not metabolised by neonates so contraindicated in neonates and labour → mepivacaine.
8. Never surface anaesthesia → bupivacaine, mepivacaine.
9. Surface anaesthesia (absorbed through mucous membrane):

Prilocaine	Pakistani
Procaine	People
Lidocaine	Like
Cocaine	Coconut
Dibucaine	During
Hexylcaine	Huge
Tetracaine	Trouble

Only LA which has
1. Maximum retention in body—etidocaine.
2. Anaesthetises gastric mucosa and reduces gastrocolic reflex—oxethazaine.
3. DOC for isobaric spinal anaesthesia and contraindicated in IV regional anaesthesia—bupivacaine.

Applied Anatomy of Central Neuraxial Blockade

Vertebral column consist of 33 vertebrae: 7 cervical, 12 thoracic, 5 lumbar, 5 fused sacral and 4 fused coccygeal vertebrae. Vertebral column has 4 curves: Thoracic and sacral spine are convex posteriorly (kyphotic) while cervical and lumbar spine are convex anteriorly (lordotic).

The tips of spinous processes are such that epidural or spinal needle should be inserted obliquely in thoracic region and straight in lumbar region.

Surface landmarks which are important while giving spinal or epidural anaesthesia are:

C7: Spinous process of 7th cervical vertebra is very prominent and easily palpable.
T7: T7 lies opposite to inferior angle of scapula.

Highest point on iliac crest corresponds to L4 and L5 interspace: It is very important to identity this intervertebral space while giving spinal anaesthesia.

Epidural Space (Extradural or Peridural Space)

It lies outside the dura mater. It extends from foramen magnum to sacral hiatus. Epidural anaesthesia is given in this space. Epidural space is triangular in shape with apex dorsomedial.

Contents

- Anterior and posterior nerve roots.
- Epidural veins
- Spinal arteries
- Lymphatics
- Fat

Epidural Veins (Venous Plexus of Batson)

These are valveless veins connecting pelvic veins to intracranial veins directly. So accidental injection of air of local anaesthetic can directly ascend to cranium. Secondly, these veins directly drain into inferior vena cava, so whenever there is obstruction to vena caval flow as in pregnancy, and abdominal tumours, these veins are engorged, reducing the size of epidural space and hence less dose of local anaesthetic is required.

Anatomy of Spinal Cord

Spinal cord extends from medulla oblongata to lower border of L1 in adults. But in infants and neonates it ends at the lower border of L3 *(Adult level is achieved by 2 years of age)*. So in infancy spinal anaesthesia should be given in L4–5 space only while in adults, it can be given L3–4 or L4–5 space (or even L2–3). Usually, it is given in L3–4 interspace.

Below L1, vertebral canal is occupied by lumbar, sacral and coccygeal nerve roots in oblique and downward direction forming cauda equina (horse tail).

Spinal cord is divided into segments by spinal nerves which arise from it. The spinal nerves are 31 pairs in number, i.e. 8 cervical, 12 thoracic, 5 lumbar, 5 sacral and 1 coccygeal. Each spinal nerve has an anterior root which is efferent and motor and a posterior root which is afferent and sensory.

Blood Supply of Spinal Cord

It is supplied by 2 posterior spinal arteries which arise from posterior inferior cerebellar arteries and 1 anterior spinal artery which is formed by branch of vertebral artery of each side.

Anterior spinal artery is reinforced by many arteries of which artery of Adamkiewicz (arteria radicularis magna) is very important which can enter anywhere between T5 and L2 and usually (75%), it enters from left side. Damage to this artery by needle can lead to cord ischemia and paraplegia.

Meninges

Spinal cord is enveloped from inside to outside by pia mater, arachnoid mater and dura mater.

Dura mater extends up to S2 in adults and up to S4 in infants while pia mater extends as filum terminale up to coccyx.

CSF (Cerebrospinal Fluid)

CSF is present between pia and arachnoid mater (i.e., subarachnoid space), that is why spinal anaesthesia is also called as subarachnoid block.

CSF is secreted by choroid plexus of third, fourth and lateral ventricles and is absorbed into venous sinuses via arachnoid villi.

500 ml is secreted in 24 hours.

Volume of CSF at one time is 140 ml, half of which is present is cranium and half in spinal canal.

Specific gravity and pH = 1.003 to 1.009 (average 1.004) and 7.35 respectively.

CSF pressure: It is same in cranium and spinal canal in lying position which is **100 to 150 mmH$_2$O** (10–15 cmH$_2$O) while in sitting position the CSF pressure at lumbar level may increase to 180 to 240 mmH$_2$O.

Advantages of central neuraxial blocks (i.e., spinal and epidural over general anaesthesia)

1. It is cheapest.
2. Lessens the risk of pulmonary aspiration.
3. Respiratory complications.
4. Systemic side effects are not seen.
5. All serious consequences of intubation can be avoided.
6. Disturbances of body chemistry are minimal.
7. Bleeding is less.
8. Decreased incidence of thromboembolism due to increased vascularity of lower limbs.

Systemic Effects (Physiological Alterations) of Central Neuraxial Blocks

Cardiovascular System

The *most prominent effect is hypotension* which is because of the following factors:

1. **Venodilatation** due to sympathetic block.
2. Decreased cardiac output
   - Decreased atrial pressure because of decrease venous return (Bainbridge reflex) and
   - Direct inhibition of cardioaccelerator fibers (T1 to T4).
3. Paralysis of nerve supply to adrenal glands with consequently decreased catecholamine release.
4. Direct absorption of drug into systemic circulation.
5. Compression of inferior vena cava and aorta by pregnant uterus, abdominal tumours (supine hypotension syndrome).

Nervous System

Autonomic fibres (mediated by C fibres) are most sensitive and they are blocked earliest followed by sensory and then motor fibres. So, sequence of block is *Autonomic → Sensory → Motor.* The recovery occurs in reverse order.

Due to this different sensitivity of nerve fibres to local anaesthetics, **autonomic level is 2 segments higher than sensory level which is 2 segments higher than motor level.** This is called as differential blockade and the segments where one modality is blocked and another is not forms the *zones of differential blockade.*

Autonomic level is tested by temperature, sensory by pin prick and motor by toe movement.

Respiratory System

In patient of COPD whose expiration is dependent on abdominal muscles and cannot bear loss of lower intercostals, there can be severe impairment of respiratory function if block is high enough to block abdominal and lower intercostal muscles.

Apnea seen after spinal anaesthesia is usually due to severe hypotension causing medullary ischemia. Other causes of apnea are:

1. **High spinal:** High enough to block phrenic nerve (C3, 4, 5) which is rare.
2. **Total spinal:** Accidental intrathecal injection of large volume of drug during epidural anaesthesia.

Gastrointestinal System

Sympathetic block and parasympathetic overactivity produces contracted gut with relaxed sphincters.

Genital System

Flaccid (paralysis of nervi erigentes) and engorged penis is one of the signs of successful block.

Endocrinal System

- Stress response to surgery (by blocking adrenals) is inhibited.
- The response to insulin is augmented and there can be hypoglycemia.
- Usual increase in ADH during surgery is suppressed.

Renal

Renal functions not impaired unless mean arterial pressure falls below critical pressure of kidney for autoregulation (which is 55 mm Hg).

Urinary System

Urinary retention is due to blockade of sacral parasympathetic fibres (S2, 3, 4).

Thermoregulation

Vasodilatation causes heat loss which is compensated by vasoconstriction above the block and shivering (a very common occurrence after spinal anaesthesia).

Site of Action of Local Anaesthetic

Local anaesthetic mainly acts on spinal nerves and dorsal ganglia but a small concentration can be detected in substance of spinal cord.

Durgs are

1. **Xylocaine:** Concentration used is 5%. The solution used for spinal is hyperbaric (or heavy) by addition of 7.5% dextrose. Hyperbaric solution tries to settle down because its specific gravity is more than that of CSF.
   Specific gravity of hyperbaric xylocaine is 1.0333 (CSF = 1.044).
2. **Bupivacaine (Sensoricaine):** Concentration used is 0.5% and it is made hyperbaric by addition of 8% dextrose.
   Specific gravity is 1.0278.
3. **Tetracaine:** Concentration used is 1% and made hyperbaric by addition of 5% dextrose.
4. **Procaine:** 10% in 5% dextrose.
   - Opioids and others like ketamine, are also used.

Table 10.4: *Local anaesthetics for spinal anaesthesia*

Drug	Concentration	Specific gravity
Lignocaine	5% in 7.5% dextrose	1.0333
Bupivacaine	0.5% in 8% dextrose	1.0278
Tetracaine	1% in 5% dextrose	1.0203
Procaine	10% in 5% dextrose	1.0203

Factors Effecting the Height of Block (i.e., Level of Block)
1. **Volume (dosage) of drug:** Greater the volume, higher the level of block.
2. **Baricity:** Baricity is the ratio of specific gravity of an agent at a specific temperature (body temperature) to specific gravity of CSF at same temperature.
3. **Hyperbaric technique:** This is the most commonly used method. The outcome of hyperbaric spinal anaesthesia is governed by position of the patient during spinal anaesthesia and after injection till drug gets fixed to neuronal tissue, which normally takes 10 to 15 minutes for xylocaine and 20 to 30 minutes for bupivacaine.

Subarachnoid block/intrathecal block/spinal anaesthesia (SA): One of the most popular form of anaesthesia. It is the commonest used anaesthetic technique. **First** discovered by **Bier in 1899. Commonest** site for LP → **L3–4**. In adults, spinal cord extends up to L_1 **vertebrae** and in children + neonates up to L_3 **vertebrae**. Injected in **subarachnoid space** between L2 and 3/L3 and 4 below the lower end of spinal cord. It acts primarily at the nerve root in the cauda equina anaesthetising **lower abdomen** and **hind limbs**. Level of LA falls rapidly after injection and gets **fixed** after **10 min**. Higher segments are at low concentration of LA.

Bell-Magendie's law: Sensory (Afferent)—root is posterior/dorsal. Motor (Efferent)—root is anterior/ventral.   **SA ME**

Postural headache with classic features due to LP is that the incidence of headache decreases with increasing age of the patient and decreasing needle diameter. Caffeine 500 mg IV is the treatment.

Extent of SA: LA in adults →**L3–4**. LP in infant →**L4–5**. LP is done in left/right lateral position and in sitting with head below flexed knees (commonest approach is midline).

Most sympathetic fibres leave the spinal cord between T1 and L2. Sympathetic blockade is several spinal segment higher, since preganglionic sympathetic fibres are more sensitive to be blocked by low concentration of LA. Thus, as the level of sympathetic block ascends, actions of parasympathetic fibres are increasing by dominant and compensatory mechanisms of inblocked sympathetic nervous system. Most sympathetic fibres leave the cord at T1 and hence, blockade of cervical level is also involved. Thus, the degree of sympathetic block is related to the weight of sensory anaesthesia.

Twe Lve~12

Level of **S**ympathetic block is 2 segment higher and level of **M**otor paralysis 2 segment lower than **C**utaneous **A**nalgesia due to **sensitivity order:**

S > CA > M = SCAM Autonomic preganglionic fibre > Somatic Sensory fibre > Somatic Motor fibre. A > SS > SM = ASS-SM

0.2–0.4 mg Adrenaline to LA prolongs spinal anaesthesia by ⅓ due to reduction in spinal cord blood flow/α_2 actions (analgesic). Adrenaline causes ↓ bleeding, ↑ LA, ↓systemic concentration of LA (except cocaine due to its vasoconstriction). Adrenaline in spinal anaesthesia acts on α = receptors which inhibit substance P release and reduce sensory nerve firing. Clonidine agents LA effect and produces analgesia. Decreased systemic absorption, increased LA uptake by nerve and α activation by adrenaline prolong LA effect by 10–50% (not used in SA due to ischemia of cord).

Most important effect of sympathetic block on CVS is hypotension due to vasodilation, so IVF 1000 ml before SA with E (DOC) is given (phenylephrine is also used). Respiratory arrest is due to medullary ischemia secondary to hypotension. High concentration of LA can cause irreversible block.

Spinal dural space is filled with semiliquid fat through which nerve roots travel. During spinal anaesthesia, nerve fibres which are:

1. **First** to be blocked →**Type B.**
2. **Last** to be blocked → α **fibres.**
3. **Last** to recover→sympathetic **type C.**

Women during pregnancy has **IVC compression** resulting in engorgement of vertebral system and reduction in capacity of subarachnoid space. Hence, LA is needed.

Uses of Spinal/Intradural/Subarachnoid Anaesthesia

Operation of all pelvic, perineal, uterine and upper abdomen (lower limb, lower abdomen, pelvis, prostatectomy, fracture setting, obs and gynae).

Barbotage: It is a process of alternatively spinal fluid withdrawal and reinjection under pressure.

Complication of Spinal Anaesthesia

1. **Respiratory paralysis:** Apnoea is rare and occurs due to paralysis of external abdominis and intercostal muscle (but diaphragm due to phrenic nerve supply maintains breathing) and hypotension.
2. **Hypotension (commonest)** and ischaemia of respiratory centre and diffusion of LA to higher centre cause respiratory failure.
3. Hypotension is mild in all and systolic BP, 90 mm Hg in 33% and is:
   A. Due to blockade of sympathetic flow to heart leading to **vasodilatation** hence low venous return. Most ADR is due to sympathetic block.
   B. Also due to skeletal muscle paralysis of lower limb.
4. Post spinal headache occurs after 12–24 hrs. Typically pain increases on sitting and relieves on lying down. It lasts 7–10 days in 90% cases and is relieved in all cases in 3 weeks. Single most important factor is needle size. Most often, headache is relieved by epidural blood path, position, analgesics and adequate hydration. **Headache** is due to CSF leakage lasting 2–3 days (10 ml/hr).
   Epidural bood patch: 10 to 20 ml of autologous blood is given in the same epidural space in which spinal is given. Blood will clot and seal the rent. Ist blood patch is effective in treating headache in 95% patients and 2nd blood patch in 99%. The blood patch should be applied only if other measures fail (15–20 ml of blood is not likely to cause significant hematoma but can cause transient rediculopathy).
5. Nausea and vomiting (most commonly due to hypotension causing central hypoxia). Nausea and vomiting due to **reflexes** initiated by traction of abdominal viscera in abdominal operations.
6. **Cauda equina syndrome** due to damage of nerve roots/chronic arachnoiditis leading to uncontrolled bladder and bowel sphincter.
7. Paralysis of all CN—6th (**commonest**) and **I, X, and IX (least).** Cranial nerves likely to be **not effected** in spinal anaesthesia is **I and X.**
   Cranial nerve palsy: Most common 90% cranial nerve effected in spinal anaesthesia—**VI nerves** due to longest course of it.

8. During LP, **infection** may cause meningitis.
9. Bradycardia and cardiac arrest.

Order of block of SA: **A**utonomic preganglionic sympathetic B fibres → **T**emperature → **P**rick → **P**ain → **T**ouch → **P**ressure → **M**otor → vibration (**P**roprioception).

> ATP Pays Total Precious Muscle Power

Most common SA used in USA is lidocaine, tetracaine and bupivacaine.

CI of spinal anaesthesia: Hypotension and increase ICT, non-cooperative patient, sepsis and shock, vertebral abnormalities (kyphosis, lordosis), haemorrhage (subarachnoid), severe HTN.

Spinal Anaesthesia in Children
- Should be given in lower space (L4–5).
- Preloading is not required as children less than 8 years are virtually free of haemodynamic side effects.
- Use of narcotics is contraindicated.
- Chances of systemic toxicity is high.

Saddle Block
It is the spinal given in sitting position and the patient remains seated for 5 minutes. Only sacral segments are blocked. Used for perianal surgeries like haemorrhoids, fistula in ano, fissure. The advantage is that haemodynamic fluctuations are minimal (because only few segments are effected).

Caudal Block (Epidural Sacral Block)
It is a type of epidural block.

Uses: Mainly used in **children** for perianal surgeries, genital surgeries (like circumcision), urethral surgeries (urethroplasties) and for providing pain relief.

In children, it is easy to perform caudal block because sacral hiatus can be easily identified.

Complications and contraindications are same as for epidural. In addition, any infection in perianal region is contraindication for caudal.

Level of Block Required for Common Surgeries

Surgery	Level
Cesarean section	Up to T6.
Prostate	Up to T10.
Testicular surgeries	Up to T10.
Hernia	Up to T10.
Appendix	Up to T8.
Hysterectomies	Up to T6.
Perianal surgeries	Sacral segements.

Maximum blood level in regional anaesthesia decreases according to the site of administration in the following order: intercostal (highest) > caudal > epidural > brachial plexus > sciatic nerve (lowest).

Extradural/peridural/Epidural anaesthesia (EA): Sympathetic nervous system (T1–T2) involves neuraxial (spinal/epidural) blockade most commonly. Hypotension is due to vasodilation but cardiac sympathetic nervous system is also blocked. LA is

injected into **spinal dural space** which is filled with **semiliquid fat** giving the way for nerve roots at which LA mainly acts—**3 categories:**
1. **Thoracic:** Injection of small amount in mid-thoracic region.
2. **Lumbar:** Large volume of LA (abdomen, pelvis, lower limb).
3. **Caudal:** Injection through sacral hiatus, into sacral canal producing anaesthesia for pelvic and perineal region, **mostly used in** anorectal genitourinary operation and vaginal delivery. **Lidocaine and bupivacaine** (with adrenaline for prolonged action) are used. **Intrathecal** space is not entered hence neurological complication is less. **Greatest separation** between motor and sensory blockade is obtained by the use of bupivacaine (0.25%). EA was first used by **Corning**. Epidural analgesia (narcotic) is preferred over EA. Epidural LA provides the most effective pain relief.

U:
1. All surgeries performed under spinal anaesthesia are performed under EA.
2. Mainly used to control postoperative pain.
3. Pain of cancer.
4. Pain of chronic condition.
5. Acute occlusive vascular conditions.
6. Blood patch for post spinal headache.
7. Fentanyl + bupivacaine is the commonest used combination for analgesia. Morphine (epidural/spinal) binds to opioid receptors of substantia gelatinosa of dorsal horn cells of spinal cord, causing only sensory block. Morphine produces delayed respiratory depression (after 6–12 hrs) after epidural anesthesia.
8. EA is better choice than spinal for cardiac and hypertensive patient.
9. Combined epidural and spinal anaesthesia is now commonly used for surgery and epidural for postoperative pain.

Complication of EA
1. Late medullary depression (**maximum** by morphine 10 mg IM but not by alfentanil and buprenorphine).
2. Vth nerve palsy. Inadequate (patchy) block (L5 and S1 segment are the most difficult to be blocked due to their large size).
3. Cauda equina syndrome.
4. Horner's syndrome (**Anhidrosis, Miosis, Ptosis ... AMP**)
5. Hypotension and apnoea.
6. Muscle spasm by fentanyl.
7. Urinary retention.

Signs of needle: The commonest used epidural needle is Tuohy's needle **in epidural space (space between vertebral canal and dura mater).** Loss of resistance, negative pressure, Gutierrez's sign (**maximum** in cervical region due to maximum negative pressure. **Minimum** negative pressure is in sacral region). Westphal's sign (absence of knee jerk) and Durrann's sign (rapid injection in epidural space of unconscious patients enhance rate and depth of respiration) are signs of EA.

Intravenous regional anaesthesia: Procedure first discovered by **Bier**. Injection of LA in a vein of torniquet occluded limb is given for the retrograde diffusion from peripheral vascular bed to nonvascular tissue used for upper limb and orthopaedic surgery. Due to cardiac toxicity, bupivacaine is not used. Pressure to occlude the

Pharmacology Review

Table 10.5: *Comparison between spinal and epidural anaesthesia*

	Spinal	Epidural
1. Cost	Cheaper (Quincke Bab-cok type needle cost around ₹ 50 to 60)	Expensive (epidural set cost around ₹ 600 to 700)
2. Onset of effect	Early (within 2 to 3 minutes with xylocaine and 5 to 6 minutes with bupivacaine)	Delayed (effect take place in 15 to 20 minutes)
3. Technically	Easier	Difficult
4. Duration of effect	Less (with xylocaine effect last for 45 min to 1 hour and with bupivacaine 2 to 3 hours)	Prolonged and with epidural catheter longer duration surgery can be performed by giving top up doses
5. Quality of block	Excellent	Patchy block is very common (due to inconsistent epidural space)
6. Change of level of block	Not possible once the drug is fixed	Level can be changed by increasing the dose through epidural catheter
7. Complications • Post spinal headache	Seen	No post spinal headache (but can occur if dura is punctured accidentally)
• Epidural haematoma	Less incidence	More incidence
• Total spinal	Rare	High chances if drug is injected in subarachnoid space by accidental dural puncture
• Intravascular injection	Chances are rare	High chances (epidural space has venous plexus of Batson)
• Drug toxicity	Less chances	High (because large volume is given)
• Catheter complications	Not seen	Present
8. Block failure rate	Less	High
9. Uses	Used for performing surgeries	Used mainly for providing postoperative analgesia
10. Site	Performed only at lumbar level (otherwise there are chances of cord injury)	Can be performed at any level (cervical, thoracic)

limb → 40 mm Hg > systolic BP. It is most often used for surgery of forearm and hand.

    Lignocaine in upper limb   – 20 ml.
    Lignocaine in lower limb   – 30 ml.

Intravenous Regional Block (Beir's Block)

First given by August Beir.

Technique

After applying tourniquet 30 to 40 ml, 0.5% xylocaine or prilocaine is injected into a vein. Adequate tourniquet functioning is most vital in Beir's block. Deflation or leak can cause drug toxicity and death. Bupivacaine is not recommended for Beir's block because it is highly cardiotoxic. Rupivacaine has been used safely. Patients with cardiac arrest following bupivacaine toxicity are very difficult to revive.

Xylocaine with adrenaline should not be used for Beir's block.

Injection of the drug should be as distal as possible. This has been shown to decrease the blood levels.

Disadvantage

- *Accidental deflation or leak of tourniquet can cause* severe drug toxicity and can be even fatal.
- Compartment syndrome.
- Tourniquet can not be released before 30 minutes (even if the surgery finishes before it).

Contraindications

- **S**ickle cell disease.
- **R**aynaud's disease.
- **S**cleroderma.

SRS

Oxygen (boiling point)	=	–189°C
Oxygen—pressure	=	2000 pounds/inch^2
Colour of cylinder	=	Black with white shoulder
CO_2—pressure	=	50 pounds/inch^2
Colour of cylinder	=	Grey
Inflammable anaesthesia	=	Ether, ethylchloride, ethylene and cyclopropane

Blocks of Head and Neck

Commonly performed blocks of head and neck are:
- Trigeminal nerve block.
- Basserian ganglion block, for trigeminal neuralgia. It is approached through foramen ovale.
- Cervical plexus block, for carotid endarterectomy.
- Stellate ganglion block, for upper extremity sympathetic dystrophies.

Stellate Ganglion Block

Stellate ganglion is formed by fusion of lower cervical and first thoracic ganglion. It is blocked anterior to the tubercle of transverse process of C6 *(Chassaignac tubercle)* vertebra.

Signs of Successful Block
Horner syndrome which consist of:
1. Flushing of face.
2. Conjunctival congestion.
3. Injection of tympanic membrane *(Müller's syndrome)*.
4. Increased skin temperature.

Trigeminal Nerve Block
Trigeminal nerve has three main branches, ophthalmic, maxillary and mandibular. Maxillary and mandibular branches are blocked for pain syndromes.

Phrenic Nerve Block
Sometimes applied for intractable hiccups. Nerve is blocked 3 cm above the clavicle just lateral to the posterior border of sternocleidomastoid. Bilateral phrenic nerve block should never be performed.

Blocks of Upper Limb
Brachial Plexus Block
This is the second most commonly practised block (after central neuraxial block).

Ulnar nerve is usually spared with this approach.
Supraclavicular Approach
This is very commonly practised approach.

Axillary Approach
It is also very commonly used approach. 20 ml of xylocaine 1 to 1.5% is injected around axillary artery in axilla.

Musculocutaneous nerve and intercostobrachial nerve are spared so arm surgery can not be performed in axillary approach.

Peripheral Nerve Blocks
Radial, ulnar and median nerves can be blocked separately at elbow and wrist.

Blocks of Lower Limb
Blocks of lower limb are no more popular because most of the surgeries of lower limb can be performed under spinal and epidural anaesthesia.
Usual blocks are:
- **Psoas compartment block**
  To block lumbar plexus.
- **Perivascular block (3 in 1 block)**
  Drug injected in fermoral canal while maintaining distal pressure, will result in upward spread of drug, blocking femoral, sciatic and obturator nerves simultaneously (that is why called as 3 in 1 block).
- **Femoral nerve, sciatic nerve and obturator nerve block**
  These nerves can be blocked separately.
- **Ankle block**
  In ankle block, deep peroneal, superficial peroneal and saphenous nerve are blocked with subcutaneous infiltration at the dorsum of foot, posterior tibial posterior to medial malleolus and sural laterally between lateral malleolus and Achilles tendon.

Xylocaine with adrenaline should not be used for ankle block.
- **Beir's block for lower limb**
Not commonly performed as it requires very large volumes (60 to 80 ml).

Blocks of Thorax and Abdomen
- **Intercostal nerve blocks**
Intercostal nerve blocks are performed for postoperative analgesia, rib fractures and Herpes zoster. Usually performed in mid or posterior axillary line at the inferior border of rib.

Complications
1. Pneumothorax is the biggest problem.
2. Highest blood level of local anaesthetic is achieved per volume of drug injected after intercostal block.
- **Celiac plexus block**
Usually given for pain relief in gastric and pancreatic malignancy. Most common complication is hypotension.
- **Lumbar sympathetic chain block**
Performed for lower limb sympathetic dystrophies especially Buerger's disease. Lumbar sympathetic chain is blocked anterior to lumbar vertebral bodies.
- **Ilioinguinal and iliohypogastric nerve block**
For hernia repair, these are blocked at a point 3 cm medial to anterior superior iliac spine.
- **Penile block**
Pudendal nerve is blocked by injection of 10 to 15 ml of local anaesthetic at the base of penis. Xylocaine with adrenaline is contraindicated for penile block.

General Anaesthesia
The term anaesthesia was given by Oliver Wendell Holmes.

The basic components (triad) of general anaesthesia are:
1. Narcosis (and amnesia)
2. Analgesia
3. Muscle relaxation

With the advancement of anaesthesia more stress on abolition of autonomic reflexes and maintenance of homoestasis is put to make it balanced anaesthesia and the concept of balanced anaesthesia was coined by John Lundy in 1926. The four components of balanced anaesthesia are:
1. Narcosis (and amnesia)
2. Analgesia
3. Muscle relaxation
4. Abolition of reflexes with maintenance of physiologic homoeostasis

This balanced anaesthesia can be achieved by combination of different techniques like general anaesthesia with different agents, premedication and regional anaesthesia.

General Anaesthesia Protocol
(For normal healthy patient)

Premedication

Benzodiazepines
Lorazepam or diazepam night before surgery and 1 tablet in the morning 2 to 3 hours before surgery or midazolam intramuscularly (IM) 30 to 60 minutes before or on operation table intravenously (IV) just before induction.

Uses of benzodiazepines are to induce sedation and produce **amnesia.**

Opioids
Fentanyl is given IV just before induction (if fentanyl is not available, pethidine/pentazocine) can be used. Opioids are used to produce analgesia.

Antisialagogues
Glycopyrrolate preferred over atropine and is given just before induction (optional).

Antiemetics
Ondansetron or metoclopramide IV just before induction (optional).

Preoxygenation
This is very important part in general anaesthesia. Preoxygenation is done for 3 minutes because 99% of denitrogenation take places in 3 minutes.

The aim of preoxygenation is to increase the oxygen reserve of body which is in the form of functional residual capacity (FRC) in lungs.

The oxygen content of the FRC filled with air is 500 ml (21% of 2.5 litres) which will last for 2 minutes only (oxygen consumption is 250 ml/min). With preoxygenation for 3 minutes the whole of air of FRC can be replaced with 100% oxygen increasing the oxygen content of FRC to 2.5 litres which can last for 8 to 10 minutes.

Induction
Intravenous induction is done with thiopentone or propofol.

Muscles Relaxation for Intubation
It is achieved by succinylcholine.

Intubation
Done with cuffed endotracheal tube. Position of the tube is to be verified with auscultation and capnography. Tube is fixed with adhesive. Once position is confirmed, start intermittent positive pressure ventilation (IPPV).

Maintenace of Anaesthesia
Anaesthesia is maintained with oxygen (minimum 33%) + nitrous oxide (66%) + inhalational agent (most commonly halothane) + long acting muscle relaxant of non-depolarizing type like pancuronium, vecuronium or atracurium.

Reversal
Non-depolarizing muscle blockade is reversed with neostigmine + atropine or glycopyrrolate.

Extubation
Extubation is done after thorough suctioning of oral cavity.

Stages of Anaesthesia

Stage of surgical anaesthesia (stagte III) is plane 3 in which the laryngeal reflexes to go and intubation can be performed.
- First reflex to go is eyelash reflex, so loss of consciousness is tested by absence of eyelash reflex.
- Last reflex to go is carinal reflex (tested by touching the carina with suction catheter which should initiate cough).

Initial pupillary dilatation seen in stage II, is because of sympathetic stimulation.

The return of reflexes is in opposite sequence, i.e. first to come is carinal reflex and last is eyelash. So theoretically, it is cough which should come first but swallowing comes earlier than coughing because coughing also requires diaphragm and respiratory muscles effort.

Onset of surgical anaesthesia (stage III) is best indicated by onset of regular respiration.

Mechanism of GA: MAC (minimal alveolar concentration) is the **lowest** alveolar concentration of anaesthesia needed to produce **immobility** in 50% cases in response to stimulus. It is a valid measure of **inhalational** GA constant for given species in varying condition. **2–4 MAC** is often lethal. It is dissolved in membrane lipid, effects the **protein** of membrane and blocks the **ion channel.** GA depresses synaptic transmission and CNS globally and reversibly, has low therapeutic indices and hence, is dangerous to administer it. An entire specialty of medicine has grown around the administration of this class of drugs. IV and inhalational GAs depress spontaneous and evoked activity of nerves in brain and target ligand-gated ion channels such as $GABA_A$, glycine, $5-HT_3$, neural nicotinic and subtypes of glutamate (NMDA, AMPA and kainate) receptors. $GABA_A$ and glutamate receptors are found throughout with specific pathways of interconnecting nuclei. ACh, NMDA and 5-HT stimulate ligand-gated K^+ channels. GA interacts with fast neurotransmitter gated channel family. IV and inhalational GAs depress hippocampal neurotransmission to produce amnesia. Inhalational GAs hyperpolarise nerves, inhibit excitatory synapses, reduce E, NE, ACh, 5-HT and enhance inhibitory synapses, GABA and adenosine. Inhaled GA hyperpolarises the membrane via its activation of ligand-gated K^+ channel of CNS involving ACh, DA, NE and serotonin and reduces the opening duration of nicotinic receptor activated cation channel (less excitation of ACh). Most IV GAs act predominantly by enhancing inhibitory neurotransmission at glutaminergic synapses. GA enhances sensitivity of $GABA_A$ receptors to GABA and facilitates GABA action to enhance ion flux. Inhalational GA activates glycine receptors (glycine-gated Cl^- channel) enhancing inhibitory neurotransmission in spinal cord and brainstem and inhibit neuronal nicotinic receptors. Ketamine, N_2O and xenon have no effect on $GABA_A$ and glycine receptors, but inhibit NMDA receptors (glutamate-gated Ca^{2+} channel) causing unconsciousness. Ketamine binds phencyclidine site on NMDA receptors and inhibit it. N_2O and xenon are potent and selective inhibitor of NMDA activated current. Inhalational GA activates K^+ channel and hyperpolarises nerves, needs protein complex (syntaxin, SNAP-25, and synaptobrevin) involved in synaptic neurotransmitter release resulting in presynaptic inhibition in hippocampus to cause amnesia. Most IV GAs act predominantly through $GABA_A$ receptors and perhaps through some interactions with other ligand-gated ion channels. Haloginated inhalational GAs are complete GAs (all components are present) due to a variety of molecular targets. ACh and glutamate receptors are blocked by volatile agents, barbiturates and ketamine. ACh, glutamate and GABA control cholinergic nerves in basal forebrain and pedunculopontine projections.

The most acceptable theory is volume expansion or fluidization theory which states that inhalational agent incorporates in lipid molecules of (hydrophobic action) causing fluidization of membrane blocking the ion channels; especially sodium channel thus preventing depolarization. Potassium and cholride conductance is increased causing hyperpolarization.

Site of Action of Inhalational Agents
- These agents mainly act on central nervous system (producing unconsciousness, amnesia and muscle relaxation) and dorsal horn cells of spinal cord (producing analgesia).
- Mainly acts on synapses (in high doses can block axonal transmission).
- Acts at both pre- and postsynaptic level.

Meyer Overton Rule
Anaesthetic potency is directly propotional to lipid solubility.

BZD facilitates GABA action but has no direct actions on $GABA_A$ receptors even at high concentration in the absence of GABA. Cells of substantia gelatinosa of dorsal horn of spinal cord are very sensitive at low concentration in CNS interrupting sensory transmission of spinothalamic tract, including transmission of nociceptive stimuli and hence contributing to **stage I** or analgesia. The disinhibitory effects of GA **(stage II)** occur at higher concentration and result from blockade of small inhibitory nerves Golgi type II cells together with facilitation of excitatory neurotransmitters. Depression of ascending pathways in reticular activating system occurs during **stage III** together with suppression of spinal reflex activity which contibutes to muscle relaxation. At higer concentration, nerves of respiratory and vasomotor centres of medulla are depressed leading to cardiorespiratory collapse **(stage IV)**.

1. **Inhalation GA, BZD, barbiturates and propofol** stimulate **GABA R.** (inhibitory transmitter GABA is potentiated).
2. **Fluorinated GA and barbiturates** additionally inhibit neuronal **cation** channel-gated by **nicotinic R.**

Ketamine selectively inhibits excitatory NMDA type of **glutamate R.** (Volatile GA has little action on this R.)

Objective of GA: Amnesia, analgesia, blunting of consciousness, suppression of autonomic reflexes, muscle relaxation. **All CNS drugs** inducing GA are either **lipid soluble** or **cross the barrier** by active transport. GA has no R for anaesthesias and no specific antagonist. At low concentration CNS is depressed more and at high concentration **all excitable cells** are depressed.

Triad of GA: Amnesia, analgesia and muscle relaxation (sleep).

Stages of GA: John snow described certain signs to determine the depth of GA (ether/chloroform) in 1848–1858.

Most anaesthetic protocols for major procedures now consists of a continuation of inhaled and IV agents. Higher functions are lost first than lower functions in CNS but in the spinal cord, lower segments are affected **first** than higher segments. In the **last,** vital centres located in the medulla are paralysed. **Guedel** (1920) described ether anaesthesia. Guedel's 4 stages of ether are:

Stage I/Stage of analgesia (from inhalation to loss of consciousness): Pain abolished, eye and ear normal, reflex and respiration normal, used for minor operation.

This stage is due to reduction in activity of cells of **substantia gelatinosa (cells most sensitive to GA)** in dorsal horn of spinal cord.

Stage II/Stage of delirium (from loss of consciousness to beginning of regular respiration): Patient's struggle, hold breathing, muscle tone elevated. Jaws closed, breathing jerky. Vomiting, retching micturition and defaecation occur. ↑ HR and ↑ BP, pupil dilated. No surgery is done. This stage occurs due to **"release of lower centres"** from ihibitory control of higher centre. If eyelash reflex and swallowing movement present→stage II not reached.

Stage III/Stage of surgical anaesthesia (from onset of regular respiration to cessation of spontaneous breathing): 4 planes of this stage are:

Plane I   : Reflexes (eyelid, cojunctiva, pharynx, vomiting) lost. Eye fixed. Revolving movements of eyeballs are present.
Plane II   : Corneal and laryngeal reflexes lost, eyes fixed and skeletal muscle relaxed. Most abdominal surgery is done.
Plane III   : Pupil dilated. Light reflex lost. ↓ BP.
            Most of the operation done in plane II and III.
Plane IV   : Fully dilated pupil, not responsive to light, intercostal paralysis, ↓ muscle tone, ↓ BP and ↑ HR, ↓ respiration (in depth and frequency).

The most reliable indications that stage III has been achieved are loss of eyelash reflex and establishment of a respiratory pattern that is regular in rate and depth.

Stage IV/Medullary paralysis (from cessation of breathing to circulatory failure and death): muscle flabby, Pupil dilated, ↓BP.

Signs of deep anaesthesia→cardiac and respiratory depression.

Most reliable indication for achieving stage III (surgical anaesthesia)→loss of lid reflex and rhythmic respiration.

Inhalational Agents

Inhalational agents are mainly used in anaesthesia for maintenance but these can also be used as induction agents especially in children (inhalational induction) and also as a sole agent for small procedures (especially ether).

Potency of Inhalational Agents

The agent with minimum MAC will be most potent. MAC for different anaesthetic agents is:

Agent	MAC
Methoxyflurane	0.16%
Trilene	0.2%
Halothane	0.74%
Chloroform	0.8%
Isoflurane	1.15%
Enflurane	1.68%
Ether	1.92%
Sevoflurane	2.05%
Desflurane	6.0%
Cyclopropane	9.2%
Nitrous oxide	104%

It can be concluded from the above Box that methoxyflurane with minimum MAC of 0.16% is the most potent inhalational agent and nitrous oxide with very high MAC of 104% is the least potent agent.

Factors Effecting MAC

1. **Age:** Maximum MAC in human beings is at the age of 6 months thereafter decreasing steadily throughout the life (except a slight increase at puberty).
2. **Temperature:** Decreasing the temperature decreases the MAC (e.g., 5% decrease in halothane MAC/°C decrease in temperature). Increasing temperature also decreases the MAC up to 42°C after that there is increase in MAC.
3. **Barometeric pressure:** Increasing pressure increases the MAC (pressure reversal theory of anaesthesia).
4. **Anaemia:** Decrease MAC.
5. **Hypoxia (pO_2 <40), hypercarbia (pCO_2 >95 mmHg):** Decreases the MAC.
6. **Alcohol:** Acute intoxication decreases while chronic intoxication increases MAC.
7. **Pregnancy:** There is decrease in MAC so inhalational anaesthetics should be used in lower concentrations.
8. **Intravenous anaesthetics:** Decrease the MAC.
9. **Local anaesthetics:** Decrease the MAC (except cocaine).
10. **Electrolytes**
    - *Sodium:* Hyponatremia decreases while hypernatremia increases the MAC.
    - *Magnesium:* Hypermagnesemia decreases the MAC.
11. **Thyroid diseases:** Both hypo- and hyperthyroidism have no effect on MAC.
12. **Sex:** MAC is same for males and females.

Uptake and Distribution of Inhalational Agents

The concentration in brain determines the effect of inhalational agent.

After equilibrium is achieved between brain and blood, alveolar concentration reflects the concentration in brain.

Blood Gas Partition Coefficient (B/G Coeff.)

This is the most important factor determining the uptake of agent and so the speed of induction and recovery. Agents with low blood gas partition coefficient will have high alveolar concentration e.g., nitrous oxide with blood gas partition coefficient of 0.47 means concentration or partial pressure in blood is 47% of alveolar concentration. Since alveolar concentration determines the induction and recovery, induction and recovery will be fast with agent with less B/G partition coefficient and induction and recovery wil be slower with agents with high B/G partition coefficients.

B/G partition coefficient of different agents are

Agent	Blood gas partition coefficient
Desflurane	0.42
Cyclopropane	0.44
Nitrous oxide	0.47
Sevoflurane	0.69
Isoflurane	1.38
Enflurane	1.8
Halothane	2.4
Chloroform	8
Trilene	9
Ether	12
Methoxyflurane	15

It can be concluded from the above Box that induction will be fastest with desflurane with B/G coefficient of 0.42 and slowest with methoxyflurane with B/G coefficient of 15.

Cardiac Output

Increasing cardiac output increases the uptake, decreasing the alveolar concentration and induction is delayed (it is contrary to what one thinks that increasing cardiac output should fasten the induction).

In low cardiac output states like shock, the agents with high B/G partition coefficient can achieve dangerously high alveolar concentrations if inspired concentrations are not decreased but the alveolar concentration of agents with low B/G coefficient will not be so high. That is why in shock, agents with low B/G coefficient like nitrous oxide are safe.

Alveolar to Venous Partial Pressure

Increasing ventilation will increase the alveolar concentration of agents with high B/G coefficient (increased uptake will decrease alveolar concentration so more room for inspired agent). Agent with low B/G coefficient least affected with increasing ventilation. Earliest recovery will be with desflurane (B/G coefficient of 0.42) and most delayed will be with methoxyflurane (B/G coefficient of 15).

Metabolism

All inhalational agents undergo oxidation (dealkylation or dehalogenation) in liver (halothane also undergoes reduction) by cytochrome P450 enzymes in phase I reaction and by conjugation in phase II reaction.

All enzyme inducers like isoniazid, phenytoin, phenobarbitone, ethanol, diazepam increases the metabolism of inhalational agents.

Nitrous oxide does not undergo any metabolism in human body.

PK of Inhalation GA

1. **H**alothane, **C**hloroform and **M**ethoxyflurane sensitise the myocardium to **CA** (so, adrenaline is not used). **MCH**

    Ether and cyclopropane cause release of CA. All the inhaled GA enhance $PaCO_2$ level **except** ether.

2. **Alveoli ⇌ Blood ⇌ Brain.**
These series of tension gradient from alveoli to brain depend on:
— **PP of GA** which is directly proportional to concentration of inspired gas mixture.
— **Pulmonary ventilation** and depend on blood solubility of agents (which are **most important** property determining induction and recovery). Most inhaled GA reduces arterial BP.
— **Most of GAs** are equally soluble in blood and lean tissue but more in adipose tissue (hence more **in white matter than grey matter**, i.e. GA concentration is greater in white matter than in grey matter). GA lowers the core temperature set point at which thermoregulatory vasoconstriction is activated to defend heat loss. Potency of IV GA is the free plasma concentration at equilibrium that produces loss of response to surgical incision in 50% of subjects. Solubility which is one of the most important factors determines the transfer of GA from alveoli to arterial blood, expressed as "blood/gas partition coefficients" (relative affinity of GA for blood as compared to air).

Halothane and methoxyflurane have higher solubility in blood (higher blood/gas partition coefficient), disolve more in blood, so higher amount of GA is needed to raise but N_2O has low solubility (low blood/gas partition coefficient) hence less amount is needed to raise arterial tension of GA.

Anaesthetic partition coefficients (blood: gas; blood: fat; brain: blood) are the ratio of anaesthetic concentration in two tissues when the partial pressures of GA are equal in two tissues. One of the most important factors governing rate of recovery is blood: gas partition coefficient.

Induction is slower with more soluble gases. For a given concentration or partial pressure of the two anaesthetic gases in the inspired air, it will take much longer for the blood partial pressure or the concentration of the gases in the brain, can rise no faster than the concentration in the blood, the onset of anaesthesia will be slower with the halothane than with N_2O. During induction phase, tissues that exert greatest influence on arterial-venous anaesthetic concentration gradient are those which are highly perfused and include liver, heart, kidneys, brain and spleen receiving >75% of cardiac output.

Muscle and skin (50% of body mass) accumulate GA more slowly than the richly vascularised tissues, since they receive 20% of cardiac output. Most anaesthetic gases are highly soluble in adipose tissues, low blood perfusion rates to these tissues delay accumulation, and equilibrium is unlikely to occur with most anaesthetics during the time usually needed for surgery.
— CO_2 inhalation with GA which is **cerebral vasodilator** accelerates induction and recovery.
— When administration is discontinued, gradients are **reversed** changing absorption channel into elimination channel. But GA of **adipose tissue** due to high lipid solubility and low blood flow is delayed in elimination. **Most GAs** are eliminated unchanged but halothane is **20%** metabolised in liver. Initial tension of induction in all tissues is zero.

Inhalational GA follows gas laws

1. **Dalton's law:** Partial pressure (PP) of GA is directly proportional to percent of anaesthesia in the mixture.
2. **Fick's law:** Anaesthesia diffuses down its concentration gradient.

3. Amount of anaesthesia dissolved in liquid is directly proportional to partial pressure (PP) of anaesthesia in the mixture. Induction depends on **blood solubility** and high blood soluble anaesthesia is **most readily hastened by hyperventilation. Final distribution** of anaesthesia depends on **tissue blood partition coefficient** which is **one** for **most anaesthesia** in **most tissue**.
4. A decrease in pulmonary blood flow increases and an increase in pulmonary blood flow decreases the rate of rise of arterial tension of inhaled anaesthetics.
5. During GA, PP of inhaled GA in brain equals to PP in lungs when steady state is reached.

Colour of cylinder:			
N_2O	—	Blue	
Cyclosporine	—	Orange	
O_2	—	Black with white shoulder	
Halothane	—	Amber (purple-red)	
Thiopentone	—	Yellow	
CO_2	—	Grey	
Entonox	—	Blue with blue-white shoulder	

Pin Code Index:
O_2 = 25
N_2O = 35
CO_2 >7.5% concentration = 16
CO_2 <7.5% concentration = 26

Systemic Effects of Inhalational Agents (Including Side Effects)

Respiratory System

1. **Ventilation:** Initially, all agents decrease the tidal volume and increase the frequency but with increasing dose, frequency also decreases so finally decreasing minute volume (except trilene and ether). Maximum depression of respiration is seen with enflurane.
   Ventilatory responses (to increased CO_2 and hypoxia) are blunted with inhalational agents (except nitrous oxide and minimum with ether). Maximum inhibition to ventilatory response is with halothane.
   Except N_2O, all inhaled GAs reduce tidal volume and enhace respiratory rate. All inhaled GAs are respiratory depressants. Isoflurane and enflurane cause maximum ventilatory depression. All inhaled GAs enhance resting level of $paCO_2$ (PP of CO_2 in arterial blood).
2. **Bronchial muscles:** All inhalational agents are bronchodilators. Maximum bronchodilation is asthmatics in seen with halothance, that is why, halothane is the agent of choice for asthmatic patients (while in non-asthmatics, maximum bronchodilation is produced by sevoflurane).
   Bronchodilatation is not only because of direct effect of agents on bronchial muscles but also by (and this is the main mechanism) inhibition of central pathways for bronchoconstriction.
3. **Effects on hypoxic pulmonary vasoconstriction (HPV):** All agents blunt HPV response; maximally inhibited by halothane.
4. **Effect on ciliary activity:** All agents (except ether) inhibit the ciliary activity thereby reduction capability of patient to cough out secretions in postoperative period. All respiratory depressant effects are overcome by controlling ventilation by ventilator.

Cardiovascular System

Nitrous oxide has negligible effect on cardiovascular system.
1. **Cardiac output:** All agents decrease the cardiac output (except ether and cyclopropane which maintain the output by sympathetic stimulation). Cardiac output is best maintained with isoflurane (by reflex tachycardia) [also well maintained with desflurane].
   Maximum decrease is seen with enflurane.
2. **Systemic vascular resistance (SVR):** SVR is decreased by all agents (except cyclopropane and ether). **Maximum hypotension is caused by isoflurane, therefore, isoflurane is the inhalational agent of choice for controlled hypotension.**
3. **Myocardial contractility:** There is significant inhibition of myocardial contractility with halothane.
4. **Baroreceptor reflex:** All protective cardiovascular responses are blunted by inhalational agents (except ether), maximum with halothane.
   It can be concluded that cardiovascular stability in decreasing order is isoflurane (most cardiovascular stable) > desflurane > sevoflurane > halothane > enflurane.
   So, isoflurane is the agent of choice for cardiac patients (except patients with myocardial ischemia) because of its minimum effect on baroreceptor reflex and maintenance of cardiac output.
   Halothane and enflurane reduce cardiac output thereby decreasing mean arterial pressure. Sevoflurane, isoflurane and desflurane cause endothelial mediated decrease in systemic vascular resistance thereby decreasing mean arterial pressure. All inhaled GAs enhance right atrial pressure in dose related fashion which reflects depression of myocardial function.
5. **Sensitization of heart to adrenaline:** Heart is sensitized to adrenaline (both exogenous and endogenous, more prominently with exogenous) by:
   - Halothane
   - Trilene
   - Cyclopropane
   - Methoxyflurane
   - Chloroform
   - Enflurane

Liver

All agents produce some degree of hepatotoxicity by decreasing the blood supply to liver (indirect effect). Direct hepatocellular damage is seen with:
- Halothane
- Chloroform
- Methoxyflurane

Renal System

All inhalational agents depress renal function by decreasing the renal blood flow, GFR and effective renal plasma flow and enhance filtration fraction.
   Direct renal toxicity has been attributed to inorganic fluoride (F) produced by fluorinated compounds. Inhalational agents are fluorinated to decrease their flammability. All GAs enhance renovascular resistance.

Renal threshold beyond which fluoride levels are toxic is 50 μm and the fluoride level produced by different agents is:

Agent	Fluoride (F⁻) level (produced after 2.5 to 3.0 MAC hours)
Methoxyflurane	50 to 80 μm
*Sevoflurane	30 to 50 μm
Enflurane	20 to 25 μm
Isoflurane	4 to 8 μm
Halothane	Produces fluoride only in anaerobic conditions
Desflurane	Does not produce fluoride

*Sevoflurane although produces fluoride level up to renal threshold level but still does not causes nephrotoxicity because of its low blood gas coefficient (0.69) which allows its rapid elimination from body.

The nephrotoxicity produced by fluorinated agents is vasopressin resistant polyuric renal failure.

Brain
Most inhaled GAs enhance cerebral blood flow by decreasing cerebral vascular resistance.

At low doses, all halogenated agents have similar effects to enhance cerebral blood flow. At higher doses, enflurane and isoflurane increase cerebral blood flow less than halothane. Halothane, isoflurane and enflurane have similar effects on EEG up to doses of 1–1.5 MAC.

Uterus
Halogenated agents are potent uterine muscle relaxants.

Spinal Cord
Nitrous oxide by inhibiting the production of thymidate can impair myelin formation which can lead to subacute degeneration of spinal cord.

Neuromuscular System
All inhalational agents produce some degree of muscle relaxation (except nitrous oxide). Maximum relaxation is produced by ether.

Teratogenicity
Exact data and conclusive evidence to prove teratogenicity of inhalational agents is not yet available.

Inflammability of Inhalational Agents
Inflammable agents are:
1. Ether
2. Cyclopropane
3. Enflurane (at concentration of more than 5%)
4. Ethyl chloride
    - Agents can be made non-inflammable by adding fluorine atoms.
    - Cautery should not be used in vicinity of inflammable agents up to 25 cm.

Analgesia

Inhalational agents have analgesic properties which is maximum with trilene, moderate with ether, methoxyflurane. While agents nowadays in common use like halothane, isoflurane are not good analgesics.

Reaction of Inhalational Agents with Soda Lime

- **Trilene** can produce toxic compound, PH_3 and dichloroacetylene with soda lime.
- **Methoxyflurane** and **halothane** can react with rubber tubing of closed circuit and can be used if rubber tubing is replaced by plastic tubing.
- **Desflurane, isoflurane** and **enflurane** can produce **carbon monoxide** by reacting with soda lime and barylime.

Metabolic

Hyperglycemia is seen with:
- Ether (causes hyperglycemia by mobilizing liver glycogen).
- Cyclopropane (mild hyperglycemia).
- Chloroform (causes most profound hyperglycemia).

Second gas effect: Initially, diffusion of N_2O from alveoli into blood is **higher** (1 L/min, i.e. higher than minute volume for N_2O given at 70–80% concentration). When another potent GA, e.g. **halothane** 1–2% is given, initially it also be delivered at higher rate than minute volume resulting in **faster induction.** When gas is discontinued after prolonged anaesthesia, initially **reverse diffusion** occurs faster due to low blood solubility of N_2O diluting oxygen of alveoli **(diffusion hypoxia)**. Hence, **100% O_2** is inhaled just after discontinuation for a few minute. This hypoxia is insignificant with other anaesthesia because of administration at low concentration and less dilution of alveolar oxygen. **Most inhalational GA** makes **50%** cases immobile at **MAC**, often **fatal at 2–4 MAC** and **all individuals** immobile at **1/3 increase over MAC. Saline** in closed system delivery absorbs CO_2, when the patient rebreathes the exhaled gas. MAC value of N_2O greater than 100% shows that it is the least potent.

Nitrous Oxide

N_2O: Gas anaesthesia was discovered by **Magill and Rowbothom**. Laughing gas (N_2O) was discovered by **Priestley (1776)**. Anaesthetic properties was first suggested by S.H. Davy in 1790. It is the **most widely used gas anaesthesia** and colour of cylinder is **blue.**

Properties of N_2O: Colourless, odourless, boiling point = –89°C. (BP of O_2 = –189°C), nonflammable, nonexplosive, nonirritating, 1.5 times heavier than air, sweet smelling, good analgesic, poor muscle relaxant, critical temperature is 36.5°C which is above room temperature, therefore, it is kept in liquefied state in blue colour cylinders. 35 times more soluble than N_2. Cheap, used as carrier and adjuvant to other GA as it is not complete GA. MAC is 104%, so impossible to deliver. O_2 is given to check hypoxia. **Mixture is 70% N_2O + 25–30% O_2 + 0.2–2% other GA** for **most surgery**. It is **the least potent** (MAC >100%) inhaled anaesthesia and cannot produce surgical anaesthesia by itself. **Only N_2O** shows **second gas effect and diffusion hypoxia** due to low blood solubility and is removed from lungs. It is prepared by heating ammonium nitrate between 245 and 270°.

Other gas used as GA—xenon and cyclopropane (the most widely used GA for 30 years—1929 to 1959).

> **N₂O:** 5Ps
> Priestley discovered in 1776.
> Poynting effect.
> Practically, safest anaesthesia.
> Poor muscle relaxant relieves pain only.
> Pneumo condition as pneumothorax, etc. (not used).

PK: It is completely eliminated by the lungs with some minimal diffusion through the skin. 99.9% absorbed N₂O is eliminated unchanged. It is degraded by interaction with vitamin B_{12} in intestinal bacteria resulting in inactivation of methionine synthesis and hence, signs of vitamin B_{12} dificiency and bone marrow depression causing anemia on chronic use >6 month of N₂O.

B/G coefficient is 0.47 making it agent with faster induction and recovery. When given with other inhalational agents, it enhances the alveolar concentration of that agent (second gas effect) and its own (concentration effect). Sudden stoppage of its delivery reverses the gradient making it gush to alveoli replacing O_2 from there (diffusing hypoxia) which can be prevented by giving 100% O_2 for 5–10 minutes. It is not metabolised in the body. Excreted unchanged via lungs (small amount via skin).

ADR of "Nitrous oxide" Net effect on respiratory system is almost normal minute ventilator and arterial oxygen tension. It depresses ventilatory response to hypoxia, hence arterial O_2 saturation must be monitored.

ICT and cerebral blood flow are enhanced. Increases cerebral metabolic rate.

Tidal volume is decreased.

Respiratory rate is increased.

Opioid and N₂O together cause decrease BP and cardiac output. Halogenated inhalational GA and N₂O together cause increase BP, cardiac output and HR. It is safely used in shock and cardiac patients. Other effects are: It reacts with O_2 to form nitric oxide which is destructive to ozone, but, pneumothorax, pneumoperitoneum, middle ear cavity, pneumoencephalum develop high pressure following N_2 inhalation.

Urine formation, gut and liver functions are unaffected.

Systemic effect is enhanced tone of peripheral and pulmonary veins. Hence, N₂O is avoided in pulmonary hypertension.

Oxygen
Inhalation
Deficiency

Exacerbates hypoxia. Impurities (NO_2, NO, NH_3, nitrogen and carbon monoxide) cause laryngospasm, pulmonary edema and methaemoglobinaemia. Effects chemotaxis and leukocyte motility. Bone marrow depression causes aplastic and megaloblastic anemia (vitamin B_{12}) and deficiency also causes demyelinating lesion degeneration of spinal cord (posterior column and lateral spinothalamic tract).

Hypoxia, methaemoglobinaemia (treated by ascorbic acid + IV methylene blue), BMD, respiratory depression, megaloblastic anaemia and peripheral neuropathy.

U: Effects of N₂O are analgesia at 20% and sedation at 30–80% but usual dose is 50% and >80% N₂O is not used because this limits the delivery of adequate amount of oxygen. It also reduces the dose of inhalational GA. Used as Entonox = **N₂O 50% + O₂ 50%**. Entonox is blue colour cylinder stored at 10°C otherwise low temperature separates O_2 and N_2O delivering more N_2O. To prevent this, the cylinder is invested 2–3 times to ensue good mixing and stored horizontally.

Uses are
- As a supplement to anaesthesia (not a complete anaesthesia).
- As a carrier gas for inhalational agent.
- As analgesic in obstetrics, dental pain, acute trauma and burn dressing.
- N_2O, desflurane, isoflurane are the most commonly used in USA among inhaled GA.

Ether (C_2H_5-O-C_2H_5)/diethyl ether: **First** used by **William Morton in 1846** for the removal of jaw tumour. It was **the first useful GA** and is **the most potent GA**. Widely used in India. Colour of cylinder is **orange**. It is pungent swelling liquid, decomposes in the presence of light, air and heat so stored in amber coloured bottles. Blood: Gas coefficient is 12 and MAC is 1.92. It is very good analgesic and muscle relaxant. **Safest** GA in unexperienced hand is ether. **Most effective** muscle relaxant (better than halothane).

Properties: Elevates BP by elevating sympathetic tone, liquid, volatile, explosive, irritating, inflammable, good muscle relaxant. Boiling point is 35°C. It causes↓**ACh output** from nerve end (hence competitive neuromuscular blocker is reduced to about **1/3**). **Atropine** is premedicated to prevent secretions (salivation, resp. secretion). Analgesic, blood soluble, cheap, BP and respiration maintained due to reflex stimulation and ↑ sympathetic tone. It is **complete anaesthesia** because it causes:
1. Muscle relaxation.
2. Analgesia
3. Unconsciousness.
4. But maintains respiration and circulation.

Effects of ether: Elevates BP and HR due to sympathetic stimulation. It is not cardiac depressant. Baroreceptor reflex is preserved, so it is safely used in shock. Tracheobronchial secretion is markedly increased, so it is premedicated with atropine. Highest incidence of nausea and vomiting among inhalational GA. Hyperglycemia due to catecholamine release so not used in DM. Elevates ICT. Respiration is stimulated at low doses and inhibited at high doses. It is bronchodilator and the only inhalational GA preserving ciliary activity. It crosses placenta to depress respiration in fetus. Ventilatory responses to hypoxia and hypercarbia are preserved.

Concentration of ether in inspired air required for induction of anaesthesia is **10–15%,** for maintenance of surgical anaesthesia is **5%** and for maintenance of analgesic stage is **1.2%**. It is metabolised to nontoxic products (alcohol, acetaldehyde and acetic acid).

Advantage: Not sensitise the myocardium to CA. Non-depolarising and curari-mimetic muscle relaxation. The only complete GA is cheap, safe, and easy to use.

Disadvantage: Slow induction, flammability, respiratory irritation, soreness of trachea, congestion of eye, burns on face, crosses placenta, convulsion (treated by thiopentone, cooling and artificial respiration).

CI of Ether: `EDD`

Diathermy as it is inflammable, **D**M as it releases CA and produces hyperglycaemia.

Xenon: It is an inert gas, first identified as anaesthetic agent in 1951 (Cullen and Gross, 1951). It is very expensive agent and virtually ideal anaesthetic gas. It is insoluble in blood and other tissues providing for rapid induction and emergence from anaesthesia. 30% O_2 + 70% xenon is given for surgery.

Most importantly, ADR is minimum (effects on CVS, pulmonary, liver and kidney functions are absent). It is not metabolised in the body.

Halothane (Fluothane): First used as GA by **John Stone** in 1956. The **first** useful halogenated hydrocarbon anaesthesia with induction **I = 2.3. One of the most popular GA** due to nonirritant, noninflammable, pleasant and rapid action. It is light-sensitive compound subject to spontaneous break down, hence marketed in amber bottles with 0.01% thymol added as preservative.

Concentration of halothane needed for induction of anaesthesia in inspired air is 2–3% and for maintenance of anaesthesia is 1–2%.

Properties: Nonirritant and **noninflammable.** Volatile liquid and no analgesia. Boiling point +50°C. Halogenated anaesthesia. **Soluble** in blood. Poor analgesia and muscle relaxant action compensated by the use of N_2O/opioid and neuromuscular blocker. **Direct cardiac depressant** by reducing intracellular Ca^{++} concentration **Sympathetic action fails** (↓CO and ↓BP). ↓HR due to direct depression of SA nodal automaticity and lack of baroreceptor activation even after BP falls. CO_2 in blood rises due to respiratory depression. Vasodilatation of hypoxic alveoli accentuates **ventilation perfusion mismatch.** Tissue: Blood ratio maximum in fat. It has high blood: Gas (2.4) and blood: Fat partition coefficient, hence induction is slow. Pleasant to smell to excellent for induction in children. Nonirritant, so induction is very smooth. Halothane has highest fat/blood coefficient (51) and is deposited in fat. Its MAC is 0.74. It is not good analgesic. Postoperative shivering and hypothermia is maximum with halothane among inhalational GA. Trichloroacetic acid, fluorine produced anaerobically, bromine and chlorine are found in urine and formed by oxidation and reduction of GA. Vasodilator, bronchodilator, uterine dilator (best uterine **relaxant**). Laryngeal and pharyngeal reflexes are abolished, coughing suppressed, bronchi dilated, hence prefered for **asthmatics (anaesthesia of choice)** and for hypotensive anaesthesia (bloodless field). It also inhibits **uterine and intestine** contraction hence used for external and internal version in late pregnancy. ↓BP→↓GFR→↓urine formation. **Hepatitis** in susceptible individual. Trifluoroacetic acid binds to protein covalently which causes liver necrosis. In low O_2 it is metabolised into chlorotrifluoroethyl free radical. Rarely **malignant hyperthermia** is due to Ca^{++} release (Ryanodine R) from SR causing persistent muscle contraction and ↑ heat production and is treated by **cooling, HCO_3** infusion, O_2, **dantrolene IV 1–10 mg/kg (DOC).** GA for malignant hyperthermia susceptible patient is IV propofol and opioids.

PK: 20% hepatic metabolite (trifluoroacetic acid) by CYP450, rest exhaled out unchanged via lungs.

> John Lundy: IV Anaesthesia discoverer.
> Stiggard Anderson: Plasma HCO_3.
> Oliver Wandel Homes: Termed anaesthesia.
> Bier: IV regional block.
> Thomas Morton: First demonstration of anaesthesia.
> Allen's test: For patency of transpalmar arch.
> Breur Lockhard reflex: Bronchospasm at different sites due to parasympathetic effects.

Contraindications
1. History of previous halothane hepatitis.
2. Patients with intracranial lesions and head injury.
3. Severe cardiac disease like aortic stenosis (as it causes decrease in cardiac output).
4. Pheochromocytoma (as it sensitizes myocardium to adrenaline).

Drug Interactions
1. β blockers and calcium channel blockers can produce severe depression of cardiac function with halothane.
2. Aminophylline can produce serious ventricular arrhythmias with halothane.
3. All cytochrome P450 enzyme inducers enhance its metabolism.
4. Action of nondepolarizing muscle relaxants is potentiated.

CI: Maximum arrhythmogenic, so contraindicated with **adrenaline**.

ADR of "HALOTHANE"

Hypotension (most predictable) due to cardiac depression and vasodilation in skin and brain.

Arrhythmia. It sensitises the heart to E (more predominantly exogenous), so maximum dose of E is 1.5 mg/kg. It blanks baroreceptor reflex.

Labour prolonged and loss of blood increased due to relaxation a smooth muscle but it is AOC for external version and removal of placenta. Also relaxes bronchial smooth muscle (hence AOC in status asthmaticus) and some skeletal muscle. Tidal volume and minute volume of lung decrease. Dose of muscle relaxant decreases by 25%.

One in 10,000 develops "halothane hepatitis" (fever, centrilobular necrosis, rash, eosinophilia, anorexia, emesis). The most probable mechanism is immunological. The most important risk factor is multiple exposure. Reductive metabolite is more dangerous than oxidative metabolite. An interval of 3 months must be given between the exposures.

Tension (ICT) due to increased cerebral blood flow.

Hepatic failure with 50% death due to antibodies against hepatic proteins in trifluoroacetylated form (CF_3CO proteins) and reactive metabolites.

Administration of dantrolene on development of malignant hyperthermia (muscle contraction + hyperthermia + increased metabolic rate) which is due to increased release of stored Ca^{2+} from sarcoplasmic reticulum causing O_2 demand 3 times of normal and temperature 43°C.

Nephrotoxic (reversible) due to decreased GFR and renal blood flow by 50% at MAC.

Elevation of arterial CO_2 (>50 mm Hg at 1 MAC).

Disadvantage: Hepatitis, arrhythmia, malignant HTN, relaxes uterus so avoided in pregnancy. Shakes and post-anaesthetic chill, dissolves rubber, hepatotoxic. Psychomotor performance and mental ability depressed for several hrs. Most commonly used in children for induction and maintenance.

AOC (anaesthesia of choice): Version, uterine tetanic contraction.

Enflurane: Properties **same** as halothane, halogenated anaesthesia, nonirritating with mild odours, low lipid soluble, costly and epileptogenic.↓BP due to ↓peripheral resistant, muscle and uterine relaxant, volatile, nonflammable, flammable at >5%.

PK: Slow induction and recovery is due to high blood: Gas partition coefficient, 2–8% is metabolised by CYP450 2E1 in the liver, producing fluoride ions as by-product. INH enhances its metabolism and induces defluorination. Induction in 10 minutes with 4% GA in oxygen. Maintenance with 3% GA in oxygen. It sensitises the heart to E less than halothane.

ADR of "ENFLURANE"

Enhanced ICT due to cerebral vasodilation. It reduces cerebral metabolic oxygen consumption like other inhalational GA.

Nephrotoxicity is present and insignificant but hepatic and splanchnic blood flow is reduced.

Fluoride ions increase due to enflurane metabolism (not nephrotoxicity at clinical dose).

Low BP due to depressed myocardial contraction and peripheral vasodilation.

Urine volume is decreased due to decreased GFR and renal blood flow.

Respiratory depression (minute volume is decreased—pCO_2 is 60 mm Hg at 1 MAC).

Appears to precipitate siezures. At high dose, it produces spike and more pattern EEG which culminates into tonic–clonic siezures.

Nondepolarising muscle relaxants increase the effects of enflurane.

Effective bronchodilator like other inhalational GA. Relaxes smooth muscles.

Uses: Same as halothane hence used as a substitute of it.

CI: Epilepsy (Enflurane) and renal disease.

ADR: Nephrotoxicity.

Chloroform: Like ether—explosive and diabetogenic

Most
- emetic
- hepatotoxic
- cardiotoxic

Death due to malignant HTN

Good for renal failure: Halothane, Isoflurane and Sevoflurane **HIS**

Isoflurane (Isomer of enflurane): It is fluorinated methyl ethyl ether.
1. Causes coronary steal syndrome (diversion of blood flow from poorly perfused to well perfused areas).
2. Properties **similar** to enflurane.
3. **Least** CVS effect.
4. **1½ times** more potent. MAC = 1.15. B/G coefficient = 1.38.
5. Pungent etheral odour, so induction is not smooth. Vapour pressure is similar to halothane (240 mm/kg).
6. Volatile and blood soluble. Non-flammable and nonexplosive in air or O_2. It is colourless.
7. Expensive: Good in CVS, CNS, renal and liver diseases.
8. ↓BP is due to **vasodilatation** (stimulation of β R).
9. **Safer** in patient with myocardial ischaemia.
10. Uterine and skeletal **muscle relaxants.** Given in myasthenia gravis.
11. Halothane, enflurane and isoflurane cause **hypotension.**

PK: Blood: Gas partition coefficient of isoflurane is lower than that of halothane or enflurane. Induction and recovery are rapid. >99% is excreted unchanged via the lungs. 0.2% is metabolised by CYP450 2E1. Isoflurane at 2 MAC can cause electrical silence in the brain. Metabolites are trifluoroacetic acid and fluride. Fluoride is not high enough to cause nephrotoxicity. It is avoided in myocardial ischemia.

ADR of "ISOFLURANE"

ICT is increased due to cerebral vasodilation which is less than enflurane and halothane (minimum among inhalational GA) hence preferred agent (AOC) of neurosurgery. Oxygen consumption of brain is also reduced.

Systemic vascular resistance is decreased due to vasodilation in most vascular beds causing maximum hypotension. But transient change in GA concentration causes isoflurane induced sympathetic stimulation leading to tachycardia and hypertension. It is inhalational AOC for controlled hypotension. Baroreceptor reflex is preserved so cardiac output is best maintained among all inhalational GA.

Oxygen consumption of myocardium is decreased and coronary blood flow is increased due to coronary vasodilation.

Flow of blood from poor to well perfused areas ("coronary steal").

Liver and splanchnic blood flow is reduced.

Urine volume is decreased due to decreased renal blood flow and GFR.

Relaxes uterine and some skelatel muscle (via its central effects).

Airway irritant stimulating airway reflexes during induction cousing caugh and laryngospasm. Depression of ventilation. Bronchodilator much less than halothane.

Normal respiratory rate but decreased tidal volume causing decrease ventilation and increase CO_2 tension.

Enhances the effects of nondepolarising and depolarising muscle relaxants more effectively than halothane.

Advantage: Lower toxicity and better adjustment of depth of GA.

U: Commonest used inhalational GA in US. Induction is achieved in <10 minutes with 3% GA in O_2 for induction and 2% GA in O_2 for maintenance. Opioids and N_2O reduce the concentration of GA.
1. Neurosurgery (AOC) due to less cerebral vasodilation.
2. Day care surgery.
3. Cardiac patients (AOC).

Methoxyflurane: It is the only agent with boiling point (104°C) more than water.
1. Halogenated anaesthesia so highly nephrotoxic.
2. Has highest amount of fluoride content.
3. The **most potent** inhalational anaesthesia (**volatile liquid**) for clinical use but nephrotoxic thus seldom used.
4. It is **best analgesic** anaesthesia.
5. MAC of N_2O >100% (so, **least potent**). MAC of methoxyflurane 0.16% (so, **most potent**). Reacts with soda lime.

Desflurane: Fluorinated congener of isoflurane (chlorine atom of isofluorine is replaced by fluorine atom). Fast induction and recovery. **Less potent** than isoflurane, airway irritant, exhaled unchanged. It is nonflammable and nonexplosive in air and oxygen. It is volatile also.

Desflurane, Isoflurane and Sevoflurane DIS are **similar in**: Respiratory depression, muscle relaxation, ↓ BP and vasodilatation, well maintained cardiac contractility and coronary circulation **without seizure** provoking potential, **arrhythmogenicity,** liver and kidney toxicity.

It has pungent odour, so induction is not pleasant. It boils at room temperature (BP = <23°C) causing vapour pressure of 681 mm Hg.

PK: Desflurane has low blood: Gas partition coefficient and less soluble in fat. Rapid induction and rapid changes in depth of GA following changes in the inspired concentration is due to the fact that the alveolar concentration reaches 80% of the inspired concentration within 5 minutes. It is the fastest acting induction agent (B/G coefficient = 0.42). Potency is medium (MAC is 6%). >99% of absorbed GA is eliminated unchanged via lungs. A small amount is metabolized by hepatic CYP450 enzymes. Low concentration of trifluoroacetic acid is detectable in serum and urine.

ADR of "DESFLURANE"

Dilates respiratory smooth muscle (bronchodilator) like other inhalational GA.

Elevated arterial CO_2 tension due to depressed minute ventilation at >1 MAC.

Sympathetic nervous system stimulation at >1 MAC (>6%) causes transient tachycardia.

Fluoride absent but trifluoroacetic acid is seen in serum. It undergoes minimum metabolism among all inhaled GA.

Low BP due to decreased systemic vascular resistance similar to isoflurane but coronary steal is absent.

Under condition of normocapnia and normotension, it increases cerebral blood flow and ICT.

Respiratory rate is increased but tidal volume, minute volume and ventilator response decreased. Relaxes skeletal muscles.

Absent nephrotoxicity.

Negative inotropic effect.

Excessive respiratory secretion, laryngospasm, breath holding and coughing due to airway irritation. Enhances the effects of depolarising and nondepolarising muscle relaxants.

Uses: Alternative to routine surgery, outpatient surgery. It is colourless, volatile, nonflammable and nonexplosive. Odour is sweet so induction is smooth.

U: Outpatient surgery and children (AOC). The most effective bronchodilator GA.

PK: Less soluble in blood and tissues. It is metabolised by CYP450 2E1 producing fluoride and hexafluoroisopropanol.

Sevoflurane (the latest polyfluorinated GA) is **intermediate** between isoflurane and desflurane and is fast acting. It is degraded by **soda lime** hence not used in closed circuit.

> **Cyclopropane:**
> **Most potent** anaesthetic agent
> **AOC** in haemorrhagic shock
> Orange cylinder

IV GA was discovered by **John S. Lundy.** This causes loss of consciousness in **one-arm brain circulation time (~11 sec)** hence used for **induction** due to rapidity of onset of action. Maintenance of anaesthesia is done by inhalational agent.

Muscle relaxant + analgesia + IV GA = Complete anaesthesia.

Propofol: Along with thoipental, it is the commonest used IV GA. Disodium EDTA or sodium metabisulfite is added to the formulation to inhibit bacterial growth. Patients "feel better" in the immediate postoperative period. It has antiemetic action. It is ued for inductional and maintenance. Acidosis in children is due to RTI.

Physical and Chemical Properties

It consists of a phenol ring with isopropyl group attached (2, 6 di-isopropylphenol).

It is oil based preparation containing soya bean oil, egg lecithin and glycerol. So injection is painful and should be preceded by lignocaine injection. The colour of solution is milky white and available in 1% and 2% concentration. It is preservative free so should be used within 6 hours after opening the vial because there have been death reports following the use of contaminated solution of propofol (as egg lecithin is a good media for bacterial growth).

Anaesthetic Properties

Induction is achieved in one arm brain circulation time, i.e. 15 seconds. Consciousness is regained after 5 to 10 minutes due to redistribution.

Advantages of Propofol Over Thiopentone

1. Rapid and smooth recovery.
2. Completely eliminated from body in 4 hours so patient is ambulatory early.
3. Antiemetic.
4. Antipruritic.

Disadvantages

1. Apnea is more profound and longer.
2. Hypotension is more severe.
3. Injection is painful.
4. Solution is less stable (6 hours).
5. Chances of sepsis with contaminated solution are high.
6. Myoclonic activity can be produced.
7. Sexual fantasies and hallucinations are additional side effects.
8. Expensive than thoipentone.
9. Allergic reactions can occur in individuals having allergy to egg lecithin.
10. Propofol addiction has also been reported.

Unconsciousness in 15–45 sec and lasts 15 min.

PK: Distribution t½ — 2–8 min
Elimination t½ — 30–60 min

ADR: Respiratory depression. Induction apnoea for 1min. ↓ BP due to vasodilation.

Dose: 2 mg/kg bolus IV for **induction** and 9 mg/kg/hr for **maintenance**.

Uses: Outpatient surgery/day care surgery, sedation in ICU.

ADR of "PROPOFOL"

1. **P**ressures of all types decrease (BP, IOP, ICP).
2. **R**apid action produces muscle twitching and myoclonic activity (convulsion).
3. **O**ooo

4. Provokes anaphylaxis and histamine release. Vasotonic, antiemetic and antipruritic.
5. Oooo
6. Foetus safe in pregnant (but GA crosses placenta).
7. Oooo
8. Low cerebral blood flow.

Etomidate: It is a carboxylated imidazole supplied as active D-isomer. It is techniques of balanced anaesthesia. Induction anaesthesia (dose = 0.2–0.4 mg/kg). Causes myoclonia. Duration of action 5–10 min.

PK: Hepatic metabolism. Elimination is both renal (78%) and biliary (22%).

It causes minimal CRS and respiratory depressure effects. It has biphasic plasma concentration curve showing distribution half-lives of 3 and 29 minutes.

ADR of "ETOMIDATE"

1. Effects similar to
2. Thiopental (cerebral blood flow, metabolism, IOP, ICP).
3. Output (cardiac) and BP unchanged.
4. Myoclonus (incidence is 30–60%).
5. Induces hiccups. Injection is painful.
6. Decreases IOP and ICP. Deficiency of vitamin C.
7. Adrenocortical suppression (hence it is no more used).
8. Transient ↓ in cortisol even on single dose. Thrombophlebitis.
9. Emesis and nausea (incidence is 40% which is highest among all IV anaesthesia).

U: IV AOC for aneurysm surgery and patients with cardiac disease.

ADR: CVS and respiratory depression (minimal). Motor restlessness and rigidity, nausea and vomiting, myoclonia.

BZD: Used for maintaining, inducing and supplementing anaesthesia.

Althesin:	Steroidal anaesthesia.
CI:	Bronchial asthma and porphyria (like thiopentone).

Ketamine is an arylcyclohexylamine related to **hallucinogen and is a congener of phencyclidine.** It was synthesized by Stevens in 1962 and first used in humans by Domino and Corsen in 1965.

It is a **"dissociative anaesthesia"** because it causes:

1. Feeling of dissociation from **one's own** surrounding and body without actual loss of consciousness.
2. Light sleep.   3. Analgesia.   4. Amnesia.
5. Immobility.   6. Catatonia (↑ muscle tone).

S-isomer is more potent and less toxic than R-isomer.
Primary site of action is thalamoneocortical projection.

Ketamine inhibits cortex (unconsciousness) and thalamus (analgesia) and stimulates limbic system (emergence reaction and hallucination). It also acts on medullary reticular formation and spinal cord.

Pharmacology Review

    Site of action   – Cortex and subcortical areas.
    Analgesic action   – 40 min (profound analgesia).
    Anaesthetic action   – 15 min.
    Muscle tone elevated. It is glutamate antagonist.

Cardiac stimulant due to **sympathetic stimulation** and NA reuptake inhibition.

ADR of "KETAMINE"

1. **K** (c) atelectic state (nystagmus, dilated pupil, salivation, lacrimation, spontaneous limb movement)
2. **E**mergence delirium (vivid dream, hallucination, illusion). Most frequent in the first hour of emergence. Delirium and hallucination is treated by lorazepam (DOC).
3. **T**one of muscles increased.
4. **A**mnesia, arrhythmia.
5. **M**yoglobinemia.
6. **I**nvoluntary movement in 50% patients.
7. **N**egative inotropic and vasodilator, but central and peripheral CA reuptake inhibition is dominant.
8. **E**nhances all pressure (BP, IOP, ICP).

Uses of Ketamine

Sympathetic stimulation by ketamine causes:
Cardiac stimulation.
Bronchodilation (AOC for bronchial asthma).
Enhances all pressure (AOC in shock).
Enhances muscle tone (AOC in skin graft).
Enhances salivation.

Advantage and Uses in Anaesthesia

1. Induction agent of choice for:
   - Asthmatics
   - Shock
   - Children (by intramuscular route) as an alternative to inhalational induction [Inhalational (sevoflurane) is the method of choice for induction in children].
   - Constrictive pericaditis, cardiac tamponade (in these conditions cardiac output is dependent on tachycardia and ketamine causes tachycardia), right to left shunt like tetralogy of Fallot (ketamine by causing hypertension increases the afterload thereby decreasing the right to left shunt fraction).
2. Can be used as sole agent for minor procedures (like incision and drainage), burn dressings.
3. Can be safely used at remote places and in inexperienced hands since it does not depress respiration and heart.
4. Preferred agent for patients with full stomach (pharyngeal and laryngeal reflexes are preserved).
5. Shock anaesthesia: DOC. Head and neck operation especially in asthmatic due to bronchospasm (it is bronchodilator hence best sucked). Burn dressing: **Ketamine + diazepam** in cardio-catheterization, trauma surgery and angiography. Pediatric surgery: Poor-risk geriatric patients.

Disadvantages
1. Incidence of hallucinations and emergence reactions is very high which are not pleasant to patient attendants and other patients. Patients given ketamine can be found shouting, weeping, singing or even abusing badly in postoperative rooms.
2. Increases muscle tone.
3. Pharyngeal and respiratory secretions are increased which can cause laryngospasm.
4. Increases myocardial oxygen demand.
5. All pressures like intraocular intragastric, intracranial are markedly raised.

Contraindications
1. Head injury (as it increases intracranial tension).
2. Patient with intracranial space occupying lesion.
3. Eye injury or other ophthalmic pathology (ketamine increases intraocular pressure).
4. Ischemic heart disease (it increases myocardial oxygen demand).
5. Vascular aneurysm (it causes hypertension).
6. Patients with psychiatric diseases and drug addicts (more incidence of hallucinations and emergence reaction).
7. Hypertensives.

Dose: IV→1 mg/kg, IM→5 mg/kg, 10 mg/kg rectally.
Effects within a **min** and last **10–15 min.** Also given orally and intrathecally.

PK: Hepatic metabolism of ketamine to norketamine which has reduced CNS activity. Norketamine is further metabolised and excreted in urine and bile.

It is lipophilic drug distributed into highly vascular organs including brain. Increase in plasma E and NE levels occur after 2 minutes of IV ketamine and return to control level 15 minutes later. In most patients, it decreases respiratory rate for 2–3 minutes.

Droperidol
It is butyrophenone structurally related to haloperidol. It is dopamine antagonist. It is a potent **antiemetic** and sedative. Rarely used in anaesthesia as a sole agent. Can be used as a premedicant.

Droperidol produces
- Hypnosis (sedation).
- Mental detachment.
- Catatonia (absence of voluntary movements).
- Antiemetic effect.
- Hypotension (due to a blockade).

Side effects of droperidol
Prolonged somnolence and detachment which can be reversed by physostigmine.
Extrapyramidal side effects like dyskinesia, grimacing, trismus, torticollis and oculogyric spasms.
Treatment: Diphenhydramine and benztropine. Hallucinations and bizzare sensation of weightlessness and loss of body image.
Malignant neuroleptic syndrome.

Treatment: Bromocriptine

It is used in combination with fentanyl to produce neuroleptanalgesia, characterized by analgesia, sedation and variable amnesia.

The combination contains droperidol and fentanyl in ratio of 50:1 (droperidol 2.5 mg + fentanyl 0.05 mg).

Fentanyl

It is more potent (100 times) than morphine. Nowadays very commonly used opioid in anaesthesia. The advantages of fentanyl are:

1. Rapid onset (2 to 5 min) and rapid recovery (1 to 2 hours).
2. It can be given by IM, IV, transmucosal (fentanyl lollipop), transdermal (fentanyl patch), intrathecal and epidural route. Fentanyl patch provides postoperative analgesia for 72 hours.
3. Opioid of choice for hepatic and renal diseases.
4. Forms an excellent combination with propofol for total intravenous anaesthesia.
5. With bupivacaine used epidurally for painless labour.
6. Better than morphine in preventing stress response to laryngoscopy, intubation and surgery.
   - Systemic effects are similar to morphine except that it has negligible effect on GFR and urine output.
   - Fentanyl can produce significant muscle rigidity (Wooden chest syndrome).
   - IV fentanyl can be sequestrated by stomach up to 20% resulting in second peak and respiratory depression after 3 to 4 hours.
   - **Dose:** 2 to 5 µg/kg.

Fentanyl produces
- Analgesia
- Bradycardia
- Respiratory depression
- Muscle rigidity

Neuroleptanalgesia

The effect of neuroleptanalgesia is simply additive effect of droperidol and fentanyl.

Uses of Neuroleptanalgesia

1. As an induction agent (very rarely).
2. As a premedication.
3. As sedation for certain minor procedures like gastroscopy, bronchoscopy, burn dressing.
4. Surgeries associated with high incidence of postoperative nausea and vomiting like middle ear surgery.
5. Neurosurgical procedures requiring arousable patient like stereotactic brain surgery, removal of seizure foci (other agents useful for such procedures are methohexitone, etomidate, low dose propofol).

Fentanyl + Droperidol = Neuroleptanalgesia. Neuroleptanalgesia + N_2O 65% + O_2 35% = Neuroleptanaesthesia. Fentanyl (opioid analgesic) + Droperidol (neuroleptic) contain a

Fixed ratio = (10.05 mg/ml) + (2.5 mg/ml), respectively.
— Fentanyl 1 part + Droperidol 50 part.
— 5 ml IV for 10 min diluted in glucose solution.
— **Effects:**
   1. Neuroleptic analgesia (without unconsciousness).
   2. General quiescence.
   3. Respiratory depression.
   4. ↓BP due to **α blockade** by droperidol.
   5. ↓HR due to **vagal stimulation** by fentanyl.
   6. ↑ chest muscle tone and rigidity cause respiratory depression.
   7. Muscle dystonia.
   8. ↓ Psychomotor function.
   9. Intense analgesia with loss of consciousness.

The state lasts for **30–40 min. Naloxone** is used in respiratory depression and mental clouding.

HR decreases but is not sensitised to **adrenaline.**

General anaesthesia produced by neuroleptanaesthesia (droperidol + fentanyl + a inhalational agent) is somewhat similar to that produced by ketamine.

Uses: It is used when GA (IV/inhalational) is contraindicated. Minor surgery: Endoscopy, bronchoscopy, angiocardiography, angiography.

Myelography: Burn dressing.

Alfentanil: Not available in India. 20 times more potent than morphine. Onset is early (1.4 minutes) and recovery is also rapid. It provides adequate analgesia for 30–60 minutes. Alfentanil is still considered as opioid of choice for day care surgery (although remifentanil is shortest acting opioid.

Alfentanil + Propofol: Total intravenous anaesthesia (TIVA) of choice (but in India, propofol + fentanyl is still combination of choice because alfentanil is not yet available).

Sufentanil: Not available in India. Most potent opioid (500 times of morphine). Quick onset and recovery. Respiratory depression and bradycardia more profound than fentanyl and alfentanil. Agent of choice for inhibiting stress response to laryngoscopy and intubation.

Remifentanil: Ultrashort acting agent. Duration 5–10 minutes. Metabolised by ester hydrolysis by non-specific esters in blood and tissues. Onset is fastest (1.1 minutes) and recovery is also most rapid among opioids but its short duration of analgesia (5–10 minutes) may not be sufficient and a long acting opioid may be required after its discontinuation even for day care surgery.

Alternative of fentanyl = Alfentanil, remifentanil, and sufentanil.

Alfentanil is shortest-acting opioid analgesic.

Esterases of tissue and plasma metabolise remifentanil.

(**Fentanyl is 100 times** more potent than morphine. Action lasts for about **30 min.** Action of **droperidol** lasts for about **2–3 hrs**).

Methoxyflurane
Physical Properties
- Sweet odour.
- Non-irritant.
- Non-inflammable.
- Boiling point more than water (107°C).
- Highly soluble in rubber tubings of closed circuit.
- Undergoes maximum metabolism among all inhalational anaesthetics.

Anaesthetic Properties
- Most potent inhalational agent (MAC 0.16%).
- Slowest induction and recovery (blood gas coefficient 15).
- Good analgesic.
- Good muscle relaxant.

Systemic Effects
Cardiovascular system: Sensitizes heart to adrenaline. Causes bradycardia and decreased cardiac output.

Liver: It is hepatotoxic.

Renal: Methoxyflurane yields highest concentrations of fluoride (F) which can damage the tubules and can cause vasopressin resistant to high output (polyuric) renal failure.

Contraindications
- Not to be used with closed circuit (reacts with rubber tubing of closed circuit).
- Renal diseases.

Cyclopropane
- It is a liquid agent stored in orange-coloured cylinders at 75 psi and delivered as gas.
- Highly inflammable and explosive.
- It is pleasant smelling.
- Induction is smooth and fast (blood gas coefficient 0.44).
- It is carried in blood attached to RBC.
- Concentration to produce deep anaesthesia is 20 to 30%.

Systemic Effects
Cardiovascular system: It stimulates sympathetic system and blood pressure is well maintained so it is inhalational agent of choice for patients in shock. It sensitizes myocardium to adrenaline.

At emergence when cyclopropane is discontinued patient can go in shock due to withdrawal of sympathetic stimulation, called as cyclopropane shock. Therefore, cyclopropane should be closed slowly.
- Nausea and vomiting is also very common following its use.
- May increase bleeding tendency.
- Can cause bronchospasm.

ADR:
1. Oxalate—renal stone formation.
2. Nephrotoxicity causes vasopressin resistance. 70% of drug is metabolised in liver releasing fluoride ions to cause nephrotoxicity.
3. Polyuric renal insufficiency.

Chloroform: **Discovered by James Simpson** in 1849 in Scotland. Not used now.
ADR: **C**ardiotoxic **H**epatotoxic **D**iabetogenic **CHD**

Chloroform

- It is very toxic compound. Numbers of cardiac arrest and death have been reported due to ventricular fibrillation. Use of adrenaline with chloroform anaesthesia is contraindicated.
- Prolonged use of concentrations above 2% can produce respiratory arrest.
- Chloroform is hepatotoxic.
- Chloroform causes profound hyperglycemia. Therefore, it should be avoided in diabetic patients.
- It is non-irritant and induction is smooth.
- Produces good muscle relaxation.
- Non-inflammable, non-explosive.

Trichloroethylene (Trielene)

It is the anaesthetic agent with **least effect** on myocardial contractility.

Physical Properties

- It is colourless liquid.
- Odour is sweet.
- Mildly irritant.
- Non-inflammable, non-explosive.
- Can decompose to phosgene and HCI at temperature above 125°C, e.g. by cautery.

Anaesthetic Properties

- Second most potent inhalational agent (MAC 0.2%).
- Most potent analgesic.
- Induction is slow (blood gas coefficient 9).
- Mild irritation.
- Normally used concentration is 0.5%.

Systemic Effects

Cardiovascular system: It sensitizes myocardium to arenaline. Blood pressure is well maintained.

Respiratory system: Stimulates respiration causing tachypnea.

Reaction with soda lime: It can react with soda lime producing *dichloroacetylene* which is *neurotoxic* effecting cranial nerves [most commonly involved are *V and VII* (commonest is V) but III, IV, VI, X and XII can slso be involved] and *phosgene* which is pulmonary *toxic* (can cause ARDS).

Uses

It was used for **labour analgesia** (painless labour). The parturient *self inhales* trilene vapours through a portable trilene inhaler.

Contraindication

Trilene is contraindicated with soda lime (closed circuit).

Fluroxene
Fluorine containing ether. Good analgesic and potent agent. Fluroxene can cross the palcenta and can be deposited in foetal tissues.

Ethyl Chloride
- It is highly inflammable and explosive.
- Decreases cardiac output significantly.
- No more used as an anaesthetic. Nowadays ethyl chloride is used as spray to produce local analgesia by blocking nerve conduction through cooling.
- Undergoes maximum metabolism among all inhalational agents.

Drug IA of GA
1. Opioids, neuroleptics and MAO inhibitor **stimulate** GA.
2. **GA + antihypertensive** = ↓BP markedly.
3. Halothane, cyclopropane, and trichloroethylene **sensitize** heart to adrenaline.
4. **GA + corticosteroid** cause CV collapse and adrenal insufficiency. Hence, hydrocortisone is given intraoperatively.
5. GA increases **insulin** need in DM.

In terms of the extent of metabolism of inhaled anaesthetics, the rank order is methoxyflurane > halothane > enflurane > sevofluran > isoflurane > desflurane > N_2O.

Table 10.6: Summary of anaesthetic properties of inhalational agents

Agent	Induction		Analgesia	Muscle relaxation	Amnesia
	Onset	Smoothness			
Halothane	Intermediate	Very smooth	+/0	++	++
Isoflurane	Intermediate	Slightly irritable	++	++	++
Enflurane	Intermediate	Slightly irritable	++	++	++
Nitrous oxide	Fast	Not used for induction	+++	–	+/0
Sevoflurane	Fast	Very smooth	++	++	++
Desflurane	Fastest	Slightly irritable	++	++	++
Ether	Slow	Highly irritable	+++	+++	++
Trilene	Slow	Smooth	++++	+	+
Methoxy-flurane	Slowest	Smooth	+++	++	++
Cyclopropane	Fast	Smooth	++	++	++
Choloroform	Slow	Smooth	+	++	++

Complications
(A) During GA
1. Respiratory and cardiac depression.
2. Respiratory secretion.

Pulmonary aspiration is a major cause of death associated with anaesthesia. Mortality after aspiration is 5 to 70% depending on the volume and pH of aspirated material and time interval between detection and management.

Incidence: 1 in 3,000.

Predisposing factors
- **Full stomach:** It is single most important factor. Therefore adquate fasting should be there.
- Depressed level of consciousness.
- Conditions decreasing the tone of LES.
- Pregnancy (acid aspiration in late pregnancy was described by Mendelson called it as Mendelson syndrome).

3. Asphyxia

4. Anaphylactic Reaction
Anaphylactic reaction can occur with any of the drug used for general anaesthesia.

Treatment
- Maintenance of airway (if laryngeal edema or bronchospasm develops).
- Adrenaline 1:10,000.
- Steroids (hydrocortisone).
- Histamine antagonist like diphenhydramine.

5. Eye Complications
 a. **Delirium**
 b. **Convulsion**

Convulsions
May be due to:
- Hypoxia
- Drugs like local analgesics, methohexitone, enflurane, atracurium
- Cerebrovascular accidents
- Laryngospasm and Explosion
- GIT

Nausea and Vomiting
This is the most common complication (40%) in recovery room.

Causes
Hypotension, hypoxia, drugs, idiopathic.

Treatment
- Phenothiazines (Stemetil)
- Metoclopramide
- Hyoscine
- Ondansetron (5-HT_3 antagonist)
- Clonidine (has role in opioid induced nausea and vomiting).

B. After GA
 1. Sedation
 2. Nerve palsy
    - Most common type is auditory.
    - Usually seen when oxygen, nitrous oxide and opioids are used for maintenance of anaesthesia.

Peripheral Neuropathies

Most common nerve injured during anaesthesia is ulnar (34%), followed by brachial plexus (24%). Lateral popliteal nerve is most frequently damaged nerve in lower limb.
- **Tourniquet palsies:** Pressure in tourniquet should not exceed more than 50% above systolic pressure and duration in upper limb should be less than 1 hour and in lower limb, less than one and half hour.
- Prolonged hypotension causing nerve ischemia.

3. Organotoxicity
4. Delirium
5. Respiratory insufficiency
6. Hypothermia and shivering.

Table 10.7: *Vital capacity reduction in different positions*

Position	Reduction in vital capacity (%)
Lithotomy	↓ by 18%
Trendelenburg	↓ by 15%
Right lateral	↓ by 12%
Left lateral	↓ by 10%
Prone	↓ by 10%

Hypothermia and Shivering

Shivering occurs as a protective mechanism as inhalational agents, spinal/epidural block causes vasodilatation leading to heat loss. Shivering can be abolished by inhibition of hypothalamus. Most commonly shivering is seen after halothane.

Treatment of Shivering
- Pethidine/pentazocine.
- O_2 consumption may increase to 4 times (400%) during shivering. So oxygen inhalation during shivering is mandatory.

Malignant Hyperthermia

It is the clinical syndrome observed during general anaesthesia associated with rapidly increasing temperature as great as 1°C/5 min.

Etiology

It is due to abnormality of Ryanodine receptor mutation in gene loci corresponding to skeletal muscle. Ryanodine receptor which is calcium releasing channel of sarcoplasmic reticulum. The abnormality leads to excessive accumulation of calcium which causes sustained contraction of muscle.

It is associated with conditions like Duchenne muscular dystrophy, arthrogryposis multiplex congenita, osteogenesis imperfecta, congenital strabismus, central core diseases.
- Patient with history of neuroleptic malignant syndrome are at high risk of developing malignant hyperthermia.
- Patients who develop masseter spasm after succinylcholine are very prone to develop malignant hyperthermia.

Incidence

1 in 2 lakhs. If only volatile anaesthetics and succinylcholine is considered, incidence is 1 in 62,000.

Causative Agents

Muscle relaxants: Succinylcholine is most commonly implicated drug.
Inhalational agents: Halothane is most common inhalational agents. Others are:
- Isoflurane
- Enflurane
- Desflurane
- Sevoflurane
- Methoxyflurane

Local anaesthetics: Lignocaine.

Other Drugs

- Tricyclic antidepressants.
- Monoamine oxidase (MAO) inhibitors.
- Phenothiazines.

Clinical Features

- Hyperthermia (temperature may rise to more than 109°F). The heat production is due to increased muscle metabolism (both aerobic and anaerobic), glycolysis and hydrolysis of high energy phosphates involved in the process of contraction relaxation.
- Increased end tidal CO_2 is most sensitive early sign of malignant hyperthermia.
- Hypoxia and cyanosis.
- Tachycardia, hypertension, cardiac arrhythmias.
- Severe metabolic acidosis (pH <7.0).
- Hyperkalemia, muscle rigidity, increased creatine phophokinase, increased myoglobin.
- Renal failure, DIC, pulmonary and cerebral edema.
- Death.

Treatment

- Stop all anaesthetics immediately.
- Hyperventilation with 100% oxygen.
- Control temperature by:
  - Ice cooling.
  - Correct acidosis: Sodium bicarbonate 2 to 4 mEq/kg.
- Correct electrolyte imbalance (hyperkalemia).
- Maintain urine output.
- **Specific:** Dantrolene 2 mg/kg to be repeated every 5 minutes to a maximum of 10 mg/kg.

Screening

The most reliable test for susceptibility is muscle contracture test. Creatine phosphokinase level is the basic screening tool. Individuals having high creatine phosphokinase levels should not be subjected to causative agents.

Anaesthesia for Patients Susceptible for Malignant Hperthermia
1. Local or regional anaesthesia is preferred technique (but lignocaine should not be used).
2. Safe drugs for general anaesthesia are barbiturates, propofol, narcotics, benzodiazepines, nitrous oxide, nondepolarizing muscle relaxants.

Other Causes of Hyperthermia in Anaesthesia are
1. Hypermetabolic states like thyrotoxicosis and pheochromocytoma.
2. Neuroleptic malignant syndrome due to phenothiazines.
3. Anticholinergics (atropine).
4. Injury to hypothalamic temperature regulatory centres.

Premedication of GA: Aims are for antianxiety (lorazepam DOC) amnesia, analgesia, ↓vagal stimulation and secretion, antiemesis, ↓acidic volume of gastric juices.

Drugs are: Antiemetics (metoclopramide/ondansetron). Metoclopramide + H_2 blockers more effective. H_2 blocker (ranitidine) or omeprazole. Neuroleptic (CPZ/haloperidol). Atropine/hyoscine BZD and barbiturates, morphine/pethidine but it depresses respiration and precipitates asthma.

Flammable agents are
- Ether
- Cyclopropane
- Ethyl chloride
- Ethylene
- Fluroxene
- Bowel gases which contain hydrogen and methane

Use: Preoperative pain (mostly).

Antanalgesics are thiopentone and promethazine. Inhalational agents used as gas in anaesthesia and stored in cylinder in liquid form are: N_2O, CO_2 and cyclopropane.

Other Intravenous Anaesthetics
Propanidid
- It is a eugenol derivative and water insoluble.
- It is metabolized by pseudocholinesterase.
- It is no more used because of severe allergic reactions.

Steroid Anaesthetics
1. **Althesin:** It is combination of two steroids, alphaxolone and alphadolone. It raises the intracranial tension significantly. No more used because of severe hypersensitivity reactions.
2. **Eltanolone** (also called as pregnanolone): It is naturally occurring metabolite of progesterone. Eltanolone is new agent under clinical trials.
3. Miniaxolone.
4. **GABA:** It is closely related to naturally occurring GABA neurotransmitter.

1. **Oxygen-Hb dissociation curve**

   Left shift = Loading of O_2 in Lungs. Right shift = Release of O_2 from Hb. Increased oxygen affinity occurs in Low (Left shift) 2, 3-DPG, Temperature, PCO_2, H^+ DTPH = Dil To Pagal Hai and in Fetal Hb (binds O_2 Forcefully). OxyHb is **R** form (Relaxed form).

2. **Treatment of ventricular fibrillation** (MEDicines for Low BP) = $MgSO_4$, Epinephrine, Defibrillation, Lidocaine, Bretylium, Procainamide.

3. **ARDS** (diagnostic criteria): Acute onset, Ratio (paO_2/FiO_2) <200, Diffuse infiltration and **SGWP** <19 mmHg.

4. Carotid **SinuS** measures pre**SS**ure. Carotid b**O**dy measures **O**xygen.

5. Alkalosis and Acidosis: ROME

   Respiratory = Opposite: pH is high, pCO_2 is low (alkalosis); pH is low, pCO_2 is high (acidosis).

   Metabolic = Equal: pH is high, pCO_2 is high (alkalosis); pH is low, pCO_2 is low (acidosis)

6. Components of **APGAR** = **A**ppearance, **P**ulse, **G**rimace, **A**ctivity, **R**espiration

7. Components of Glasgow Coma Scale = **VI**bratory (**6**), **V**erbal (**5**), **EYES** (4 letters).

8. Arrhythmia (Heart/Cardiac Muscle Tremor) Causing GA: **H**alothane, **CHCl₃**, **M**ethoxyflurane, **T**rilene and **C**yclopropane.

9. Day care GA for maintenance is **D**esflurane, **I**soflurane and **S**evoflurane; for induction is **T**hiopentone, **E**tomidate, **M**ethohexitone and **P**ropofol and for analgesia is alf**E**ntanil and **R**emifentanil DISTEMPER

- Meperidine reduces shivering, an ADR during emergence from GA.
- Barbiturates are precipitated when mixed with muscle relaxants.
- Clonidine and dexmedetomidine (α_2 agonists) are used for sedation anxiolysis, hypnosis and sympatholysis. Clonidine is analgesic also. Dexmedetomidine reduces the MAC of inhalational GA by as much as 90%, a property referred to as "anaesthetic sparing". It also causes less respiratory depression but infusion of longer than 24 hrs causes rebound hypertension. It causes unconsciousness via actions in locus ceruleus. Alpha agonists are antagonised by atipamezole. Althesin and Alphaxalone (steroid) were used for sedation and anaesthesia in 1971 but it was subsequently banned.
- Sodium thiopental is the commonest used barbiturates for induction and formulated as sodium salt with 6% $NaHCO_3$ and reconstituted in water or isotonic saline to produce 2.5% (thiopental), 2% (thiamylal) and 1% (methohexital) with pH of 10 to 11. Thiamylal is equipotent with and in all aspects very similar to thiopental. Thiopental often evokes garlic taste just prior to induction. Thiopental, thiamylal and methohexital are used in pediatric patient by rectum at 10 times the IV dose and decrease BP, IOP and ICP and cause histamine release and porphyria. α agonists increase the depth and α inhibitors increase the amount of GA.

  Opioids have the greatest use in the treatment of postoperative and chronic pain. Presynaptic opioid receptors inhibit the release of substance P and other neurotransmitters while postsynaptic opioid receptor decreases the activity of certain dorsal horn nerves in spinothalamic tract.

"Conscious sedation" is drug-induced alleviation of anxiety and pain, together with altered level of consciousness, but with retention of the ability of the patient to maintain a patent airway and to respond to verbal commands. The drugs are BZD and opioids. Deep sedation" is a controlled state of GA involving decreased conciousness from which the patient is not easily aroused. The drugs are thiopental, ketamine, propofol and certain opioids. The commonest used BZD in the perioperative period is midazolam followed by diazepam and lorazepam. Midazolam is typically administered IV (0.4 mg/kg) but can be given IM, orally or rectally.

Parenteral GAs are the commonest used drugs for anaesthetic induction of adults. Thiopental and propofol are the two commonest used parenteral anaesthetics. Propofol is advantageous for procedures where rapid return to a preoperative mental status is desirable. Etomidate is usually reserved for patients at risk for hypotension and/or myocardial ischemia. Ketamine is best suited for patients with asthma and/or for children undergoing short, painful procedures. With the exception of ketamine, neither parenteral nor inhalational GA are effective analgesics. The order of potency (relative to morphine) to perioperative opioid analgesics are: sufentanil (1000X) < remifentanil (300X) > fentanyl (100X) > alfentanil (15X) > morphine (IX) > meperidine (0.1X). All opioids cause sphincter of Oddi spasm.

Hypotensive Anaesthesia (Controlled/Deliberate Hypotension)

Definition

It is the technique of deliberately reducing the systolic blood pressure to 80 to 90 mmHg or mean arterial pressure to 50 to 65 mmHg in order to reduce the intraoperative bleeding. The clinical criteria is to reduce the blood pressure by one-third of preoperative value. Continuous measurement of BP by invasive BP monitoring is mandatory.

Techniques

A. **Vasodilators**
1. **Sodium nitroprusside (SNP)**
   It produces hypotension by arteriolar dilatation. The matter of concern is cyanide toxicity with its prolonged used which is diagnosed by continuous fall of oxygen saturation (histotoxic hypoxia) and maximum safe dose of SNP is 1.5 mg/kg.
2. **Nitroglycerin (Glyceral trinitrate; NTG)**
   - Its solution can be absorbed by polyvinyl chloride so preferably glass bottles should be used.
   - NTG and SNP infusions are most commonly applied techniques to produce deliberate hypotension.

B. **Inhaled anaesthetics**
   - Isoflurane is the inhalational agent of choice for producing deliberate hypotension.

- Halothane
- Enflurane

C. Spinal/epidural block.
D. Ganglion blockers (trimethaphan).
E. α blockers (phentolamine).
F. β blockers (esmolol or propranolol).
G. α + β blockers (labetalol).
H. Calcium channel blockers.
I. Prostaglandins: PGE.

Contraindications
- Cerebrovascular disease.
- Coronary vascular disease.
- Atheroma.

11. Sedative–Hypnotics

All sedative–hypnotics and antianxiety drugs have **anticonvulsant** activity.
Common mechanism is increased inhibitory effect of **GABA** in CNS.
The most important use—treatment of insomnia.
Sedation: Reduced responsiveness to any stimulus due to reduced motor activity.
Hypnotic is drug inducing sleep.
Hypnosis: It is a sleep like condition produced in a person so as to obey suggestions.
Order of CNS depression is Sedation < Hypnosis < GA. High doses of all hypnotics produce GA. The oldest hypnotics→opium and alcohol.
Sleep (unconsciousness from which person is aroused): It depends on **age** and **individuals. Total sleep time—highest** in infancy. **Coma** is unconsciousness from which person is not aroused.
Two types of sleep: **REM** (rapid eye movement), **NREM/SWS** (slow wave sleep = Brain wave is slow, i.e. **70–75%** of total sleep time). Somnambulism, Enuresis and Night Terror occur in **stage IV NREM sleep SENT**. But **nightmare** is in REM sleep. **Maximum GH secretion** occurs during NREM sleep. **Most sleep** is SWS type which is deep restful type during **the first hour** of sleep. 10–30% decrease in BP, RR, BMR in REM sleep occurs periodically in **every 90 minutes. Paradoxical sleep** is in REM sleep (25% of sleep time of young adult) associated with **vivid dream. Nocturnal angina** occurs in REM sleep because of ↑ BP and ↑ HR. **Cholinergic excitation** (erection of penis) is **maximum** in REM sleep. **The most conspicuous stimulation** area for causing almost nocturnal sleep is the **raphe nuclei** in the lower half of pons and in the medulla which secrete **serotonin**. Others are stimulation of the nucleus of **tractus solitarius of pons and medulla.**

Stage of Sleep

1. **Stage 0/Awake:** EEG shows α activity when eyes **closed** and β activity when eyes opened.
2. **Stage 1/Dozing:** α activity interspersed with θ waves.
3. **Stage 2/Unequivocal sleep:** θ waves and κ complexes evoked on sensory stimulation. **Sleep spindle** also present **50% of time (greatest proportion of sleep).**
4. **Stage 3:** EEG shows **θ, δ and spindle** activity, **κ complexes** evoked with strong stimuli only.

5. **Stage 4/cerebral sleep:** α **activity** predominates in EEG, κ complexes not evoked. **Eyes** are **fixed.** Subject not aroused. Night terror may be there. **10–20% of sleep time.**

Stages 2, 3, 4 have steady HR, BP and respiration.

Brain waves (EEG):

D	T	A	B
3,	7,	14,	35

1. Alpha (α) = 8–14 cps →high amplitude and frequency.
2. Beta (β) = 15–35 cps →low amplitude and **highest frequency.**
3. Theta (θ) = 4–7 cps →low amplitude and low frequency.
4. Delta (δ) = <3 cps →high amplitude and **lowest** frequency.
5. κ complex = deep negative waves followed by positive waves.
    - Characteristic EEG pattern seen when person is awake—α wave.
    - Characteristic EEG pattern seen in deep sleep (δ sleep)—δ wave.

REM (features): Rapid pulse/respiratory rate, Erection, Muscle paralysis/mental activity increase. dREaM during REM sleep. DElta waves during DEepest sleep (stages 3 and 4, slow wave).

Insomnia (inability to sleep)
— Transient (<1 week)
— Short-term (week)
— Chronic/long-term (month–year).

A. Classification of barbiturates
1. **Long-acting barbiturates** (8 hrs or more)
    a. Phenobarbitone
    b. Mephobarbitone
2. **Intermediate acting barbiturates** (4–8 hrs)
    a. Pentobarbitone
    b. Amylobarbitone
    c. Butobarbitone
3. **Short-acting barbiturates** (<4 hrs)
    a. Secobarbitone
    b. Hexobarbitone
4. **Ultrashort acting barbiturates**
    a. Thiopentone
    b. Methohexitone

B. Classification of BZD (benzodiazepine) based on use:
Hypnotics:
- **D**iazepam
- **F**lurazepam
- **F**lunitrazepam
- **N**itrazepam
- **T**emazepam
- **T**riazolam
- **M**idazolam and estazolam

To This Mid-Night Famous Film: Darr

Antianxiety
- **D**iazepam
- **C**hlordiazepoxide
- **O**xazepam
- **L**orazepam
- **A**lprazolam

> A COLD

Anticonvulsant
- **D**iazepam
- **C**lonazepam
- **C**lobazepam

C. **Newer non-BZD hypnotic:** Zopiclone, zolpidem.
D. **Others:** **O**pioids, anti**D**epressant, some anti**C**holinergic, some anti**H**istaminic, and some **N**euroleptic have sedative action.

> ON CHD

BZD classification (based on duration of action)
1. **Long-acting:** Diazepam, nitrazepam, flurazepam, prazepam, chlorazepate, chlordiazepoxide.
2. **Short-acting:** **T**emazepam, **O**xazepam, **T**rizolam, **A**lprazolam, **L**orazepam.

> TOTAL

Barbiturates

Barbiturates (acidic drug): Derivatives of **barbituric acid (malonylurea)**. Barbituric acid = urea + malonic acid. Used as **sodium salt** due to water solubility. Barbiturates were used up to 1960 (precipitate **porphyria** in susceptible individual). They are **depressant for all excitable cell.**

> Malonic acid → Barbituric acid → Barbiturates.

ACTION OF BARBITURATES

1. CNS is **most sensitive (dose dependent). All areas** are effected but reticular activating system is **the most sensitive** (hence lack of wakefulness). **Order of effects are: Sedation → Sleep → Anaesthesia → Coma.**

   Hypnotic dose (short-acting–150 mg) causes disruption of **REM-NREM sleep cycle**—reduced stages 3 and 4, reduced time taken to fall asleep, elevated sleep duration, reduced night awakening and reduced REM. **Sedative dose** causes learning, judgment and short-term memory impairment and euphoria in addicts. These cause **hyperalgesia** and **anticonvulsant** property is present. Rebound increases in REM and nightmare due to discontinuation. Thiopentone has instantaneous entry into CNS due to **high lipid solubility.**

2. **CNS and respiratory system** are depressed. Dose for cardiac arrest is **3 times more than that for respiratory failure.**

   Tone and mobility of **smooth muscle** are reduced. Skeletal muscle contraction is decreased due to neuromuscular junction depression. **Urine flow** is reduced due to ↓BP and ↑ **ADH release.**

Mechanism of Action of Barbiturates

1. Interfere with **Na⁺K⁺ transport** across cell membrane.
2. Inhibit **mesencephalic reticular activating system and poly-synaptic transmission** in CNS. Block glutamate effect.

3. Potentiate **GABA action** without binding BZD R and GABA R.
4. At clinical doses it is GABA facilitatory but at higher doses, it has GABA-mimetic action (but BZD has GABA-facilitatory action only and inhibit Ca^{2+} dependent release of neurotransmitters at higher concentration. Facilitate GABA and glycine effects.

It inhibits the function of synapses. Transmission of excitatory neurotransmitters like acetylcholine is inhibited and that of inhibitory neurotransmitters like GABA is enhanced.

> **Barbiturates** facilitate GABA action by increased **DURATION** of Cl^- channel opening. BarbiDURATe = ↑ DURATion.

PK:
1. Enzymes induced by barbiturates are:
   — Microsomal → **CYP450**
   — Mitochondrial → **δ-ALA synthetase**
   — Cytoplasmic → **Aldehyde dehydrogenase**
   — **Hepatic glucuronyl transferase**
2. Well absorbed orally from GIT.
3. Widely distributed in the body, lipid soluble.
   Cross CNS and placenta.
4. **Long-acting: t½ →** 80 to 120 hrs **(longest duration of action).**
   — **Lowest lipid solubility.**
   — Hepatic metabolism.
   — Plasma protein binding of phenobarbitone 35%. It induces **bilirubin conjugation** and hastens **jaundice clearance** in congenital non-hemolytic anemia and kernicterus.
   — Excreted unchanged in urine (phenobarbitone: 30% renal clearance).
   — **Alkalinised urine (most significant for long-acting)** enhances ionisation and excretion.
5. **Short-acting:**
   — t½ of elimination phase →**15–50 hrs.**
   — Plasma t½ → 20–40 hrs.
   — **Intermediate** lipid soluble.
   — Effect lasts 8 hrs and consciousness is regained in 15–20 min due to redistribution.
   — Metabolised in liver by **oxidation, conjugation** and **dealkylation.**
6. **Ultrashort-acting:**
   — t½ of elimination phase →**9 hrs.**
   — **Highly** lipid soluble (Thiopental-highesT).
   — Effect lasts 15–20 min due to **redistribution.**
7. Metabolism by **side chain oxidation** accounts for clearance of **all barbiturates** from body but phenobarbitone has **30% renal** clearance.
8. **Mephobarbitone (methyl phenobarbitone)** $\xrightarrow{\text{Liver}}$ Phenobarbitone.

ADR of barbiturates

1. Phenobarbitone → **cheapest** and **least** toxic (rash, megaloblastic anemia, osteomalacia).
2. Confusion, traffic accident, impaired performance.

3. **Idiosyncracy** common in elderly (excitement, porphyria).
4. **Hypersensitivity: Alcohol + Barbiturate cause rapid death.**
5. **Tolerance** on repeated use due to enhanced metabolism from stimulation of MFO and reduced effect on CNS.
6. **Dependence** and **abuse liability.**
7. **Withdrawal syndrome:** excitement, hallucination, delirium, convulsion, death.
8. Binding to plasma protein is **highest** for highly lipid soluble barbiturates.

U of barbiturates: Only **phenobarbitone** in epilepsy (sedative action is drawback) and **thiopentone** in induction of **GA** are used now:

Indications are: As sedative hypnotic, anticonvulsant, preanaesthetic medication in mania and delirium. Phenobarbitone induces **bilirubin** conjugation to clear jaundice of congenital nonhaemolytic type. Febrile seizure: Phenobarbitone **(DOC—diazepam).** Grand mal epilepsy: Phenobarbitone **(DOC—phenytoin).**

Thiopentone sodium: It is sodium ethyl thiobarbiturate discovered by Water and Lundy in 1934. Solution strength = **2.5%.** pH = **10.4.** First IV GA introduced in 1935. **The commonest** used ultrashort-acting barbiturates for induction of anaesthesia (**the commonest** IV inducing agent). **The last weapon** for status epilepticus. Anticonvulsant and antipsychotic. Unconsciousness in **15–20 sec.** Regaining of consciousness in 10–20 min. Distribution phase t½—3 min. Highly water soluble and produces **alkaline** solution, hence freshly prepared before injection. Undissociated form is highly **lipid soluble.** Poor analgesic (hence **N_2O/opioid** is used). Poor muscle relaxant: Action is reduced due to rapid distribution into **fat and muscle.**

Physical and Chemical Properties

- Available as yellow amorphous powder as 0.5 g and 1.0 g vial to which 20 ml of sterile water for injection is added yielding a concentration of 2.5% and 5% respectively (5% solution is further diluted to make it 2.5% solution). The solution is not stable and should be used within 48 hours (or till precipitate appears). It should not be prepared with Ringer lactate otherwise it will be precipitated due to acidic pH of Ringer lactate solution.
- It is sulphur analogue of pentobarbitone. **Sulphur is added to increase the lipid solubility.**
- The ultrashort duration of thiopentone is because of methyl group added to it.
- It is available as sodium salt to make it water soluble but this increases the alkalinity of solution. pH of sodium thiopentone (2.5%) solution is 10.4 (highly alkaline).
- 6% anhydrous sodium carbonate is added to powder to prevent the formation of free acid by carbon dioxide from atmosphere.
- It is prepared in the atmosphere of nitrogen.

Anaesthetic Properties and Pharmacokinetics

Unconsciousness is produced in one arm brain circulation time, i.e. 15 seconds and induction is very smooth (but sometimes may be associated with intial excitatory responses). Its such rapid induction is because of its high lipid solubility and high degree of non-ionization.

The **elimination half life of thiopentone is 10.4 hours** but consciousness is regained after 15 to 20 minutes which is because of redistribution which means that drug is redistributed from brain to tissues with less vascularity like muscle or fat but repeated doses saturates these tissues and regaining of consciousness after repeated doses depends on its metabolism and elimination.

At induction, it causes **mild hypokalemia**.

Protein binding: In blood, **80 to 90%** of thiopentone is bound to plasma proteins, mainly to albumin.

Systemic Effects

Central nervous system
- Unconscious is produced in 15 seconds but maximum depth is achieved in 60 seconds.
- **Sleep:** It increases stage 2 and decreases stages 3, 4 and REM sleep.
- Cerebral oxygen consumption (CMO_2), cerebral metabolic rate (CMR) and intracranial tension (ICT) are decreased. So, it is the agent of choice for cerebral protection.
- **Anticonvulsant action:** It is because of phenyl group and convulsions not responding to other anticonvulsants are controlled with thiopentone.
- **Antanalgesic action:** At subanaesthetic doses, it is antanalgesic.
- **Acute tolerance:** Tolerance is seen if initial dose is high.

Cardiovascular system: It causes **hypotension** which is more because of venodilatation but also because of direct depression of vasomotor centre.
- It is also direct myocardial depressant.

Respiratory system
- If a painful stimulus is given at inadequate depth, severe **laryngospasm** and bronchospasm may occur. Laryngospasm is treated with small dose of succinylcholine (25 to 50 mg).
- **Transient apnoea** is a very common finding, it usually requires no treatment but if prolonged (>15 seconds), gentle IPPV with bag and mask should be given.
- At higher dosage, thiopentone depresses respiration significantly (depth affected more than rate), so it is mandatory that tools for airway management should be kept ready.

Eye: Thiopentone decreases the intraocular pressure.

Pregnancy: It crosses the placental barrier and achieves high concentration in brain of fetus. Thiopentone crosses the placenta most readily and the equilibrium with maternal circulation is achieved within 3 to 5 minutes.

Kidney: It stimulates ADH action.

Thyroid: Thiopentone has got **antithyroid** activity.

Muscular system: It is a poor muscle relaxant.

Dose and Recovery

Dose of thiopentone is 5 mg/kg body weight. Males requiring more than females, obese more than thin and young more than old. Although consciousness is regained after 15 minutes due to redistribution, the drug is eliminated after 10 to 12 hours ($t½$—10.4 hours) so patients should not be allowed to carry out important work like driving for 24 hours.

PK of Thiopentone Sodium
1. Ultimate disposal by kidney→hepatic metabolism by **CYP450 14%/hr**.
2. Elimination t½—10.5 hrs.
3. Residual CNS depression persists >12 hrs.
4. t½ of distribution phase—3 min.
5. Dose 5 mg/kg for induction.
6. Effect lasts 15–20 min due to **redistribution**.
7. Plasma protein binding **75%**.

ADR (Thiopentone Sodium)
1. **Thrombophlebitis:** Due to chemical irritation produced by alkaline solution.
2. Necrosis.
3. Intra-arterial injection causes **thrombosis and pain** (first symptom).

    Intra-arterial injection: This is a very dreadful complication which can lead to gangrene and loss of limb if not diagnosed and managed timely.

    This complication is commonly seen when thiopentone is injected in antecubital vein because in 10% of the cases, brachial artery divides above elbow giving a very superficial abnormal ulnar artery which lies just deep to antecubital vein.

    Symptomatology: With injection, patient complains of severe burning pain down the injection site which is followed by pallor, cyanosis, edema and finally gangrene of limb.

    Pathophysiology: Because of its high alkalinity, the thiopentone gets precipitated in acidic pH of blood forming crystals leading to thrombus formation which blocks the microcirculation. Thiopentone also causes the endothelial damage. Both these processes produce vasospasm leading to ischemia and gangrene of limb.

    Treatment: Imediate heparinisation, ganglionic block, surgical removal of clot.

    Inject papaverine 40 to 80 mg in 10 to 20 ml of saline (it will produce local vasodilatation).

    Other vasodilators like tolazoline, phenoxybenzamine can be used.

    If none of the above is available, 10 ml of 1% xylocaine should be injected.

    Urokinase infusion.

    Brachial plexus or stellate ganglion block should be given as early as possible (this will relieve the vasospasm).
4. Respiratory depression.
5. Intense pain, CVS collapse in case of hypovolemic shock and sepsis.
6. Euphoria, vertigo, postoperative disorientation.
7. Gangrene due to alkalinity of injected drugs (IM, SC, IV).
8. Troubles related to swallowing (coughing and hiccups).
9. Reduced cerebral blood flow: Shivering and delirium.
10. **Median nerve:** If the solution is directly injected into nerve.
11. **Laryngospasm** (hence **Atropine + SCh** given as premedication but SCh and **thiopentone** are not mixed in the same syringe due to chemical reaction).

CI (Thiopentone Sodium)

1. Thiopentone sensitive to anaphylaxis (absolute).
2. Hypotension and shock.
3. Increased uncontrolled BP more prone to hypotension, on injection.
4. Obstructive cause to bronchospasm: Apnoea, bronchial asthma.
5. **Porphyria:** Acute intermittent porphyria precipitation.
6. Enhanced K^+ loss (familial hypokalemic periodic paralysis).
7. Liver necrosis or kindney disease.
8. Oral cavity, jaw and neck (burns, quinsy).
9. **Enzyme:** Thiopentone induces enzyme amino-levulenic acid synthetase which stimulates the formation of porphyrin in susceptible individuals. So it is contraindicated in acute intermittent and variegate porphyria (can be used safely in porphyria cutanea tarda).

Uses of thiopentone sodium: Induction of anaesthesia. In patient with raised ICP because it reduces ICP (disadvantage: CVS and respiratory depression).

Methohexitone sodium: Similar to thiopentone sodium but **quicker and briefer** action and **3 times** more potent.
- Used as 1% solution with pH of 11.1.
- **Dose:** 1.5 mg/kg.
- Elimination half life is 4 hours.
- It can be given intramuscularly and per rectally to produce sedation in children.
- It induces seizures (while thiopentone is anticonvulsant) and can produce myoclonus. So it is the agent of choice for electroconvulsive therapy (ECT).

Secobarbitone and Pentobarbitone

Can be used as premedication to produce sedation by oral, IM or rectal route.
- **Acute barbiturate poisoning:** Mostly suicidal. If a person, after taking hypnotics, fails to fall asleep, gets confused and takes the drugs again and again, then develops acute poisoning, called **drug automation.**
- **Lethal dose: 3 gm,** more lipid soluble agents; **5–10 gm,** less lipid soluble agents.

Manifestations of Barbiturate Poisoning

1. ↓BP due to ganglionic blockade.
2. Vasomotor centre depression.
3. Respiratory failure.
4. CVS collapse.
5. Renal shut down.
6. Excessive CNS depression.
7. Miosis initially.

Fatal dose
Short-acting = 1–2 gm
Medium-acting = 2–3 gm
Long-acting = 3–5 gm

ABCDEFGH

Treatment: **A**irway maintenance.
Breathing maintenance.
Circulation maintenance.
Drugs: Vasodepressor (DA) and forced alkaline diuresis with **mannitol and $NaHCO_3$**.
ECG monitoring.
Fluid infusion.
Gastric lavage: Activated **charcoal,** no specific antidote.
Haemodialysis and **H**aemoperfusion.

CI (barbiturates): Obstructive sleep apnoea, liver and kidney disease, bronchial asthma, severe pulmonary insufficiency (emphysema, etc.). Acute intermittent porphyria: Barbiturates induce microsomal enzyme (**d-aminolevulinic acid synthetase**) to synthesize porphyrin.

IA of barbiturates (due to induction of hepatic microsomal enzymes CYP450):
1. Barbiturates induce metabolism of **steroids, warfarin, tolbutamide, theophylline, chloramphenicol, griseofulvin** and potentiate **CNS** depressant (alcohol, opioid and antihistaminics).
2. Phenobarbitone reduces **griseofulvin** absorption from GIT and interferes with **phenytoin, sodium valproate** and **imipramine** metabolism.

Sodium. Valproate enhances phenobarbitone concentration in plasma.

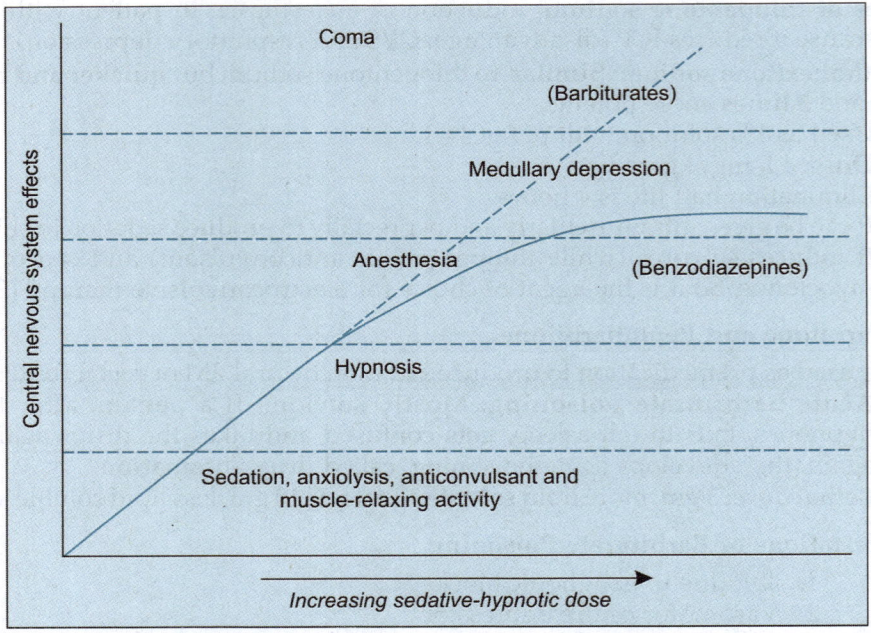

Fig. 11.1: Relationship between doses of BZD and barbiturates and their CNS effects

Benzodiazepine (BZD)

BZD: 1. BZD has **5 aryl substituent.**
2. **BZD ring** fused with **seven membered diazepine ring.**

Advantage of BZD over barbiturates
1. **High therapeutic index (hence less suicidal potential).**
2. No effect on **body systems** (CVS, respiration). **On IV injection,** cardiac contractility and BP decrease. BP falls by diazepam and lorazepam →**due to ↓ CO.** BP fall by flunitrazepam and midazolam →due to **↓ TPR.** IV diazepam dilates **coronary artery** and causes **analgesia.** Diazepam reduces **natural gastric secretion** and prevents stress ulcer.

3. Lower abuse liability, mild tolerance, less marked dependence and **withdrawal syndrome**.
4. **Hastens** onset of sleep, reduces intermittent awakening, enhances total sleep time, shortens REM phase but nitrazepam enhances REM sleep and reduces night terror. **Most subjects** have a feeling of refreshing sleep after wake up.
5. **Skeletal muscle** is relaxed without impairing voluntary action.
6. BZD has **low ceiling CNS depressant effect** due to GABA **facilitatory but not GABA mimetic action**.
7. BZD acts on **midbrain** ascending reticular formation (which maintains wakefulness) and on limbic system (thought and mental function).

   BZD advantage over barbiturate: Less abuse. High TI (low suicidal potential). Less ↓ in REM sleep. *Withdrawal* syndrome milder but prolonged. Less pronounced induction of MFO. Flumazenil reverses BZD effects.

Mechanism of BZD: It acts as **GABA agonist**. Overall action of all BZD is the same.

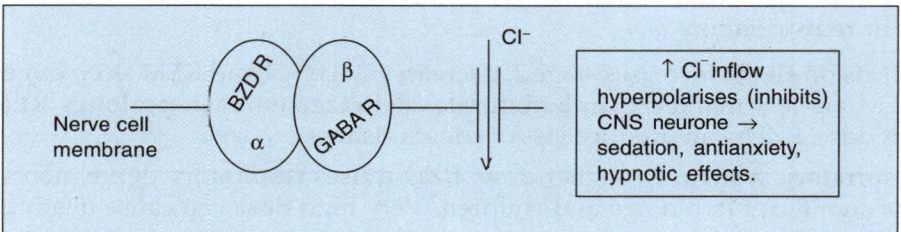

BZD-GABA$_A$R-Cl$^-$ channel complex

GABA$_A$-BZD R-Cl$^-$ channel complex is formed of **α, β, γ and δ subunits**.
1. Empty GABA R → inactivated Cl$^-$ channel closed.
2. GABA binding with GABA R → Cl$^-$ channel opening → **hyperpolarization**.
3. BZD binding with BZD R(α) → ↑ GABA binding with GABA R (β) → ↑ Cl$^-$ **entry**.
4. **Cl$^-$ entry** hyperpolarises cell (postsynaptic potential away from threshold) making it more difficult to depolarise and hence **reduces neural excitability**.
5. BZD → facilitates GABA R binding in brain → ↑ GABA activity → cell hyperpolarisation → **CNS depression**.
6. BZD **cannot** act without GABA. Facilitates **inhibitory GABAergic** transmission.
7. BZD R is only in CNS especially in **midbrain** ascending reticular formation and on **limbic system**.
8. BZD-inverse agonist **(DMCM)** inhibits GABA mediated Cl$^-$ channel opening. **Flumazenil** inhibits both BZD and DMCM.
9. **Barbiturate R** facilitates GABA and directly opens Cl$^-$ channel. **Bicuculline** blocks GABA$_A$ R while **picrotoxin** directly inhibits Cl$^-$ channel. **Muscimol** is GABA$_A$ R agonist.
10. BZD potentiates **adenosine**.
11. Diazepam produces **brief initial phase of strong action** followed by **mild prolonged effect** due to **2 phases plasma concentration decay curve**.

BZD Facilitates GABA action by ↑ Frequency of Cl$^-$ channel opening.

BZDs bind to specific receptors in brain which facilitates GABA receptor binding which in turn increases the membrane conductance to chloride ion causing hyperpolarization of membrane (GABA facilitatory).

Systemic Effects

CNS: Mainly acts on reticular activating system (RAS) and amygdala (limbic system) producing sedation, anxiolysis and amnesia.

Also acts on medulla producing muscle relaxation and on cerebellum producing ataxia.
- BZDs are *anticonvulsants*.
- They are *not analgesics*.
- Produce *muscle relaxation* by acting at medullary and spinal cord level (central action) and not at neuromuscular junction.
- Reduces cerebral metabolic rate, brain oxygen consumption and intracranial pressure.
- Initial regain of consciousness is seen after 10 to 15 minutes, which is because of redistribution.

Effects on sleep: Increases stage 2, decreases stage 3, 4 and REM sleep but effects on REM are less marked than barbiturates. **Nitrazepam even prolongs REM.** At higher dose, BZDs can produce loss of consciousness.

Respiratory system: At higher dose, BZD causes respiratory depression which can be significant in old age and children. Very high dose can cause death due to respiratory depression.

PK of BZD: GABA $\xrightarrow{\text{GABA-Transaminase}}$ **succinic semialdehyde.**

- Hepatic metabolism by **dealkylation** and **hydroxylation**, differs in lipid solubility, widely **distributed in the body, crosses placenta.**
- Only lorazepam is regularly absorbed from IM sites.
- Some **cross BBB** and diazepam undergoes **hepatic circulation.**
- BZDs and their phase I metabolites excreted as **glucuronide conjugates** in urine and gut.
- Diazepam (rapidly absorbed) → **desmethyl diazepam and oxazepam** (active metabolites).

Elimination t½	—	30–60 hrs
Distribution phase t½	—	1 hr
Dose	—	7 mg

- BZDs having common active metabolite →**desmethyl diazepam,** are diazepam, prazepam, chlorazepate and chlordiazepoxide.
- BZDs not having active metabolites are **temazepam, oxazepam** and **lorazepam.** The fastest acting BZD is midazolam.
- **Triazolam** is not accumulated on repeated use.
  t½ — 3–5 hrs (**shortest** among BZD), peak effect in 1 hr.
- **Midazolam:** Peak effect in 20 min. →abuse liability present.
- **Clonazepam:** Orally absorbed, **85% plasma protein bound. Completely** metabolised in liver, excreted in urine, t½—24 hrs.

Sedative–Hypnotics

- **Clobazam** is **1,5-BZD** (others are **1,4-BZD**). Oral bioavailability **–90%**. Most sedative–hypnotics are lipid soluble.
  Elimination t½—**18 hrs** but its active metabolite has t½ — **> 35 hrs**.
- **Chlordiazepoxide:** Slow oral absorption, t½—5–15 hrs.
- **Oxazepam :** Slowly absorbed. Plasma t½—10 hrs.
  Slow penetration into brain.
- **Lorazepam :** Slow penetration into brain, t½—10–20 hrs.
- **Alprazolam :** Plasma t½—12 hrs. No residual effect like diazepam.

Table 11.1: *Pharmacokinetics of commonly used benzodiazepines*

	Diazepam	*Midazolam*	*Lorazepam*
Route of administration	• Oral • IM or IV	IM or IV	Oral IV or IM
Onset of action after:			
IV	30 to 60 sec	30 to 60 sec.	1 to 2 min
Oral	1 to 2 hours	—	1 to 2 hours
IM	30 min	30 min.	30 min
Preparation (intravenous)	Oil based so injection is painful	Water based so injection is painless	—
Elimination half life	30 to 60 hours	2 to 3 hours	15 hours but clinically duration of effect is longer because of strong binding to receptors
Dose for sedation	0.05 to 0.2 mg/kg	0.01 to 0.1 mg/kg	0.03 to 0.04 mg/kg

ADR of BZD

1. **Long-acting** BZD—**withdrawal symptoms** develop after 4–6 days.
   Short-acting BZD—**withdrawal symptoms** appear within 1–2 days.
2. **Prolonged reaction** time.
3. **Vertigo, ataxia, dizziness, light headedness.**
4. **Disorientation, amnesia, confusion.**
5. **Nightmares** and **behavior alteration** (nitrazepam).
6. **Cross tolerance** with other CNS depressants.
7. **Altered sexual** function.
8. **Floppy baby syndrome** due to use of BZD to mothers before delivery.
9. **Less dependence.**
10. **Mild withdrawal syndrome** (insomnia, anxiety, restlessness, malaise, loss of appetite, bad dreams).
11. **Flaccidity and respiratory depression** in neonates on administration during labour.
12. Clonazepam (**sedation and dullness-most important**) →lack of concentration and ataxia, irritability, etc.
13. **Failure to ovulate.**
14. **Weight gain** due to increase appetite.

IA of BZD: BZD **synergises** other CNS depressant. It causes **psychosis** with sodium valproate. **Cimetidine, INH and OC** retard BZD metabolism.

CI of BZD: All hypnotics aggravate **apnoea**.

Uses of BZD: One of the most frequently used drugs (**chlordiazepoxide** was the first clinically used BZD).
1. As hypnotic—**DOC** (in all types of insomnia).
2. Sedative: Flunitrazepam in "**date rape**" (rapid amnestic).
3. Anxiolytic (BZD–**DOC**): Chlordiazepoxide is given.
4. Anticonvulsant (diazepam 100 mg/d max.). **Diazepam** is not used in long-term therapy of epilepsy due to **sedative action.**
   Rectal instillation of diazepam for febrile convulsion in children.
5. As centrally acting **muscle relaxant.**
6. **Preanaesthetic medication** (for amnesia of anterograde and to prevent hallucination by ketamine) and **IV anaesthesia.**
   Agent of choice for preoperative sedation is lorazepam.
7. In **alcohol withdrawal.**
8. With analgesic, antiulcer, NSAID and spasmolytic.
9. Clonazepam in **absence seizures** and adjuvant in myoclonic and akinetic epilepsy.
10. Adjuvant to **antiepileptic drug.**
11. **Tension syndrome and neurosis** → lorazepam.
12. **Diazepam is DOC in:** | **The SPASM** |
    — Delirium **T**remens
    — **S**tatus epilepticus (IV)
    — **P**ostoperative delirium
    — **A**lcohol withdrawal syndrome
    — Febrile **S**eizures
    — Preanaesthetic **M**edication (lorazepam is better DOC).

Alprazolam is BZD of choice in | **APE** |
    — **A**goraphobia (fear of being alone or in open space).
    — **P**anic disorder
    — **E**lderly individual

> **Uses of DIAZEPAM:** **D**elirium tremens (in alcohol withdrawal), **I**nsomnia and neurosis, **A**nxiety, before cardiac catheteri**Z**ation, sedation before surgery, **E**pilepsy, **P**reanaesthetic medication, IV **A**naesthesia, As Adjuvant with Antiemetics, **M**uscle relaxation.
>
> Therapeutic effects of **DIAZEPAM:**
> **D**rowsiness, **I**ncreased reaction time, **A**taxia, di**Z**ziness (hangover), **E**pigastric distress, **P**aradoxical CNS stimulation, **A**buse liability (due to dependence), **M**emory loss (amnesia).

13. Choice of BZD for **anxiety** is based on **pharmacokinetics.** Relieves anxiety at low doses without producing CNS **depression,** is more selective for **limbic system** than barbiturates. This is **one of the most widely used** class of drugs due to **milder withdrawal syndrome and safe in overdose.**
    BZD is stored in **the smallest** possible dose.

Diazepam

Now, not preferred benzodiazepine in anaesthesia because of the following reasons:
1. Preparation is oil base so injection is painful.
2. Sleep is not smooth (incidence of dysphoria is highest among BZDs).
3. Elimination half life is prolonged (30 to 60 hours). So chance of postoperative respiratory depression are there.

Midazolam

It is 3 times more potent than diazepam. Midazolam is now very commonly used BZD in intraoperative period.
1. Water based preparation so injection is painless.
2. Elimination half life is 2 to 3 hours so midazolam can be safely used for day care procedures.
3. Reversal with flumazenil is complete (no resedation).

Disadvantages

Incidence of apnea and respiratory depression are higher and more profound than diazepam.

Zopicolone: It is **cyclopyrrolone** hypnotic, acts as **BZD** in sleep.
Mechanism: Potentiates **GABA** by binding to a different site other than BZDs.
PK: $t_{1/2}$ →5–6 hrs. In **overdose,** drug is safe as BZD.
ADR: Metallic taste, dry mouth, psychological disturbance, impaired judgement and alertness.
U: Insomnia.

Zolpidem: It Iis **imidazopyridine** hypnotic, reduces **sleep latency** and **sleep duration in insomnia,** safer in overdose like BZD.
PK: $t_{1/2}$—2 hrs. Interacts with BZDR (BZ_1 or ω_1 subtypes).

Flumazenil: It is specific BZD R antagonist.
Mechanism: Competes with BZD R **agonist and inverse agonist** for BZD R to reverse their **depressant/stimulant** effects respectively. Action lasts for 1–2 hrs.

It antagonises hypnosis, respiratory depression and sedation but amnesia is minimally reversed.

The disadvantage for flumazenil is that its half life is short (1 to 2 hours) while that of diazepam (36 hours) and lorazepam (15 hours) is long. So, it gives effective protection for 1 to 2 hours only and chances of resedation are high but this problem is not seen with midazolam which has similar elimination half life to flumazenil.

Antagonism is most difficult with lorazepam because of its highest receptor hinding a affinity.

ADR: **A**gitation, **A**nxiety, **C**oldness, **D**iscomfort, **T**earfulness.

A CAT and Dog

PK: Absorbed orally, hepatic metabolism, bioavailability 16%, elimination $t_{1/2}$—1 hr.
U: IV 0.3–1 mg reverses BZD anaesthesia in 1 min.
Maximum 5 mg IV (0.2 mg/min) controls BZD intoxication in **all patients** in 5 min.

Chloral hydrate (prodrug): The **oldest** synthetic hypnotic. It is liquid, irritant to gastric mucosa and skin with **burning horrible taste. Low TI** (therapeutic index).

Chloral hydrate $\xrightarrow{\text{alcohol dehydrogenase}}$ **Trichloroethanol (active moiety).**

> **Chloral hydrate** is colourless with pungent odour.
> Fatal dose = 5–10 gm, fatal period = 8–12 hrs.
> It is called "*Knockout drops*" due to its rapid action for the purpose of rape/robbery.
> Mickey Finn = Alcohol + chloral hydrate.

Trichlophos: It is **monosodium salt of phosphate ester of trichloroethanol** (active moiety of chloral hydrate).

Paraldehyde: It is condensation product of **3 molecules of acetaldehyde** in the form of cyclic ester $\xrightarrow{\text{hepatic metabolism}}$ Acetaldehyde $\to CO_2 + H_2O$ (20% exhaled in breath) → **Soreness** of respiratory tract.

ADR: It is a volatile liquid with **pungent** smell and **disagreeable burning taste, inflammable and irritant.**

U: It is **potent hypnotic** with sharp and short lasting actions. Uses are:

Convulsion of **S**tatus epilepticus, **E**clampsia, **T**etanus, **D**elirium and to calm down **A**gitated patients.   **DATES**

Methaqualone: Causes excessive **dreaming**, has **all disadvantages of barbiturates**, is drug of abuse due to **paresthesias, euphoria and feeling** of "**high**".

Drugs with increased absorption with food are **D**iazepam, **T**hiazides, **P**ropranolol, **H**alofantrine, **L**ithium and **G**riseofulvin.

DTPH and Love Guru

12
Anti-Seizure Drugs

Seizures **are paroxysmal event due to uncontrolled excessive hypersynchronous discharges from an aggregate CNS neurones.**

Major types
1. **Focal/partial (local brain part):**
   a. **Simple (SPS) cortical lobe epilepsy:** Lasts 1 min, involves a group of muscle, no loss of consciousness.
   b. **Complex (CPS)/psychomotor/temporal lobe epilepsy:** Lasts 1–2 min, bizarre behaviour (staring, roaming). It is associated with attention in consciousness coupled with automation (chewing, aimless walking, etc.).
2. **Generalised (large part of the body):**   **I AM FAST**
   a. **Infantile spasm:** Intermittent muscle spasm with mental retardation.
   b. **Atonic seizures (akinetic epilepsy):** Unconsciousness without relaxation of **all muscle** due to excessive inhibitory discharge.
   c. **Myoclonic:** Momentary muscle contraction.
   d. **Febrile seizures (6 months to 6 yrs):** Due to >101.8°F temperature.
   e. **Absence/Petit mal:** Brief impairment of consciousness, involves mainly **children,** lasts ½ min, **EEG** →3 cps (spike and wave pattern).
   f. **Status epilepticus:** Continuous clinical menifestations of epileptic disease without intermission.
   g. **Tonic-clonic/grand mal/major epilepsy: Commonest,** lasts 1–2 min.
      Aura→ cry →unconsciousness → tonic spasm of all muscle → clonic jerk →sleep and depression of all CNS function due to extreme neural discharge in **all areas** of the brain.

Syncope: Loss of consciousness due to hypoperfusion in the brain.
Faintness: Presyncope is called faintness.
Epilepsy is recurrent seizure due to chronic underlying process.
Maximum electric shock induces convulsion **similar** to tonic-clonic seizures.
Pentylenetetrazol induces convulsion **similar** to absence seizures.

Classification: **SHOIAB DON**

Oxazolidinediones	— Trimethadone
Hydantoin	— Phenytoin, mephenytoin
Iminostilbene	— Oxcarbazepine, CBZ
Succinimide	— Ethosuximide, phensuximide

Aliphatic carboxylic acid — Valproic acid/sodium valproate
BZD — Diazepam, clonazepam, clobazepam
Barbiturates — Phenobarbitone, mephobarbitone
Deoxybarbiturates — Primidone
Others — Phenacemide, acetazolamide
New drugs
— Lamotrigine, Gabapentin, Felbamate,   **FT V**
   Levetiracetam, Progabide,   **LPG**
   Vigabatrin, Topiramate, Tiagabine

Primidone

Primidone is a deoxybarbiturate.
Primidone $\xrightarrow{\text{Liver}}$ **Phenobarbitone and PEMA** (phenylethyl malonamide/active metabolite).

PK: t½—10 hr, ⅓ excreted unchanged by kidney.

ADR: Same as phenobarbitone plus anemia, leukopenia, lymphadenopathy and psychotic reaction.

Phenytoin

Phenytoin/diphenyl hydantoin: It limits the spread of tonic phase of maximal electroshock seizure (**the most outstanding action**). It is **the oldest nonsedative antiepileptic drug** used. Antiepileptic drugs suppress seizures but **do not cure** the disorder. Hence, the aim of treatment is to **control and totally prevent all seizures activities at an acceptable level of ADR.**

Mechanism

1. Antiepileptic drugs block **initiation of electrical discharge** from focal area or more commonly prevent spread of abnormal electrical discharge to adjacent brain area.

   Mechanism of phenytoin: Use dependent blockade of Na⁺channel.

2. Phenytoin **stabilizes** neuronal membrane by blocking repetitive detonation of normal neurone during depolarising shift and prolonging Na⁺ channel inactivation (intracellular Na⁺ is reduced).
3. **At higher concentration,** phenytoin reduces Ca^{++} influx during depolarisation, inhibits **glutamate** and facilitates **GABA** responses.

> **Mechanism of action of antiepileptics**
>
> 1. Inhibition of **GABA—Transaminase** by **vigabatrin** and **valproic acid.**
>   **VIGABATRIN = GABA TRansaminase INhibition (irreversible).**
> 2. ↑ **GABA release** in brain by **GABApentin** (not act as $GABA_A$ R agonist).
> 3. Facilitation of GABA mediated Cl^- **channel opening** by BZD, barbiturates, valproate, vigabatrin, gabapentin.
> 4. Induction of **T type Ca^{++} current** by **valproate, trimethadione and ethosuximide.**
> 5. Prolongation of **Na⁺ channel inactivation** by **phenytoin, valproate, carbamazepine and lamotrigine.**

4. Phenytoin in the **heart** blocks inactivated Na⁺ channel and has short recovery time. Cardiac electrophysiological actions are **similar** to those of lidocaine. **Depression of automaticity** in PF and ventricular fibres without effecting that in SA node. **Suppression** of digitalis induced **after-depolarization.** It promotes **AV conduction** slowed by digitalis. It reduces **AP difference and ERP** in hypokalemia and digitalis toxicity.

PK
— **Poor water solubility** hence slow oral absorption.
— **Widely distributed in the body** and 80–90% bound to plasma protein.
— Hepatic metabolism by **hydroxylation and glucuronide conjugation.** "Capacity limited" kinetic of metabolism changes from **first order to zero order** over therapeutic range (small dose increments cause high plasma concentration).
— Due to saturation of metabolising enzymes, **>10 mg/ml rise in plasma concentration of drug** increases t½ from **20 to 60 hrs.**
— 5% unchanged drug is excreted by kidney. Elimination follows **zero order kinetics.** Fosphenytoin is its water soluble parenteral prodrug.

ADR of phenytoin
A. At therapeutic level
— **Gum hypertrophy (commonest): 20%** incidence, more in younger. Nifedipine, cyclosporin, OC, also cause gum hypertrophy.
— **Acne, coarsening of face, hirsutism and hypertrichosis.**
  Drugs causing hypertrichosis are: Phenothiazine, cyclosporin A, minoxidil, diazoxide, hexachlorobenzene.
— **Hypersensitivity reaction** (SLE, rashes, lymphadenopathy). Other drugs causing SLE are HIP **H**ydralazine, **I**soniazid, **P**rocainamide (**commonest** cause of drug induced SLE).
— **Cardiac arrhythmia** and VF plus reduced BP.
— **Megaloblastic anaemia:** Reduces folate absorption and enhances excretion.
— Injury to **injected vein.**
— **Inconsistent efficacy** of oral phenytoin is ischaemic VES/VT.
— **Osteomalacia** due to desensitization of tissue to vitamin D and interference of Ca⁺⁺ metabolism by drugs.
  Heparin, Corticosteroid, and GnRH-analogues cause osteomalacia. HCG
— **Hyperglycemia** due to inhibition of insulin release.
— **Foetal hydantoin syndrome** due to **arene oxide metabolite** (microcephaly, harelip, hypoplastic phalanges, cleft palate).

> **Drugs and hormones countering effect of insulin**
> 1. Glucagon, GH, TH, and glucocorticoids
> 2. Vinblastine, thiazide, somatostatin, CA and phenytoin inhibit insulin release.

B. At higher dose
— **Cerebral and vestibular effect** (ataxia, vertigo, diplopia and nystagmus) →most characteristic feature.

- **Hallucination**, mental confusion and abnormal behaviour.
- **Epigastric pain,** nausea, vomiting.
- ↓BP and arrhythmia.

ADR of PHENYTOIN: P450 interaction, **H**irsutism, **E**nlarged gum, **N**ystagmus, **Y**ellow-brown skin, **T**eratogenic, **O**steomalacia, **I**nterference with B_{12} metabolism leading to anemia, **N**europathy (vertigo, ataxia, headache).

IA:
- **Sucralfate** reduces phenytoin absorption by binding it in GIT.
- **Acidic drugs** displace phenytoin from protein binding sites.
- Inhibits **tolbutamide** metabolism.
- Enhances degradation of **digitoxin, theophylline, doxycycline and steroids** by microsomal enzyme induction.
- **Warfarin, dicumarol, cimetidine, INH** and **chloramphenicol** inhibit phenytoin metabolism.
- **Valproate** displaces protein bound phenytoin and reduces its metabolism (hence free phenytoin in plasma is enhanced).
- **CBZ and phenytoin** enhance each other's metabolism.
- **Phenobarbitone** inhibits competitively phenytoin metabolism but both enhance each others metabolism by enzyme induction.

U: Best and most reliable screening test of thyroid function in patient on phenytoin is measurement of **TSH**. Phenytoin is one of the **most widely** used antiepileptic drugs.
- **Grand mal (DOC)** and **focal seizures:** 400 mg/d (max).
- **Trigeminal neuralgia:** 2nd choice, **DOC**–carbamazepine.
- **Cardiac arrhythmia** (especially digitalis induced) (DOC–lignocaine).
- **Status epilepticus** (**DOC**–IV diazepam).

Precaution: Dilantin (special solvent) dissolves phenytoin but it should not be diluted in IV use due to drug precipitation.

Carbamazepine (CBZ): Has **antidiuretic** action.
Mechanism: Prolongs inactivated state of Na^+ channel.
PK: Poorly water soluble. **75% plasma protein bound.** Hepatic metabolism by:
1. **Oxidation** –10–11 epoxy CBZ (active metabolite).
2. **Hydroxylation and conjugation** to inactive form.
   Plasma t½ is reduced from **30 to 15 hrs** due to **autoinduction** of metabolism on chronic medication.

ADR:
1. **Neurotoxicity** (sedation, vertigo, ataxia, diplopia).
2. **CVS collapse, convulsion, coma.**
3. **Hypersensitivity reaction** (rashes, hepatitis, photosensitivity).
4. **Water retention** and hyponatremia in elderly due to **ADH action.**
5. With **valproate,** it doubles teratogenic frequency.
6. **Aplastic anemia** (rare and severe).

IA: Induces **valproate, phenytoin and phenobarbitone** by enzyme induction. **Erythromycin** induces CBZ metabolism. Reduces efficacy of **OC and haloperidol** by enzyme inducton.

U: The **most effective** in CPS. GTC and SPS—**DOC** (phenytoin also **DOC**). **Trigeminal neuralgia–DOC.** Alternative to Li in acute **mania. DI** of pituitary origin (reduces urine volume).

Ethosuximide is a succinimide.

Mechanism: Raises seizure **threshold,** acts on **thalamocortical system** which generates absence seizures. **Thalamic neurone** exhibits **T (transient) current**—a low threshold Ca^{++} current due to Ca^{++} influx through T type Ca^{++} channel. Ethosuximide and trimethadone selectively **suppress** T type Ca^{++} current without effecting other type of Na^+/Ca^{++} current.

PK:
1. Slowly and completely absorbed.
2. **Evenly distributed** in the body.
3. Hepatic metabolism by **hydroxylation** and **glucuronidation**.
4. Excreted in urine (¼th in the unchanged form).
5. t½—**48 hrs in adult (32 hrs in children).**

ADR: BMD, GIT intolerance, mood change, headache.

U: Absence seizure **(DOC).**

Trimethadione (Troxidone): Both troxidone and ethosuximide are oxazolidinedione derivative. Troxidone is **the first drug** found to be effective in absence seizures.

Mechanism: Mechanism and action same as of ethosuximide.

ADR: Kidney damage, hepatitis, exfoliative dermatitis, blood dyscrasias, **hemeralopia** (inability to tolerate bright light).

U: Absence seizure.

Valproic acid is a branched chain **aliphatic carboxylic acid** and **broadspectrum** longer acting anticonvulsant.

Mech: Prolongs Na^+ channel inactivation. Suppresses Ca^{++} **mediated T current** like ethosuximide. Inhibits **GABA transaminase →** GABA is enhanced to be released. Hyperpolarises nerve (↑ K^+ permeability).

PK: Orally absorbed, **90%** bound to plasma protein, complete hepatic metabolism by **oxidation** and **glucuronide conjugation,** excreted in urine, t½ →**10–15 hrs,** highest risk of fetal (<2 yrs) liver damage.

ADR:
— Ataxia, tremor, anorexia, vomiting.
— Alopecia and curling of hair.
— Enhanced blood NH_3.
— Fulminant hepatitis (rare but serious).
— **Neural tube defects** in the offspring.
— **Drugs causing fatty liver are:** **SMART**

Sodium valproate, **M**ethotrexate, **A**miodarone, aspa**R**aginase, **T**etracycline.

Causes of fa**T**ty li**V**er: **T**etracycline and **V**alproate (microvascular), **M**TX, **A**miodarone and **C**orticosteroid (**MAC**rovascular).

ADR of **VALPROATE**: **V**omiting, **A**lopecia, **L**iver toxicity, **P**ancytopenia/pancreatitis, **R**etention of fat (weight gain), **O**edema (peripheral), **A**norexia, **T**remor, **E**nzyme inducer (liver).

U: Myoclonic and atonic seizures **(DOC).** Absence seizure **(DOC).** GTCS and partial seizure (SPS, CPS)—**alternative.** Mania—alternative to Li.

CI: Concurrent administration of **valproate and clonazepam** precipitates **absence status.**

IA: Concurrent administration of **valproate** and **CBZ** causes foetal abnormalities. Both also induce each other's metabolism. **Valproate** also inhibits **phenobarbitone** metabolism and enhances its plasma level. It also displaces **phenytoin** from protein binding site and reduces its metabolism (**phenytoin toxicity**).

Lamotrigine: Efficacy **similar** to CBZ. It is phenyltriazine.
Mech: Blocks voltage sensitive Na^+ **channel** and stabilises **presynaptic membrane.** Inhibits release of excitatory neurotransmitter (**glutamate** mainly) but does not block **NMDA type glutamate R.**
PK: — Orally absorbed, **complete** hepatic metabolism.
— t½—**24 hrs** but reduced to 16 hrs due to receiving phenytoin, phenobarbitone and CBZ.
ADR: Sleepiness, Ataxia, Diplopia, vomiting.   **SAD**
IA: **Valproate** reduces lamotrigine clearance but lamotrigine lowers its level.
U: Reduces partial seizure frequency.
Gabapentin: It is **lipophilic.** GABA derivative (cyclic GABA analogue).
Mech: It crosses brain and enhances **GABA release.**
PK: Well absorbed orally, excreted unchanged in urine, t½—7 hrs.
ADR: Unsteadiness, tiredness, sedation.
U: Partial seizure.
Vigabatrin (gamma vinyl GABA)
Mech: It is **inhibitor of GABA transaminase** which degrades GABA.
Anticonvulsant action is due to increase in synaptic GABA concentration.
PK: Well absorbed orally, excreted unchanged in urine, t½—7 hrs.
ADR (behavior change, psychosis, depression) →**most important.**
U: Partial seizure

Treatment of epilepsy: A single drug at low dose is started to the **maximum** tolerated dose, then combination is used when **all reasonable monotherapies** get failed. **All drugs** withdrawal should be **gradual,** otherwise **status epilepticus** can precipitate. **Most antiseizure drugs** cause birth defects and mental retardation due to **hypoxia** during seizures, when mothers during pregnancy take them.
1. **GTC and SPS:** Phenytoin and CBZ—**DOC** (efficacy—**highest**).
   Valproate—**2nd choice** (but hepatotoxic in young children).
   Complete control in **90%** with generalised seizures.
2. **Absence seizures:** Valproate and ethosuximide **equally** effective.
   Valproate superior in mixed GTCS and absence.
3. **Infantile spasm** (hypsarrhythmia): Corticosteroid for symptomatic relief.
   Valproate and clonazepam—adjuvant.
4. **Status epilepticus:** Diazepam—DOC; phenobarbitone and clonazepam—alternative; general measures.
5. **Atonic seizure:** Valproate—**DOC.**
6. **Febrile convulsion** (mainly under 5 yrs): **The best treatment**—rectal **diazepam** 0.5 mg/kg at the onset of convulsion, paracetamol, external cooling.
7. **CPS:** CBZ, valproate, phenytoin.

Common features to most antiepileptic
— None of these are **curative**.
— Highly bound to **plasma protein**.
— Usually cleared by **hepatic metabolism** (inhibit metabolism of other drugs, induce metabolism of other drugs).
— It is important to measure serum anticonvulsant concentration.
— **Common ADR:** CNS depression, skin rashes, nystagmus and teratogenicity.

Choice of antiepileptic drugs

Types of seizures	DOC (drugs of choice)	Second choice
1. GTC/SPS	CBZ, phenytoin, valproate	Phenobarbitone, primidone
2. Trigeminal neuralgia	CBZ	
3. Hypsarrhythmia	ACTH / corticosteroids	
4. Psychomotor seizure (CPS)	CBZ, valproate, phenytoin	Phenobarbitone, primidone
5. Absence	Valproate, ethosuximide	Clonazepam, clobazepam
6. Myoclonic	Valproate	Clonazepam, clobazepam
7. Atonic	Valproate	Clonazepam, clobazepam
8. Febrile	Rectal diazepam	
9. Status epilepticus	Diazepam (IV) Clonazepam (IV)	Phenytoin (IV) Phenobarbitone (IV)

Topiramate: Broad spectrum anticonvulsant.
Mech: Weak carbonic anhydrase inhibitor. Prolongation of Na^+ channel inactivation, antagonism of glutamate receptors and potentiation of GABA by postsynaptic effects.
ADR: **W**eight loss, **O**verbalanced psychology with paresthesia, **R**enal stone, **D**ifficulty in word finding, **S**edation, **A**taxia. **WORDS A**bsent
U: As alternative in GTCS, SPS and CPS.

Tiagabine: Anticonvulsant.
Mech: Tia**GAB**ine depresses **GAB**A transporter **GAT-1** →removal of synaptically released GABA into glial cells and nerves →inhibition of GABA mediated nerves.

ADR: 4A = **A**mnesia, **A**sthenia, **A**bdominal pain and **A**bnormal consciousness.
U: To supplement partial seizures.

Levetiracetam: Anticonvulsant.
Mech: Suppresses kindled seizures only.
ADR: Somnolence, **A**sthenia (loss of strength), **D**izziness.   `SAD`
U: To supplement refractory partial seizures.

13 Alcohol

It is **hydroxy** derivatives of aliphatic hydrocarbon.

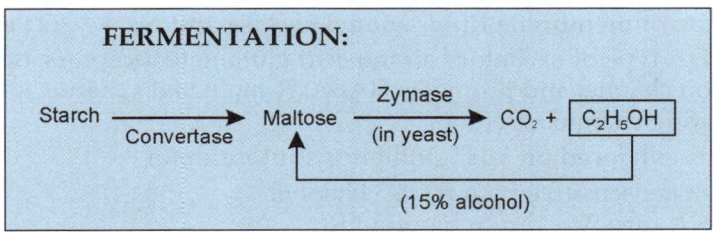

Source of commercial alcohol—**mollases**.

Alcoholic beverages

1. **Malted liquor:** 3–6% alcohol produced by germinated **cereal** fermentation.
2. **Wines:** 9–22% alcohol, produced by **fruit** fermentation.
   All alcohol fermented — dry wine
   Some left — sweet wine
3. **Spirit:** 40–55% alcohol
   Fermentation →distillation →spirit formation
   Proof sprit — explosive.
   Rectified sprit — 90% W/W ethanol
   Absolute alcohol — 99% W/W ethanol
   100% proof spirit is 49.29% W/W or 57.1% v/v alcohol.

Actions of alcohol (ethanol)

1. It is **neural depressant**. The **most sensitive areas** are **cortex and reticular activating system. Anticonvulsant** actions present.
2. It produces **cooling** by evaporation and causes irritation, burning, necrosis and fibrosis on **skin**. It produces permanent **nerve damage** after injecting around nerves.
3. **At low doses,** it causes ↑ HDL, ↓ LDL, ↑ adrenaline release, cutaneous and gastric **vasodilatation** (hence sense of warmth), tachycardia and ↑ BP due to **sympathetic stimulation,** ↑ gastric secretion and ↑ muscular activity.
4. **At high doses,** it causes ↓BP, myocardial and vasomotor centre **depression,** ↓ gastric secretion, **hypoglycaemia** and temperature regulating centre depression.

5. **Chronic alcoholism** causes **cardiomyopathy, impotency, gynaecomastia** and **megaloblastic anemia** due to interference with folate metabolism.
6. It **stimulates** respiration due to irritation of buccal and pharyngeal mucosa.
7. It metabolises **peripheral fat** to enhance fat synthesis in the liver. Alcohol metabolism produces **acetaldehyde** which damages **hepatocyte. Enhanced lipid peroxidation, glutathione depletion** and **nutritional deficiency** takes place. These cause alcoholic **cirrhosis**. Wernicke-Korsakoff syndrome commonest in alcoholics.
8. **Diuresis** occurs due to inhibition of ADH secretion and more water ingestion with drinks.
9. Loss of restraint and inhibition causes **aggressive sexual behavior (Aphrodisiac)**. Uterine contraction is reduced.

Mechanism of action of alcohol (ethanol)

1. Alters the state of **membrane lipid, adenyl cyclase and Na^+K^+ ATPase.**
2. Inhibits NMDA type of excitatory amino acid glutamate receptors, operating through cation channel and promotes $GABA_A$R-mediated synaptic inhibition through chloride channel opening.
3. 5-HT action is enhanced on $5-HT_3$ inhibitory autoreceptor.
4. It inhibits voltage sensitive neural Ca^{++} channel.
5. It enhances NA turnover through opioid R.

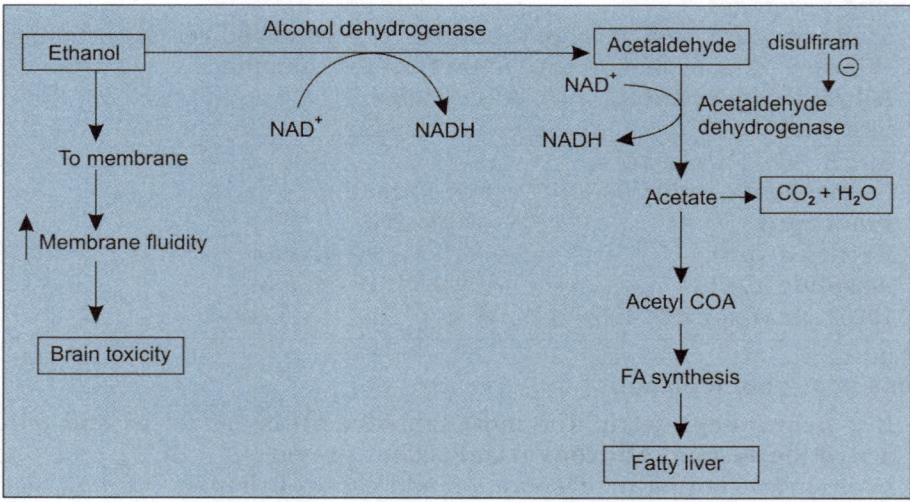

PK: Metabolism is rapid and needs no digestion yielding energy **(7 cal/gm)** that is not stored. Metabolism follows **zero order kinetics** (10–15 ml/hr constantly). Absorption from stomach depends on concentration and stomach contents and determines absorption rate because intestinal absorption is very fast. Widely distributed in the body, crosses placenta, 98% oxidised in liver, excreted by lungs and kidney.

ADR:
1. 150–200 mg/dl → Ataxia
   200–300 mg/dl → Stupor
   >300 mg/dl → Coma, medullary paralysis and death.

2. Fatty liver
3. Brain toxicity
4. Excitement→stupor→coma:
   Contracted pupil dilates
   (McEvan sign).

Causes of cardiomyopathy
Alcohol
Beriberi
Cocaine, Coxsackievirus
Doxorubicin
ABCD

Toxicity: On moderate drinking: Traffic accident and flushing. At 100 mg/100 ml–alcohol gaze nystagmus.

(A) Acute alcoholic intoxication: Causes **hypoglycaemia** hence glucose is given.

Treatment
1. Airway maintenance.   **ABCDEFG**
2. Breathing maintenance.
3. Circulation maintenance.
4. Drip (fructose + insulin) accelerates its metabolism (**most** patients recovered by supportive therapy).
5. ECG monitoring and electrolyte balance.
6. Fluid maintenance.
7. Gastric lavage.

(B) Chronic alcoholism: Develops tolerance and dependence (physical and psychic), nutritional deficiencies (due to malabsorption and neglected food), neuropathy (polyneuropathy, pellagra, seizure, tremors, **Korsakoff's psychosis**, Wernicke's encephalopathy), cirrhosis, HTN, myopathy (skeletal and cardiac), CHF, arrhythmia, ↓immunity, withdrawal syndrome (anxiety, sweating, confusion, hallucination, delirium), convulsion and collapse. Peripheral neuropathy (commonest).

Treatment
— Psychological and medical supportive measures.
— CNS depressant preferably BZD (diazepam, chlordiazepoxide), others are barbiturate, chloralhydrate, phenothiazines. Naltrexone inhibits relapse of alcoholism (reducing alcohol craving and frequency).

IA of ethanol
— Aspirin causes gastric bleeding with alcohol.
— Enhances generation of toxic metabolite of paracetamol.
— Enhances hypoglycemia.
— Acute ingestion inhibits and chronic ingestion induces phenytoin and tolbutamide metabolism.

- Alcohol with Cephalosporin/Sulfonamide/Metronidazole causes bizarre somewhat disulfiram like reaction. **MSc**
- It synergises with hypnotics, antihistaminics and opioid and causes CNS depression with motor impairment.

CI of ethanol
- Epilepsy, hyperacidity, peptic ulcer, liver disease.
- Pregnant mother: Causes foetal alcohol syndrome (low IQ, growth retardation, immunological impairment), LBW and miscarriage.
- Unstable personalities. Consumption of >3 drinks/day leads to ADR (hence avoid drinking). Safe limit for woman is lower than that of man. One drink = 50 ml of spirit =150 ml of wines = 400 ml of beer has about 20 gm alcohol.

U of ethanol
1. **Antiseptics:** 100% ethanol is more dehydrating but poorer antiseptic than 80% because antiseptic action which is enhanced from 20 to 70% remains constant from 70 to 90% and is reduced above that is not due to dehydration of bacterial protoplasm. Spores are not killed by ethanol.
2. Bedsores.
3. Counter-irritant and rubefacient.
4. After shave lotions due to astringent actions.
5. Methanol poisoning.
6. To reduce body temperature in fever.
7. Reflex stimulation in fainting/hysteria.
8. As appetite stimulant and carminative (40 ml of 8% alcohol).

Disulfiram

Mech: Inhibits **aldehyde (acetaldehyde) dehydrogenase irreversibly,** enhances acetaldehyde concentration in the body, causes **aldehyde syndrome** which reinforces not to drink. It also inhibits **alcohol dehydrogenase**, DA β-hydroxylase, CYP450 isoenzymes, and prolongs t½ of many drugs.

ADR
1. **Causes aldehyde syndrome lasting 1–4 hrs, characterised by:** Flushing, fainting, burning sensation, throbbing headache, confusion, visual disturbances, tachycardia, hyperventilation and CV collapse.
2. Metallic taste, abdominal upset, nervousness, malaise and rashes.

U: Not to drink alcohol (citrated calcium carbimide is similar to disulfiram but is rapid acting + short lasting).

Dose of disulfiram		
1 gm	—	Ist day
¾ gm	—	2nd day
½ gm	—	3rd day
¼ gm	—	Subsequently

OR ½ gm per day for 14 days followed by ¼ gm (max)/day. Effects start after 2–3 hrs of first dose and lasts for 7–14 days after stopping it. Fresh enzyme synthesis continues the activity.

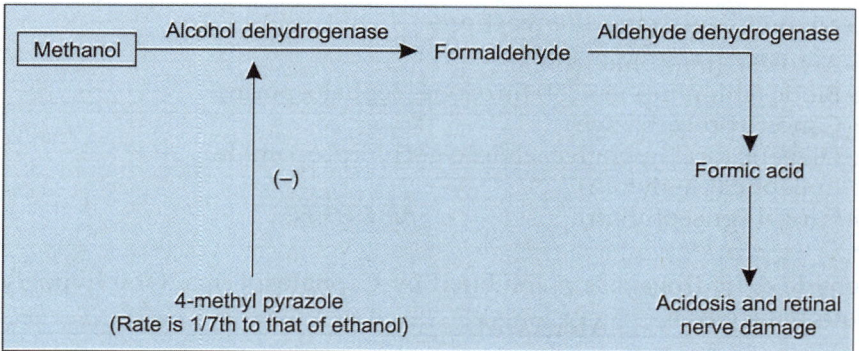

Methanol (Wood Alcohol): **Less potent** CNS depressant than ethanol.
PK: Follows **zero order kinetics, t½ →20–60 hrs.**
Methanol + rectified spirit = unfit for drinking.
ADR: It is due to formic acid. Fatal dose = 75–100 ml, fatal period = 1 day, 15 ml causes blindness.
— Dyspnoea, bradycardia, hypotension, headache, epigastric pain. Formic acid causes acidosis, retinal damage (blindness) and death due to respiratory failure.

Treatment of methanol poisoning: **ABCDEFGH**

1. **A**cidosis treatment by **IV NaHCO₃ (the most important measure).** **A**irway maintenance.
2. **B**reathing maintenance.
3. **C**irculation maintenance.
4. **D**rugs—4-methylpyrazole.
5. **E**ye protection from light. Ethanol (specific antidote) 100 mg/dl in blood saturates alcohol dehydrogenase and reduces methanol metabolism.
   Dose: 0.7 ml/kg/hr then 0.15 ml/kg/hr drip.
6. **F**olate therapy (Ca leucovorin) reduces blood formate level by enhancing its metabolism.
7. **G**astric lavage by NaHCO₃.
8. **H**aemodialysis (treatment of choice) clears methanol and formate. Hypokalemia due to alkali therapy is treated by IV KCl.

Fomepizole: Approved by FDA in late 1997. Orphan drug due to rare use and increased cost (₹ 2 Lakh/patient).

Mech: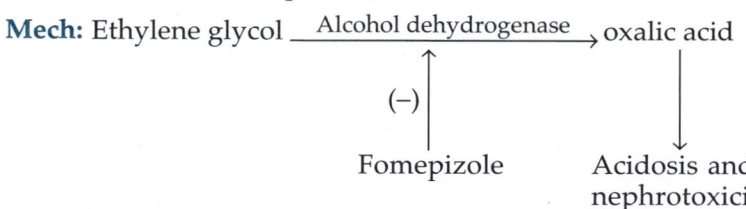

ADR: 1. Headache, nausea, dizziness are most common, 2. Allergy.
U: Ethylene glycol poisoning (1 gm/ml IV). Antidote is methanol.

Pharmacology Review

Drugs causing disulfiram like reactions

Anti-**A**moebic (metronidazole).
Anti-**B**iotic (chloramphenicol, furoxone, cephalosporin)
Anti-**C**ancer (procarbazine)
Anti-**D**iabetic (oral hypoglycaemic, e.g. chlorpropamide)
Anti-**E**pileptic (phenytoin)
Anti-**F**ungal (griseofulvin).   **ABCDEF**

Aldehyde dehydrogenase is inhibited by **C**ephalosporins, **O**ral hypoglycaemic and **M**etronidazole   **Ald. COM**

14. Drugs for Mental Illness: Psychotropic Drugs, Psychopharmacological Agents

The simplest way to describe a psychiatric disorder is as a disturbance of *Conation* (action), *Cognition* (thought), and *Affect* (feeling).

At present, there are 2 major classifications in psychiatry: ICD-10 (WHO) and DSM-IV. These drugs effect **Psyche** (mental process), hence used in psychiatric disorder.

Psychoses: These mean **disorientation** of thought, behavior, perception (delusion, hallucination) and capacity to recognise reality, are:
  a. **Acute and chronic** organic brain syndrome (cognitive disorder), i.e. delirium, dementia.
  b. **Functional disorder** (undefined cause, i.e. memory and orientation retained but emotion and thought behavior altered):
     Schizophrenia (split mind)   =   **Bipolar** (manic-depressive).
     Paranoid state (false belief)   =   **Unipolar** (mania/depression).

Affective disorder: It is mania and depression.

Neuroses are anxiety, phobic state, obsessive and compulsive disorder (limited abnormality of thought and behavior not to be removed on voluntary effort), reactive depression (due to bereavement, etc.), hysterical (dramatic symptoms like serious illness). **Schizophrenia and mania** are due to **dopaminergic overactivity** whereas **depression** is due to **monoaminergic (NA, 5-HT) deficit, with 3 types (endogenous, reactive, bipolar affective).**

Causes of schizophrenia
1. Age 15–25 years for **Male** and 25–35 years for **Female**.
   12% children on **one parent loss,** 35% children on both **parents loss.** 50% monozygotic twin.
2. **Dopaminergic overactivity:**

Classification of schizophrenia
1. Simple (**worst** prognosis)
2. Hebephrenic
3. Catatonic (**commonest** type, **best prognosis**).

Commonest symptom →auditory hallucination.
  Bleuler's 4 As of "**schizophrenia**":
  — Ambivalence
  — Autism

— Blunted Affect
— Loose Association

Major depressive episode is characterised by **5 of the following for 2 weeks** including depressed mood or anhedonia:
— **S**leep disturbances
— **I**nterest loss   **SIG Energy CAPSules**
— **G**uilt
— **E**nergy loss
— **C**oncentration loss
— **A**ppetite change
— **P**sychomotor retardation
— **S**uicidal ideations

Manic episode: Distinct period of abnormally and persistently **elevated** expansive or irritable mood lasting at least **1 week**.

During mood disturbance, **3 or more of the following occur:**
— **D**istractibility
— **I**nsomnia   **DIG FAST**
— **G**randiosity
— **F**light of ideas
— Increase in goal directed **A**ctivity (psychomotor agitation)
— Persistent **S**peech
— **T**houghtlessness

Treatment is symptomatic, not disease specific and **drugs are:**
Psychotomimetic, antipsychotic, antianxiety, antidepressant and antimanic.

Tranquilizer reduces mental tension and produces calmness without inducing sleep or depressing mental faculties.

Classification of antipsychotic drugs

1. Butyrophenones — Droperidol
   BOAT in Pond   — Haloperidol
                      — Penfluridol
   MRP — Six Lacs — Trifluperidol   **DTPH = Dil To Pagal Hai**
2. Others: Pimozide, Sulpiride, Loxapine, Reserpine, Molindone.
3. Atypical: Clozapine, Olanzapine, REsperidone.   **CORE**
4. Thioxanthenes: Chlorprothixene, Flupenthixol, Thiothixene.
   CFT = Complement Fixation Test
5. **Phenothiazines**
   Aliphatic side chain: Chlorprom**azine**, Triflupromazine.   **CAT**
   Piperi**D**ine side chain: Thiori**D**azine.
   Piperazine side chain: Trifuoper**azine**, Thioproper**azine** and Fluphen**azine**.

   Fertilization of Two ova in Two different cycles (superfeTation)

Chlorpromazine

Chlorpromazine (CPZ) (as prototype) has **aliphatic side chain.** It is antipsychotic with **2nd highest** anticholinergic action.

Actions

> Chlorpromazine is the prototype **ANTIPSYCHOTIC**. Its actions are:
> Antipsychotic effect in psychotic patients (therapeutic effect).
> Neuroleptic syndrome in normal persons (unpleasant).
> Temperature control is disturbed.
> Increased chances of epileptic fits due to decreased seizure threshold.
> Prolactin release increases—galactorrhoea and gynecomastia.
> Side effects: Extrapyramidal, e.g. Parkinsonism, dystonias, akathisia, dyskinesia.
> Yellowness, i.e. cholestatic jaundice.
> Cholinergic antagonism leading to dry mouth, etc.
> Hypotension
> Obesity
> Tolerance to some effects like sedation.
> Inhibition of gonadotropin secretion and D_2 R mainly.
> Certain spastic conditions are relieved.

1. CNS is effected differently in **normal and psychotic persons:**
   A. **Normal person:** Produces **neutral and unpleasant** effects, different from sedative action of barbiturates and neuroleptic syndrome (indifference to surrounding, psychomotor slowing, emotional quietening, loss of sleep).
   B. **Psychotic person: Suppresses** delusion, hallucination, hyperactivity, relieves anxiety, **normalises** altered thought and behavior, **reduces** irritational behavior, agitation, aggressiveness and **controls psychotic** symptoms.
   All phenothiazines + thioxanthenes + butyrophenones have same antipsychotic efficacy. Aliphatic and piperidine side chains (phenothiazines) produce **more sedation immediately** (antipsychotic effects take weeks to develop). **Tolerance** is due to sedative action, not due to antipsychotic action. **Vigilance** is impaired. CPZ reduces **seizure threshold** causing fits in untreated epileptics. It produces **poikilothermic effect** (fall in body temperature in cold surrounding).
   Neuroleptics, **except** thioridazine, have potent **antiemetic** action exerted through **CTZ**.
2. Neuroleptics are **α blocker** in the order:
   CPZ= triflupromazine > thioridazine > fluphenazine > haloperidol > trifluoperazine > clozapine > pimozide
   Anticholinergic in the order: **Thioridazine > CPZ > triflupromazine > trifluoperazine = haloperidol.**
   Phenothiazines are **weak H_1 blocker** and **5-HT blocker**. Neuroleptics do not affect **spinal reflexes**.
3. CPZ is as potent as procaine but is **irritant**.
4. They reduce skeletal muscle **spasticity** (**site of action**—basal ganglia and medulla oblongata).
5. They cause **hypotension** through **α** blockade (central and peripheral action). CPZ reduces heart action and produces ECG changes (**Q-T prolongation and T-wave suppression**).
6. They enhance **prolactin release** by blocking inhibitory action of DA on pituitary **lactotropes** → **galactorrhoea and gynaecomastia**. Reduce **gonadotropin**

secretion, GH release, ADH release (↑ urine), ACTH release (↓corticosteroid level).

Mech: All antipsychotics (except clozapine like) are D_2 blocker.
Clozapine
— Weak D_2 blocker
— Selective D_4 blocker
— 5-HT_2 blocker
— α_1 blocker

Phenothiazine and thioxanthene are D_1, D_2, D_3 and D_4 blockers. Blockade is mainly in **limbic system and mesocortical area**. **DA theory** for schizophrenia = **DA over activity in limbic area**. Antipsychotic actions depend on **specific profile of action of drugs** on several neurotransmitter receptors. Most phenothiazines have antiemetic actions.

Dopaminergic blockade causes extrapyramidal symptoms in basal ganglia and antiemetic action in CTZ. **All antipsychotics** have dopaminergic blocking action. **Tolerance** is due to **sedative** and **hypotensive** actions but not due to antipsychotic and extrapyramidal actions. **Physical dependence** is **absent** in neuroleptics.

PK: Brain concentration > plasma concentration. Volume of distribution—20 L/kg. Hepatic metabolism into many metabolites. Duration of action—6–8 hrs. Elimination t½—**30 hrs (variable)**. Drug **cumulates**. Excreted in **urine and bile** for months after discontinuation. Dose of CPZ = 100–800 mg/day. Long t½ of most antipsychotics allows OD intake.

ADR of neuroleptics

A. Hypersensitivity reaction (not dose related)
— Skin rashes, urticaria, contact dermatitis, photosensitivity = 5%.
— Cholestatic jaundice = 4%.
— Agranulocytosis (common with clozapine) = 0.8%.

B. Dose related   ACE Blockade
— **A**nticholinergic (dry mouth, constipation, urinary hesitency, blurred vision).
— **C**NS (confusion, drowsiness, tolerance and ↑ appetite).
— **E**ndocrine (amenorrhoea, infertility, gynaecomastia due to ↑ prolactin and ↓gonadotropin).
— Extrapyramidal disturbances (least with clozapine, risperidone, thioridazine, and more with potent drugs).
— α **B**lockade (postural hypotension, palpitation, inhibition of ejaculation).
— Blue pigmentation of exposed skin and retinal degeneration.

Extrapyramidal ADR

1. **P**arkinsonism (rigidity, tremor, hypokinesia, **m**ask-like facies, shuffling gait) within **1 month**.   SMART Person
2. **A**cute **M**uscular dystonia: Bizarre muscle spasm **mostly** involving linguofacial muscle (grimacing, torticollis, locked jaw) **mostly** in the **first week** of therapy. Common in girls <10 yrs, incidence—2%.
   Treatment: Benztropine, promethazine, hydroxyzine.
3. Aka**t**hisia/**Not to sit** (**r**estlessness, feeling of discomfort, apparent agitation, manifested as compelling desire to move about but without anxiety), incidence 20%. **Commonest** extrapyramidal ADR. **2 mg benztropine (IM)** differentiate akathisia from psychosis (only akathisia responds).
   Treatment: Dose reduction/alternative neuroleptic.

4. Malignant neuroleptic **S**yndrome (rigidity, immobility, fever, fluctuating BP and HR) occurs rarely. **Treatment:** Bromocriptine, dantrolene.
5. **Tardive dyskinesia: Common** ADR of phenothiazine on chronic use. **Most severe extrapyramidal ADR.** It is purposeless involuntary facial and limb movements, constant chewing, pouting, puffing of cheeks, lip licking, choreoathetoid movements. It occurs late in therapy.

    It is **commonest** in **elderly women** due to **neuronal degeneration** along with supersensitivity to DA. **Antiparkinsonian anticholinergics** accentuate and neuroleptics temporarily suppress it. Incidence = 10–20% (uncommon with clozapine and risperidone).
    Treatment—unsatisfactory.
6. **Rabbit tremor** occurs after years with neuroleptics and responds to central anticholinergic drugs.

Evolution of ADR	
4 hours	Acute dystonia
4 days	Akinesia
4 weeks	Akathisia
4 months	Tardive dyskinesia

IA of neuroleptics

1. Enzyme inducers **(anticonvulsants, barbiturates) reduce blood level of neuroleptics.**
2. CPZ reduces antihypertensive action of **clonidine and methyldopa** and abolishes antihypertensive action of **guanethidine** by blocking its active transport into adrenergic terminal.
3. Neuroleptics block action of **levodopa and direct DA agonist** in parkinsonism and **potentiate all CNS depressant** (alcohol, hypnotic, anxiolytic, opioid, analgesic, antihistaminic).

Uses of neuroleptics (intensity of antipsychotic action is poorly correlated with plasma concentration):

1. **Neuroleptics DOC in**
    — Schizophrenia (DOC–CPZ). (**Fluphenazine** in patient not taking CPZ–DOC).
    — **Delirium, mania, manic phase** of manic—depressive illness, **psychosis.**
    — **Gilles de la Tourette's** (haloperidol–DOC).
    — **Neuroleptanalgesia** (fentanyl + droperidol).
    — **Intractable cough** (DOC–CPZ).
2. **Anxiety**
3. **As antiemetic**
4. **Preanaesthetic medication.**
5. **To potentiate:** Hypnotic, analgesic and anaesthetics.
6. **Tetanus:** For skeletal muscle relaxation.
7. **Rare indication:** Alcoholic hallucination, Huntington's disease.
8. **Psychoses:** Neuroleptics control **positive symptoms** (hallucination, delusion, insomnia, disorganised thought, anxiety, restlessness, aggression) better than **negative symptoms** (apathy, loss of volition and insight, poverty of speech, affective flattening, social withdrawal) and restore cognitive, affective and motor disturbances **(90% cure rate). Treatment** is symptomatic and lifelong.

Disorders	DOC
1. Hypomania and mood elevation	Haloperidol, thioproperazine
2. Negative symptoms and resistance cases	Clozapine
3. Withdrawn and apathetic	Trifluoperazine, fluphenazine.
4. Agitated, violent and combative	CPZ, triflupromazine
5. Extrapyramidal ADR	Risperidone, clozapine, thioridazine
6. Elder patients	One potent drug

Neuroleptics are for rapid control of **mania** and for short-term basis to control **organic brain syndrome. Maximum therapeutic effect** in chronic schizophrenia occurs in **2–4 months** therapy.

DISTINCTIVE FEATURES OF OTHER NEUROLEPTICS

Molindone: It is indole compound, has less marked antidopaminergic and sedative actions. Hypotensive and antiemetic actions absent.

Olanzapine

Mech: Blocks muscarinic, H_1 and monoaminergic (α_1, α_2, D_2, 5-HT_2) receptors (antipsychotic action means D_2 and 5-HT_2 blockade).
    PK: Metabolised by CYP1A2 and glucuronyltransferase.
           Half-life = 24–30 hours.
    ADR: **WE ARE** ADR
           Weight gain
           Extrapyramidal
           Anticholinergic (constipation, dry mouth, etc.)
           Raised prolactin
           Epileptogenic
    U: Schizo-Affective disorder
           Olanzapine + Lithium/Valproate in **M**ania/Bipolar disorder.
           Schizophrenia (positive and negative). **SMS**

Risperidone is D_2 blocker, α blocker ($\alpha_1 + \alpha_2$), 5-HT_2 blocker, H_1 blocker.

Antiemetic action **absent. All antipsychotics** have sedative, antiemetic, hypotensive and extrapyramidal effects. Molindone, risperidone, clozapine have **no antiemetic** action. Molindone has **no hypotensive** action.

Clozapine is **atypical** antipsychotic.

Mech: Only weak D_2 blocker, suppresses schizophrenia and refractory to typical neuroleptic respond. *Selective D_4 blockade*, M blocker, α_1 blocker, H_1 blocker, 5-HT_2 blocker.

    ADR: Agranulocytosis (0.8%)—**major limitation, sedation** and **salivation, increase HR, unstable BP, urinary incontinence, myocarditis.**

    U: Resistant schizophrenia (**2nd choice**).
    Reserpine: The **first** psychoactive drug used in schizophrenia.
    Mech: Acts by depleting brain **DA, NA and 5-HT.**

ADR: Mental depression, suicidal tendency.
Loxapine is **dibenzoxazepine** with **CPZ like** DA blocking and antipsychotic action.
Sulpiride: Selective D_2 blocker.
U: Controls **florid +ve symptoms** of schizophrenia **at high doses.**
Dose: 1000 mg BD for **+ve symptoms.**
  300 mg BD for **–ve symptoms.**
Pimozide is DA blocker, α blocker, cholinergic blocker.
ADR: Arrhythmia.

Triflupromazine
ADR: Acute muscle dystonia in children.
Thioridazine: Central anticholinergic action (**highest** among antipsychotics).
ADR:
  — **Lowest** incidence of extrapyramidal ADR.
  — Male sexual dysfunction.
  — Cardiac arrhythmia (**highest** cardiotoxic antipsychotic).
  — Brawning of vision (drugs causing cardiomyopathy—**L**i, **E**metine, **T**hioridazine, **S**ulfonamide, **S**ympathomimetics).   **LET'S**
Haloperidol: Action resembles piperazine substituted phenothiazine.
U: Acute schizophrenia, Huntington's disease, Gilles de la Tourette's syndrome. (**weight gain** is ADR with all antipsychotics **except haloperidol**).
Droperidol: Used **mostly in GA.**
Penfluridol: Exceptionally long-acting neuroleptic.
U: Chronic schizophrenia, affective withdrawal, social maladjustment.
Chlorprothixene: Resembles CPZ.

Anxiolytic drugs: Classification   **BIG**
1. BZD 2. β blocker 3. **Azapirone: B**uspirone, **I**psapirone, **G**epirone. 4. Other sedatives: Meprobamate, hydroxyzine.

Anxiety is **universal phenomenon** and is emotional state, unpleasant in nature, associated with uneasiness, discomfort and fear about some defined or undefined future threat and may be pathological or a part of normal life. **Anxiolytic drugs** are **mild depressant (CNS),** resembling sedative–hypnotic, have **anticonvulsant** property, produce physical **dependence** and carry **abuse liability.**
Buspirone: It is the **first azapirone** and is different from **BZD** because:
1. Sedation/cognitive/functional impairment is **absent.**
2. It does **not** interact with BZD R/modify GABAergic transmission, not produce tolerance/dependence, not suppress BZD/barbiturate withdrawal syndrome.
3. Muscle relaxant and anticonvulsant activity **absent.**

Mechanism: Weak D_2 blocker, selective $5\text{-}HT_{1A}$ R partial agonist-antagonist. Anxiolytic effects take a week to develop.
Non-BZD, nonsedative.
PK: Rapdily absorbed, extensive first pass metabolism, bioavailability < 5%, t½— 3 hrs, excreted in urine and faeces.
ADR: Dizziness, nausea, headache, light headedness.
Meprobamate was **the first tranquilliser** with centrally acting muscle relaxant property.

Hydroxyzine is H_1 **blocker** with sedative, antiemetic, antimuscarinic and spasmolytic properties.

DRUGS FOR AFFECTIVE DISORDERS

Affective disorders (pathological change in mood state) have **2 extremes** (bipolar cycle of mood siwings) **mania ⇌ depression.**

Drugs are:
1. Antimanic (mood stabilizer): Li_2CO_3
2. Antidepressant: TCA, MAO inhbitor.

MAO inhibitors
A. Isoenzyme selective
 1. MOA-**A**: **C**lorgiline, **M**oclobemide.   **MCA**
 2. MOA-B: Selegiline (deprenyl).
B. Nonselective
 1. **H**ydrazine: **P**henelzine, **I**socarboxazid.   **HIP**
 2. Nonhydrazine: Tranylcypromine.

TCA (Tricyclic and related antidepressant)
1. **N**onselective (NA: 5-HT) RI: **A**mitriptyline, **D**oxepin, **D**othiepin, **I**mipramine, **C**lomipramine, **T**rimipramine.

   Never **ADD ICT** (hypotension)

2. **PreD**ominantly **NA** (NA >5-HT) reuptake inhibitors: **P**roptriptyline, **D**esipramine, **N**ortriptyline, **A**moxapine.
3. **Selective 5-HT reuptake inhibitors (SSRI):** Fluoxetine, Fluvoxamine, Paroxetine, Sertraline, Citalopram.

   First For Prophylaxis + Severe Case

4. **Atypical: M**ianserin, **B**upropion, **C**ongener of trazodone (nefazodone), **A**mineptine, **T**razodone, **M**ianserin, **T**ianeptine, **V**enlafaxine.

   Monica + Bill Clinton **AT MTV**

5. **Newer compound:** Maprotiline (DA R inhibitor).

MAO

MAO is **mitochondrial enzyme** for **oxidative deamination of biogenic amines** (Adrenaline, NA, DA, 5-HT). **2 isoenzyme** forms of **MAO: MAO-A** and **MAO-B**.

MAO-A deaminates **5-HT and NA**. **MAO-B** deaminates **phenylethylamine.** Both isoenzymes degrade **DA equally.**

Distribution: Peripheral **A**drenergic nerve ending, and **A**limentary (intestinal) mucosa including human placenta contain **MAO-A mainly.** Brain and Blood platelet contain **MAO-B mainly. Liver** contains **both** MAO-A and B.

Mechanism of MAO inhibitors: Inhibit MAO **irreversibly** and **noncompetitively** allowing **NA, DA, 5-HT** to accumulate in their respective neurones in brain and periphery. **Selegiline** selectively inhibits MAO-B at doses 5–10 mg/day, and is metabolised to **amphetamine. At high doses,** it becomes **nonselective** (exhibits antidepressant and excitant properties).

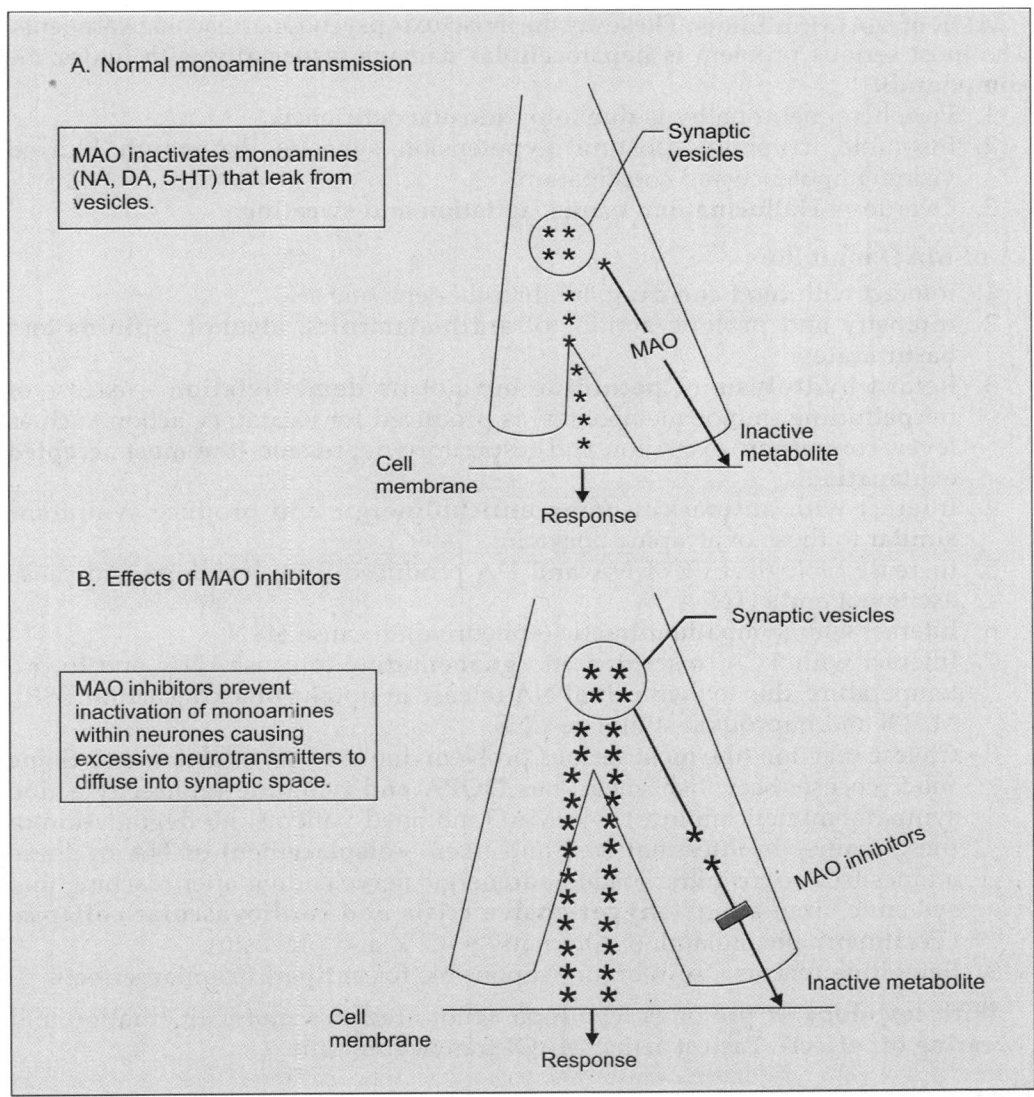

A. Normal monoamine transmission

MAO inactivates monoamines (NA, DA, 5-HT) that leak from vesicles.

B. Effects of MAO inhibitors

MAO inhibitors prevent inactivation of monoamines within neurones causing excessive neurotransmitters to diffuse into synaptic space.

MAO-B inhibitor suppresses the production of **neurotonic substances in nigrostriatal dopaminergic tract** (thus retards the disease process). Selective (only alters **basic pathology** of parkinsonism).

Nonselective MAO inhibitors are mood elevators in depression. MAO inhibitor causes **postural hypotension** due to ↓ **central sympathetic outflow**, inhibition of nerve impulse coupled **release of NA** from adrenergic nerve ending and interference with **ganglionic transmission**. Drugs themselves stay in the body for relatively short period but their effects last **2–3 weeks** after discontinuation. Tissue monoamine level **remains elevated** long after the drug has been largely eliminated.

Return of MAO actively depends on **fresh enzyme synthesis** hence drug is called "hit and run drug".

ADR of MAO inhibitors: These are the **most toxic** psychopharmacological agents. The most serious problem **is hepatocellular damage (especially with** hydrazine **compound).**
1. Peripheral neuropathy **is due to** pyridoxine deficiency.
2. Insomnia, irritability, postural hypotension, syncope, dry mouth, blurred vision, impotence and constipation.
3. Overdose: **Hallucination, mania, agitation and sweating.**

IA of MAO inhibitors
1. Interact with **food and drug.** Inhibit other enzyme also.
2. Intensify and prolong actions of **antihistaminics, alcohol, opioids and barbiturates.**
3. Retard **hydrolysis** of **pethidine** but not its **demethylation** →excess of **norpethidine** (minor metabolites) is produced for excitatory action such as fever, convulsion, excitation and respiratory depression **(the most accepted explanation).**
4. Interact with **antiparkinsonian anticholinergic** and produce symptoms **similar** to those of atropine poisoning.
5. Increase biological t½ of **NA and DA** produced from levodopa and cause excitment and HTN.
6. Interact with **sympathomimetic** (ephedrine) to cause HTN.
7. Interact with **TCA, reserpine** and **guanethidine** to cause HTN and to rise temperature, due to their **initial NA release or uptake blocking action.** SSRI, MAOI and bupropion stimulate CNS.
8. **Cheese reaction** (the **most serious** problem due to MAO inhibitor use). **Some food** (cheese, beer, fish, meat) has **DOPA and tyramine** (indirectly acting sympathomimetic amines) →in MAO inhibited patients, **no degradation** of these amines in intestinal wall and liver →**displacement of NA** by these amines from transmitter loaded adrenergic nerve ending after reaching into systemic circulation →**hypertensive crisis and cardiovascular collapse.** **(Treatment:** phentolamine. Alternative—CPZ and prazosin).
9. **Selegiline** retards DA in brain (responsible for **antiparkinsonian effect).**

With **levodopa,** it prolongs levodopa action, reduces motor fluctuation and "wearing off effect". **Fastest** acting MAOI-tranylcypromine.

Uses of MAO inhibitors
1. Major **depression** (not responding to TCA and ECT **contraindicated** patient).
2. **Narcolepsy** (by inhibiting REM sleep).
3. **Neurotic problem** (phobic state, obsessive compulsive behaviour).
4. Adjuvant to levodopa (reduce levodopa dose up to **30%** and benefit **50–70%** patients). **ON-OFF effect** worsens, as clinical benefit of selegiline is short lived (6–26 month).

CI: Selegiline contraindicated in **convulsive disorder.**

Moclobemide: It is **reversible selective MAO-A inhibitor** and only weakly potentiates the pressor action to ingested tyramine **(no dietary restriction).** It is **safer in overdose** and **lacks** sedative, anticholinergic and cardiovascular effects of typical TCA.

U: Alternative to TCA for major **depression** and **social phobia.**

TCA

TCA: Imipramine (prototype) is a **dibenzazepine** and **analogue** of phenothiazine in which **sulfur** atom of central ring is replaced by **ethylene** bridge (structure **similar** to phenothiazine). Some **atypical and selective 5-HT** reuptake inhibitor in the past 20 years is **the most significant development** in psychosis treatment.

Basis of TCA: Drugs improve mood in depressant patient but not in normal subject.

Actions of TCA (imipramine)

1. TCA inhibits monoamine uptake and acts on R (**M, D_2, α, H_1, $5\text{-}HT_1$**, and **$5\text{-}HT_2$**). All antidepressants potentiate 5-HT and NA.
2. In **normal person,** it causes peculiar **clumsy** feeling, **light headedness, sleepiness,** difficulty in concentrating and thinking, **unsteady gait,** and no **euphoria or mood elevation.**
3. In depressed patients, it causes **mood elevation, interest in self and surrounding,** more communication, **suppressed REM sleep, reduced awakening,** EEG effect **similar** to hypnotic at low doses but **desynchronisation** at high doses, lowering seizure threshold (hence **convulsion**).
4. In **overdoses,** only imipramine and amitriptyline depress **respiration.**
5. Bupropion, maprotiline, clomipramine have **the highest** seizure precipitating potential.
6. Causes **tachycardia** due to **anticholinergic and NA** potentiating action. Postural hypotension is due to **cardiovascular reflex inhibition and α_1 blockade.** T-wave suppression/inversion is **the most consistent change in ECG.**
7. Most TCAs (except fluoxetine, fluvoxamine, trazodone and bupropion) are anticholinergic.

Mechanism of TCAs

1. Inhibit active uptake of **amines** (NA, 5-HT) into neurons and **potentiate** them. **Only bupropion and maprotiline** inhibit **DA uptake. Cocaine and amphetamine** (both are CNS stimulant) inhibit **DA uptake. Amoxapine and maprotiline** block DA R (possess antipsychotic or neuroleptic activity). Hence, **amine** concentration is **enhanced** in the **synaptic cleft** in CNS and periphery.
2. Reason for stimulant action—**DA uptake inhibition.**
   Reason for sedative action—**5-HT uptake inhibition.**
   Reason for antidepressant action—**NA and 5-HT uptake inhibition.**
3. Initially, increased NA/5-HT in the synaptic cleft activates **presynaptic α_2 and $5\text{-}HT_1$ auto R** resulting in **reduced firing of raphe (serotonergic) and locus coeruleus (noradrenergic) neurons.** After long-term administration, adaptive changes in the **number** and **sensitivity** of pre- and postsynaptic NA/5-HT R and in **amine turnover** of brain enhance serotonergic transmission.

PK: Average dose **2 mg/kg/day** for all **except** fluoxetine and paroxetine (maximum 1 mg/kg/day).

Tolerance develops gradually. No abuse potential. **Slow** oral absorption. **Hepatic** metabolism.

Imipramine $\xrightarrow{\text{demethylation}}$ Desipramine (active metabolite).

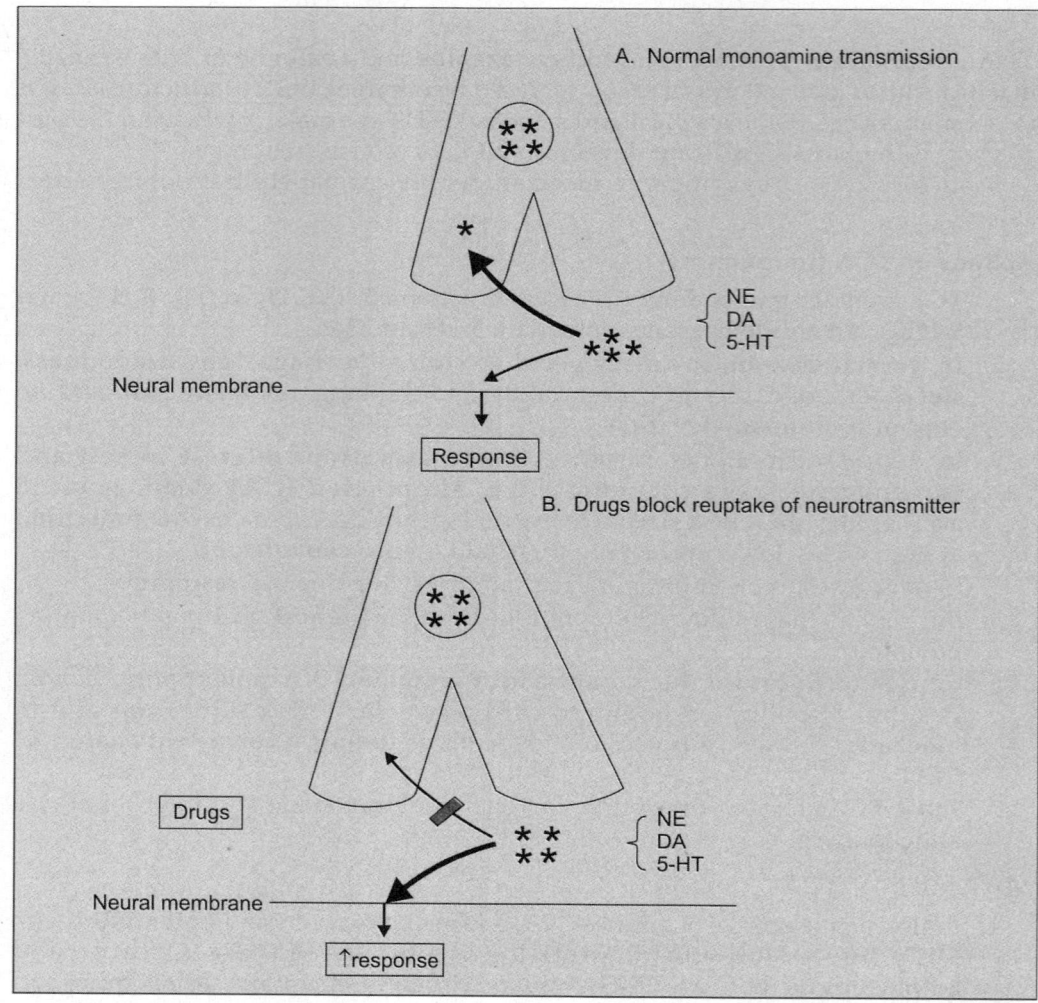

Amitriptyline $\xrightarrow{\text{demethylation}}$ **Nortriptyline** (active metabolite).

Oxidation and glucuronide conjugation inactivate metabolites. Excretion in urine over **1–2 weeks**.

Plasma t½ of imipramine, amitriptyline, doxepin = 16–24 hrs and fluoxetine = 2 days.

Therapeutic window (optimal antidepressant effect exerted at a narrow band of plasma concentration) is shown by imipramine, amitriptyline, nortriptyline = **50–200 hg/ml.**

Beneficial effect is **suboptimal** both above and below this range.

ADR: It is due to sedative, anticholinergic and antiadrenergic actions.

ADR of **SSRI** = **S**erotonin syndrome (causes **HARM** = **H**yperthermia, **A**utonomic instability, **R**igidity, **M**yoclonus), **S**timulates CNS, **R**eproductive dysfunction in male, **I**nsomnia.

ADR of **TCAs** = **T**hrombocytopenia, **C**ardiac (MI, stroke), coma, convulsion, **A**nticholinergic, **S**eizures.

Desipramine is least sedating

1. **Mania,** hypomania, **fine tremor, sweating, lower seizure threshold, postural hypotension, caridac arrhythmia.**
2. **Weight gain** and ↑ **appetite** occur by **most** TCA **except** bupropion and SSRI.
3. Sedation, mental confusion, weakness.
4. **Anticholinergic effect** (dry mouth, blurred vision, bad taste, epigastric distress, urinary retention, constipation).

Acute poisoning: Symptoms of atropine poisoning, convulsion and coma, muscle spasm, decreased BP, increased HR, depressed respiration, ECG change, ventricular arrhythmia.

Treatment:
1. HCO_3^- for acidosis.
2. Physostigmine to reverse anticholinergic and cardiac effects.

IA of TCA

1. **Reserprine/guanethidine/TCA** with **MAO inhibitors** casue ↑ temperature, ↑ BP, excitement due to their initial **NA releasing/uptake blocking** action.
2. **MAO inhibitors** cause dangerous hypertensive crisis with hallucination and excitement.
3. **Potentiate** CNS depressants (**alcohol** and **antihistaminics**) and directly acting **sympathomimetic amines, inhibit** indirectly acting sympathomimetic, **abolish** antihypertensive action of **clonidine** and **guanethidine** by preventing their transport into adrenergic neurons.
4. **P**henytoin, **P**henylbutazone, C**P**Z and **A**spirin displace **TCA** from protein binding sites and cause **toxicity.**

> Where there is sins **(PAPZ),** there is toxicity (to **TCA).**

5. **Phenobarbitone** competitively inhibits imipramine metabolism.

Limitation of TCA: **L**imited efficacy, **L**ow therapeutic margin,
Lag time of 2–4 weeks before response
ADR (**A**nticholinergic, **C**ardiovascular and **N**eurological).   **3Ls CAN**

U of TCA

1. **Depression:** TCA **most effective** in severely depressed patients. Response appears after **3 weeks.**
2. **Attention deficit hyperactive disorder in children** (alternative to amphetamine like drugs).
3. **Obsessive—compulsive** and **phobic states** (clomipramine), also to reduce compuslive eating in **bulimia.**
4. **Enuresis** in children >5 yrs.
5. **Peptic ulcer**
6. **Pruritis**
7. **Migraine:** Amitriptyline as prophylaxis.

> Antidepressants have low TI and effects emerge after 2–3 weeks of treatment.

Amoxapine: Inhibits **NA uptake** and blocks D_2. Has **mixed** antidepressant and neuroleptic properties. **Seizures** occur with overdose.

Mianserin: Blocks presynaptic α_2 R ($\uparrow$ NA release and turnover in brain)→ antidepressant action. Blocks 5-HT and H_1 →sedation.
ADR: Seizures occur in overdose, blood dyscrasias, liver dysfunction.
Tianeptine: 5-HT uptake enhancer.
ADR: Flatulence, dry mouth, epigastric pain, insomnia, bodyache.
Venlafaxine: It is a novel antidepressant, sedation absent.
Mech: 5-HT and NA reuptake inhibitor but does not interact with cholinergic, adrenergic and histaminergic R. It enhances BP.
ADR: **R**aised BP, **A**nxiety, **I**mpotence, inhibitor of CYP450, **S**weating, **E**nhanced nasal secretion (nausea), **D**izziness.

RAISED BP

U: Resistant cases (Dose: 150 mg maximum daily). Antidepressant action similar to TCA, faster onset of action.
Mirtazapine: It is noradrenergic and specific serotonergic antidepressant.
Mech: It blocks α_2 autoreceptors NA nerves and heteroreceptors on serotonin nerves (increased release of both NA and serotonin). Enhanced NA also increases firing of serotonergic nerves through α_1 receptors. It blocks $5\text{-HT}_{1,2,3}$ and H_1 receptors.
U: Similar to TCA in mild and severe depression (benefit after one week only).
Trazodone: Blocks **5-HT uptake and α R** and antagonises **5-HT_2** weakly.
Sedation: Postural hypotension and **priapism** (painful penile erection) due to α blockade.
Amineptine: Antidepressant action is due to increased serotonin uptake (similar to tianeptine).
ADR: Postural hypotension, **A**nticholinergic ADR, **C**onductive disturbance of the diseased heart, **T**achycardia. **PACT**
Nefazodone: Trazodone congener.
It selectively blocks 5-HT_2 receptors and 5-HT reuptake. It also blocks α_1, and X_1 receptors, and CYP450.
ADR: Sedation, priapism, postural hypotension.
U: Severe depression (similar to imipramine).
Recurrent depression (prophylaxis).
Sertraline and citalopram: Both SSRIs lead to lower propensity to cause drug interactions when taken together.
Mech: SSRI.
PK: CYP inhibition with longer acting active metabolite and half-life 26 hrs (sertraline). No active metabolite but death in overdose with half-life 33 hrs (citalopram). SSRI + MAOI cause **serotonin syndrome.**
Fluoxetine: SSRI inhibits drug metabolising enzyme **CYP2D6** and enhances **TCA** and **haloperidol** level.
ADR: Dyskinesia, nervousness, anorexia, diarrhoea.
U: Prophylaxis of recurrent depression.
Mirtazapine
Blocks α_2 R, H_1 R, 5-HT R.
Enhances NA and 5-HT release.$\uparrow$ NA enhances firing of **serotonergic raphe neurones** via α_1R.

Li₂CO₃/Mood stabiliser/Antimanic drug: Li^+ is small monovalent **cation which** stabilises **the mood in** bipolar **MDI (Manic Depressive Illness) on prolonged use.**

Mech: Possibly related to inhibition of phosphoinositol cascade.

It **reduces** NA and DA release in the brain, **replaces** body Na^+ and is **equally** distributed inside and outside the cell. It inhibits **hydrolysis** of inositol-1-PO_4^{3-} → reduced free inositol for regeneration of membrane phosphatidyl inositides (**the source of IP₃ and DAG**)→hyperactive neurone for mania is effected. It inhibits **ADH action** on DCT and causes **DI**. It has some **insulin like** action on **glucose metabolism** and also reduces **thyroxine synthesis** by interfering with **iodination of tyrosine.** It also enhances **leucocyte count.**

PK: Well absorbed orally, neither protein bound nor metabolised.

Order of distribution → ECF first → cells → CNS → uniformly in total body water **(0.8 L/kg).**

Most of the filtered Li^+ reabsorption occurs in **PCT**. Renal excretion is rapid for 10–12 hrs (⅕th of creatine clearance). t½—16–30 hrs.

Maintenance dose in MDI → 0.5–0.8 mEq/L.

Episodes of mania →0.8–1.2 mEq/L. **>1.5 mEq/L** →**toxicity.**

Excreted in sweat and saliva and secreted in breast **milk.**

ADR

1. Nephrogenic DI.
2. Thirst and polyuria by **most patient.**
3. Tremors and seizures.
4. CNS toxicity (ataxia, motor incoordination, nystagmus, slurred speech, hyperreflexia, muscle twitch, convulsion, coma).
   Treatment: No specific antidote for Li^+, osmotic diuretic and $NaHCO_3$ infusion, haemodialysis (>4 mEq/L).
5. **Goitre** due to interference with iodination of tyrosine →↓ thyroxine synthesis.

Treatment: Thyroxine administration inhibits TSH and reverses thyroid enlargement.

ADR of LITHIUM: Leukocyte Increased, Tremor, Hypothyroidism, Increased Urine, Moms alerted due to teratogenicity.

CI: Pregnancy→foetal goitre, **sick sinus syndrome.**

IA:
1. Li^+ potentiates **neuroleptics.**
2. **SCh** and **pancuronium** cause prolonged paralysis with Li^+.
3. Li^+ causes insulin/sulfonylurea induced **hypoglycaemia.**
4. Li^+ reduces pressor response to NA.
5. **ACE inhibitors, indomethacin** and **tetracycline** cause Li^+ retention.
6. **Diuretics** promote reabsorption of Na^+ and Li^+ from PCT by causing Na^+ loss→plasma level of Li^+ rise. Na^+ and Li^+ handled by the kidney are the **same.**

U: As carbonate salt (less hygroscopic and less gastric irritant than (LiCl). **10 mg/kg/day** starting. **25 mg/kg/day** (maximum for maintenance).

1. **Acute manic episode: Maintenance** Li therapy for 1 year (maximum) to prevent recurrences.

2. **Prophylaxis of MDI:** Bipolar MDI (**commonest** indication of Li$^+$). Recurrent unipolar depression.
3. **Recurrent:** Neuropsychiatric illness, cluster headache.
4. **Inappropriate: ADH secretion syndrome** to counteract water retention.
5. Cancer chemotherapy induced **leukopenia and agranulocytosis.**

Alternative to Li$^+$: Verapamil and clonidine, Li$^+$ and CBZ for acute mania and bipolar MDI, Li$^+$ and valproate.

Newer drugs for schizophrenia are **sertindole** and **quetiapine** having varied heterocyclic structure. All atypical drugs except sertindole block histamine R. Sertindole prolongs QT interval. **Mesoridazine** is a piperidine.

SSRI + MAOI cause **serotonin syndrome** (hyperthermia, muscle rigidity, myoclonus, rapid changes in vital signs and mental status).

Toxic value for most commonly monitored drugs (Magic of 2)

Digitalis (0.5–1.5)	DDLJ	= Toxicity (**2**)
Lithium (0.6–1.2)		= Toxicity (**2**)
Jogger/stimulant drugs (theophylline) (10–20)		= Toxicity (**20**)
Dilantin/phenytoin (10–20)		= Toxicity (**20**)

15. CNS Stimulants, Cognition Enhancers, Hallucinogens and Psychostimulants

Hallucinogens: These alter mood, thought, behaviour and perception-like psychosis **(a dream-like state). On closing the eyes,** an unending series of colourful, very realistic and fantastic images is seen. **Laughing** is uncontrollable. One can **read but cannot understand. High doses** cause **sinking sensation. Reverse tolerance** and **psychological dependence** present but physical dependence **absent. All are drugs of abuse.**

Drugs are: PCP, LSD, $^9\Delta$THC, Dronabinol.

Phencyclidine (PCP) is **"angel dust" similar** to anaesthesia **Ketamine.** It causes **"drunken like state"** at low doses and **"amphetamine like state"** at high doses. Most dangerous hallucinogen.

LSD (lysergic acid diethylamide): It is **indole amine,** was synthesized by **Hofmann (1938)** from **ergot** alkaloids. It is **the most potent psychedelic,** 25–50 mg produces **all the effects,** stimulates **central sympathetic** to involve serotonergic neurone system in brain. No physical dependence with LSD/cocaine. It is psychedelic and mind-revealing.

Cannabinoids: $^9\Delta$ Tetrahydrocannabinol ($^9\Delta$THC) is **the active principle of** *Cannabis indica* **(Marijuana) obtained from hump plant.** It is **the most popular recreational and ritualistic intoxicant** used for **millennia.** It is abused by **smoking.** Its different forms are:

1. **Bhang** (dried leaves) acts slowly.
2. **Ganja** (dried female influorescence) is smoked and acts instantaneously.
3. **Charas/Hashish** (dried resinous extract from flowering tops and leaves) is the **most potent** and smoked with tobacco.

PK: $^9\Delta$THC $\xrightarrow{Liver}$ 11–OH–$^9\Delta$THC (active metabolite) $\rightarrow$ 8,11–OH$_2$–$^9\Delta$THC (inactive metabolite).

ADR: Loss of sense of time and vivid dream-like state.

Dronabinol (A $^9\Delta$THC) is **antiemetic** used in cancer.

CNS stimulants

Mostly produce a generalised action which results in **convulsion.**

Classification
1. **Convulsants:** Strychnine, picrotoxin, bicuculline, PTZ (pentylene tetrazol).
2. **Psychostimulants:** Amphetamine, Cocaine, Methylphenidate, Pemoline, Methylxanthine.   **CAMP**
3. **Analeptics:** Doxapram, nikethamide, ethyl and propyl butamide.

Cocaine: Smoked as **crack** in free form, has **the most rapid onset** and induces **the most pleasurable effects. Vasoconstrictor.**

ADR: Gangrene, convulsion, perforation of nasal septum. Cocaine and amphetamine are the **commonest abused CNS stimulant →Euphoria. Tactile hallucination/cocaine bug or Magnan's symptom** present.

Strychnine: It is an **alkaloid** from seeds of **Strychnos nux-vomica,** causes reflex, tonic-clonic and symmetrical **convulsions** (glycine R antagonist).

Mech: Stimulates the **whole cerebrospinal axis** by blocking **post-synaptic** inhibition produced by inhibitory transmitter **glycine.** The site is **Renshaw cell-motorneurone junction** in the spinal cord through which inhibition of antagonistic muscle occurs. Any nerve impulse becomes generalised resulting in excitation and convulsion **due to loss of synaptic inhibition.**

Treatment of poisoning: Similar to status epilepticus.

Picrotoxin: Obtained from *A. cocculus*; causes clonic spontaneous asymmetrical **convulsion** due to stimulation of vomiting, vasomotor, respiratory centre of medulla (GABA R antagonist).

Mech: Acts by blocking **presynaptic** inhibition mediated through **GABA** at the distal site of **GABA R** to prevent Cl⁻channel opening.

Treatment of poisoning: Diazepam—DOC.

Bicuculline: It is **synthetic** convulsant and **competitive GABA R** (intrinsic Cl⁻ channel R) **antagonist.**

U: As a research tool.
Pentylene tetrazol (PTZ, metrazol, leptazol):
Mechanism: Same as picrotoxin.

U: For testing anticonvulsant drugs (**commonest**). **Shock therapy** for psychosis and depression (ECT preferred).

Analeptic: It is **stimulant of respiration** and has **resuscitative value** in coma or fainting.

U: Hypnotic drug poisoning. Suffocation on drowning. Acute respiratory insufficiency. **Apnoea** in premature infant. Failure to ventilate after GA. **Respiratory failure** due to high O_2 concentration.

Drugs are
1. Ethyl propyl butamide.
2. **Nikethamide and doxapram:** At low doses, these are selective for **respiratory centre** by stimulating respiration through **carotid and aortic body chemoreceptors** and raising the falling BP.

CNS Stimulants, Cognition Enhancers

Psychostimulant has **cortical action (psychic** effect is more than effects on medullary vital centres).

Methylphenidate similar to amphetamine.

Mechanism: Both release **NA and DA** in the brain. Methylphenidate is **superior** to amphetamine for **hyperkinetic children** (attention deficit disorder) because it causes lesser **tachycardia and growth retardation.**

PK: Well absorbed orally, hepatic metabolism, excreted in urine, t½—1–2 hrs.

ADR: Bowel upset, insomnia, anorexia.

U: Narcolepsy, hyperkinetic person.

Pemoline: Similar to methylphenidate, t½—10 hrs.

Cognition enhancers (cerebroactive drugs)

Dementia: Global impairment of intellect memory and personality (cognitive function) in the absence of gross clouding of consciousness. Alzheimer's disease (**commonest** cause of dementia): Progressive neurodegenerative disorder effecting older individuals. **Atrophy of cortical and subcortical area** is due to deposition of **β-amyloid** protein and formation of **neurofibrillary tangles** with cholinergic deficiency in the brain. APP gene on chromosome-21 has been tried for vaccine preparation.

Mech: ↑ **CBF** (cerebral blood flow), direct support of neuronal metabolism and improvement in memory.

U:
1. **Dementia** of Alzheimer's type (DAT) and multi-infarct dementia (MID).
2. **Memory disturbances.**
3. Mental retardation in children, learning defects.
4. **Hyperkinetic disorder.**
5. **Organic psychosyndrome.**

Classification

1. Nootropic (cognition enhancer): Piracetam.
2. Metabolic enhancer: Dihydroergotoxine (codergocrine).
3. Cholinergic activator: Tacrine, rivastigmine, galantamine, donepezil
4. Vasoactive cerebral protector: Ginkgo biloba.

Piracetam

Mechanism: It has antithrombotic effect, stimulates synaptic transmission and improves ATP/ADP ratio in **telencephalon.**

ADR: Discomfort, insomnia.

U: Dementia and confusion (most noticeable change—alertness). Mental retardation and learning defect.

Piribedil (a dopaminergic agonist): It improves memory, concentration and vigilance in elderly.

Tacrine: Centrally acting reversible anticholinesterase.

Mechanism: ↑ ACh in cortex.

ADR: Polyuria due to peripheral cholinergic activity, increased serum transaminase, hepatitis.

U: Alzheimer's dementia.

Ginkgo biloba: It is **dried extract** of this Chinese plant containing **ginkgo flavon glycoside** (e.g. **ginkgolide B**) which has **PAF antagonistic action.**

Mech: PAF antagonist and antiaggregation of platelet.
U: MID, cognitive and behavioural disorder in elderly.
Pyritinol (pyrithioxine): It consists of **2 pyridoxine molecules** joined through a **disulfide bridge.**

Mech:
1. ↑ blood flow in ischaemic area.
2. ↑ cerebral cholinergic transmission.
3. ↑ glucose transport across BBB.

U:
1. Delayed milestone.
2. Organic brain syndrome.   **COPD**
3. Prolonged anaesthesia.
4. Cardiovascular accident.

> Alzheimer's/A7hiemer's diseases (significance of 7): 7% familial, 7 years time for progress, 7 × 2 and 7 × 3 chromosome involved, occurs after 7 × 7 yrs.

Tobacco

Cigarettes give **nicotine** (active substance) which causes:
1. **CNS stimulation** (arousal, relaxation and mild euphoria).
2. **Stimulation of sympathetic nervous system** →vasoconstriction → ↑BP.

Tars and CO inhaled enhance **COPD, cancer** and **heart disease. Physical and psychological dependence** occurs. **Abstinence** leads to anxiety, insomnia and appetite loss.

Approaches to abstaining from cigarettes
1. **Bupropion** (TCA).
2. Behavioural modification.
3. Nicotine available in gum, patch and inhaler.

Smoking

N. tobacum/Tobacco/cardiac poison (the **most** common species) is the native plant of America, where addiction was introduced to Columbus by American. The **oldest** insecticide known. Cultivated all over the world. Used by **all classes** of people. **All** parts are poisonous except seeds. Dried leaves (tambaku) contain 1–8% nicotine. Anabasine equally toxic to nicotine. Nornicotine is less toxic. Cigarettes are 20th century phenomena. Lobeline of Indian tobacco is less toxic.

Nicotine ($C_{10}H_{14}N_2$) is colourless, volatile, bitter and hygroscopic liquid used as insecticides, worm powder, etc. 2 active principles are nicotine (pyridine bases are collidine and lutidine) and nicotianine. Ptomaine of human body is similar to nicotine but non-poisonous. Tar is carcinogen, nicotine causes premalignant changes, nicotine and CO cause CHD (the most noxious component of smoke). Pan (betel leaf + arecanut + tobacco + slake time) and khaini (tobacco + lime) are most common tobacco chewing in all classes of people. 10% of leukoplakia caused by pan develops into oral cancer. Death rate due to lung cancer (most common, 51% in developed country and 75% man at present) has increased by 75% in male and 135% in female (reported by WHO 1960–80). Every 3rd person is addicted to smoking before the age of 20 years and every 3rd of lung cancer death occurs below the age of 65 years in India. Death rate in developed country, is 91% male and 62% female and in developing country 76% male and 24% female. The largest preventable cause of disease.

Mech: The most prominent effects relate to stimulation of adrenal medulla, CNS, CVS (CA release), GIT (parasympathetic stimulation), salivary and bronchial glands and the medullary vomiting centre, subsequently blockade of autonomic ganglia and NM junction transmission, inhibition of CA release from adrenal medulla, and CNS depression. **First** stimulates vagal nerve and all autonomic ganglia through the body, after that, depresses and lastly paralyses them. Similarly, cerebral and spinal centres are stimulated first and paralysed on later stage. It rivals cyanide as a poison capable of producing rapid death.

PK: Nicotine is major active metabolite of tobacco. Burning acrid taste. Soluble in water alcohol, etc. **(alkaline reaction)**. No absorption from stomach (here, no poisoning). Rapidly absorbed from all mucous membrane, lungs and skin. 80–90% hepatic metabolism. $pKa = 8.5$. Renal excretion in 16 hours. Half-life = 2 hours. Concentration in smoking mother is 0.5 mg/L milk. 10–50% nicotine absorbed during mouth puffing and 80–100% during deep lung inhalation. Single cigarette puff delivers 0.05–0.15 mg nicotine. Filtred cigarette delivers 0.2–1 mg and nonfiltered one 1–2.5 mg nicotine. All mucous membrane except stomach absorbs nicotine. At pH ≤ 5.5, 23% excreted unchanged and at pH 2, 2% renal excretion. Half-life of cotinine = 10–20 hours. Nicotine in liver is changed into nicotine –1'–N–oxide and cotinine (72% renal excretion of both in 4 days).

Fatal dose (FD) = 60–100 mg = 1–2 drop = 1 mg/kg = 30 gm crude tobacco.

1 cigarette = 1 gm tobacco (½ of FD) = 15–30 mg nicotine and 17–27 mg tars.

1 cigar = 15–40 mg nicotine. Smoking provides 1–2 mg nicotine absorption per cigarette.

Chewing tobacco = 2–8 mg/gm. Tobacco leaf = 1–6% nicotine/leaf.

Fatal period = 15 min.

ADR: Indian filtered cigarette is completely unsafe.

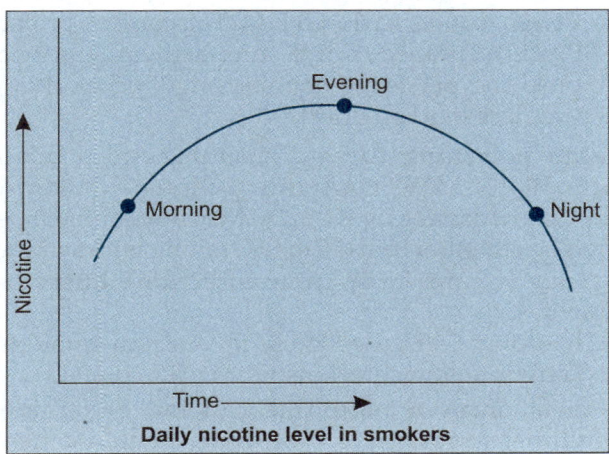

Daily nicotine level in smokers

A. **Acute poisoning:** Green tobacco sickness occurs during processing and extracting tobacco (child **most** effected). Nicotine poisoning manifests in 15 min (GIT first).

Psychological habituation to smoking is complete and so far largely insoluble problem for most smokers. Nicotine overdose causes PMN leukocytosis and glycosuria. Smoking elevates serum thiocyanate level.

1. **Gut:** Disturbance and hypersalivation.
2. **CVS:** Early (tachycardia, hypotension, tachypnoea) and late (bradycardia, hypotension and respiratory depression even death too).
3. **CNS:** Early (confusion, headache, sweating, ataxia, agitation, restlessness, hyperthermia) and late (lethargy, miosis in early stage followed by mydriasis in late stage, convulsion and coma).

B. **Chronic poisoning:** Cough, wheezing, dyspnoea, anorexia, vomiting, diarrhoea, anemia, faintness, impaired memory, amblyopia, blindness, tobacco heart (extrasystole and angina pectoris), bronchitis due to pyridine base, peptic ulcer, angiospasm, CHD twice in smoker than nonsmoker, lung cancer due to smoke (polonium-210, CO_2, CO, HCN, Ni, As, cresol, aromatic hydrocarbon, aldehyde, H_2S, NH_3, ciliotoxin, pyridine base) which declines after discontinuation in 10 years, carboxy Hb, oral cancers (50% tongue, 25% cheeck, 15% floor, and 10% gums), smoker's hypertrichosis of lips and palate (self-limited after discontinuation). Tobacco is the most important factor in the development of lung, URT, GIT, GUT cancers. 8–17 times more risk of cancer of uterine cervix. Alteration of α-antiprotease: Elastase of lung.

Withdrawal symptoms: Peak at 1–3 days lasting up to 3–4 weeks. Features are irritability, drowsiness, anxiety, hunger, increased appetite, sleep disturbance, decrease CA, bradycardia, intense urge to smoke, impaired concentration and memory, headache, depression, muscle cramp, diaphoresis, rapid respiration, weight gain due to increased appetite and loss of nicotinic stimulation of metabolism, constipation (to the best of author's knowledge and approach). Nicotinic replacement therapy is gum, inhaler, etc. 2 gm nicotine as gum for 30 min releases 90% of it.

Primary effects of smoking are: Pleasure, arousal, increased vigilance, improved task performance, decreased hunger (decreased weight), relief of anxiety, skeletal muscle relaxation, increased (CA, ADH, GH, ACTH, cortisol, prolactin, β-endorphin, BMR, FFA, HR, BP, CO), cutaneous and coronary vasoconstriction. Nicotine is stimulant at small dose and persistent depolarising blocker at large dose. Tea and coffee have similar but less marked effect.

Treatment of acute poisoning: Airway, breathing and circulation maintenance. **W**ash **W**ith **W**arm **W**ater **(4W)** containing charcoal, tannin and KI. Urine acidification, BZD. Gastric lavage by $KMnO_4$. Mecamylamine (specific antagonist). $NaSO_4$, atropine and hexamethonium (50 mg SC) along with symptomatic treatment. Clonidine 30 mg/day (weans away from addiction), buspirone, 5-HT uptake inhibitor, doxepin, vit. C.

The smoker **PUTS** down 4 diseases (these favour non-smokers): **P**re-eclampsia, **U**lcerative colitis, **T**remor agitans (parkinsonism), **S**arcoidosis.

IA:
1. Alters metabolism of antipyrine, caffeine, glutethimide, propranolol, theophylline, imipramine, lidocaine, pentazocine, phenacetin and warfarin.
2. DA modulates dependence of nicotine.
3. It enhances antipsychotic drug level after cessation of smoke.
4. It enhances the level of NE, E, and serotonin.

Passive smokers are at higher risk where bidi, chutta (cigar), chilum, hookah (hubble-hubble), betel quid (pan) and khaini are used by all classes of people.

U: Clinical use is absent except as a quick remedy for **ringworm**.

CNS Stimulants, Cognition Enhancers

1. For **addiction** (respiratory and CNS stimulants).
2. **Infanticide** (mainly in Agra and Gwalior).
3. **Malingering:** 2 cheroots in water/cigar water in axilla at night for 6–8 hours to develop symptoms.
4. **Medicolegal:** Nicotine resists **putrefaction**.

Unsafe ingredients of tobacco products: Ground cloves, ground coriander, eucalyptus oil, ginger, lemon, licorice, menthol, quinine ascorbate, thymol, $AgNO_3$.

Cigarette is a roll of tobacco with a flame at one end and a fool at the other end.

Therapeutic drug abuse and rehabilitation

1. **Non-narcotic drugs (soft drugs):** Barbiturates, BZD, amphetamine, TCA, hallucinogens (PCP, LSD, cocaine, cannabis).
2. Narcotic (hard) drugs: Opium

Actions of drug of abuse are three:
   1. Alter peception
   2. Stimulate the brain
   3. Depress the brain

TCA structurally and pharmacologically similar to phenothiazines.

Classification

1. **Nonselective:** Amitriptyline — **ADDICT**
   Doxepin
   Dothiepin
   Imipramine
   Clomipramine
   Trimipramine
2. **Predominantly NA RI:** Protriptyline
   Desipramine
   Nortriptyline
   Amoxapine
3. **SSRI:** Sertraline, citalopram, peroxetine, fluoxetine.
   Reason for antidepressant action = 5-HT and NA RI.
   Reason for sedative action = 5-HT RI.
   Reason for stimulant action = DA RI.

- **FD** — 2–5 gm.
- **PMA** — Nonspecific like amphetamine
- **MLI** — Suicidal (easily available and taken by depressed person).

ADR of "ANTIDEPRESSANTS"

Agitation
NA blockade →HTN
Toxic to heart by unknown mechanism
Increased HR
Dilated pupil
Extension of plantar response
Pulmonary system depression
Retention of urine due to anticholinergic ADR

Eye—blurred vision.
Siezure (myoclonic jerk).
Suppression of BP.
Acidosis (metabolic).
NA and 5-HT inhibition causes mood elevation.
Tremor
Serotonin syndrome causes **HARM** (**H**yperthermia, **A**utonomic instability, **R**igidity, **M**yoclonus).

Treatment
ABCD

1. **A**dequate O_2, activated charcoal,
   Antidote—physostigmine 2 mg IV for 5 min.   **SLUD**
   Watch out **S**alivation **L**acrimation, **U**rination, **D**efecation, central effect present.
2. **B**icarbonate ($NaHCO_3$) 50 mEq IV.
   Lidocaine/phenytoin may be used.
3. **C**orrection of hypotension and acidosis.
4. **D**iazepam for convulsion.

BZD: It has 5 aryl substituent. BZD ring is fused with 7 membered diazepine ring.

One of the most important psychotropic drug. Used as hypnotic, sedative and tranquilliser.

MOA: Acts as GABA agonist → ↑Cl^- inflow hyperpolarises CNS nerves → sedation, antianxiety and hypnotic effects.

Classification

Hypnotics	— Diazepam, flurazepam, flunitrazepam, nitrazepam, temazepam, midazolam, estazolam.
Antianxiety	— Chlordiazepoxide, oxazepam, lorazepam, alprazolam, diazepam.
Anticonvulsant	— Clonazepam, clobazepam, diazepam.

Absorption, distribution and excretion

Metabolised by dealkylation and hydroxylation. Distributed in the body, cross placenta. Some cross BBB.

ADR of BZD: **D**iplopia, **D**ysarthria, **I**ncreased reaction time, **A**taxia.

1. **Acute:**   Di**z**Ziness   **DIAZEPAM**
   Epigastric pain
   Paradoxical CNS stimulation
   Abuse liability due to dependence
   Memory loss.
2. **Chronic:** Anxiety, intolerance, tremor and muscle spasm.

Treatment of BZD intoxication
Airway, breathing and circulation stabilisation by O_2, intubation.
Diazepam 5 mg IV for withdrawal then tappered off.
Electrolyte balance (NS, RL).
Flumazenil 5 mg IV at the rate of 0.1 mg/min.

MLI: Suicidal attempt (death is rare)

Barbiturates

Derived from barbituric acid/malonylurea (urea + malonic acid)
Malonic acid → barbituric acid → barbiturates.

Classification

LA (8 hrs, FD 4–7 gm/10 mg%): Phenobarbitone, mephobarbitone
IA (4–8 hrs, FD 2–3 gm/7 mg%): Pentobarbitone
SA (<4 hrs, FD 2 gm/4 mg%): Secobarbitone
USA (FD 2 gm): Thiopentone, methohexitone

MOA

Blocks Na^+ K^+ transport and glutamate effect potentiate GABA-mimetic action and glycine.

Absorption, distribution and excretion

Absorbed from gut, distributed all parts of the body, cross placenta and BBB. Enzymes induced are CYP450, δ-ALA synthetase, aldehyde dehydrogenase, and hepatic glucuronyl transferase. Lowest lipid soluble is LA and highest—USA. With CPZ → dangerous. Synergistic with all sedative, tranquilliser, hypnotic, anti-convulsant and analgesics. Metabolism by side chain oxidation.

ADR of "BARBITURATES"

BP↓ due to medullary and myocardial depression. **Arrhythmia** → death. Peripheral blood pooling. **Respiratory**, CVS, CNS depression due to ↓ BP. **BZD** and alcohol Intensify toxicity. It is cumulative.
Tone of muscle lost.
Unsteady gait, unconsciousness, urine and stool incontinence.
Rapid toxicity by USA (a few sec to min).
Ataxia, absent reflex (plantar and flexor), Babinski +ve
Temperature ↓, somnolence.
Eye → miosis, thereafter mydriasis.
Skin cold, calmy and cyanotic, barbiturate blister.

Gradation of coma: Category I (cloudy consciousness)
↓
Category II (stupor)
↓
Category III (coma)

PMA

1. **External**
   - Cyanosis of extremities.
   - Froth at mouth and nostril
   - Bullous lesion of skin (barbiturate blister)
2. **Internal**
   - Gut, liver, kidney, brain congested
   - Pulmonary and cerebral edema
   - Presentation: Routine viscera, brain and urine.

MLA
- Suicidal (most common) but less commonly prescribed now due to safer alternative BZD.
- Accidental (automatism—repeated intake due to forgetfulness).
- Homicidal
- Addiction
- "As truth serum" → thiopentone IV → a state of drowsy disorientation → truth revealed (e.g. ABUSALIM).

Treatment of Barbiturate poisoning "ABCDEFGH"

- Airway ⎫
- Breathing ⎬ Stabilisation by O_2, IVF and antishock measure by NA and DA.
- Circulation ⎭
- Do not revive CNS/respiratory depression with analeptics (amphetamine 20 mg IV, cardiazol 5 mg IV, amiphenazole 15 mg IV, picrotoxin, nikethamide) due to ↑ O_2 demand, ↑ temperature and ↑ siezures.
- Extremely hard **concretion** in stomach → stomach wash up to 8 hrs post-ingestion.
- Forced **alkaline** diuresis in case of LA. The **most** useful is mannitol 200 ml of 25% then 500 ml of 5% in next 3 hrs then 5% dextrose in 1 day for 10–20 L urine excretion.
- Gastric lavage with activated charcoal (1 mg/kg), $KMnO_4$, tannic acid, $MgSO_4$ for purgation.
- Gradual withdrawal in chronic use with symptomatic treatment due to physical and psychological dependence.
- Hemodialysis and haemoperfusion.

Amphetamine/phenylisopropylamine

First synthesized in 1887 but used in 1930 for fatigue abolition and appetite suppression.

Activity more with D-isomer than L-isomer.

Metabolism: Methamphetamine
↓
Amphetamine
↓
Norephedrine/Benzoic acid

MOA: Synaptic ↑ of NA/DA by direct release or inhibition of reuptake → CNS and CVS stimulation → ↑ alertness and self-confidence.

FD = 250 mg

Diagnosis: Intensified bowel sound in coma.

ADR of "AMPHETAMINE"

Arrhythmia and HTN, ↓appetite.
More extrovert behaviour.
Pupil dilated, paranoid delusion, profuse sweating.
Hyperactivity, hallucination.
Excitability, euphoria, eye blink and jaw jerk (Gills de la Tourette's).

Trismus (spasm of muscle of mastication), bruxism (teeth grinding).
Mucous membrane dry, and rhabdomyolysis.
Insomnia, ↑ temperature, ↑ tremor.
No specific finding on autopsy.
Except
Subarachnoid or cerebral heamorrhage
Due to HTN and congestion of gut, lung and abdominal viscera.

Treatment of Amphetamine poisoning

"ABCDE"

Acidification of urine for renal excretion.
Beta-blocker for HTN (nitroprusside 2–8 µg/kg/min IV, nifedipine)
CPZ 50 mg QID for psychosis).
Diazepam and symptomatic treatment.
Electrolytes 500 ml NS and 50 ml D_5W.

MLI

1. **"Pe pill"** by student during exams, **"Speed"** (methamphetamine) and **speed ball** (amphetamine + barbiturates) for **"rush"** (stimulation) followed by depression.
2. Psychological dependence and tolerance present.

Other derivatives: Methamphetamine, methylphenidate, phentermine, dextroamphetamine and fenfluramine.

Synthetic amphetamines

- Love drug: MDA or methylenedioxyamphetamine
- Ecstasy: MDMA or methylenedioxymethamphetamine
- Eve: MDEA or methylenedioxyethamphetamine

Uses

1. By athletes to improve performance.
2. Designer drug in rave party to dance whole night.
3. Narcolepsy
4. Obesity
5. Attention deficit disorder in children.
6. Hypotension (mephentermine)
7. Epilepsy
8. Parkinsonism

Lysergic Acid Diethylamide/LSD/Acid/Microdot/Purple haze/White Lightning

The **most** powerful hallucinogen (psychedelics)/indole alkaloid derivative of magic mushroom (Mexican mushroom—*P. mexicana* and *P. corymbosh*).

1. Natural product of ergot fungus C. purpurea
2. Synthesised by Hofmann (1938) from ergot alkaloid.
3. 25–50 µg produces all psychedelic and mind revealing effects.

ADR of "HALLUCINOGENS"

Hypertension, hyperthermia.
Acute mania, arrhythmia.

LSD effect re-experienced without exposure (flashbacks).
Limb aplasia, anophthalmia, cerebral malformation in pregnancy.
Under UV light, it shows blue fluoroscence.
Changed mood and perception (colour heard and music palpated).
Increased temperature (cotton fever) and bad trip (MC).
No abstinence syndrome but psychic dependence present.
Orally taken usually, myositis ossificans due to repeated puncture.
Gynaecological—teratogenic.
Erection of hair, eye—mydriasis.
Nausea.
Syndrome (body packer and body stuffer syndrome), slow passage of time, salivation.

MOA: 5-HT antagonist (also mimics its action).

PK: Absorbed from gut, found to blood protein, highest concentration in lung, liver, kidney, brain. Found in bile also. For psychotropic effect ("take a trip") 100–200 µg.

FD = 14 mg. Half life = 3 hrs

Treatment: Diazepam 20 mg IV
Electrolyte, glucose, multivitamins
Psychotherapy

MLI

Homicidal, suicidal, accidental.

Phencyclidine/PCP/Angel Dust/Peace Pill/Hog T/Snort/Flakes/Goon/Rocket fuel/Cadillac

Analogues TCP, PHP, PCPP, PCE.

The **most** dangerous hallucinogen used as anaesthetic till 1970 but banned threafter. Angel dust has 50–100% drug concentration (MC). First synthesized in 1926. Marketed by P. Devis in 1950 as anaesthetic. Abused with tobacco/marijuana (sniffed, smoked, injected).

MOA

Blocks NMDA/δ/DR/Cholinoceptor. Stimulates α R.

ADR of "ANGEL DUST"

Analgesia like opioid, amphetamine like at high dose.
Numbness, nystagmus, a feeling of dissociation.
Generalised siezure, sweating, salivation, dystonia.
Euphoria, miosis, visual hallucination.
Low sugar level.
Distorted perception and body image, diaphoresis.
Urine (feature of ARF).
Similar to vitamin K (ketamine), catatonic syndrome (violent, bizarre, nudism).
Temperature raised

FD = 1 gm; FP = Non-specific.

Treatment

Acidify urine, NH_4Cl_3 mEq per kg.

"ABCD"

Breathing stabilisation by O_2
C vitamin 2 gm IV
Diazepam, Diphenhydramine
MLA: Suicidal, homicidal, violence, psychosis.

Chloral hydrate/dry wine

The **oldest** synthetic hypnotic. Irritant liquid to gastric mucosa and skin with burning horrible taste. Low therapeutic index.

Chloral hydrate $\xrightarrow{\text{Alcohol dehydrogenase}}$ Trichloroethanol (active)
$\downarrow$ Glucuronic acid
Urinary excretion

ADR of "CHLORAL" hydrate

Convulsion, mental retardation.
Habitual use—tolerance and physical dependence.
Like barbiturates, it manifests.
Ocular—pin-point pupil before death.
Albuminuria
Loss of life due to paralysis of respiratory centre.
FD = 10 gm. FP = 12 hrs.

Treatment of "ABCDEF"

→ Airway—intubation
→ Breathing—O_2
→ Cardiac stimulant
→ Drugs—flumazenil 0.1 mg (max 3 mg), diazepam
→ Electrolyte—glucose, NS and RL IV
→ Forced alkaline diuresis

PMA

1. Like $NaNO_3$, it rapidly deteriorates after death.
2. Brain and lungs congested. Hepatorenal damage.
3. Gastric mucosa—soft, red, eroded with smell of drug.

MLI

1. **Micky finn**—chloralhydrate + alcohol.
2. **Knock out drops**—given in food and drink to render a person helpless for rape and robbery.

Cannabis indica/Indian Hemp/Dagga

History traces its use in China 5000 yrs ago. It is the **most** popular recreational and ritualistic intoxicant obtained from *C. sativa* (dioecious plant, 15 feet).

Order of drug concentration

Flower > leaves > stem > seed > root.

Various preparations are

1. **Bhang:** Dried leaves and fruit shoots—15% concentration.
2. **Majun/Sweaterneat:** Bhang + flour + milk + butter.

3. **Ganja:** Resin of female flower—25% concentration. Mixed with tobacco and smoked in pipe.
4. **Charas/Hashis:** Resin of leaves and stems. Most powerful (40% concentration). Smoked with tobacco.
5. **Sinsemilla:** Seedless marijuana.

The term **Marijuana/Marihuana** is used in America. **Reefers/Weed** = Cigarette of Indian hemp.

Active principle is soluble oleoresin **cannabinol**.

FD:
- Charas = 2 gm/kg
- Ganja = 8 gm/kg
- Bhang = 10 gm/kg

U:
- Banned all over the world but used as anaesthetic, hypnotic, aphrodisiac, etc.
- Dronabinol (THC) as antiemetic in chemotherapy.

Metabolism

Cannabinol $\rightarrow$ ΔTHC $\xrightarrow{\text{Liver}}$ 11–OH–^{9} ΔTHC
(active)
8, 11–(OH)$_2$ – ΔTHC

ADR of "CANNABIS INDICA"

CNS—higher centre depression with loss of preception of time and space.
Anaesthetic effects
Numbness and tingling
Nausea and dizziness
Aphrodisiac, talkative and rarely **Running amok.**
Breathing paralysis →death
Increased appetite with intake of food with great relish, weight ↓
Sign and symptom similar to alcohol (excitement →narcosis).
Impotence (↓sperm, ↓DHT), irresistible desire to destroy life + property.
Nude beautiful women dancing before abuser—perception.
Dilated pupil
Insomnia, hashish insanity, mood deterioration.
Confusion
Anorexia

Treatment

"ABCDEFGH"

→ Airway—intubation
→ Breathing—O$_2$
→ Circulation—RL, NS, D5W
→ Drugs—Diazepam 10 mg IV, naloxone 2 mg, thiamine 100 mg IV, strychnine hypodermic injection.
→ ECG monitoring
→ Fluid with 100 ml of 50% glucose
→ Give strong tea and coffee orally
→ Haloperidol for psychosis

PMA: Not specific, finding of asphyxia.

MLA
- Errors of judgement.
- **Run amok** (impulsive desire for murder and suicide).
- Used by **Sadhu/Fakir** to free from worldly attachments and to participate with divine spirit.

Cocaine (Coke, Snow, Cadillac, White Lady)

Obtained from leaves of *E. coca* and *E. novogranatonse*
Properties: LA and vasoconstriction.
Synthetic: Cocaine is LA (xylocaine, novocaine and nupercaine).
Crack = cocaine + baking soda + H_2O for smoke.
Speed ball = cocaine + heroin.
Route: Snorting (nasal mucosa), IV line smoking.
MOA: Inhibits reuptake of **NA, DA and 5-HT** and **Na^+** current →stimulation of cortex followed by depression. Desensitises terminal nerve. Procaine is half, butacaine twice and dibucaine 5 times toxic than cocaine.
PK: Absorbed from mucosa and subcutaneous tissues.

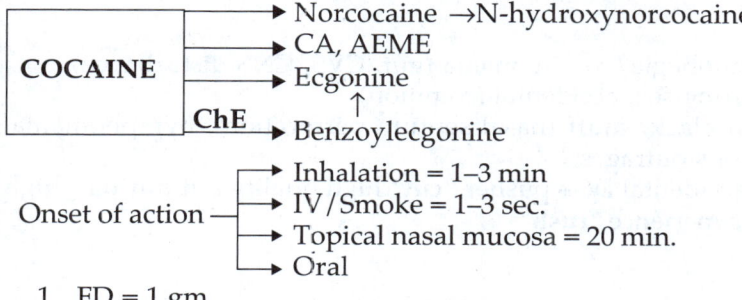

1. FD = 1 gm
2. FP = 2 hrs

Stage of Excitement of Cocaine

Cortex and medulla stimulation, convulsion, cord degeneration.
Ocular—mydriasis
Cyanosis, colour of skin—pallor
Absense of fatigue and depression
Increased HR, RR, temperature, physical and energy and ↓BP.
Numbness of extremities, nose and throat, nausea.
Excited, restless and talkative.

Stage of Depression "WHITE LADY"

Within an hour
Heart failure, respiratory depression and vascular collapse.
Irritability
Tactile hallucination **(cocaine bugs),** tachycardia, tachypnea.
Eye—mydriasis
Loss of interest in family, food and sex.
Abnormal behaviour (paranoid, mania, depression).
Dysphoria (depression, insomnia)
Young of upper class more effected due to high cost.

Treatment
ABCDEFGHI

Airway
Breathing } O_2, RL, NS, intubation.
Circulation

Drugs—Diazepam/chloroform for convulsion. Barbiturates for stimulation.
Naloxone 2 mg IV, thiamine 100 mg IV.
Ice bath for hyperthermia.
Ensure ligature above the part if injected.
For chronic case—amphetamine, Li, bromocriptine.
Gastric lavage by warm H_2O containing charcoal, $KMnO_4$ and tannic acid. Wash out nose and throat with H_2O.
Inhalational **amyl NO_3** is antidote.

PMA
- Finding of asphyxia and heart failure.
- Edema of lung, liver, kidney, brain.
- Brain and blood (+F^-) preserved.

MLA
- Cocainism/cocainophagia/cocainomania (gut, CVS, CNS disturbance)
- By prostitutes, during sex, accidental (common)
- Tongue and teeth black, snuff (nasal septum perforation), nymphomania, shameless libidinous outrages.

The greatest risk of accidental IV→ pusher **"cut"** high quality but during ↓high quality → ↑ amount to experience **"rush"**

OPIUM/AFIM

It is part of health care since 300 BC and is obtained from dry juice of poppy (*P. somniferum*) cultivated in India and Eastern countries under licence.

- **Size:** 1 metre in height, 5–8 capsules/plant, white flower.
- **Extraction:** Unripe capsule —Incision→ white juice —evaporation→ opium.
  It is **alkaline** and had **bitter** taste.
  Ripe and dried capsule has **trace** of opium for sedation and narcosis.
- **Khas khas** (poppy seed) is white, harmless demulcent used for food. Oil is used for cooking.

Crude opium has 25 alkaloids with meconic, lactic and sulfuric acids.

Classification
(A) Two groups are
1. **Phenanthrene (narcotic)**
   Morphine   10% → Isolated by **Serturner** and called as
   Codiene   0.5%   God's own medicine by Sir W. Osler.
   Thebaine   0.3%
2. **Isoquinolone**
   Papavarine 1%
   Narcotine   6% (analgesic but no narcosis).

(B) Basis—origin
1. **Natural:** Morphine, codiene
2. **Semisynthetic:** Pholcodiene, oxycodone, hydromorphone, oxymorphone, hydrocodone, oxycodone, heroin.
3. **Synthetic:** Pethidine, methadone, tramadol, dipipanone, levorphanol, dextromoramide, fentanyl, alfentanil, sufentanil, remifentanil, ethoheptazone, dextropropoxyphene.

(C) Basis—Function
1. **Strong stimulant:** Morphine, heroin, fentanyl, sufentanil, methadone, meperidine.
2. **Moderate agonist:** Codeine, propoxyphene.
3. **Mixed agonist-antagonist:** Nalorphane, pentazocine, levallorphan, butorphanol, buprenorphine.
4. **Pure anatagonist:** Nalmefene, naloxane, naltrexone.

Mech: AC – Gi activation ⟶ ↑ K^+ efflux→hyperpolarisation
↓ Ca^{2+} influx ↠↓ neurotransmitter release.

Actions of receptor type (spinal and supraspinal)
1. **μ:** Hormone changes
Analgesia
Respiratory depression
DA release **HARD ARMC**
ACh release
Reinforcements euphoria
Motility of gut ↓
Cough and appetite suppression
2. **κ:** ↓ dysphoria, ↓ Gl motility
↓ appetite ↓ respiration, analgesia
Psychoses, sedation, diuresis.
3. **δ:** Hormone changes, DA release ↓ appetite.
4. **σ:** Cardiac stimulation
Hallucination **CHD**
Dysphoria

Genetics: >3000 male twin pairs showed genetic influence to opium dependence.

Actions of morphine   **MORPHINES**

Miosis
Orthostatic hypotension and fainting, vasodilation blood shift from pulmonary to systemic circuit.
Respiratory depression, cough, temperature and vasomotor centre depression.
Pain suppression→inhibits substance P release from substantia gelatinosa.
Histamine release, harmones (↓ CRF, LH, TRH, FSH, ACTH, steroid and ↑ Prl, GH, ADH).
Increased ICP due to ↑ CO_2 →vasodilation.
Nausea
Euphoria

Sedation, stimulant at CTZ, vagal centre ($\downarrow$HR), EW nucleus of III CN (miosis), cortical area and hippocampal cells (convulsion and muscle rigidity→GABA release inhibition). Sympathetic stimulation and anticholinergic action. Spasm of sphincter of Oddi→biliary colic. ↑ tone of sphincter of UB→urinary urgency. All GIT secretion decrease. Depresses all centres except oculomotor, sweating and vomiting.

1. **FD:** Opium 2 gm, morphine 0.2, codiene 0.5 gm
2. **FP:** 6–12 hrs.

Absorption, distribution, excretion

Onset of action
- Oral — ½ hrs
- Inj — 4 min

Route: Mucosa, dermal, inhalational, concentration in liver, kidney and spleen more than that in plasma. Renal and fecal excretion. Crosses BBB partially and placenta freely.

Hepatic metabolism by glucuronide conjugation. Morphine-6-glucuronide is active metabolite. Drugs recovered from bile, blood and urine.

Three stages of opium poisoning

1. **Stage of excitement**
   - ↑ mental activity
   - Freedom from anxiety, hallucination
   - Maniacal condition
2. **Stage of stupor**
   - Nausea, vomiting, motionless
   - Miosis, cyanosis, itch
   - Sense of weight in limbs
   - Pulse and RR normal
3. **Stage of coma:** Pinpoint pupil, reflex absent, resp. paralysis, all secretion $\downarrow$ except sweat, $\downarrow$temp, blisters, Cheyne-Stokes respiration.

Diagnosis: 3 ml H_2SO_4 + 3 drops formalin + solution →purple-red →violet →Blue (Marquis test)

Treatment of acute poisoning

ABC maintenance

ABCDEFG

Amphenazole 30 mg IV
Breathing supported by O_2
Coma cocktails treated by 100 ml of 50% glucose, 100 mg thiamine.
Drugs: Naloxone **(specific antidote)** 10–20 mg IV, methadone (long action), nalmefene 1 mg IV, physostigmine 0.04 mg/kg IV
Ephedrine, caffeine, amphetamine
Fluid maintenance
Gastric lavage by $KMnO_4$, $NaSO_4$ and charcoal.

PMA

Signs of asphyxia
Cyanosis of face and nails
Froth on mouth and nostrils
Internal organs edematous and congested.

MLI of poisoning

It is included in DSM–IV and used for painless death of suicides.
Rarely for homicide due to bitter taste, smell, etc.

Chronic poisoning of OPIUM (Morphinism/Morphinomania)

Opium addicts tolerate up to 6 gm/day.
Pleasurable feeling of relief and well being then depression.
Irritation, insomnia, impotence, intellectual deterioration.
Ultimate results to foetus—life-threatening.
Miosis, mental fatigue, memory loss, moral deterioration.

Treatment

1. Gradual withdrawal and psychiatric counselling.
2. Methadone 40 mg/day than tapered off. Codiene/dihydrocodiene for less severely opiate depress out.
3. Propranolol 80 mg for anxiety and craving.
4. Naltrexone, tranquillisers, flumazenil 0.2 mg/min (max 3 mg).

Substitution therapy in opioid dependence

One mg oral methadone is substituted for
- Heroin 2 mg.
- Morphine 4 mg.
- Pethidine 20 mg.

HMP
2 4 20

Tolerance — PK (↑ metabolism).
         — PD (cellular).

Cross-tolerance present.

Effects for high degree tolerance: Sedation   **SMEAR**
                                        Mental clouding
                                        Euphoria, dysphagia
                                        Analgesia, antidiuresis
                                        Respiratory depression

Dependence: Physical and psychological.

Minimal tolerance
   Constipation
   Antagonism
   ConvuLsion   **CALM**
   Miosis

Dimorphine/heroin/brown sugar/diacetylmorphine

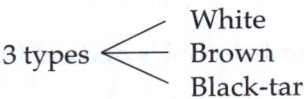

3 types — White
        — Brown
        — Black-tar

- Sweat heroin/Smack/Junk/Dope is diluted with quinine/lactose/mannitol, etc.
- It is **most** dangerous among all drugs of addictions.
- **Route:** Smoked, injected, snuffed.

- More lipid soluble, more euphoriant, 3 times more potent than morphine but similar duration of action to it.
- **Causes of death:** Infection and respiratory depression.

Metabolism

Heroin → monoacetyl morphine/acetyl morphine → morphine.
Chemical analysis detects morphine not heroin. Renal excretion.

Treatment

1. Methadone 40 mg/day
   80 mg/day for euphoria then tapered off by 20%.
2. Never give 20 mg methadone at one time.
3. Narcotic antagonists:
   Naltrexone
   Naloxone
4. Haloperidol
   Clonidine
   Cyclozocine
5. Cold turkey

PMA

Lungs congested with foreign body and granuloma.
Liver—chronic triaditis.

Meperidine/pethidine

Colourless powder with bitter taste.

Action: Analgesic; antispasmodic, sedative.

Route: IV/IM   **Drug** ⟨ Hydroylsis → meperidinic acid (major)
                              Demethylation → norpethidine (minor)

Glucuronide conjugation
Renal excretion

1. **FD:** 2 gm
2. **FP:** 1 day.

Signs and symptoms: Similar to morphine except it causes:
- More dizziness, greater elation.
- Impaired ability, addiction more in **Doctors**.

IA: MAO inhibitors/phenothiazines + drugs.
Treatment: Acidification.

Alcohol

It is the **commonest** drug encountered in FM. The word alcohol is derived from the Arabic for "Something subtle".

Properties of C_2H_5OH

- Transparent
- Colourless
- Volatile

- Spirit odour
- Burning taste
- Weakly charged molecule.

20% of average physician's patients suffer from alcoholism. **80% population suffer from alcoholism** involving all cultures and all socioeconomic strata. It accounts **half of all traffic accident** and **half of all homicides**.

Fermentation: It is **as old as** civilisation.

$$\text{Starch maltose} \xrightarrow{\text{Convertase}} \text{Maltose} \xrightarrow[\text{(Yeast)}]{\text{Zymase}} C_2H_5O + CO_2$$

(15% alcohol)

Mollases—commercial source.

Alcoholic beverages

1. Malted liquor—6% alcohol from cereal.
2. Wine—9–22% alcohol from fruits. All alcohol fermented → dry wine. Some left → sweet wine.
3. Spirit—40–55% alcohol. Proof spirit → explosive. Rectified spirit → 95% alcohol. Absolute alcohol → 99.95%.
   100% proof spirit is **49.29%** W/W or **57.1%** V/V alcohol.

- Underproof/weak spirit.
- Overproof/strong spirit.

Industrial methylated spirit/denaturated alcohol = 95% alcohol + 5% wood naphtha.

Rum	≥50%
Whisky, gin, brandy	40–45%
Port/sherry	20%
Wine	10–15%
Beers	4–8%

Included in DSM–IV.

Safe Limit

♂ — 210 gm/w
♀ — 140 gm/w

Absorption

Absorbed from **mucosa** by simple diffusion without digestion.
20% from stomach.
80% from small intestine.
60% is absorbed in 30 min and 90% in 60 min.
Detected in blood in 2–3 min.
Maximum concentration in 45–90 min.
Carbonated alcohol enhances absorption due to bubble (increased surface area).

Absorption **most** delayed by fat and protein. Warmed alcohol absorbed > iced alcohol due to vasodilation. Absorption is **most** rapid at 10–20% concentration. Absorption of >40% alcohol reduces due to pyloric spasm motility and irritation. Drinker absorbs more rapidly than nondrinker.

Distribution

Insoluble in fat. RBC has less alcohol than plasma. Evenly distributed throughout body water. Crosses BBB.

Female has increased concentration due to small aqueous compartment. Venous blood alcohol in absorption phase is 10% lower than arterial blood alcohol after 1 hour equilibrium is attained.

Excretion

Excreted by **all** routes of excretion. 5% by lungs and 5% urine. **Peculiar** odour is due to excretion by skin glands.

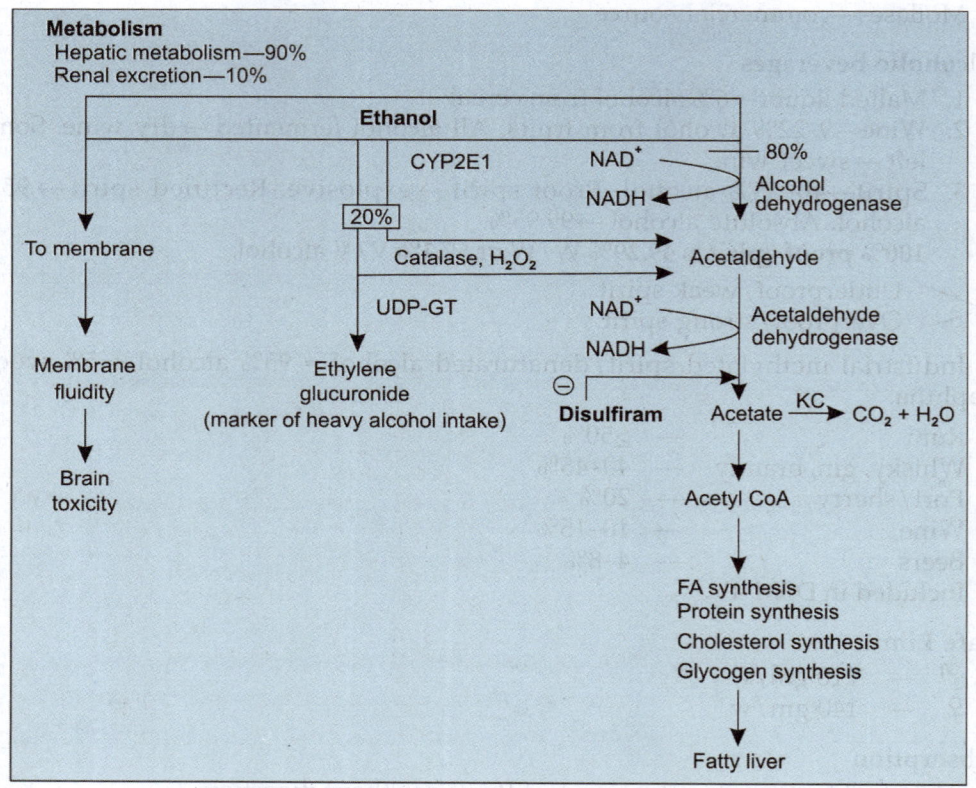

Acetaldehyde causes
- ↓ Glutathione
- ↓ Vitamins
- ↓ Trace metals

Enzymes increase on regular use of alcohol → alcohol consumption is doubled. **Fructose** enhances the metabolism. **15 ml/hrs** is rate of disappearance (15 mg/100 ml blood/hr). Alcoholic → 50 mg/100 ml blood/hr. 10% metabolised alcohol is deposited as cholesterol and natural fat. 7 cal per gm energy (not stored). Zero order kinetic (15 ml/hr—constantly) is followed.

Genetics: Asian has **less** ALDH activity.

Offspiring of alcoholics need increased alcohol for same effect. Runs in family with 60% genetic contribution. **4-fold** increased risk in twin adopted at birth without knowledge of biological parents.

Physiological Effects

100 – 150 mg%	—	Memory loss, slow reaction time.
150 – 300 mg%	—	Muscular incoordination, ↓ pain response.
300 – 400 mg%	—	Stupor, ↓ response to stimuli.
≥400 mg%	—	Anaesthesia, respiratory failure, coma, death.

Actions

Traces of alcohol **(<0.001 mg%)** in all persons are present due to (N) metabolism and bacterial action. Depresses **RAS,** cerebral cortex (altered judgement) midbrain and medulla; first two is most sensitive.

Order of Sensitivity

Frontal lobe (mood change) > occipital lobe (visual disturbance) > cerebellum (loss of coordination).

Similar to hypoxia, it reduces nerve cell activity. Heat loss, hypnosis, diaphoresis. ↑ HDL, ↓ LDL, ↑ adrenaline release, vasodilation, sympathetic stimulation, ↑ tPA, ↑ gastric secretion, ↑ muscle action. Two standard drink → 2 mm Hg ↑ BP due to ↓ NO release.

At high doses: ↓ BP, cardiac depression, ↓ gastric secretion, ↓ glucose, ↓ temperature.

Chronic user: Cardiomyopathy, "Holiday heart" (increased HR) syndrome = French paradox (no IHD), impotence, gynaecomastia, megaloblastic anemia (decreased folate metabolism), pancreatitis, osteoporosis.

Stellate Cells seen

Mallory body formation present.

TNF α & TG β
↓
Collagen deposition and necrosis
↓
Fibrosis of liver

Diuresis due to ADH inhibition.
Increased anion gap.
Aphrodisiac: Aggressive sexual behaviour
    Decreased Leydig cell function
    Decreased orgasm
    Increased ejaculation

Mech of Action

— Alters membrane lipid, AC, Na^+K^+ ATpase.
— Inhibits NMDA R, voltage sensitive Ca^{2+} channel, adenosine uptake, PK translocation.
— Stimulates $GABA_A$ R, $5-HT_3$ R and NA turnover through opioid R, kainate R.
— Increased steroid and ACTH, decreased oxytocin and T_3 and T_4.

Sign and Symptoms

Most patients have no symptoms.
Most common problems are
- Marital
- Job related
- Legal

1. **CAGE question is positive, i.e.**
   Cutting down/feel the need
   Annoyed on criticism
   Guilty of drinking
   Eye—open on drinking in the morning.
2. **Three stages are**
   - Stage of excitement
   - Stage of incoordination
   - Stage of coma

1. Stage of EXCITEMENT

Excitation and well-being.
Concentration and confidence decreased. Lack of self-control.
Inhibition low
Time of reaction impaired, prolonged intercourse without ejaculation.
Motor coordination, cognitive function, sensory perception reduced.
Emotion, action, speech less restrained.
Nystagmus (alcohol gaze nystagmus)—Jerky movement.
Time and space perception altered.

Decreased visual acuity
- At 20 mg% in abstainers
- At 20–33 mg% in moderate drinker
- At 40–70 mg% in heavy drinker

2. Stage of incoordination

Loss of inhibition at 150–250 mg%/100 ml
Ill-tampered, irritable
Impaired fine and skilled movement
Flushed face, rapid pulse
Blurring of consonant is the earliest sign of incoordination.

3. Stage of coma/"STAGE OF COMA"

Sensory and motor cells deeply affected.
Temperature subnormal
Asphyxia → death
Gut disturbance
Eye: Miosis changed to mydriasis (McEvan sign)
Oxidation and excretion of alcohol → so low level in coma.

Five hours or more duration of coma → **worst** prognosis. Recovery leads to irritation, depression, headache (hangover).
Consciousness lost during urination (micturition syncope).

Overactivity of muscle→muscle paralysis.
Munich Beer Heart (cardiac depression, hypertrophy)
After irreversible damage to vital centres→death.
- FD: 150–250 ml absolute alcohol in 1 hr.
- FP: 12–24 hrs.

Tolerance: 3 types of tolerance occur:
1. **Metabolic/Pharmacokinetic:**
   30% hepatic metabolism.
2. **Cellular/Pharmacodynamic:**
   Neurochemical changes cause physical dependence (nerves need alcohol to function optimally).
3. **Behavioral:** Adapts behavior to work normally.

Tolerance is lost by those "out of practice" (restricted by liver damage). Barbiturate + alcohol→hepatic metabolism of both→barbiturate remains active for longer time.

Dependence
1. Physical (nerves need drug to function optimally).
2. Psychological (psychologically uncontrollable without drug).

Consent for Exam
Even in unconscious patients, dector should wait for consent till consciousness arrives.

Treatment (acute care)   **ABCDEFGH**
Alkaline solution to wash bowel
Breathing—O_2
Caffeine and strychnine for nerve stimulation.
Drip (fructose + insulin)—**most** patients are recovered.
Electrolyte balance, EGG monitoring, 100 mg thiamine
Fluid—1L (NS) with 10% glucose. Coramine 5 ml.
Gastric lavage by $NaHCO_3$ 2 gm per 250 ml water.
Haemodialysis

PMA

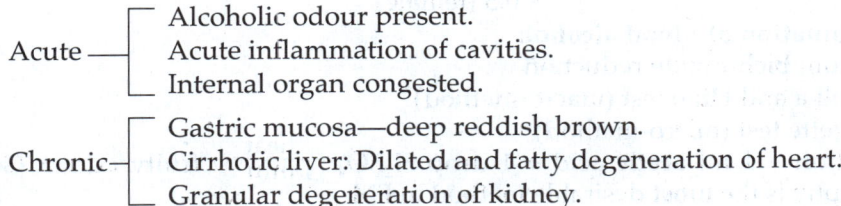

Precaution for sample collection
Sample collected from femoral/subclavian arteries and heart. In embalmed bodies, sample from vitreous/muscle.

Treatment of chronic case
Acamprosate 2 gm per day/Naltrexone 100 mg/day
BZD: 1 mg lorazepam, vitamin B_1 100 mg.

Clonidine 100 mg IV/hr, CPZ 50 mg QID, chlormethiazole. Conditioned reflex treatment: Alcohol + drug →↑ ADR →Abstinancy.

Disulfiram 250 mg/day → 100 mg/day.   **ABCD**

Side effects of DISULFIRAM (starts after 3 hrs)

Dangerous → CV collapse
Increase pulse and hyperventilation
Sweating
Upset—abdominal
Loss of vision
Flushing, fainting
Increased throbbing headache
Anxiety
Metallic taste, malaise
Hence, patients dislike drinking due to increased acetaldehyde.

Investigations

1. **Blood: Most** suitable and **most** direct evidence of concentration of alcohol to brain is blood.
   10 ml blood + 100 mg NaF + 30 mg K oxalates → no freezing due to RBC break down. PM blood is valid for 36 hrs after death.
2. **Urine:** It has 25% higher concentration than blood. 50 mg phenyl mercuric nitrite/Na azide as preservative for 10 ml urine/blood.
3. **Widmark formula:**   a = CPR for blood.

$$a = \frac{3}{4} QPR \text{ for urine}$$

   a = Alcohol in gm in urine/blood.
   c = Concentration in mg/kg in blood.
   p = Body weight in kg.
   q = Concentration in mg/kg in urine
   r = Constant — 0.6 (male) / 0.5 (female)

4. **Determination of blood alcohol:**
   Potassium bichromate reduction
   a. Kozelka and Hine test (macro-method)
   b. Corvette test (micro-method)
   1 ml solution + 1 ml acetic acid + 1 drop H_2SO_4 $\xrightarrow[1 \text{ min}]{\text{heat}}$ fruity odour. Gas chromatography is the **most** desirable method in FM.

5. **Breathalyser**
   Infrared light absorbed by vapour (100 ml) is α alcohol concentration in vapour. 2100 ml vapour has same amount as 1 ml blood. Breath + bichromate—H_2SO_4 → green (80 mg%). For every unit of alcohol in blood, there is 1.2 units of alcohol in vitreous.

6. **Lab diagnosis**
   ↓K, Mg, Zn, PO_4^{3-}, RBC, WBC
   ↑ Uric acid, TG

Abnormal LFT.
For screening, 2 tests (70–80% sensitive and specific) are:
1. GGT (>30 U) or gamma glutamyl transferase.
2. CDT (>20 U/L)/carbohydrate deficient transferin.

Hazards of alcoholism
— Decreased resistance to hypoxia.
— Saturday night palsy (radial nerve pressure)
— Alcoholic blackout/palimpsests:
Loss of memory and amnesia →committed crimes not recalled.

Traffic accidents
- 2 times risk at 60 mg%
- 12 times risk at 100 mg%
- 25 times risk at 150 mg%
- Offence at 20 mg% in Poland
- Offence at 50 mg% in Norway
- Offence at 80 mg% in UK, France
- Offence at 100–150% in USA
- Offence at 30 mg% in India

In India, Section 185 Motor Vehicle Act, 1988 punishes
₹ 2000/6 month for first time.
₹ 3000/2 year for 2nd time.

Alcohol withdrawal syndrome
— Tremor, seizures typically single after 6–48 hr
— Shakes and Jitter (earliest sign 10 hr after drink)
— ↓HR, nausea, emesis.
— 33% delirium tremens.

Treatment
- 20 mg chlordiazepoxide
- 100 mg diazepam
- 20 mg/day haloperidol
- Relapse prevention

Pathology
1. Delirium tremens is due to temporary excess/sudden withdrawal. Typically begins 3–4 day after last drink.
   Disorientation to time and place.
   Tremors
   Restlessness
   Enhanced HR, BP, temperature
   Memory loss
   Excess fear
   No control on violence
   Suicidal tendency, visual and auditory hallucination, death—5–15%.

   Delirium TREMENS

2. Alcoholic polyneuritis and Korsakoff's psychosis
3. Paranoia

4. Hallucination
5. Epilepsy
6. Wernicke's encephalopathy
7. Cardiac dysrhythmia
8. **Marchiafava's** syndrome: 1% degeneration of corpus callosum.
9. Mallory-Weiss syndrome
10. Peptic ulcer, CA breast 1.5 times on 1.5 drink/day.
11. Cirrhosis, myocarditis, pancreatitis
12. Inhibition of tryptophan to 5-HIAA (5-HT metabolites)
13. ADH inhibition, $T_3 > T_4 \downarrow$
14. Fetal alcohol syndrome

Triad ⟨ Growth retardation / CNS dysfunction / Craniofacial abnormality

Sudden Death

Catecholamine released during struggle →HR and cardiopulmonary arrest → death.

Alcohol concentration
1. >0.2% →consumption prior to death
2. <0.2% →alcohol production due to putrefaction

AGRICULTURAL POISONS

>1000 insecticides/pesticide

Classifications

1. **Virtually harmless:** Cu oxides as fungicides.
2. **Comparatively harmless:** H_2SO_4 as weed-killers. Na chlorate as mass herbicide for road and rail track.
3. **Mild toxic:** DDT, aldrin, gammaxane.
4. **Highly toxic:** As, Pb, Ca compounds.
   — Nicotine, sulfate, tennates, KCN, Na CN, DNP, DNOC. Insecticides of veg. origin are nicotine, pyridine and rotenone.
1. **Chemical insecticides:** Sb, P, As, Ba, Hg, Th, Zn, F
2. **Synthetic chemical insecticides**
   — Carbamates, phosphate ester, chlorinated HC.
   — Indane derivatives (aldrin, dieldrin).
   — DDT, BHC.

Organophosphate poisoning

⎡ Alkyl and aryl phosphates
⎢ Chlorinated compound (DDT, endrin)
⎣ Coaltar product (naphthalene)

Aliphatic chain —H→ alkyl compound

 e.g. HETP (hexaethyl tetraphosphate)
 TEPP (tetraethyl pyrophosphate)
 OMPA (octamethyl pyrophosphoramide)
 Melathion.

Aromatic HC —H→ aryl compound, e.g. parathion.

Routes: Oral, dermal, inhalational

Mech: Inhibits **irreversibly AChE** (true ChE of RBC, nerve and skeletal muscle) and **pseudo ChE** (plasma, liver, heart, pancreas and brain) →↑ **ACh** at parasympathetic, sympathetic and somatic sites.

Phosphorylated AChE loses alkyl group→enzyme is not hydrolysed→Enzyme permanently inactivated after 24–36 hrs.

- Mild poison →> 20% ChE activity + present.
- Moderate poison →>10% ChE activity present.
- Severe poison → <10% ChE activity present.

Symptoms are **similar** to overactivity of cholinergic drugs.

Sings and Symptoms

ChE level ≤30% of normal activity.

Order: Inhalational (most rapid) > oral > dermal. Involuntary muscle and secretory gland (first) > voluntary muscle > vital brain centres.

Actions:
- Muscarinic
- Nicotinic
- CNS

1. Muscarinic "MUSCARINIC"

Miosis
Urination↑.
Secretion (salivation, respiration, sweating, lacrimation—red due to porphyrin)
Cardiospasm (epigastric and substernal tightness)
Abdominal cramps, anorexia
Resp. obstruction due to ↑ secretion, bronchoconstriction, froth at nose and mouth.
Involuntary defecation and diarrhoea
Nausea, vomiting
Increased expiration
Cyanosis

2. Nicotinic/"NICOTINIC"

Nicotinic stimulation causes
Initially
Contraction then muscle paralyzes.
Occasional HTN (sympathetic ganglia stimulation)
Tachycardia
Increased BP
Increased cramp
Cyanosis

3. CNS

Irritability
Tremor   **ITS Coma**
Stupor
Coma

Initially, headache, malaise, constriction of chest and decreased vision due to miosis.

2–8 hrs: Nausea → abdominal cramp → vomiting/diarrhoea → sweating → salivation,→ muscle twitching and red tears/chromogenic tears→ convulsion, pulmonary edema, death due to CVS collapse, respiratory depression and muscle paralysis.

5 weeks: Delayed peripheral neuropathy, paresthesia and cramps of calves then ataxia and toe drop → flaccid paralysis similar to GB syndrome.

2–3 months: Muscle wasting.
Complete recovery in 10 days.

Diagnosis

5 ml heparinised blood is frozen→ ChE activity falls by 22–88%. Confirmed by adding 2 mg atropine→ symptoms relieved without atropinisation.

Treatment ABCD

ABC maintenance and removal of the source. BZD/phenytoin for convulsion. Activated charcoal 1 g/kg, $KMNO_4$, ChE inhibitors: DAM (diacetyl monoxime) or parlidoxime (2-PAM) competes for phosphate moiety of the poison and releases it from ChE. More action on nicotinic site. **Dose:** 1–2 gm IV (max 12 gm/day). 2-PAM + atropine → **synergistic.** Oximes reactivate ChE, remove block of NMJ, prevent formation of phosphorylated E and detoxify poison. **Obidoxime** is more potent and toxic (D: 250 mg IV/1 m).

Drugs of other type

Atropine inhibits muscarinic and CNS but no nicotine effects.
Cathartic (sorbitol/mannitol).
Cholestyramine for endrin →faecal excretion increased.
Antibiotics

Prophylaxis

Covering the whole body by white cotton. <2 hr spray per day by the worker.

PMA: Signs of asphyxia, congested face. Cyanosis of lips, fingers and nose. Stomach content—smell of **kerosene** and its mucosa—congested with submucous petechial hemorrhage. **Internal** organs—edematous and congested. Poison detected in putrefied body.

Carbonates

Carbonic acid → carbonates
Trade name: Tennic (aldicarb)
Matacil (aminocarb)
Baygon (aprocarb)
Sevin (carboryl)

Difference	
Carbamates	**Organophosphates**
1. Hydrolysed from ChE in 1–2 days	✗
2. Not penetrate into CNS	✓

Treatment

Atropine (specific antidote), pralidoxime.
Organochlorates
Four groups
— DDT
— BHC, lindane
— Cyclodienes: Aldrin; endrin (plant penicillin)
— Toxapine

Route: Oral, dermal, inhalational.
PK: DDT is least absorbed. Lipid soluble, partial hepatic metabolism. Renal excretion.
Chlorates: Toxicity Na salt > K salt. FD: 25 gm. Attacks all body cells, lyses RBC and forms met Hb.
Treatment: Methylene blue and vitamin C.

PARAQUAT

Weed-Killer

Mech: NADPH dependent formation of free radical →cell death.
Distributed to all organs. Gut erosion.
FD: 3–5 gm
FP: 2–7 days
Treatment: Emetic contraindicated.
— Fuller's earth   — Activated charcoal 2 gm/kg.
— Mannitol   — Bentonise

Pyrethrins

Extracted from Crysanthemum plant.
FD: 1 gm/kg
Mech: Binds **Na$^+$ channel** and prolongs its inactivation in open state.

Symptoms and Signs "PYRETHRINS"

PYRExia—hyperthermia
Throat—sore.
Hyperactive muscle →convulsion
Rash
Inhalational (rhinorrhoea)
Nausea
Skin bluster

Treatment

Activated charcoal
Atropine and oxime contraindicated
Skin washed with soap and water

Aluminum Phosphide

It's solid fumigant pesticide, insecticide and rodenticide. Trade name: Celphos, Alphos, Quickphos, Phostoxin, Phosphotox. Each weighing 3 gm $\xrightarrow{\frac{H_2O}{HCl}}$ 1 gm phosphine (PH$_3$).

ALUMINIUM PHOSPHIDE

Mech: PH_3 is systemic poison, effects all organs. Inhibits ETC (cytochrome oxidase).

PK: Garlic odour, absorbed orally, hepatic metabolism. $PH_3 \rightarrow$ hypophosphite (renal excretion). Also excreted unchanged from lungs.

FD: 1–3 gm; **FP:** 1 hr to 4 day.

Signs and Symptoms
- ARDS
- Lung—edema
- Urine formation disturbed due to ARF
- Massive GIT bleeding
- Irritation of mucosa
- Nausea and vomiting
- Incoordination
- Ultimate cause of death—cardiogenic shock
- Muscular weakness
- Paresthesias
- Heart failure—CHF
- Overactivity of muscle—tremor
- Severe convulsion—coma
- Paralysis
- Higher than 0.3 PPM PH_3—severe illness
- Increased HR
- Dizziness
- Easy fatigue

PMA: Garlic odour of gastric content.
Blood stained froth at mouth and nostril.
GI mucosa congested.
Internal organs congested and hemorrhagic necrosis of liver.

Diagnosis: 5 ml of gastric aspirate + 15 ml H_2O in flask with mouth covered with $AgNO_3$ (0.1 N) paper $\xrightarrow[20\ min]{50°C}$ black.

Treatment ABCDEFGH
- Activated charcoal 100 mg, antacid
- Breathing—O_2
- Circulation—50% NS
- DA 6 mg/kg for 1 min
- Elevation of pH—$NaHCO_3$
- Fluid
- Gastric lavage—$KMnO_4$
- Hydrocortisone, Haemodialysis

MLI: Suicidal, rarely accidental/homicidal

16
Analgesics (Opioid)

Algesia/Pain is ill-defined unpleasant sensation evoked by stimulus (external/internal)—**the most important symptom** giving warning signal and primarily protective in nature. Pain and fever are not our enemies but these are our friends because they foretell that something is going on wrong in the body. Opioids are the most powerful analgesics.

Analgesics: 1. Opioid/narcotic/morphine like.
2. Non-opioid/non-narcotic/antipyretic/anti-inflammatory analgesics.

Opioid analgesics: Morphine is extracted from **opium** poppy in which 10% of alkaloid content is morphine and 1% is codeine.

Morphine = 10% opium.
Codeine = 1% opium.

Both are **phenanthrene** derivatives. Opium is **dark brown resinous material** obtained from **poppy capsule of *P. somniferum*.** It is **Benzo-isoquinoline** derivative of **Papaverine/Noscapine**.

Opioid **P**revents substance P release.

Classification (Basis–origin)

1. **Natural opium alkaloid:** Morphine, codeine.
2. **Semisynthetic opiates:** Pholcodeine, oxycodone, hydromorphone, oxymorphone, hydrocodone, oxycodone, heroin (diacetyl-morphine).
3. **Synthetic: P**ethidine (meperidine), **m**ethadone, **t**ramadol fentanyl, ethoheptazone, **d**extropropoxyphene, alfentanil, remifentanil, sufentanil, dipipanone, levorphanol, dextromoramide.

FED To My Patient

Classification (Basis—function)

1. **Strong stimulant:** Morphine, heroin, fentanyl, methadone, meperidine, sufentanil.
2. **Moderate agonist:** Codeine, propoxyphene.
3. **Mixed agonist-antagonist** (activates some R and blocks others): Nalorphine, Nalbuphine*, Pentazocine, Levallorphan*, Butorphanol, Buprenorphine
   (* Not used as analgesic).

Pure antagonist: Nalmefene (nonhepatotoxic, longer-acting, high oral bioavailability).

4. **Antagonist:**
   — Naloxone (**competitive** inhibitor of opioid).
   — Naltrexone (**17 times** more potent than naloxone).

Opioid receptors (4 types)

1. **μ (mu)** (endomorphin 1 and 2 and physical dependence present):
   — μ_1 (supraspinal analgesia)
   — μ_2 (spinal analgesia, respiratory depression and constipation)
2. **κ (kappa):**
   — κ_1 (spinal analgesia)
   — κ_3 (lower ceiling supraspinal analgesia)
3. **δ (delta):**
   — spinal analgesia found in dorsal horn of spinal cord.
   — Effective component of supraspinal analgesia, respiratory depression.
   — Affective behavior
4. **σ (sigma):**
   — Cardiac stimulation
   — Hallucination
   — Dysphoria

```
                  Drug binding to μ, κ, δ R
                     AC + Gi activation
          ┌──────────────┬──────────────┐
        (−)            (−)            (+)
         │              │              │
        (κ)          (μ, δ R)       (μ, δ R)
         ▼              ▼              ▼
    N type Ca++        cAMP
     channel                      K+ channel    ↑ K++
         │              │      ──opening──────▶ efflux
         ▼              ▼         (−)             │
    ↓ Ca++ influx ──▶ ↓ Ca++ ◀────                ▼
                        │                  Hyperpolarisation
                        ▼
              ↓ neurotransmitter release
                              AC = adenylcyclase
                              Gi = coupling protein
```

κ R has affinity for **Dynorphin A** and **Ketocyclazocine**. **Norbinoltorphimine** is selective **κ** blocker.

σR has affinity for **Leu/Met enkephalin**. Endogenous ligand for μ R is **endomorphin 1 and 2**.

Receptors for **antitussive action** is distinct because they bind codeine and morphine.

Actions of µR: Respiratory depression
Analgesic at supraspinal level
Physical dependence and Euphoria

RAPE

Agonists stimulate µ, κ and σ R.
Antagonists inhibit µ, κ and σ R.
Mixed agonist-antagonist stimulates κ R and inhibits µ R.
Supraspinal binding site for opioid: Locus ceruleus, thalamic nuclei, nucleus raphe magnus, hypothalamus.

Transducer mechanism for opioid R

All are G protein coupled R situated mostly on **prejunctional** neurones and reduce release of junctional transmitter **monoamines** (NA, DA, 5-HT), GABA and Glutamate (NMDA).

R stimulation → ↓ cAMP intracellularly
↓
Open K⁺ channel (µ, δ R) or suppress voltage gated N type Ca⁺⁺ channel (κ R)
↓
1. ↓ Ca⁺⁺ intracellularly
2. Neural hyperpolarisation due to κ channel opening
↓
↓Neurotransmitter release by CNS and myenteric neurones

Codeine is **methyl morphine**, partly converted to morphine. It is **1/8th** analgesic of morphine. 60 mg codeine = 600 mg aspirin as analgesic. More selective **cough suppressant.**

PK : Given orally
ADR : Constipation
U : Diarrhoea

Morphine:

Opium poppy:

Morphine = For More Pain

10% opium → Morphine
1% opium → Codeine

They are phenanthrene derivative of *P. somniferum*. Pure active morphine was isolated from opium by **Serturner**. Morphine is called **God's own medicines** by Sir William Osler. Morphine and pethidine are **anodyne hypnotics**.

Mechanism of action of opioid: It causes **hyperpolarisation** of nerve cell, inhibition of nerve firing and presynaptic inhibition of transmitter release. Effects of **MORPHINES:** **M**iosis, **O**rthostatic hypotension, **R**espiratory depression, **P**ain suppression, **H**istamine release and hormonal alteration, **I**ncreased ICP, **N**ausea, **E**uphoria, **S**edation.

Actions

1. Binding sites for morphine are endorphin, dynorphin and enkephalin R (µ, κ, δ R). It has site specific **depressant** and **stimulant** action and is agonist at **all R (µ, κ and δ R)**, but much more at µ R.

2. **Stimulant action** is due to stimulation at **CTZ** (nausea, vomiting), **vagal centre** (↓HR), **Edinger-Westphal nucleus** of III nerve (miosis), **cortical area and hippocampal cells** (causing proconvulsion due to inhibition of GABA release, muscular rigidity).
3. **Depressant action:** Analgesia is strong and has **spinal** and **supraspinal** components. It acts in the **substantia gelatinosa** of dorsal horn to inhibit release of excitatory transmitter (**substance P**) from primary afferents carrying pain impulses. It causes **sleep** (but no convulsion), feeling of detachment, **calming effect,** inability to concentrate, **respiratory depression** (even death due to respiratory failure in poisoning), **temperature regulating centre depression** (hypothermia), **cough centre** depression and **vasomotor centre depression** (↓BP).
4. Dampening of **hypothalamus** activation by afferent collaterals reduces its influence on pituitary leading to ↓**FSH, LH, ACTH, sex hormones, corticosteroids and** ↑ **GH, ADH and prolactin.** But **tolerance** develops with sex hormones and corticosteroids. It has **weak anticholinergic** action and causes mild hyperglycaemia due to central sympathetic stimulation.

> **Actions of morphine:** Analgesia (due to ↓ in pain perception and ↓ in psychological response to pain →inhibition of substance P release), respiratory depression (↓ sensitivity of medullary respiratory centre to CO_2), dependence and tolerance, cough suppressant (anti-tussive), emetic, miosis (↑ parasympathetic tone to pupil), histamine release, constipation due to ↓GI mobility, ↑ tone of ureter and biliary tract.

5. It causes **spasm** of sphincter of Oddi in biliary tract → ↑ intrabiliary pressure →biliary colic (**Treatment:** Naloxone, nitrates, theophylline). It causes ↑ tone of sphincter and detrusor in urinary bladder→urinary urgency and **micturition difficulty.** It releases histamine in bronchi leading to ↑ bronchoconstriction → dangerous in **asthma.**
6. In **GIT,** it causes constipation, ↑ tone and segmentation, spasm of pyloric part, reduction in **all GIT secretion,** ↑ absorption due to stasis, inattention to/ineffective defaecation reflex.
7. It causes **vasodilation** due to histamine release, depressed vasomotor centre and depressed tone of vessels. Blood shifts from pulmonary to systemic circuit. **Postural hypotension** and **fainting** are due to vascular reflex impairment. HR is **enhanced** (reflexly due to ↓BP) or **reduced** due to vagal centre stimulation. Cardiac work is reduced due to reduced peripheral resistance.

> ↑ CO_2 → ↑ ICP → vasodilation

PK: 30% plasma protein bound. Widely distributed. Concentration in liver, kidney and spleen is higher than that in plasma. Only small fraction crosses **BBB** but freely crosses **placenta. Hepatic** metabolism by **glucuronide conjugation. Morphine-6-glucuronide** is active principle and **more potent** than morphine. t½—2–3 hrs.

ADR

1. Sedation, lethargy, idiosyncrasy and allergy. **Allergy and idiosyncrasy** (local reaction due to histamine release, swelling of lips, urticaria).

2. **Apnoea** in newborn due to drug intake by mother during pregnancy (more attainment of drug by foetus in brain). **Naloxone** 10 µg/kg injected in cord is DOC.
3. **Acute morphine poisoning:** Lethal dose—**250 mg. Manifestations**—coma, cyanosis, flaccidity, ↓BP, pinpoint pupil, death due to respiratory failure. Excitement →stupor →coma.
   Treatment: **ABCDEFG**
   — **A**irway, **B**reathing and **C**irculation maintenance.
   — **D**rugs (vosoconstrictor) and 0.6 mg/IV naloxone (DOC).
   — **E**CG monitoring and **F**luid balance.
   — **G**astric lavage with $KMnO_4$.
4. **Tolerance and dependence** (psychological and physical) present. Tolerance is partly **pharmacokinetic** (↑ rate of metabolism) but mainly **pharmacodynamic** (cellular tolerance). **Cross-tolerance** present. Effects of morphine for which **high degree of tolerance** develops are: **S**edation, **M**ental clouding, **E**uphoria and dysphoria, **A**nalgesia and antidiuresis, **R**espiratory depression.

   SMEAR

   Effect of morphine for which **minimal** or **no tolerance** develops are: Antagonistic action, **C**onstipation, convu**L**sion and **M**iosis.   **CALM**
5. **Morphine withdrawal** causes drug seeking behaviour, lacrimation, yawning, anxiety, fear, mydriasis, tremor, dehydration, weight loss, HTN. Naloxone and nalorphine precipitate acute withdrawal syndrome.
   Treatment: Substitution with methadone (orally) followed by gradual withdrawal of methadone.
6. Constipation, addiction, urinary retention, sedation, respiratory depression are ADR of **opioids**.

Precautions

— **Infants and elderly** more sensitive to respiratory depression. **Elderly** susceptible to urinary retention.
— Diseases of liver, kidney and thyroid.
— Unstable personalities.

Contraindication

— **Respiratory insufficiency** (cor pulmonale, respiratory fibrosis, emphysema) which results in death.
— **Bronchial asthma** due to histamine release.
— **Head injury** (due to CO_2 retention → ↑ ICP, respiratory depression, vomiting, miosis, altered mentation).
— Undiagnosed acute **abdominal pain.**
— **Addison's** disease and **Myxoedema.**

IA

— **Phenothiazines, TCA, MAO inhibitors, amphetamine, neostigmine** potentiate morphine by reducing its metabolism.
— Morphine **retards** absorption of orally administered drugs by delayed gastric emptying. MAOI + opioid = hyperpyrexic coma.

Pholcodeine: It has **codeine like** property.
U: As antitussive.

Heroin/diamorphine/diacetylmorphine: It is **3 times** more potent than morphine, more **lipid soluble** (enters brain), more euphoriant (especially on IV injection) but duration of action is **similar** to it. It is **most popular opioid for abuse. Rush/orgasmic** feeling on IV injection.

Cause of death: Infection and respiratory depression.

Withdrawal from heroin is done by methadone, clonidine, naltrexone and cold turkey.

Pethidine/Meperidine: Same actions as morphine but chemically unrelated to it. It interacts with **opioid R** and is blocked by **naloxone**. Analgesic efficacy **near to morphine** and **more than codeine**. Onset of action is **rapid** after IM injection.

Mech: Spasmodic action on smooth muscle (miosis, constipation, urinary retention, biliary spasm) is less marked. It is **equally** sedative and euphoriant and has **similar** abuse potential and respiratory depression to morphine. It is **safer in asthma** due to less histamine release and has local anaesthetic action.

PK: Well absorbed orally. t½ →2–3 hrs. Complete hepatic metabolism.

Pethidine $\xrightarrow{\text{hydrolysis}}$ Meperidinic acid (major metabolite)

Pethidine $\xrightarrow{\text{demethylation}}$ Norpethidine (minor metabolite)

Metabolites conjugated with glucuronic acid and excreted in urine.

Acidification of urine enhances excretion of unchanged metabolites.

ADR: Similar to morphine **except** some atropinic effects (dry mouth, etc.). **Tolerance and physical dependence** slow. But **withdrawal syndrome** rapid due to shorter duration of action. **Overdose** causes excitatory effects (convulsion, mydriasis, hyper-reflexia, myoclonus) due to accumulation of norpethidine.

IA: Non-selective MAO inhibitors interfere with **hydroxylation only.** Hence, norpethidine is produced in excess and excitement occurs.

U:
— Preanaesthetic medication.
— As analgesic in biliary colic and during labour **(DOC)**.

Methadone: Pharmacologically **similar** to morphine (analgesic, emetic, antitussive, constipating, respiratory depressant, biliary action) with slow and persistent nature of action persent. **The most important feature** is high. Oral: Parenteral acitvity ratio **(1:2)** and its firm binding to tissue proteins (plasma protein bindings—90%). **Duration of action**—5 hrs, on IM injection. **1 mg of oral methadone = 4 mg of morphine = 2 mg of heroin = 20 mg of pethidine.**

PK: Plasma t½ →30 hrs. **Hepatic** metabolism by **demethylation** and **cyclization** →metabolites excreted in **urine**. By inducing metabolism, rifampin and phenytoin cause **withdrawal symptoms** in methadone dependent subjects. **Esterases** metabolise remifentanil.

ADR: Same as morphine but tolerance is slow.

Abuse potential lower than morphine. **Withdrawal syndrome** is gradual, and permits slow tapering off effects.

U: **MADS**
1. **Substitution** therapy in opioid dependence.

1 mg oral methadone substituted for
HMP—2, 4, 20
— 2 mg **H**eroin
— 4 mg **M**orphine
— 20 mg **P**ethidine

2. Opioid used for **D**etoxification of morphine addicts →methadone **(DOC)**.
3. As **A**nalgesic in labour and biliary colic.
4. Nonaddicting drug used in opioid withdrawal syndrome →clonidine.
5. **M**aintenance **therapy in opioid addicts:** methadone in sufficient dose given orally to produce high degree of **tolerance** so that subjects give up the habit in the absence of pleasurable effects of IV doses of **heroin and morphine**.

Dextropropoxyphene: **Similar** in analgesia and ADR to codeine but less constipating. Potency = Half to that of codeine.

PK : Hepatic metabolism. t½ — 4–12 hrs.

ADR : — Delirium and convulsion in **overdose**.
— Demethylated metabolite is **cardiotoxic**.
— Abuse liability **same** as codeine.

U : Analgesia (dextropropoxyphene + aspirin/paracetamol).

Tramadol: Centrally acting analgesic.
Affinity for μ R → Modest
Affinity for δ and κ R → Weak

Mech: Inhibits **reuptake of NA/5-HT and activates** monoaminergic spinal inhibition of pain. **Naloxone** is its partial antagonist. 100 mg IV **tramadol** = 10 mg **morphine** as analgesic (actionless marked than morphine).

PK : t½ →4 hrs. Effects last 5 hrs.

ADR : Sleepiness, dry mouth, sweating.

U : — Cancer pain (chronic pain).
— Pain of medium intensity and short duration due to diagnostic procedures, injury, surgery.

Ethoheptazine: Low efficacy, orally active related to **pethidine**.

U of opioids   ABC DAMPEN

1. **E**pidural anaesthesia: The **most** frequently used agent is **morphine**.
2. **C**ough (dry and irritating cough →codeine, noscapine, dextromethorphan and levopropoxyphene).
3. Acute **P**ulmonary edema—morphine.
4. **D**iarrhoea—codeine.
5. Cardiac **A**sthma (acute LVF): **morphine IV** →by reducing preload on heart due to vasodilatation and peripheral pooling of blood, shifting blood from lungs to systemic circuit (relieving congestion and edema of lung), depressing respiratory centre to allay air hunger, reducing cardiac work by blocking sympathetic stimulation.
6. Preanaesthetic **M**edication: morphine and pethidine.
7. **B**alanced anaesthesia and neurolept analgesia: Morphine, pethidine, fentanyl, alfentanil and sufentanil.
8. **A**nalgesic: In severe pain of any type—opioid analgesia but it provides symptomatic relief without affecting the cause.

Pain {Traumatic, Postoperative, Visceral, MI, Burn, Cancer} → Morphine/its parenteral congener

Morphine = For More Pain

Obstetric analgesia → pethidine.

Segmental analgesia is produced by epidural/intrathecal injection of morphine which lasts ~ **12 hrs** without sensory/motor/autonomic modalities. Opioids **ascend** through subarachnoid space to respiratory centre causing respiratory depression.

9. **Neurogenic shock** in emergency →morphine.

Nalorphine

Lethidrone/Nalorphine is N-allyl-normorphine, the **first antagonist** of morphine introduced in 1951. Narcotic antagonists have structure **similar** to morphine (**bulky substitution on "N" results in antagonistic activity**). Specific antidote for morphine, codeine, pethidine and methadone. Abuse liability less than full agonists.

Mech
— Activates κ R.
— **15 mg** nalorphine = **10 mg** morphine as analgesia.
— Antagonises (μ R action) **all morphine** effects and **reverses** respiratory depression.

ADR: — Dysphoria, hallucination, nervousness.
— No psychological dependence and no abuse liability.
— **Tolerance and physical dependence** present.
— Mild withdrawal syndrome.

U: — **Opioid poisoning** (4 mg nalorphine parenteral).
— **Neonatal asphyxia** (0.2 mg nalorphine injected in chord).

Levallorphan: Same as nalorphine. More potent.

Pentazocine: The **first agonist-antagonist** used as analgesic in 1970.

Mech

1. Of all the opioids, **least** constipation causing one →pentazocine.
2. **Weak** antagonist, **strong** agonist.
3. Analgesia caused by pentazocine →**mostly spinal**.
4. κ agonist and μ antagonist.
5. Action **same** as morphine except mostly spinal ($κ_1$) analgesia. 30 mg pentazocine = 10 mg morphine.
6. ↑ HR and ↑ BP due to sympathetic stimulation, hence avoided in MI and coronary ischaemia.

PK: t½ — 4 hrs. Dose →1.5 mg/kg/day orally. Hepatic metabolism by **oxidation** and **glucuronide conjugation**. Excreted in urine.

ADR: Tolerance and dependence present. Withdrawal syndrome present (drug seeking occurs).

CI: MI

U: Postoperative and moderately severe pain.

Nalbuphine

1. It is **pentazocine like** agonist-antagonist with stronger μ antagonistic action and pentazocine like character and ceiling of analgesia.
2. Causes no cardiovascular action.
3. Abuse liability is nearly **similar** to pentazocine.
4. Constipation and biliary spasm are **like pentazocine**.

U: Postoperative pain, MI and labour.

Buprenorphine

Buprenorphine is **synthetic thebaine** congener, highly **lipid soluble** and **25 times** more potent than morphine.

Mech: Partial agonist at μ R. Analgesia lasts 8 hrs after single dose and 24 hrs after chronic use. It is κ **antagonist**.

ADR

— Sedation, CV effects, miosis **similar** to morphine but constipation less marked, postural hypotension present.
— **Respiratory depression** and analgesia exhibit ceiling effect.
— **Tolerance and dependence.**
— Withdrawal syndrome **similar** to morphine (drug seeking present).
— **Abuse liability** lower than morphine.

PK: t½—40 hrs. Highly plasma protein bound. **Mostly** excreted unchanged in bile →**faeces**. **Only opioid** given by sublingual route →buprenorphine.

U: — Cancer pain, postoperative pain
— MI
— Premedication

Butorphanol

Butorphanol is κ analgesic **similar** to but **more potent** than pentazocine **(20 mg butorphanol = 30 mg pentazocine)**. Analgesia and respiratory depression have lower ceiling than morphine. The most outstanding feature→ it neither substitutes for nor antagonises morphine showing its very weak interaction with μ R.

U: Short lasting pain such as renal colic (duration of action **similar** to morphine).

Naltrexone: Chemically related to **naloxone** but **differs** from it in being orally active and having longer (1–2 days) duration of action.

U: 1. **Opioid** blockade therapy of post addicts 50–100 mg/day OD.
2. Relapse of heavy drinking of **alcohol**.

Naloxone is a **competitive antagonist** on all types of opioid R and is a N-allylnoroxymorphone. **NA**rcotic **AN**tagonists are **NA**loxone and **NA**ltrexone.

Mech

1. Pure **opioid antagonist**.
2. **Blocks** μ R at much lower doses than those needed to block κ/δ R.
3. Antagonises **all actions** of morphine on IV 0.6 mg →respiration is stimulated and analgesia is lost.
4. Blocks the actions of endogenous **opioid peptides**.
5. **Dependence and abstinence** syndrome are absent.
6. Blocks acupuncture, placebo and stress induced analgesia.
7. Partly antagonises **respiratory depression** produced by non-opioids.

8. Buprenorphine action is prevented but not reversed by naloxone due to binding to opioid R.
9. 0.4 mg IV precipitates morphine **withdrawal** in dependent subjects. 5 mg precipitates **nalorphine/pentazocine withdrawal.**

PK: Inactive orally due to high first pass metabolism in liver. It acts within 2–3 min on IV injection. Metabolism by **glucuronidation.** t½ = 1 hr for **adult** and 3 hrs for **newborn.**

U: **SPREAD**

1. **S**hock (endotoxic/hypovolemic/stroke/spinal injury): It elevates BP in shock.
2. **P**oisoning of morphine. 0.6 mg (max. 10 mg)/3 min.
3. To **R**everse **R**espiratory depression.
4. Acute opioid overdose: **Naloxone (DOC)** is used to treat overdose with all opioids **E**xcept buprenorphine.
5. Neonatal **A**sphyxia due to opioid use during labour. (10 µg/kg in cord).
6. **D**iagnosis of opioid dependence: It precipitates opioid withdrawal in opioid dependent subjects.

Endogenous opioid peptides: These were isolated from mammalian **brain, pituitary, spinal cord** and **GIT** having **morphine like actions and affinity to opioid R,** blocked by **naloxone.** They are derived from large precursor **polypeptide.** 3 types of opiopeptins are:

1. **Endorphine:** β endorphine/β-END is **the most important endorphine** formed of 31 aa derived from POMC, giving rise to γ-MSH, ACTH, and 2 lipotropins and is µ agonist.
2. **Enkephalin/ENK:** Methionine—ENK and leucine—ENK are **the most important** and are pentapeptides. Proenkephalin = 1 leu ENK (affinity for δ R) + 4 met—ENK (equally affinity for µ and δ R).
3. **Dynorphin/DYN:** It is more potent on κ R but also active on µ and δ R, is derived from **prodynorphin** containing 3 leu-ENK residues. DYN A and B are 8–17 aa peptides. They form **endogenous opioid systems** normally modulating pain perception, mood, hedonic (pleasure related), motor behaviour, GIT motility, emesis and pituitary hormone release. **β-END** is 20–40 times more potent analgesia than morphine when directly injected into brain. It is present in hypothalamus and pituitary having long t½. Hence, it acts as **neurohormone** (reduces LH and FSH release, enhances GH and prolactin release). **ENK and DYN** are widely distributed and have short t½ (hence act as **neurotransmitter/neuromodulator**). They regulate **pain** at spinal and supraspinal level. Morphine is also present in mammalian brain. **The smallest** peptides possessing direct opioid activity are methionine enkephalin and leucine enkephalin.

There are 4 Schedules of Controlled Drugs

A. **I** (no medical use and high addiction potential)
B. **II** (medical use and high addiction potential)
C. **III** (medical use and moderate dependence potential)
D. **IV** (medical use and low abuse potential).

Antiparkinsonian Drugs

Classification
1. Drugs affecting **dopaminergic** system.
    a. **Dopaminergic agonists:** Bromocriptine, lisuride, pergolide, piribedil, ropinirole, pramipexole.
    b. **Peripheral carboxylase inhibitors:** Carbidopa, benserazide.
    c. **DA precursor:** Levodopa (L-dopa).
    d. **Facilitate dopaminergic transmission:** Amantadine, selegiline (deprenyl).
    e. COMT inhibitors: Tolcapone and entacapone.
2. Drugs affecting brain **cholinergic** system.
    a. **Antihistaminic:** Orphenadrine, promethazine.
    b. **Central anticholinergics:** Biperiden, benztropine, benzhexol (trihexyphenidyl), cycrimine, ethopropazine, procyclidine.

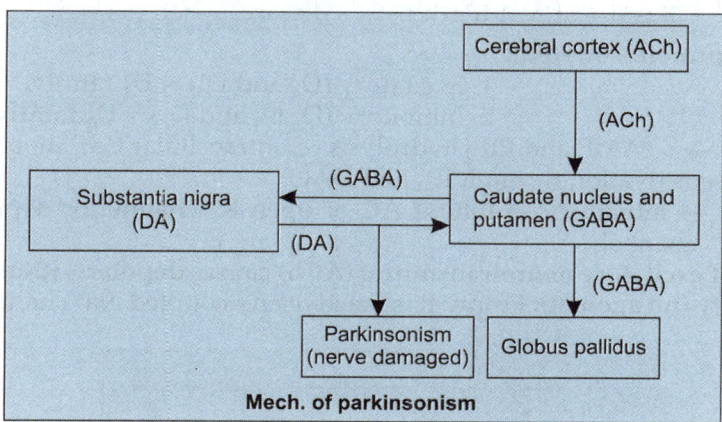

Mech. of parkinsonism

Antidopaminergic drugs are **antipsychotic**. None of the above drugs alter the basic pathology of parkinsonism but most patients get an **additional** 3–6 yrs of happier and productive life. None of the direct DA agonists are superior to levodopa. Levodopa + decarboxylase inhibitor are **the standard therapy** for the **most patients**.

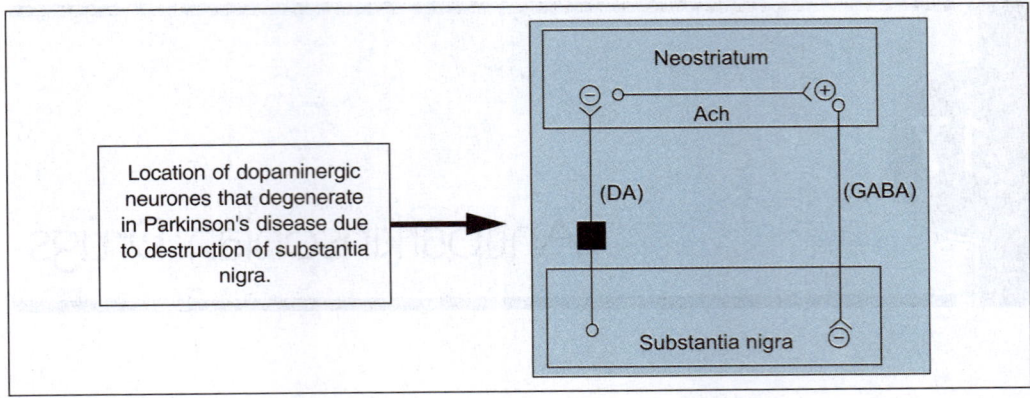

Parkinsonism

Signs: **R**igidity, **A**kinesia, **F**lat facies, **T**remor (at rest).   **RAFT**

It is due to reduction in the activity of dopaminergic inhibitory neurons in **substantia nigra and corpus striatum** (basal ganglia for motor control).

Causes

— Mostly idiopathic
— Wilson disease (hepatolenticular degeneration due to chronic Cu poisoning) is rare cause.

The lesion in parkinsonism is degeneration of neurons in **substantia nigra** and negrostriatal (dopaminergic) tract.

Enhanced DA   —   Schizophrenia.
Reduced DA   —   Parkinsonism.

Cerebellar tremor is intentional tremor. **Basal ganglion** tremor is resting tremor.

Basal = at rest (Parkinson's disease) when **park**ed

DA R (G protein coupled):

1. Excitatory (D_1 and D_5) = D_1 family.
2. Inhibitory (D_3 D_4 and D_2) = D_2 family.

D_1 **family** → ↑ cAMP and PIP_2 hydrolysis → intracellular Ca^{2+} mobilisation and protein kinase activation through IP_3 and DAG.

D_2 **family** → inhibitory → inhibit AC or open K^+ channel or depress voltage sensitive Ca^{2+} channel.

Binding of excitatory neurotransmitter (ACh) causes depolarisation of neurons.

1. **R empty (no agonist):** Empty R is inactive and coupled Na^+ channel is closed.

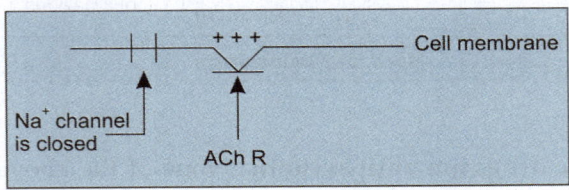

2. **R binding of excitatory neurotransmitter:** ACh binding causes Na^+ channel to open. Entry of Na^+ depolarises cell and enhances neural excitability.

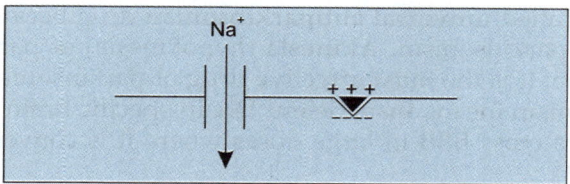

3. **R binding of inhibitory transmitter causes hyperpolarisation:** Cl⁻ influx hyperpolarises cell, making it more difficult to depolarise and hence reduces neural excitability.

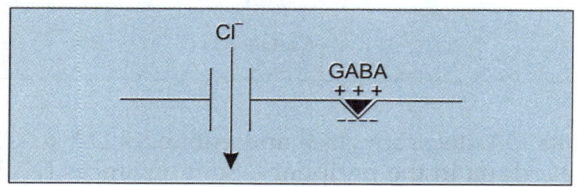

Pakinsonism was first described by **James Parkinson**. It is an **extrapyramidal** disorder characterised by:

1. **Rigidity:** **Cog wheel** rigidity — Upper limbs
   Lead Pipe rigidity — Legs + Trunk
2. **Tremor:** Frequency **4/sec.** **First** in fingers/thumb. Due to excessive **ACh**.
3. **Hypokinesia:** It is due to **DA deficiency**.

   It is associated with defective **posture, gait, sialorrhoea, dementia** mostly affecting **older** individual.
   - Degeneration of neurons in substantia nigra and corpus striatum is the **most consistent lesion** in parkinsonism and results in **DA deficiency** in striatum (which controls muscle tone) leading to imbalance between dopaminergic (**inhibitory**) and cholinergic (**excitatory**) system in the striatum →**motor defect.**
   - **DA oxidation** by MAO-B and aldehyde dehydrogenase generates **hydroxyl free radicals** in the presence of **ferrous** ion of basal ganglia, which is quenched, normally, by glutathione. These radicals damage lipid membrane and DNA resulting in neuronal degeneration.
   - **Ageing** (which induces defects in mitochondrial electron transport chain) and **Wilson's disease** cause these defects.
   - **MPTP** (a synthetic toxin) causes nigrostriatal degeneration and manifestation **similar** to parkinsonism. Its reactive species **MPP** impairs energy metabolism in dopaminergic neurons leading to **cell death.**
   - Neuroleptics, Metoclopramide (dopaminergic blockers) and Reserpine induce parkinsonism. MNR
   - **Lewy body** in neurons of brain is seen in parkinsonism.
   - **DOPA** reverses reserpine induced motor defect.
   - Tremor of parkinsonism is **best** relieved by **Benztropine**.

Levodopa: It is called **universal antiparkinsonian** drug because it improves **all manifestations** of parkinsonism. **Akinesia** (hypokinesia) of parkinsonism is **best** treated by levodopa. It is the **most effective** drug of parkinsonism.

Mech: Parkinsonism means **insufficient DA** in specific brain part. Levodopa is **inactive** but able to cross BBB in large doses where it is converted into **DA** (DA does not cross BBB).

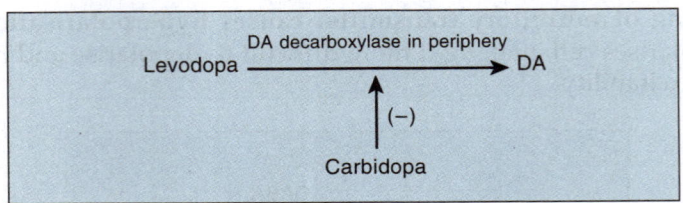

Carbidopa inhibits DA decarboxylase and enhances DA to CNS by preventing the conversion of levodopa in the periphery. So it enhances DA by **4–5 folds**. 95% levodopa is decarboxylated mainly in gut and liver. DA acts on **heart, vessels** (postural hypotension) and **CTZ** of floor of IV ventricle. 1–2% administered levodopa crosses BBB, is taken up by dopaminergic neurons and is converted to DA. DA levels are **lower** in untreated parkinsonism. Patients responding well have higher DA than those responding poorly. Benefits of dopaminergic antiparkinsonian drugs are due to D_2R stimulation (for levodopa also). D_1 R stimulates adenyl cyclase.

Actions

1. **It resolves** rigidity and hypokinesia first, tremors later.
   Secondary symptoms (gait, posture, speech, mood, self-care and interest in life) is gradually normalised.
2. It produces non-specific **awakening** effect in hepatic coma.
3. Peripherally formed DA gains access to CTZ without hindrance (enhances **nausea** and **vomiting**) which has excitatory receptor (R).
4. It reduces **sympathetic outflow** →postural hypotension, impedes **ganglionic transmission,** causes tachycardia but does not enhance BP (β stimulation).
5. It acts on **somatotropes** → ↑GH release and on **mammotropes** → prolactin release inhibition.

PK: Rapidly absorbed by **active transport** process of **aromatic amino acid** from small intestine. **1–3%** enters brain when used **alone. 10%** enters brain when used with dopadecarboxylase inhibitor. t½ →1–2 hrs.

Amino acid of food competes for the **same carrier** for absorption, hence blood level is lower.

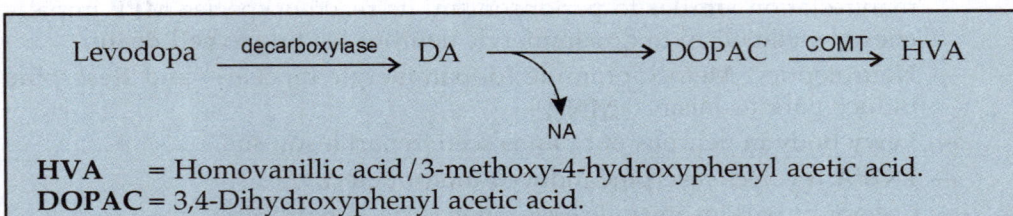

HVA = Homovanillic acid/3-methoxy-4-hydroxyphenyl acetic acid.
DOPAC = 3,4-Dihydroxyphenyl acetic acid.

Pyridoxal is a cofactor for dopa-decarboxylase. Metabolites excreted in **urine** mostly after **conjugation**.

ADR
1. Initially **CTZ stimulation** (nausea and vomiting), **CVS effects** (angina, cardiac arrhythmia, postural hypotension) and **altered taste**.
2. On **chronic** use:
   — Abnormal body movement **(most important dose limiting ADR)**.
   — **Psychosis** (due to ↑ DA).
   — **Fluctuation in motor performance.** "End of dose (wearing off) deterioration" develops into rapid **"switches or on-off effects"** then all-or-none response develops = patient is alternately well and disabled due to degeneration of DA neurons and DA synthesis in the striatum on a moment to moment basis resulting in fluctuation in motor control. **After 2–5 years** of therapy control shows fluctuation.
3. **Coombs' positive haemolysis**
4. **Priapism**
5. **Gout precipitation**
6. **Saliva discolouration**
7. ADR is more when taken with carbidopa (dyskinesias—choreoathetosis of face and distal extremities → **commonest**).

Precaution: Elderly having IHD, CVS disease, liver and kidney disease, gout, glaucoma and peptic ulcer.

IA: Anticholinergic drugs have **additive** antiparkinsonian action with low doses of levodopa.

1. 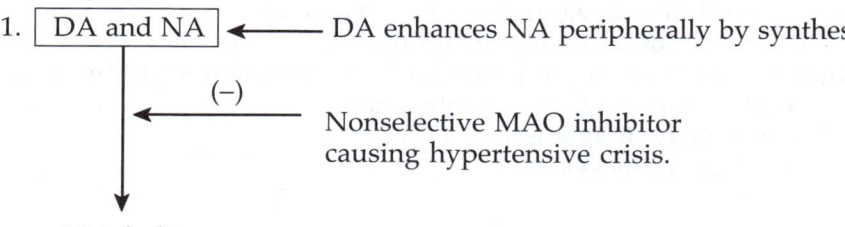 DA enhances NA peripherally by synthesis.

   Nonselective MAO inhibitor causing hypertensive crisis.

   Metabolites

2. **Pyridoxine (vitamin B_6)** enhances peripheral decarboxylation of levodopa → **reduces efficacy of levodopa** (as less levodopa is available to cross BBB).
3. **Domperidone** blocks levodopa induced nausea and vomiting without abolishing its therapeutic effect because it does not cross BBB.
4. **Reserpine** blocks levodopa action by blocking DA entry into synaptic vesicles.
5. **Butyrophenone, metoclopramide** and **phenothiazine** block DA R and reduce efficacy of levodopa.

Peripheral decarboxylase inhibitors (carbidopa and benserazide): They do not cross BBB, hence do not inhibit conversion of levodopa to DA in brain (i.e. **extrapyramidal decarboxylase inhibitor**). They enhance t½ of **levodopa** in the periphery and make more of it available to cross BBB when administered with levodopa. They reduce **"on-off effect"** as cerebral DA levels are more sustained.

Nausea and vomiting are reduced due to reduced DA in the periphery.

ADR (peripheral decarboxylase inhibitor):
Postural hypotension, behavioral abnormalities, involuntary movement.
U (levodopa and decarboxylase inhibitor):
1. Levodopa + Carbidopa = **Cocareldopa** (standard therapy for **most patients** of parkinsonism).
2. Clinical feature best treated by levodopa—**bradykinesia**.

Direct DAergic agonists
Two Classes
1. **Aporphines** (related to apomorphine): Piribedil.
2. **Ergolines** (synthetic ergot derivates): Bromocriptine, pergolide, lisurgide.

Mech: They act on **striatal DA R** even in patients having no capacity to synthesize, store and release DA from levodopa.

Piribedil
1. **It improves** memory, concentration, vigilance, giddiness in elderly.
2. It has **apomorphine like** DA agonist activity and produces **modest** improvement in parkinsonism.
3. It is **less potent** than levodopa and bromocriptine.

ADR: GIT intolerance

U: Cerebroactive drug

Pergolide:
1. **10 times** more potent than bromocriptine
2. It activates both D_1 and D_2 R.
3. It has efficiency and use **similar** to bromocriptine.

Lisurgide:
1. **5-HT and D_2 agonist** but D_1 antagonist.
2. ADR similar to bromocriptine.

Bromocriptine: It is **synthetic ergot** derivative "2-Bromo-α-ergocryptine" and is
- D_1 R partial agonist or antagonist
- Strong D_2 R agonist
- Weak α blocker

Mech:
1. Reduces **prolactin release** due to DA R stimulation on lactotrope cells (strong antigalactopoietic) of pituitary gland (selective D_2 agonist on pituitary).
2. Enhances **GH release** in **normal** person and reduces GH release in **acromegaly**.
3. **Levodopa like action** in CNS present.
4. Emetic (less potent than ergotamine). **Nausea and vomiting** due to DA R stimulation in CTZ.
5. **Hypotension** due to weak peripheral α blockade and central suppression of postural reflexes.
6. Antiparkinsonism in striatum.

Efficacy of anti-parkinsonian drugs
L-dopa > bromocriptine > amantadine > anticholinergic.
7. Weak anti-5-HT present.

PK: 1/3 abosrbed orally. t½—3 hrs. Excreted mainly in **bile**.

U: Started at low doses **1.25 mg** BD then gradually increased.

Antiparkinsonian Drugs

1. **Hyperprolactinemia (DOC)** due to microprolactinomas causing amenorrhoea, galactorrhoea, infertility in **women,** gynaecomastia, impotence and sterility in **man** (stop in pregnancy). **Dose** 10 mg (max)/day. DA and levodopa also reduce **prolactin** secretion.
2. **Acromegaly** 40 mg (max)/day.
3. **Hepatic coma.**
4. **Breast engorgement and lactation suppression.**
5. **Parkinsonism** (dose 20–80 mg/day). Response **similar** to that of levodopa. Improvement in one hour but action lasts **8 hrs**. Used in late cases as **supplement** to levodopa. Controls **"end of doses"** and **"on-off fluctuation"**. **DOC in parkinsonism** with freezing episodes → DOPS (Dihydroxy-phenylserine). Punch Drunk Syndrome is called **Boxer's parkinsonism.**

Drugs causing parkinsonism
1. DA depleting agent (reserpine, tetrabenzine)
2. DA R blocker (haloperidol and CPZ)
3. Manganese

Drugs damaging dopaminergic neurons: Methyl-phenyl-tetrahydrophysidine. Treated by **benztropine** (DOC).

Drugs causing hyperprolactinemia
1. **DA antagonist:** Phenothiazine, metoclopramide, butyrophenone (haloperidol).
2. **DA depleting drugs:** Methyldopa, reserpine.
3. **Hormone:** TRH and estrogen.

ADR (bromocriptine):
1. **Early**
   — painless Digital vasospasm
   — postural Hypotension
   — Syncope
   — Constipation
   — Nasal blockade, nausea and vomiting.

   Dynamic Hip Screw/DHS = CN/Cancellous Nail

2. **Late:** — Erythromelalgia (red painful swollen feet)
   — Psychosis
   — Abnormal movement
   — Hallucination
   — Behavioral alteration
   — Mental confusion   MALE →BPH
   — Livedoreticularis

CI: Patient with **psychotic** illness, recent **MI.**

Ropinirole and pramipexole
Mech: Selective D_2 and D_3 agonists with weak affinity for D_1 and non-dopaminergic receptors.
PK: Ropinirole is rapidly absorbed orally with 40% plasma protein bound and hepatic metabolism by CYP1A2 to inactive metabolites with half-life 6 hrs.

ADR: Low dyskinesias, motor fluctuation and on-off effect; Sedation, Hallucination, Postural hypotension   **LHS Proved**

U: Parkinsonism (Dose = 1.5 mg TDS, dose titration in 15 days for maximum benefit).

Tolcapone and Entacapone (COMT inhibitors)

Mech: Peripheral decarboxylation of levodopa blocked by carbidopa/benserazide is metabolised by COMT to **3-O-methyldopa** that step is blocked by **COMT inhibitors** →prolonged half-life of levodopa→more levodopa to brain/preserved in brain. Smooth **"wearing off"** (increased **"on"** time and decreased **"off"** time).

ADR: Hepatotoxicity (by tolcapone only→elevated serum aminotransferases), **H**allucination, **H**ypotension (postural), **D**yskinesia **D**iscoloured urine (yellow-orange), **D**iarrhoea (15%)   **3 HD**

U: Advanced parkinsonism (200 mg).

Movement disorder	Site of lesion	
Athetosis and **D**ystonia	— Basal ganglia (putamen)	**BAD**
Chorea	— Caudate nucleus	
Hemiballismus	— Subthalamic nucleus	
Parkinsonism	— Substantia nigra and corpus striatum.	

Chorea is due to excessive DA

Causes

1. **Inherited:** Huntington's disease (↓GABA). Defective gene present on **chromosome** 4, autosomal dominant, common in middle adult life.
2. **Metabolic:** Pregnancy, thyrotoxicosis, hypoparathyroidism, oral contraceptive.
3. **Vascular:** SLE and polycythemia.
4. **Drugs:** Levodopa, Li, phenytoin, OC, amphetamine, antimuscarinic.

Treatment: 1. DA R antagonist
2. DA depleting agent
3. GABA enhancing drug (Na valproate)

Treatment of hemiballismus: Tetrabenazine and haloperidol.

Wilson's disease: Autosomal recessive, disorder of Cu metabolism.

Clinical features

1. ↓Serum Cu
   ↑ Urinary Cu
   ↓Serum ceruloplasmin
2. **Commonest** manifestation of Wilson's disease in children and early adolescence—hepatic **cirrhosis** and in young adult—**extrapyramidal** features.
3. **Kayser-Fleischer ring** present in Descemet's membrane.

Treatment: Penicillamine **(DOC)** and **trientine** (DOC if patient not tolerating penicillamine).

Strategies of antiparkinsonian agents are to increase DA activity and to decrease muscarinic activity in the brain.

18. Drugs for Arthritides

Arthritides: Chronic progressive crippling disorder with a **waxing and wanning** course.

Rheumatoid arthritis (RA): It is chronic multisystem disease of **unknown** etiology characterised by persistent inflammatory synovitis usually involving peripheral joints in **symmetric** fashion. Cartilaginous destruction, bony erosion and joint deformity are hallmarks, and are **immunologically** mediated (autoimmune) events in which joint injury occurs (joint inflammation, synovial proliferation and articular cartilage destruction).

Immune complexes composed of **IgM** activate complements $\xrightarrow{(+)}$ cytokines $\xrightarrow{(+)}$ neutrophils $\xrightarrow{(+)}$ **lysosomal enzyme** causes cartilage damage and bone erosion. **PG** causes vasodilatation and pain. For symptomatic relief, **NSAID** is used first **(DOC)**.

Corticosteroid is adjuvant to others. **Except** corticosteroid, all suppress disease and produce remission. (**DMD** = Disease modifying drugs/**DMARD** = Disease modifying anti-rheumatic drugs.) Corticosteroids are **drug of last resort** in RA. Glucocorticoid is **the most potent** anti-inflammatory drug. Drugs for arthritides are:

1. **DMDs:**
   — d-penicillamine
   — Sulfasalazine
   — Etanercept
   — Chloroquine/hydroxychloroquine
   — Gold
   — Immunosuppressant (methotrexate, cyclosporine, azathioprine, chlorambucil, cyclophosphamide)
   — Infliximab and leflunomide (newer drugs)
2. **NSAID**

Gold

Gold is **the most effective** agent for arresting the rheumatoid process and preventing involvement of additional joints.

Mech

1. **Reduces** phagocytosis, chemotaxis, macrophage, lysosomal activity and monocyte differentiation.
2. Inhibits **CMI**.

PK: Heavily bound to plasma and tissue protein specially in kidney. **Accumulates** in the body for years. **Bioavailability (Auranorfin)** →25%.

ADR: HLA-DR3 allele develops ADR to gold therapy (proteinuria, thrombocytopenia and rashes) and d-penicillamine therapy (proteinuria).
1. **Commonest** (dermatitis, pruritic rash, stomatitis).
2. **Vasodilatation** and postural hypotension.
3. **Albuminuria** secondary to membranous GN in 10% patient and resolves on stopping.
4. **Pulmonary fibrosis, peripheral neuropathy, encephalopathy, hepatitis.**
5. **Eosinophilia and bone marrow depression.**
6. ADR of auranorfin: **Diarrhoea 30%**, GIT upset, **taste disturbance, alopecia.**

CI: 1. Kidney, liver and skin disease.
2. Colitis.
3. Pregnancy and lactation.
4. With bone marrow toxic drugs.

U: 1. **Psoriatic** arthropathy.
2. Rapidly **progressing** forms of RA when NSAID fails → DMD + NSAID are given. Benefit is in **70%** after 5 weeks.

Compounds of gold used are:
1. **Aurothiomalate sodium** (gold sodium thiomalate) has **50% gold** and is **water soluble. Starting dose:** 10 mg IM/week up to 50 mg IM/week (max. total dose 1 gm). **Maintenance dose:** 50 mg IM/month.
2. **Auranorfin (orally):** It is orally active, has **29% gold**. Plasma gold level and efficacy is lower than gold sodium thiomalate and is less toxic.
3. **Aurothioglucose:** Given intramuscularly.

Leflunomide
Leflunomide is isoxazole immunomodulatory agent causing cell arrest of autoimmune lymphocyte through its action on DHODH (dihydro-orate dehydrogenase). Efficacy similar to methotrexate/sulfasalazine.

Mech
It is a reversible inhibitor of DHODH. It also inhibits tyrosine kinase.

It inhibits proliferation of activated lymphocytes in RA (immunomodulator). Rapidly converted active metabolites inhibit dihydro-orate dehydrogenase and pyrimidine synthesis in dividing cells.

PK: Well absorbed orally. >90% bound to albumin. t½ →14–18 days (hence loading dose is needed). Converted to active metabolite → undergoes biliary recycling → excreted in urine and faeces.

ADR
1. *Commonest*: headache, diarrhoea, nausea.
2. Allergy (Flu-like syndrome, rash, alopecia, hypokalemia).
3. Weight loss
4. **Diarrhoea, Mental** problem (headache), **Alopecia, Rashes, Decreased WBC** and platelets, **Raised** transaminase, **Anticipation** of chest infection.

DMARD-RA

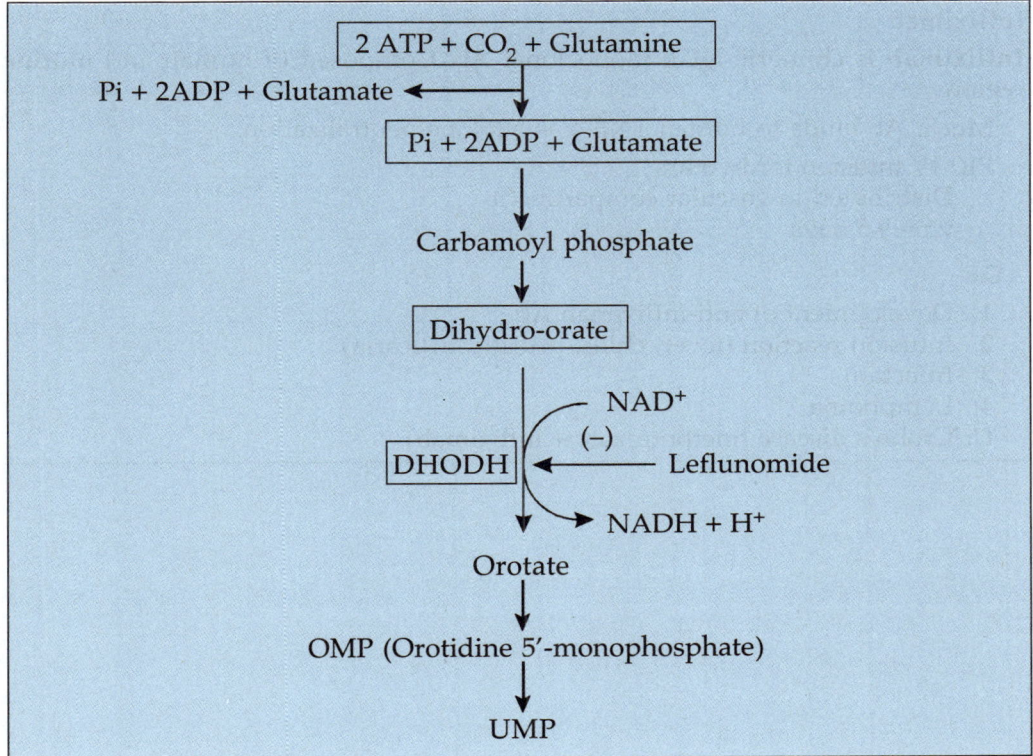

CI:
1. Pregnancy due to teratogenicity (lactating women also) and children.
2. Liver disease due to its clearance by both biliary and renal excretion.

IA:
Cholestyramine enhances its clearance.

U:
Rheumatoid arthritis (alternative to methotrexate/sulfasalazine, 100 mg OD × 3 days followed by 20 mg OD due to longer half-life of active metabolite, i.e. 15 days.

Etanercept is genetically engineered fusion protein composed of 2 identical chains of recombinant human TNF-receptor p 75 monomer fused with Fc domain of human IgG_1.

Mech: The soluble fusion protein binds two molecules of TNF and prevents them from binding to cellular receptor (TNF activity is reduced). The protein does not discriminate between TNF-α and TNF-β (lymphotoxin).

PK: Given subcutaneously, maximum serum concentration—3 days. Median t½—5 days.

ADR: Well tolerated but causes local inflammation.
U: Rheumatoid arthritis (methotrexate + etanercept).
CI: Infection.

Infliximab

Infliximab is chimeric IgGk monoclonal Ab. Composed of human and murine regions.

Mech: Ab binds to human TNF-α →cytokine neutralization.

PK: IV infusion for two hrs
Distributed in vascular compartment
t½ = 9.5 days

ADR
1. Development of anti-infliximab Ab
2. Infusion reaction (fever, chills, pruritis, urticaria)
3. Infection
4. Lymphoma

U: Crohn's disease (methotrexate + infliximab).

19

Drugs for Gout

Gout is a **spectrum of manifestations** having hyperuricemia as biological hallmark of gout. **Plasma and ECF** supersaturated with **uric acid** crystallise and result in clinical gout. It is metabolic disorder of **purine catabolism.** At high blood level, it deposits in joints, kidney and subcutaneous tissue **(tophi). Gout** is always preceded by **hyperuricemia** but **hyperuricemia** does not always lead to gout. Normal plasma urate →1–4 mg/dl. **Secondary hyperuricemia** occurs due to (i) **enhanced nucleic acid metabolism and uric acid production** in leukemia, lymphomas, polycythemia or (ii) **reduced uric acid excretion** by kidney or by drug induction (thiazide, furosemide, ethacrynic acid, ethambutol, pyrizinamide, levodopa, clofibrate).

Acute gout is **sudden onset** of severe inflammation in **small joint** due to urate crystal precipitation in joint space (**commonest**—metatarsophalangeal joint of great toe). Joint becomes red, swollen and extremely painful.

Chronic gout: Pain and stiffness **persists** in joint between attacks.

Outcomes of **GOUT** are:
— Great toe involved.
— One joint (75% monoarticular)
— Urate stone in kidney due to hyperuricemia
— Tophi (chalk like stone under skin in pinna, eyelids, nose and around joint).

GOUT

Classification
A. **Acute gout:** NSAID, corticosteroid, colchicine.
B. **Chronic gout/hyperuricemia:** Synthesis inhibitor (allopurinol). Uricosurics (probenecid and sulfinpyrazone).
   Aspirin is **contraindicated** in gout because it reduces renal clearance of uric acid and enhances hyperuricemia.

Colchicine: It is an **alkaloid** from *Colchicum autumnale* and produces polyploidy in plants. It is neither analgesic nor anti-inflammatory but superficially suppresses **gouty** inflammation and does not effect blood uric acid levels.

Mech: Urate crystal precipitation in the synovial fluid starts **inflammation**, producing chemotactic factor → **granulocyte** migration into joint → crystal **phagocytosis** and **glycoprotein release** → inflammation due to:

1. Lysosomal enzyme release causing joint destruction.
2. ↑ **lactic acid production** from inflammatory cells →↓ **local pH** → ↑ **urate crystal precipitation.**

Drug inhibits **glycoprotein release** (which aggravates inflammation) and **granulocyte migration** into inflamed joint thus interrupts **vicious cycle.** It causes **metaphase arrest** by binding **mitotic spindle** and enhanced **gut motility** through neural mechanism.

PK: Rapidly absorbed **orally,** partly **hepatic** metabolism and excreted in **bile** (**enterohepatic circulation** → ultimately excreted **in urine and faeces**).

ADR

1. Nausea, vomiting, **diarrhoea** (watery/bloody), **abdominal cramp** (due to drug accumulation in intestine and mitosis inhibition in mucosa).
2. In overdose → **CNS depression, kidney damage, intestinal bleeding. Muscular paralysis and respiratory failure** → death.
3. Chronic therapy causes **alopecia, aplastic anemia, agranulocytosis** and **myopathy** (hence chronic use avoided).

U: Acute gout:
1. **Treatment:** 1 mg orally followed by ¼ mg 2 hourly till control is achieved or diarrhoea starts.
2. **Prophylaxis.**

Probenecid: Neither analgesic nor anti-inflammatory. Highly **lipid soluble** organic acid. Inhibits renal tubular secretion of penicillin (duration of action is enhanced).

Mech: Competitively blocks active **transport** of organic acid at **all sites** (**most prominently** in **renal tubules**). Transport is **bidirectional** (reabsorption and secretion). **Uric acid** is reabsorbed by active transport but drug **promotes** its excretion.

PK: Completely absorbed orally, **90%** plasma protein bound. t½ → 9 hrs. Partly **conjugated in liver** and excreted in **urine.**

ADR: Well tolerated.
1. **Dyspepsia (commonest).** Caution needed in peptic ulcer.
2. **Toxic dose** → convulsion and respiratory failure.

IA
1. Inhibits urinary excretion of **cephalosporin, penicillin, sulfonamide, indomethacin, methotrexate** and **nitrofurantoin** (duration of action is enhanced, may not attain antibacterial concentration in urine).
2. **Inhibits biliary excretion** of rifampin.
   Ethambutol and pyrizinamide interfere with uricosuric action of probenecid.
3. **Salicylates** block uricosuric action of probenecid.

U:
1. **Secondary hyperuricemia.**
2. To **prolong** penicillin/ampicillin action.
3. **Chronic gout: 70%** cure, **lifelong** treatment needed. It should not be started in acute attack.

Dose: Starting ¼ gm BD. After week, ½ gm BD (maximum dose **1 gm** BD).

Alkalinisation and **plenty of fluid** concurrently needed to prevent crystallization of excess urate in urinary tract. NSAID/colchicine is needed in first 1–2 months to prevent acute attack.

Sulfinpyrazone

Sulfinpyrazone is pyrazole derivative related to **phenylbutazone**. But unlike phenylbutazone, it does not produce fluid retention and blood dyscrasias. Uricosuric action present but analgesic/anti-inflammatory action absent.

Mech: 1. Cyclo-oxygenase inhibitor.
$\downarrow$
Reduces TXA_2, PGI_2, and PG synthesis.
2. Inhibits tubular reabsorption of uric acid at therapeutic dose.
3. Blocks "release reaction" in platelets, enhances their survival time in thromboembolic disease, reduces platelet adhesion to collagen of vessel wall (breached vessel wall).
4. Inhibits platelet aggregation

IA: 1. Additive action with probenecid but antagonised by salicylates.
2. Inhibits warfarin and sulfonylurea metabolism.

PK: Well absorbed orally, 98% plasma protein bound. Rapid excretion mainly by active secretion in PCT.

ADR: Gastric irritation **(commonest).**

CI: Peptic ulcer.

U: Single dose action lasts 8 hrs.
1. Lowers the rate of sudden death in MI. Dose—200 mg QID.
2. Secondary prophylaxis of arterial thrombosis
3. Chronic gout

Dose: Starting 100–200 mg BD (maximum 800 mg/day).

Allopurinol

Allopurinol is substrate and inhibitor of xanthine oxidase and is the purine analogue 4-hydroxypyrazolopyrimidine.

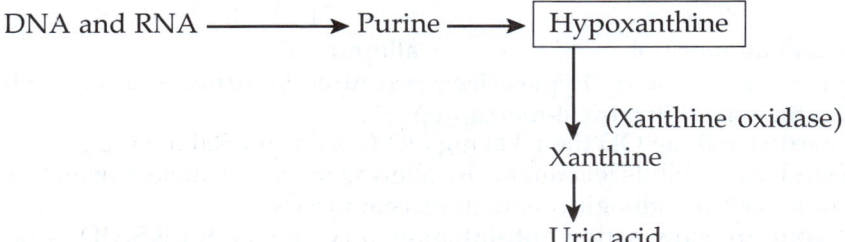

Uric acid has low water solubility especially at low pH. Phagocytosis of uric acid crystal occurs by neutrophils.

Mech: Allopurinol
          ↓
     Alloxanthine (major metabolites)

Allopurinol and alloxanthine inhibit xanthine oxidase. Allopurinol inhibits competitively and is short-acting. Alloxanthine inhibits non-competitively and is long-acting. Precursor of purine synthesis (PRPP) is also reduced by allopurinol.

PK: 80% of oral allopurinol is absorbed, hence not bound to plasma protein. Metabolised largely to alloxanthine. It inhibits its own metabolism during chronic medication and one-third is excreted unchanged, the rest as alloxanthine.

ADR

1. **Commonest:** Hypersensitivity reaction (rashes, fever, malaise, muscle pain).
2. Ampicillin + allopurinol cause skin rashes.

With long-term allopurinol therapy, tophi disappears and nephropathy is reversed.

CI: Pregnancy, lactation, hypersensitive patient.

Precaution

1. Liberal fluid intake.
2. Liver and kidney disease, children and elderly.
3. During initial 1–2 months of treatment with allopurinol and uricosurics, attack of acute gout is common, hence these drugs are not started during acute attack of gout.

IA: No displacement interaction occurs with allopurinol.

1. Inhibits theophylline and warfarin metabolism (hence potentiates them).
2. Ampicillin + allopurinol cause higher incidence of skin rashes.
3. Interferes with mobilization of hepatic iron store.
4. Inhibits degradation of azathioprine, 6-mercaptopurine (their doses are reduced to 1/3) but not that of thioguanine (because it follows a different metabolic path → S-methylation).

Azathioprine is catabolised to 6-mercaptopurine.

U

1. **Chronic gout**

                    Hyperuricemic patient

Underexcretors   Overexcretors
↓   ↓
Uricosuric and allopurinol   allopurinol

2. **Prophylaxis in secondary hyperuricemia** (caused by drugs and radiation).
3. **To potentiate azathioprine/6-mercaptopurine**
   Dose: Starting 100 mg OD then 300 mg OD (maximum 600 mg OD).
4. **Kala-azar:** Drug inhibits leishmania by altering its purine metabolism. Use as adjuvant to sodium stibogluconate in resistant cases.

Drugs for gout are slow acting anti-inflammatory agents but NSAID is rapid acting, anti-inflammatory agent.

20. Nonopioid Analgesics: NSAIDs

"No single drug is superior to all others for every patient."

NSAIDs are weak analgesics/antipyretic analgesics/non-narcotic, do not depress CNS and cause no physical dependence/no abuse liability, act on periphery and most are organic acids.

Two isoforms of cyclo-oxygenase (COX) are
1. COX-1 (function: Physiological housekeeping)
2. COX-2 (function: Inflammation)

COX-1 is constitutive and COX-2 is inducible mainly. Nearly all NSAIDs are selective for COX-1.

Mech: Most NSAIDs block PG generation by blocking COX.

Nabumetone and meloxicam inhibit COX-2 selectively.

Aspirin inhibits COX-1 irreversibly by acetylating one of its serine residues, COX activity returns after fresh enzyme synthesis. Other NSAIDs inhibit COX reversibly and competitively.

PG synthesis inhibitions cause
1. **Analgesia:** Due to blockade of pain nerve sensitising mechanism induced by bradykinin, TNFα, ILs.
2. **Antipyresis:** In febrile person (unaffected in normothermic individual) due to blockade of action of interferons, ILs, TNFα, and pyrogen.

$$\text{PG synthesis production inhibition in hypothalamus} \\ \downarrow \\ \text{Raises temperature set point}$$

3. **Anti-inflammatory:** Due to inhibition of COX (inhibition of PG synthesis) at the side of injury mainly.
4. **Inhibition of dysmenorrhoea** (which occurs due to enhanced PG level) by lowering uterine PG level.
   NSAIDs inhibit parturition by inhibiting PG synthesis.
5. **Anti-aggregatory action of platelet:** Due to inhibition of synthesis of TXA_2 and PGI_2 by NSAID.

TXA_2 action on platelets (which has antiaggregatory action in circulation and aggregatory action on injury) predominates.

NSAIDs inhibit platelet aggregation on therapeutic doses.
6. **Ductus arteriousus closure:** Due to inhibition of PG production (because PGE_2 and I_2 normally keeps ductus arteriosus patency during foetal circulation and an unknown mechanism inhibits PG synthesis, later on, resulting in closure of patent ductus arteriousus).
7. **Anaphylatic reaction** (asthma, rhinitis, urticaria, angioneurotic swelling) probably due to inhibition of COX and lipo-oxygenase.
8. **Renal Na^+ and water retention:** Due to inhibition of PG synthesis limiting renal blood flow (because PG causes vasodilatation, inhibition of ADH action and inhibition of tubular Cl^- reabsorption).
9. **Gastrointestinal damage:** Due to inhibition of synthesis of gastroprotective PGE_2 and $I_2 \rightarrow PG$ deficiency reduces HCO_3^- and mucus secretion, enhances acid secretion, promotes mucosal ischaemia.

All NSAIDs are ulcerogenic. Stable PG analogues (misoprostol, etc.) antagonize NSAID and reduce gastric toxicity.

"See box of page 261."   **LOX forms LT**
1. Thromboxane synthetase
2. Prostacyclin synthetase
3. Isomerase
4. Synthetase

HPETE: Hydroperoxy eicosatetraenoic acid (hydroperoxy arachidonic acid)
HETE: Hydroxyeicosatetraenoic acid (hydroxy arachidonic acid)

Function
LTB_4 – Chemotaxic
     – Reduced permeability
LTC_4 and D_4
     – Vasoconstriction
     – Bronchoconstriction
     – Enhanced vascular permeability
PGI_2 – Bronchodilation
     – Vasodilatation
     – Uterine relaxation
     – Potentiates edema
     – Reduced platelet aggregation

PGI = Platelet Gathering Inhibitor

TXA_2 – Vasoconstriction
     – Bronchoconstriction
     – Platelet aggregation on injury
     – Platelet antiaggregation in circulation
PGD_2 and E_2
     – Vasodilatation
     – Bronchodilation
     – Enhanced permeability
     – Uterine contraction by PGE_2

$PGF_{2\alpha}$
- Vasodilatation
- Bronchoconstriction
- Uterine contraction

$PGD_2, E_2, I_2, F_2\alpha \rightarrow$ vaso**DI**latation   **2 = DI**

$LTC_4, D_4, E_4 \rightarrow$ vasoconst**R**iction   **Fou R = Forced Restriction**

PAF → **P**latelet **A**gg. **F**actor, increases **P**ermeability due to vasodilation.

THROMBOxane A_2 = **THROMBO**sis (**A**gg. of platelet).

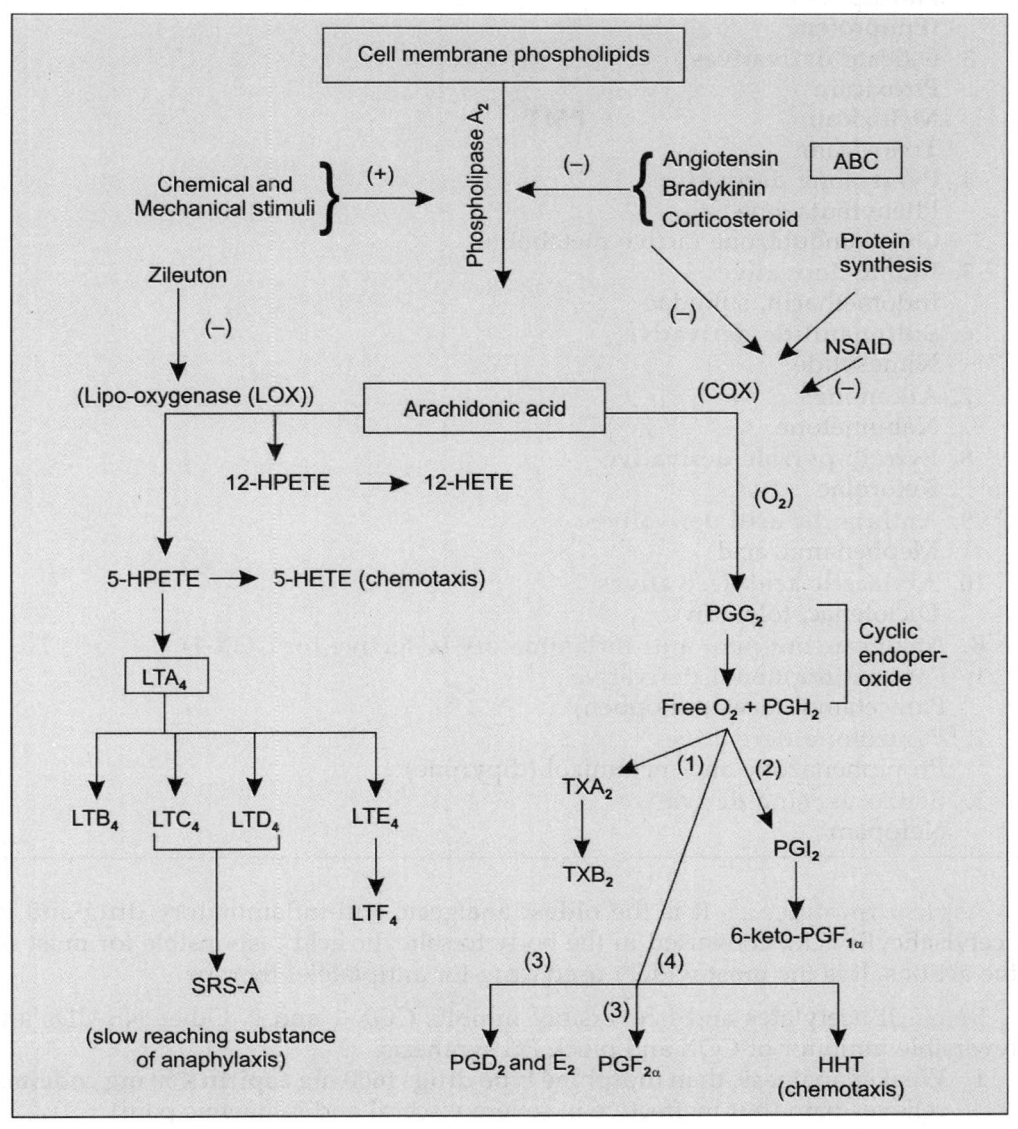

Classification

A. Selective COX-2 inhibitors
  1. Celecoxib
  2. Rofecoxib
  3. Valdecoxib

B. Analgesic and anti-inflammatory (selective for COX-1)
  1. Salicylates: **A**spirin, **B**enorylate, **D**iflunisal and **S**alicylamide. **BADS**
  2. Propionic acid derivatives
     Ketoprofen **KNIFE**
     Naproxen
     Ibuprofen
     Flurbiprofen
     f**E**noprofen
  3. Oxicam derivatives
     Piroxicam
     Meloxicam **PMT**
     Tenoxicam
  4. Pyrazolone derivative
     Phenylbutazone
     Oxyphenbutazone (active metabolite)
  5. Indole derivatives
     Indomethacin, sulindac
  6. Sulfonanilide derivative
     Nimesulide
  7. Alkanones:
     Nabumetone
  8. Pyrrolo-pyrrole derivative
     Ketorolac
  9. Anthranilic acid derivative
     Mephenamic acid
  10. Arylacetic acid derivatives
     Diclofenac, tolmetin

B. Analgesic but poor anti-inflammatory (selective for COX-1)
  1. Para-aminophenol derivative
     Paracetamol (acetaminophen)
  2. Pyrazolone derivatives
     Propiphenazone and metamizol (dipyrone)
  3. Benzoxazocine derivative
     Nefopam

Aspirin (prototype): It is the **oldest** analgesic anti-inflammatory drug and is acetylsalicylic acid, converted in the body to salicylic acid responsible for **most** of the actions. It is the **most** widely used drug for antiplatelet therapy.

Mech: It acetylates and irreversibly inhibits COX-1 and 2. Other NSAIDs are reversible inhibitor of COX and block PG synthesis.
  1. Weaker analgesic than morphine type drugs **(600 mg aspirin ≤ 60 mg codeine)** relieves pain (but ineffective in severe visceral and ischaemic pain).

Analgesic action is due to inhibition of PG mediated sensitisation of nerve endings.

Anti-inflammatory action occurs at **the dose 100 mg/kg/day.** It resets hypothalamic thermostat and promotes heat loss (sweating, cutaneous vasodilatation) to reduce fever. But it reduces no heat production.

2. Due to uncoupling of oxidative phosphorylation, cellular metabolism is enhanced causing increased heat production and glucose utilisation.

    At **toxic** doses, hyperglycemia due to central sympathetic stimulation (adrenaline and corticosteroid release) occurs.

    At **chronic** uses of large doses, negative N_2 balance due to enhanced conversion of protein to carbohydrate takes place and plasma cholesterol as well as FFA are also reduced.

3. Gastric mucosal damage due to reduced acid secretion. Nausea and vomiting due to CTZ stimulation. "**Ion trapping**" in mucosal cell enhances gastric toxicity because drug is unionised and diffusible in gastric juices but after entering the gastric mucosal cell, it ionises and hence becomes indiffusible.

    (Aspirin + $CaCO_3$ + citric acid) tablet is less ulcerogenic.

4. **Respiration** is stimulated at inflammatory doses due to enhanced CO_2 production and enhanced sensitivity of respiratory centre to CO_2 leading to hyperventilation → respiratory failure if dose is further enhanced.

    Respiratory stimulation tends to washout CO_2 → respiratory alkalosis which is compensated by renal excretion of HCO_3^- → compensated **respiratory alkalosis**.

    Most adults with a dose of 5 g/day have compensated **respiratory alkalosis.**

    Respiratory depression is due to CO_2 retention (↑ production and ↓ excretion) → **respiratory acidosis.**

    All acids (metabolic acids—acetoacetic, lactic, pyruvic, sulphuric, phosphoric and salicylic of aspirin) due to depressed renal function cause uncompensated metabolic acidosis.

    Most children have uncompensated metabolic acidosis and adult at later stages.

    Dehydration occurs due to sweating, hyperventilation and enhanced loss of Na^+, K^+, HCO_3 and water.

    > **Intially = Compensatory respiratory alkalosis.**
    > **At high doses = Respiratory acidosis.**
    > **Late effect = Compensated respiratory alkalosis.**

5. It causes **vasodilatation** and enhanced CO at large doses and vasomotor centre depression (↓BP) at toxic doses.

    CHF may precipitate due to Na^+ and water retention and enhanced CO.

    Before it is deacetylated in liver, it acetylates COX in platelets in portal circulation irreversibly and inhibits TXA_2 synthesis irreversibly. Hence, it inhibits platelet aggregation. It also reduces clotting factor synthesis.

    It acetylates and inhibits irreversibly COX-1 and 2 and TX-synthetase. So, platelet cannot synthesise new enzyme and remain inactive for rest of its lifespan (platelet forms **no enzymes** due to lack of nuclei).

Aspirin induced prolongation of bleeding time lasts 5–7 days.

Dose of 40 mg/day is effective and **maximum** inhibition of platelet function occurs at ≥160 mg/day.

It also inhibits PGI synthesis but intimal cell of vessels synthesises fresh enzyme, hence activity returns rapidly.

Low dose (40–150 mg/day or 300 mg twice weekly)→TXA_2 formation reduced.

High dose (>900 mg/day) →TXA_2 and PGI_2 production reduced.

It inhibits **ADP release** from platelets and their sticking to each other (but no effect on their adhesion to damaged vessel wall and on platelet survival time).

PK: Absorbed from GIT. Limiting factor in absorption is its poor water solubility and solubility is more at higher pH.

Alkalinisation enhances elimination

It is rapidly **deacetylated** in the liver, plasma and gut wall to release salicylic acid (active form). Both aspirin and salicylic acid are **conjugated** in the liver with glycine →salicyluric acid (major pathway) and with glucuronic acid.

80% salicylic acid is plasma protein bound.

Excretion is with glomerular filtration and tubular secretion and 1/10th is excreted as free salicylic acid.

Urate excretion

<2 gm/day—urate retention and antagonism of **all** uricosuric drugs.

2–5 gm/day—variable effects.

>5 gm/day—urate excretion.

High doses in chronic gout are tolerated by few (hence aspirin is contraindicated in gout).

Plasma t½ of aspirin →18 min

Plasma t½ of both aspirin + salicylic acid→4 hrs ⎤

t½ of anti-inflammatory dose →10 hrs   ⎬ Elimination is dose dependent

t½ of toxic dose → 30 hrs.   ⎦

ADR

1. **Gastric mucosal damage:** Gastric irritation and peptic ulcer with GI bleeding are **commonest** and **most important**, which are due to reduced production of mucus and HCO_3^-→back diffusion of H^+ in gastric mucosa and production of local mucosal ischaemia.
2. **Hypersensitivity and idiosyncrasy** (rash, asthma, angioedema, anaphylactic shock).

    Asthma is due to inhibition of PG synthesis and consequent diversion of arachidonic acid to lipo-oxygenase pathway.
3. **Salicylism:** Electrolyte imbalance, hyperventilation, and CN VIII damage (vertigo, tinnitus, dizziness, reversible hearing and vision impairment) occur at anti-inflammatory dose (100 mg/kg/day). Tinnitus is early indication of toxicity.

4. **Liver damage:** Aspirin therapy in children with RA raises serum transaminase →liver damage.
5. **Reye's syndrome:** Association between salicylate therapy and Reye's syndrome is seen in children having viral infection.
6. **Acute salicylate poisoning:** More common in children. Fatal dose in adult → 15–30 gm and lower in children.

> ADR of **ASPIRIN**: **A**sthma, **S**alicylism, **P**remature closure of PDA/**P**latelet disaggregation/**P**hosphorylation–oxidation uncoupling, **I**ntestinal bleeding due to peptic ulcer, **R**eye's syndrome, **I**diosyncracy, **N**oise (tinnitus).

Order of toxicity

Tinnitus →uncoupling of oxidative phosphorylation (↑ CO_2 →↑ respiration) → (medullary stimulation →HCO_3^- loss and respiratory alkalosis) →**acidosis** (HCO_3^- loss, fluid and electrolyte loss, respiratory depression).

Manifestations

1. **N**ausea and vomiting   **ABCDEFGH**
2. **E**lectrolyte imbalance
3. **A**cidotic **B**reathing
4. **C**oma and **C**onvulsion
5. **D**ehydration and **D**elirium
6. Death due to respiratory **F**ailure + cardiovascular collapse
7. **G**iddiness
8. **H**allucination and **H**yperpyrexia
9. **R**estlessness

Treatment

1. **A**irway **B**reathing and **C**irculation maintenance   **ABCDEFGH**
2. Forced alkaline **D**iuresis and **H**emodialysis to remove absorbed drug.
3. **E**lectrolyte balance by IV **F**luid with Na^+, K^+, HCO_3^- and **G**lucose and External cooling (most important).
4. Gastric lavage to remove unabsorbed drug.
5. **B**lood transfusion and vitamin K.

IA

1. Reduces protein bound iodine level by displacing thyroxine without causing hypothyroidism.
2. Blunts diuretic action of furosemide and thiazides and blocks the action of spironolactone. Active metabolite of spironolactone is canrenone and aspirin competes with each other in PCT for active transport.
3. Interferes tubular secretion of methotrexate and blocks tubular secretion of uric acid. Antagonises the uricosuric action of probenecid.
4. Depletes methotrexate, phenytoin, warfarin, sulfonylurea and naproxen from binding sites on plasma protein (toxicity may occur)
5. Causes bleeding in patient on oral anticoagulants due to its antiplatelet action.

U:
1. **RA (Rheumatoid arthritis):** Aspirin DOC in most cases.
2. **Osteoarthritis.**
3. **Acute rheumatic fever:** Aspirin DOC in all cases. Starting dose →100 mg/kg/day. Maintenance dose →50 mg/kg/day. Withdrawal gradually within 2–3 weeks.
4. **As antipyretics** (fever of any origin) 500 mg TDS.
5. **As analgesics** (headache, bodyache, pulled muscle, joint pain, myalgia, toothache, neuralgia, dysmenorrhoea). Menstrual cramp is due to intermittent ischaemia of myometrium. Drugs used are aspirin, ibuprofen, naproxen, piroxicam, mephenamic acid and diclofenac.
6. **Patent ductus arteriosus.**
7. **To delay labour.**
8. **Eclampsia and pre-clampsia by** suppressing TXA_2 production.
9. **Post-MI and post-stroke:** Now routinely prescribed. 325 mg OD reduces MI in male. At low doses, it inhibits TXA_2 synthesis. At high doses, it reverses the beneficial effects by inhibiting PGI_2 synthesis in vessel wall (antiaggregatory and vasodilatory). It also reduces transient ischaemic attacks and incidence of stroke. But incidence of stroke in post-MI is not reduced. New onset or sudden worsening angina is reduced to half by 300 mg aspirin daily for 12 week.

Precautions
1. Avoided in DM, CHF and juvenile RA.
2. Stopped 1 week before elective surgery.
3. In **pregnancy,** it causes LBW, prolonged labour, premature closure of ductus arteriosus, greater postpartum blood loss.

Contraindication
Aspirin is contraindicated in **gout** because it reduces renal clearance of uric acid and enhances hyperuricemia.

Phenylbutazone
The term **"NSAID"** was first used to contrast phenylbutazone from corticosteroid, both used in RA due to anti-inflammatory action and NSAID, **'like steroid'**, does not cause Cushing's syndrome. More potent anti-inflammatory than the usually tolerated dose of aspirin.

Mech
1. Anti-inflammatory action present.
2. Its **active metabolite** (phenylbutazone → oxyphenbutazone) is uricosuric causing inhibition of renal tubular reabsorption of uric acid.
3. Phenylbutazone causes retention of **Na^+ and water** by direct action on renal tubules leading to edema and plasma volume expansion after 10 days.

PK
Completely absorbed orally. **Complete hepatic** metabolism by hydroxylation and glucuronidation. 98% bound to plasma protein. Plasma $t_{1/2}$ →60 hrs.

ADR
1. More toxic than aspirin.
2. **Hypothyroidism** and goitre on long-term use (agranulocytosis, bone marrow depression, Stevens-Johnson syndrome)→dangerous edema (major limitation of use for >1–2 weeks).
3. **Hypersensitivity** (rashes, stomatitis, serum sickness).
4. Peptic ulcer.
5. CNS effects (nausea, vomiting).

Contraindications
1. **CHF and HTN**
2. Peptic **U**lcer
3. **T**hyroid disease
4. Blood dyscrasias

IA
1. Displaces sulfonamide, methotrexate, warfarin, tolbutamide, imipramine from protein binding sites.
2. Phenylbutazone + anticoagulant enhance bleeding.
3. Inhibits phenytoin and tolbutamide metabolism competitively.
4. It is an inducer of microsomal enzyme enhancing the metabolism of steroid and its own.

U
1. In **severe cases** not responding to other NSAIDs in acute exacerbation of RA and ankylosing spondylitis, rheumatic fever and to suppress attack of acute gout.
2. It inhibits swelling and inflammation after blunt injuries and fracture, etc.

Oxyphenbutazone: It is major **active** metabolite of phenylbutazone. Similar in pharmacological profile to phenylbutazone but causes less gastric irritation.

Indomethacin: It is potent anti-inflammatory, analgesic and antipyretic drug.

Mech
1. Inhibits PG synthesis and suppresses **neutrophil motility.**
2. **At toxic doses,** it uncouples oxidative phosphorylation like aspirin.

PK
Well absorbed orally, rectal absorption slowly, 90% bound to plasma proteins, partly metabolised in liver, excreted in urine, plasma t½ →2–5 hrs.

ADR
1. **50% GIT and CNS effects.** Gastric bleeding (enhanced risk due to reduced platelet aggregation). Frontal headache (very common). Hallucination, depression, psychosis.
2. **Hypersensitivity** (leukopenia, rashes, etc.)
3. **Aplastic anemia**
4. **Renal damage**

Contraindications
1. Indomethacin + Triamterene = renal failure
2. Kidney disease
3. Epileptics and psychiatric patients
4. Pregnant women and children
5. Mechinery operator and driver.

Precautions
Indomethacin + anticoagulants not given together due to bleeding.

IA
1. Reduces antihypertensive effects of thiazides, furosemide, β-blocker, ACE inhibitors.
2. Blunts diuretic action of furosemide.
3. Displaces warfarin from protein binding sites.

U
1. Closure of **patent ductus arteriosus (commonest)** → 0.15 mg/kg/12 hourly three times (70% success). Misoprostol (PGI analogue) keeps it open.
2. Malignancy associated fever
3. **Bartter's syndrome** responds dramatically
4. **Acute gout**
5. **RA not controlled by aspirin**
6. **Ankylosing spondylitis**
7. Acute exacerbation of destructive arthropathies and psoriatic arthritis.

Propionic acid derivatives
All members have similar pharmacodynamic properties but differ in potency and duration. They are analgesic, antipyretic and anti-inflammatory.

Mech
1. Inhibit PG synthesis (naproxen **most** potent) and platelet aggregation.
2. Ketotifen stabilises lysosomes.
3. Ibuprofen is the **safest**.
4. Naproxen is the most efficacious and better tolerated.

ADR
1. **Commonest** (nausea, vomiting and gastric discomfort).
2. CNS effects (blurring of vision, tinnitus, depression, headache).
3. Ibuprofen is the safest.
4. Precipitation of aspirin induced asthma.

Contraindications
1. Pregnancy and lactating mother.
2. Peptic ulcer.

PK
All propionic acid derivatives enter brain, synovial fluid, and cross placenta. Well absorbed orally. 98–99% plasma protein bound. Hepatic metabolism by

hydroxylation and glucuronide conjugation. Excreted in urine and bile. t½ →2–4 hrs (naproxen t½ →14 hrs).

IA

Reduces diuretic and antihypertensive action of furosemide, thiazide and β-blockers.

U

1. Available as an **"over-the-counter drug"**. Analgesic and antipyretic like aspirin.
2. In **dysmenorrhoea** due to PG synthesis inhibition.
3. **Musculoskeletal disorder** (RA, osteoarthritis) specially where pain is more prominent than inflammation.
4. Soft tissue injury, vasectomy, fractures, tooth extraction postoperatively.
5. Naproxen in acute gout due to potent inhibition of leukocyte migration and ankylosing spondylitis. Naproxen and piroxicam especially inhibit chemotactic migration of leukocyte into the inflamed joint.
6. Flurbiprofen is **ocular anti-inflammatory drug** (more efficacious than ibuprofen but more gastric ADR is present).

Diflunisal

Not marketed in India. Not antipyretic.

PK

Not metabolised to salicylic acid. Undergoes **"futile"** enterohepatic cycle with reabsorption of its glucuronide followed by cleavage of glucuronide, again to release the active moiety.

ADR

Pseudoporphyria.

U

As uricosuric at 500 mg BD.

Mephenamic acid: It is anthranilic acid derivative (fenamate).

Mech

1. Exerts central and peripheral analgesic actions.
2. Inhibits PG synthesis and also antagonises certain action of PG.
3. Analgesic, antipyretic and anti-inflammatory actions present.

PK

Slow but complete oral absorption. Partly metabolised and excreted in bile and urine. Plasma t½ →3 hrs.

ADR

1. Diarrhoea: **most** important dose related ADR.
2. Haemolytic anemia (rare but serious).
3. CNS effects (rashes and dizziness).

U

1. Dysmenorrhoea.
2. As analgesic in soft tissue, joint and muscle pain where strong anti-inflammatory action is not required.

Enphenamic acid

Developed in **India** and claimed not to cause Na^+ and water retention like other NSAIDs.

Nimesulide: It has analgesic, antipyretic and anti-inflammatory action.

Mech

1. Selectively inhibits **COX-2** (PG synthesis).
2. Reduces superoxide generation by neutrophils.
3. **Free radical scavanging** present.
4. Inhibits **metalloproteinase** activity in cartilage, TNF-α release and PAF synthesis.

PK:

Completely absorbed orally, 99% plasma protein bound, extensively metabolised with t½ →4 hrs, excreted in urine.

ADR

1. CNS (somnolence, dizziness)
2. GIT (diarrhoea, heart burn)
3. Skin (rashes, etc.)

U

Short-lasting painful inflammatory conditions (ENT disorder, sports injury, sinusitis, dental surgery, bursitis, low backache, osteoarthritis, postoperative pain, dysmenorrhoea).

Nabumetone

Nabumetone (prodrug) → 6-MNA (active metabolite).

Mech

6-MNA inhibits COX (COX-2 > COX-1).

ADR

Ulcer and bleeding

U

1. Soft tissue injury.
2. RA
3. Osteoarthritis

Diclofenac sodium: It is analgesic, antipyretic and anti-inflammatory drug. Efficacy similar to naproxen.

Mech: It inhibits PG synthesis and has antiplatelet action.

PK

Well absorbed orally, 99% plasma protein bound, metabolised and excreted both in urine and bile, good tissue penetratibility, concentration in synovial fluid is 3 times longer than that in plasma (extented therapeutic action in joint), plasma t½ →2 hrs.

ADR

1. GIT (ulcer, pain, bleeding)
2. CNS (headache, dizziness, nausea)
3. Skin (rashes, etc.)

IA

Enhances plasma level of digoxin and lithium.
U: Same as ibuprofen.
1. Postoperative and post-traumatic conditions (affords quick relief of pain and wound edema).
2. Dysmenorrhoea.
3. Osteoarthritis.
4. Bursitis.
5. RA
6. Ankylosing spondylitis.

Tolmetin

Analgesic-antipyretic-anti-inflammatory actions present. Order of anti-inflammatory action: phenylbutazone > tolmetin > ibuprofen.
Mech: Inhibits PG synthesis.
ADR: Mostly GIT (ulcer)

U

1. Soft tissue inflammation.
2. Arthritides.

Piroxicam

Analgesic-antipyretic-anti-inflammatory drug. Inflammatory potency similar to indomethacin.

Mech

1. Inhibits COX reversibly.
2. Inhibits platelet aggregation.
3. Lowers PG concentration in synovial fluid.
4. Reduces the production of **IgM rheumatoid factor** and lowers its plasma level in patients of RA.
5. T_H: T-suppressor ratio and chemotaxis of leukocytes are reduced.

PK

Completely and rapidly absorbed. **99%** plasma protein bound, extensively metabolised in liver by hydroxylation and glucuronide conjugation, excreted in urine and bile (enterohepatic cycling present).
Plasma t½ →2 days.

ADR
1. Edema and reversible **azotemia.**
2. Skin (rashes and pruritis).
3. GIT (heart burn, anorexia, nausea) but **less ulcerogenic.**

U
1. As **short-term analgesic and long-term anti-inflammatory** drug in:
   - Musculoskeletal injury
   - Episiotomy
   - Dentistry
   - Acute gout
2. Dysmenorrhoea
3. RA, osteoarthritides and ankylosing spondylitis.

Ketorolac
Potent analgesic and modest anti-inflammatory drug. Same efficacious as morphine in postoperative pain.

Mech
Inhibits PG synthesis and platelet aggregation.

PK
Rapidly absorbed orally and intramuscularly. 60% excreted unchanged in urine, metabolised by **glucuronidation** (plasma t½ → 6 hrs).

ADR
1. GIT (dyspepsia, ulcer, diarrhoea)
2. CNS (nervousness)
3. Skin (pruritis)
4. Fluid retention and ↑ serum transaminase.

U
1. Acute pain
2. Migraine
3. Renal colic
4. Pain due to bony metastatis.
5. Postoperative and acute musculocutaneous pain.
   30 mg (max) IM QID.
   20 mg (max) oral QID.

Nefopam does not inhibit PG synthesis.

ADR
1. Sympathomimetic (↑ HR, nervousness)
2. Anticholinergic (urinary retention, dry mouth, blurred vision)

Contraindication: Epileptics.

U
1. Musculoskeletal pain.
2. Traumatic and postoperative pain (efficacy approaches morphine).

Meloxicam: Congener of pyroxicam.
Mech: Inhibits COX-2 more than COX-1.
ADR: GIT (better gastric tolerabilities).
U: Rheumatoid and osteoarthritis.

Tenoximcam: Congener of pyroxicam with similar properties and uses.

Sulindac: Sulindac (prodrug)→active sulfide metabolite. Weaker anti-inflammatory action than that of indomethacin.
Mech: Selective extrarenal PG synthesis inhibitor.
ADR: Order of frequency of bleeding and ulceration: indomethacin> sulindac > ibuprofen.
U: As analgesic-antipyretic-anti-inflammatory drug.

Metamizol/dipyrone and propiphenazone: These are analgesic, antipyretic and poor anti-inflammatory but metamizol causes agranulocytosis. Dipyrone is a derivative of amidopyrine.

Paracetamol (Acetaminophen): It is diethylated active metabolite of phenacetin. It is used since **1950**. But phenacetin was introduced in 1887 (but banned due to analgesic abuse causing nephropathy). Paracetamol is good antipyretic. Paracetamol + aspirin is **additive**.

Mech
1. Raises pain threshold and has weaker peripheral anti-inflammatory component.
2. Inhibits PG synthesis in the periphery **poorly** but inhibits COX in the brain **more actively**.
3. Weak PG inhibitor.

PK
Well absorbed orally, 1/3 plasma protein bound, uniformly distributed in the body, conjugated with glucuronic acid and sulfate, excreted rapidly in urine.
Plasma half-life → 2–3 hrs.
Effects after oral dose last 4 hrs.

ADR
1. Analgesic nephropathy (papillary necrosis, tubular atrophy, renal fibrosis, kidney shrinkage, loss of urine concentrating ability).
2. **Paraphenatidine** and other minor metabolites produced from phenacetin but not from paracetamol cause haemolysis and methaemoglobinemia.
3. Delayed hepatic necrosis (due to glutathione depletion) forms toxic tissue adducts in liver.
Treatment: N-acetylcysteine to replenish glutathione.
4. **Acute paracetamol poisoning:** Children having "low hepatic glucuronide conjugating ability" are more susceptible.
    >150 mg/kg → serious toxicity.
    >250 mg/kg → fatal

(a) *Early manifestations*
Abdominal pain
Liver tenderness
Nausea and vomiting

(b) *After 12–18 hrs:* Centrilobular hepatic necrosis, renal tubular necrosis. hypoglycemia →coma.
(c) *After 2 days:* Jaundice

Mech of toxicity

N-acetyl-benzoquinone-imine is highly reactive arylating minor metabolite which is detoxified by conjugation with glutathione. In large doses, glucuronidation capacity is saturated and hepatic glutathione is depleted. The metabolite then, binds covalently to protein of hepatic cells and renal tubules causing necrosis. It also causes hepatotoxicity in premature infants (<2 kg), hence it is contraindicated. In chronic alcoholics, 6 gm/day results in hepatotoxicity in a few days.

Treatment

1. Gastric lavage with activated **charcoal**.
2. **N-acetyl cysteine** 150 mg/kg is infused (IV) over 15 min followed by same dose over the next 20 hrs or 75 mg/kg oral QID for 3 days to replenish glutathione stores of liver and inhibits binding of cellular metabolites to cells. Treatment is ineffective 16 hrs after ingestion.

U

1. One of the **best** antipyretics. One of the **commonest** used **"over-the-counter"** analgesic for headache, musculoskeletal pain and dysmenorrhoea, etc. if anti-inflammatory action is not needed.
2. Given in ulcer patient and in aspirin contraindicated patient.

Medications that can cause depression
Amphetamines
Antihypertensives (clonidine, propranolol, thiazides, reserpine).
Benzodiazepines
Cimetidine
Cocaine
Hormones (oral contraceptives)
Interferon
Isotretinoin
Nonsteroidal anti-inflammatory agents
Ranitidine
Steroids

ABC
SIR
INH

Celecoxib: Also called **"safe arpirin"** because it inhibits COX-2→gastric damage absent which is due to COX-1 inhibitor, approved in **1998** in USA. **Rofecoxib** was approved in **1999**. COX-2 expression causes colon cancer and Alzheimer's disease.

Mech: Selectively inhibits **COX-2 more than COX-1** (*in vivo*, celecoxib does not block COX-1). COX-2 inhibition is time-dependent and reversible (aspirin inhibits COX-1 rapidly and irreversibly). Not inhibit platelet aggregation. Spares COX-1 which helps in maintaining gastric mucosa.

PK

Readily absorbed (peak concentration 3 hrs), extensive hepatic metabolism by cytochrome P450 **(CYP2C9)**, excreted in feces and urine, t½–11 hrs (hence taken OD).

ADR
1. Abdominal pain, diarrhoea and dyspepsia are the **commonest** ADR.
2. Renal toxicity
3. Gastroduodenal ulcer

CI: Patient allergic to sulfonamide

IA
1. Inhibitors of **CYP2C9** (fluconazole, fluvastatin, zafirlukast) enhance serum level of celecoxib.
2. Celecoxib inhibits **CYP2D6**.
   ↓
   Elevates β-blocker, antipsychotic and antidepressant.

U
1. Osteoarthritis
2. Rheumatoid arthritis (it is not analgesic)

Valdecoxib: Similar to rofecoxib. Half-life = 10 hrs.

U: Dose = 10 mg OD in RA and osteoarthritis. 20 mg OD in dysmenorrhea and postoperative pain.

Unit 3
Hormones

21 An Overview of Hormones

Steroid hormones
1. Estrogen
2. Antiestrogen
3. Progesterone
4. Antiprogestin
5. Androgen
6. Antiandrogen
7. Corticosteroid
8. Inhibitors of adrenocorticoid biosynthesis
   - Spironolactone
   - KTZ
   - Mifepristone
   - Metyrapone
   - Aminoglutethimide

Function of hypothalamus
1. **T**hirst and water balance (supraoptic nucleus)
2. **A**denohypophysis control (via releasing factor)
3. **N**eurohypophysis release hormones synthesized in hypothalamic nuclei.
4. **H**unger (lateral nuclei).
5. **A**utonomic regulation (**A**nterior hypothalamus regulates parasympathetic activity). Circadian rythms (suprachiasmatic nucleus).
6. **T**emperature regulation.
7. **S**exual urges and emotions (septate nucleus).

Hypothalamus is a part of CNS and not a gland.   **TAN HATS**

Hormone (i.e. to stir up): It is a substance of intense biological activity produced by specific cells to act on its target cells and to regulate body functions for bringing about a programmed pattern of life events and for maintaining homeostasis. Hormones are local and general.

1. **Local hormones:** These are ACh, secretion of duodenal wall to cause pancreatic secretion, CCK to contract gallbladder and to cause pancreatic secretion.

2. **General hormones:** These are secreted from ductless (endocrine) gland, e.g. GH causes growth of body parts.

(A) Pituitary hormone

Posterior pituitary hormone (neurohypophysis): ADH/VASopressin from **S**upraoptic nucleus. Oxytocin from paraventricular nucleus.

Anterior pituitary hormone (adenohypophysis/master gland): Hormones are secreted from 5 cell types:
1. GH from somatotropes (acidophilic)
2. ACTH (MSH also) from corticotropes (basophilic)
3. TSH from **T**hyrotropes (basophilic)
4. FSH, LH from gonadotropes (basophilic)
5. Prolactin from lactotropes (acidophilic)

- GH is **most abundant** hormone from **most** abundant cells—somatotropes. GH is also called **somatotropin/somatotropic** hormone.
- Tissue in the body receiving **maximum** blood supply/gm tissue is anterior pituitary (0.8 ml/gm/min).
- **Commonest** symptom of pituitary tumour is headache (**most characteristic**).
- Visual field defect in pituitary tumour is bitemporal heminopia. **Commonest** X-ray feature of raised intracranial tension is erosion of posterior clinoid process.
- **All or most** of the hypothalamic (inhibitory and releasing) hormones are secreted at nerve ending in the median eminence before being transported to the anterior pituitary gland to control the secretion of this gland.

  a. TRH (thyrotropin releasing H) →↑ TSH
  b. GHRH (GH releasing H) →↑ GH
  c. CRH (corticotropin releasing H) →↑ ACTH
  d. GHIH (GH inhibitory H)/somatostatin→↓GH
  e. GnRH (gonadotropin releasing H) →↑ LH and ↑ FSH.
  f. PIH (prolactin inhibitory H) →inhibits prolactin secretion.
     - FSH causes follicle growth before ovulation and sperm formation. LH causes ovulation and sex hormone secretion. Both LH and FSH are present in ovary and testes.
     - ↑ ACTH and GH →↑ blood glucose level →↑ insulin.
     - In male, **LH** sltimulates testosterone secretion by **L**eydig cells and is called ICSH (interstitial cell stimulating hormone). Inhibin (a peptide from gonad) inhibits both LH and FSH release.
     - All anterior pituitary hormones are peptide, act at extracellular receptor located on their target cells and are controlled by hypothalamic hormones, transported via hypothalamic-hypophyseal—portal system subjected to feedback inhibition by hormones of their target cells.
     - Hormones formed in the paraventricular and supraoptic nuclei of hypothalamus are directly transported by nerve fibres to posterior pituitary.

     - α subunits →common to TSH, LH, FSH, hCG.
     - β subunits →determine hormone specificity.

- (B) **Pancreas** →insulin and glucagon.
- (C) **Parathyroid →PTH:** Controls Ca^{++} in ECF by controlling absorption from gut, excretion by kidney and release from bone.
- (D) **Adrenal:**
  1. **Medulla:** Adrenaline/Epinephrine and NA/NE.
  2. **Cortex:**   **GFR**
     — Zona **G**lomerulosa →Aldosterone (0.125 mg/day).
     — Zona **F**asciculata and Zona **R**eticularis →androgen and cortisol (10 mg/day—50% secretion in the morning).

> **GFR** corresponds with salt (Na$^+$), sugar (glucocorticoids) and sex (androgen)". The deeper you go the sweeter you find.

ACTH secretion has **circadian rhythm**. Peak concentration in plasma occurs in early morning and is lowest at midnight. In night sleep, cortisol is highest at **8 am** and lowest at 12 pm.

ADDISON'S = ADrenal cortex Deficiency **IS ON**.

Cushing's Disease = **B**asophilic **A**denoma of **A**nterior pituitary→(hyper**S**ecretion of **S**uprarenal cortex = Cushing's Syndrome).

ABCD

Rate of synthesis of adrenal steroids governs the rate of release. ACTH exerts trophic influence on cortex through cAMP, i.e. high doses cause hypertrophy and hyperplasia (absence of ACTH results in adrenal atrophy), lipolysis, ketosis, hypoglycaemia, pigmentation in Addison's disease. Precursor of ACTH is proopiomelanocortin.

ACTH/Corticotropin is a 39 amino acid single chain peptide with MW 4500, larger peptide proopiomelanocortin (MW 30,000) forms ACTH, endorphins, 2 MSH and 2 lipoproteins.

CRH R on **corticotropes** is G-protein coupled R causing ACTH synthesis and release through cAMP. ACTH secretion has circadian rhythm (peak plasma level →early morning →decrease during day →lowest at midnight).

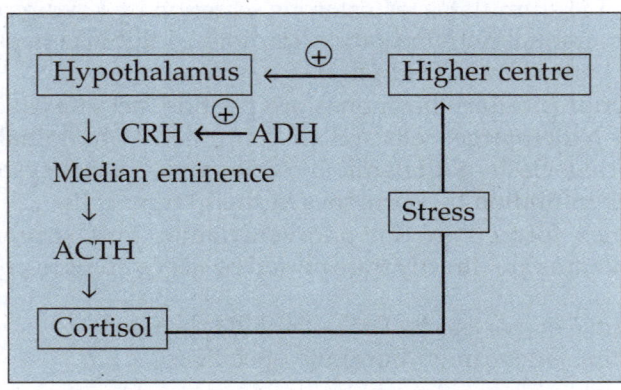

An Overview of Hormones

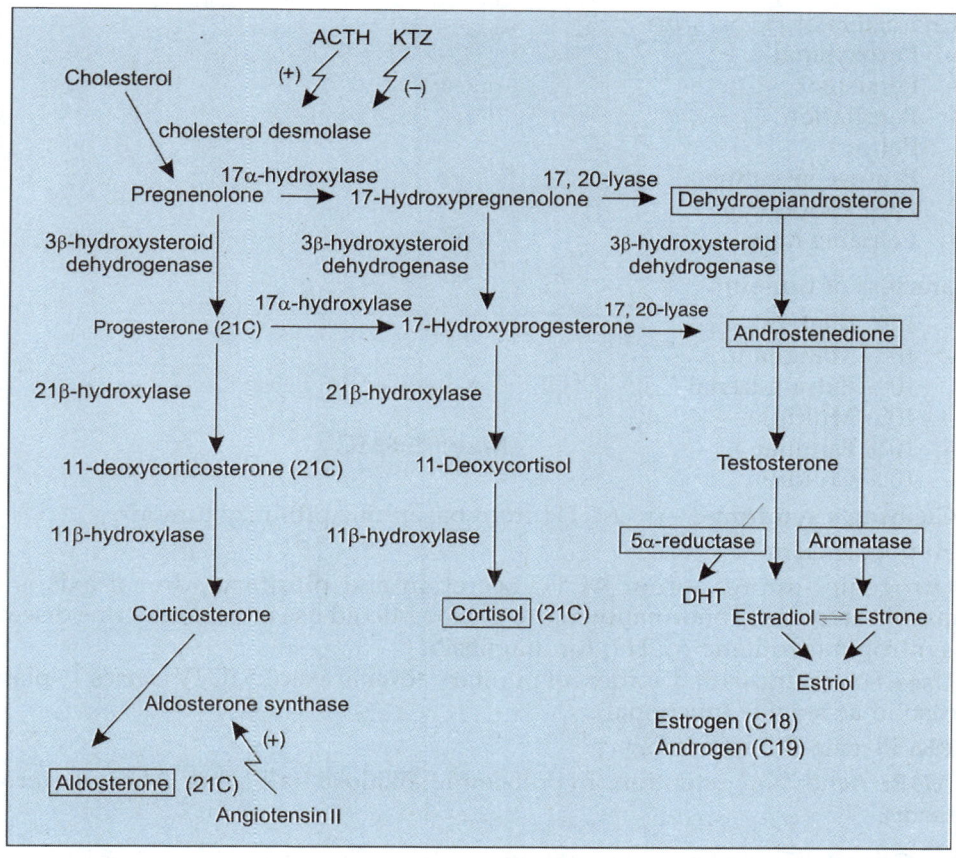

Congenital adrenal hyperplasias

- **A. 17α-hydroxylase deficiency:** Decreased sex hormones, decreased cortisol, increased mineralocorticoids. Cx = hypertension, hypokalemia; phenotypically female but no maturation.

- **B. 21β-hydroxylase deficiency: Most** common form. Decreased cortisol (increased ACTH), decreased mineralocorticoids, increased sex hormones. Cx = masculinization, **HYPO**tension, hyperkalemia.

- **C. 11β-hydroxylase deficiency:** Decreased cortisol, decreased aldosterone and corticosterone, increased sex hormones. Cx = masculinization, **HYPER**tension (11-deoxycorticosterone acts as a weak mineralocorticoid).

Pheochromocytoma (10% tumour)

Most common tumour of adrenal medulla causing HTN.

Characters of HTN: **7P**
- Paroxysmal
- Persistent
- Palpitation
- Pallor
- Profuse sweating
- Pain abdominal
- Palpable mass

Characters of tumour:
- 10% **Bilateral**
- 10% **Malignant**
- 10% **Extra-adrenal**
- 10% **Multiple**
- 10% **Familial**   May BE FMC
- 10% **Children**

Cushing's syndrome →↑ ACTH from basophilic pituitary tumour.
Hypocorticism →↓ ACTH
Iatrogenic suppression of ACTH secretion and pituitary adrenal axis is the **commonest** form of abnormality due to glucocorticoid use in nonendocrine diseases. Cosyntropin (synthetic ACTH) for diagnosis.

Uses: For diagnosis of disorders of pituitary adrenal axis (25 IU IV causes ↑ plasma cortisol if adrenal is functional).

PK: Plasma t½ → 15 min.

ADR: Ache, Na^+ retention, hypokalemic alkalosis (all other ADR of steroids present).

(E) **Gonads** (1) Testes → Testosterone
              (2) Ovaries
   a. Estrogen (develops female sex organ and secondary sex character).
   b. Progesterone (enhances **"uterine milk"** secretion and secretory apparatus development of breast).

(F) **Placenta**
   1. Estrogen
   2. Progesterone
   3. hCGH →↑ corpus luteum growth leading to ↑ estrogen and progesterone from corpus luteum.
   4. **human somato-mammotropin** (growth of foetal tissue and development of mother's breast).

Sites and mechanism of hormone and drug actions: Receptor activation by hormone is translated into response in many ways.

1. **At Nuclear R**
   Thyroid hormone penetrates nucleus → combines with its R → alters DNA-RNA mediated protein synthesis.   Nuclear Theory

2. **At Cytoplasmic R**   Civil Services

Body function	Major regulatory hormones
1. Metabolic rate	T_3 and T_4
2. Somatic growth	GH and insulin like growth factor
3. Circulating volume	ADH and aldosterone
4. Adaptation to stress	Adrenaline, glucocorticoids
5. Ca^{2+} balance	PTH, calcitonin, vitamin D
6. Availability of fuel	GH, insulin, glucagon

Steroid hormones (estrogen, progesterone, glucocorticoid, mineralocorticoid) penetrate cell membrane and combine with cytoplasmic receptors → expose their DNA binding domains → enter nucleus and bind to specific genes → DNA mediated mRNA synthesis → functional protein synthesis.

Others act on membrane R

3. **At cell membrane R (all peptide hormones)**
   - ADH and oxytocin act through IP_3/DAG generation.
   - Insulin causes direct transmembrane activation of tyrosine protein kinase → phosphorylation cascade → regulation of enzyme.
   - Hormones (TSH, FSH, LH, ACTH, PTH, calcitonin, glucagon, adrenaline, hypothalamic releasing hormone) act through cAMP → PKA activation → cell function regulation and Ca^{++} acting as third messenger.
   - Digitalis →↑ contraction.
4. **Extracellular action of drugs**
   — Osmotic diuretic (mannitol)
   — Plasma expander

22. Growth Hormone, Prolactin and Somatostatin

Growth hormone

GH (Growth hormone) is the **most** abundant hormone of somatotropes (the **most** abundant cells in anterior pituitary gland). It was obtained from cadavars.

It is a 191 amino acid, single chain peptide of MW 22000.

Physiological function

1. Enhances size and number of **all cells except** eye and brain.
2. It enhances body protein, uses up the fat stores and conserves carbohydrate.
3. Enhances all facets of amino acid uptake and protein synthesis by cells and reduces protein breakdown.
4. Fat →GH→ Acetyl CoA
   ↓ Excessive GH
   (Acetoacetic acid by liver → ketosis).
5. Causes **diabetogenic** effect by enhanced insulin secretion.
6. Causes **"pituitary diabetes"** due to reduced glucose uptake by cells and enhanced blood glucose concentration.
7. Without gonadotropin, sexual maturation is **not** caused by GH.
8. GH exerts its effects through intermediate substance (IGF or somatomedin/ insulin-like growth factor).

IGF-1/insulin enhances lipogenesis and glucose uptake by muscle. IGF-1 R is similar to insulin R.

First hormone to be reduced in pituitary disorder is GH. **Last** hormone to be reduced in pituitary disorder is TSH.

Mech

1. a. Acts on cell surface R found on **all cells** → stimulates tyrosine protein kinase → phosphorylation of proteins.
   b. R of GHRH and GHIH is G-protein coupled R (acts through cAMP formation). **GHIH** inhibits Ca^{++} channel and opens K^+ channel.
   c. 5-HT, α agonist, fasting, stress, exercise, arginine cause GH release. β agonist, glucocorticoid and enhanced plasma FFA **inhibit GH release.**
   d. Target organ of GH is liver. Target organ hormone of GH is somatomedin.
   e. ↑ GH → gigantism in children and acromegaly in adults. ↓GH → pituitary dwarfism.

2. In adult GH deficient patient, it enhances lean body mass but reduces body fat **(stature unaffected)**.
3. **Commonest** cause of short stature is constitutional growth delay.

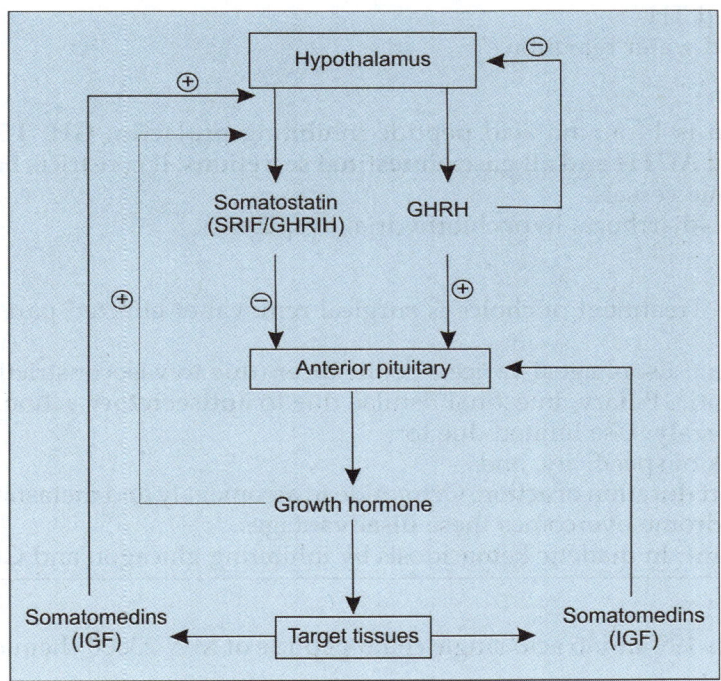

More GH of pituitary also inhibits its secretion from the glands (feedback inhibition).

GH release from pituitary is regulated by somatostatin (hypothalamic hormone)/GHRIH. **Commonest** pituitary adenoma secretes prolactin and next → GH.

GH secreting tumour is acidophil macroadenoma (>10 mm diameter). ACTH secreting tumour is basophil microadenoma (<10 mm diameter).

Challenge tests: These are available.
1. To enhance GH release including insulin, L-dopa and bromocriptine
2. To reduce GH release including glucose, somatostatin and glucocorticoids. This test is for
   GnRH →↑ LH and ↑ FSH
   CRH →↑ ACTH
   TRH →↑ TSH

Human GH produced by recombinant DNA technology are
1. Somatrem (↑ GH)
2. Somatotropin (somatrem minus methionine).
They cause IGF-1 to restore stature to near normal.

ADR
1. **Somatrem** has additional methionine residue and is more immunogenic than somatotropin.
2. GI intolerance
3. Reduced TH
4. Salt and water retention

Somatostatin

Somatostatin is 14 amino acid peptide inhibiting **prolactin, GH, TSH, insulin, glucagon and ACTH and all gastrointestinal secretions.** It constricts hepatic, renal and splanchnic vessels.

ADR: GIT (diarrhoea, hypochlorhydria, dyspepsia).

U
1. ↑ **GH:** Treatment of choice is surgical removal of effected part of pituitary gland.
2. **Bleeding:** Esophageal varices, peptic ulcer (due to vasoconstriction).
3. **Pancreatic:** Biliary, intestinal fistulae due to **antisecretory** action.
4. **Acromegaly:** Use limited due to:
    a. Lack of specificity, and
    b. Short duration of action. Octreotide in acromegaly and metastatic carcinoid syndrome overcomes these disadvantages.
5. **Adjuvant:** In diadetic ketoacidosis by inhibiting glucagon and GH secretion.

Prolactin

Prolactin: It is 199 amino acid single chain peptide of MW 23000 chemically similar to GH.

Physiological function: It causes growth and development of breast during pregnancy by promoting proliferation of ductal and acinar cells in breast, induces synthesis of lactose and milk protein and milk secretion.

Prolactin has inhibitory effect on hypothalamo-pituitary-gonadal axis.

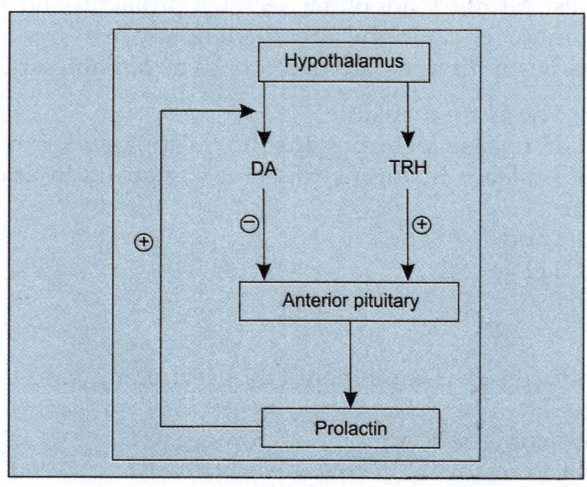

Mech: Prolactin R is similar to GHR → transmembrane stimulation of tyrosine protein kinase. Releases lymphokines from lymphocytes.

GH and placental lactogen also bind to prolactin R causing similar effect. Except PIH (DA), all hypothalamic and pituitary H are peptides.

Regulation of secretion: PRIH of hypothalamus is DA acting on pituitary lactotrope D_2 R. Dopaminergic agonists (apomorphine, bromocriptine) reduce prolactin level, but dopaminergic antagonists and DA depletors cause hyperprolactinemia.

Hypothalamus produces PRF (prolactin releasing factor). TRH has some PRF like activity. Prolactin level is more in adult female at term. Stress and exertion also stimulate prolactin release.

Earliest feature of Sheehan's syndrome (ischaemic necrosis of pituitary gland) is failure of lactation.

Hyperprolactinemia causes galactorrhoea-amenorrhoea-infertility syndrome in female and impotence, gynaecomastia and sterility in male, due to drugs and tumour (microprolactinomas) removal of inhibitory control of hypothalamus.

Feedback control inhibits secretion of **all pituitary hormones except** prolactin.

U: There is no clinical use of prolactin.

Gonadal Hormones

Gonadotropin: The human Menopausal Gonadotropin (hMG) and human Chorionic Gonadotropin (hCG) have LH and FSH activity, thus a functional pituitary gland is not needed. hCG is used to treat cryptorchidism.

Two gonadotropins (LH and FSH) from anterior pituitary are glycoproteins with 26% sugar and 2 peptide chains of total 207 amino acid. Menotropins (hMG) = LH + FSH from postmenopausal urine.

Physiological function
FSH
1. Causes follicular growth before ovulation.
2. Mainly promotes **S**permatogenesis in tubular (**S**ertoli) cells.
3. Estrogen secretion.
4. Ovarian and testicular atrophy takes place in the absence of FSH.

LH
1. Ovulation
2. Luteinization of ruptured follicle
3. Maintenance of corpus luteum till next cycle
4. Atresia of the rest follicle
5. Progesterone secretion
6. Testosterone secretion by interstitial cells in the male (then LH is called ICSH in male). Pulsatile secretion of LH from pituitary causes testosterone secretion. It is **20–200 times** more potent than natural GnRH.

Gn
1. Disturbed Gn secretion from pituitary causes delayed puberty or precocious puberty both in boys and girls.
2. Inadequate Gn secretion causes sterility and amenorrhoea in women, oligozoospermia, impotence and infertility in man.

Mech
1. LH and FSH have G-protein coupled R producing cAMP on activation → gametogenesis and cholesterol conversion into pregnenolone (first step in progesterone, testosterone and estrogen synthesis).
2. FSHR is on **S**eminiferous (**S**ertoli) cells and LHRS on interstitial (Leydig) cells in the testes.

Gonadal Hormones

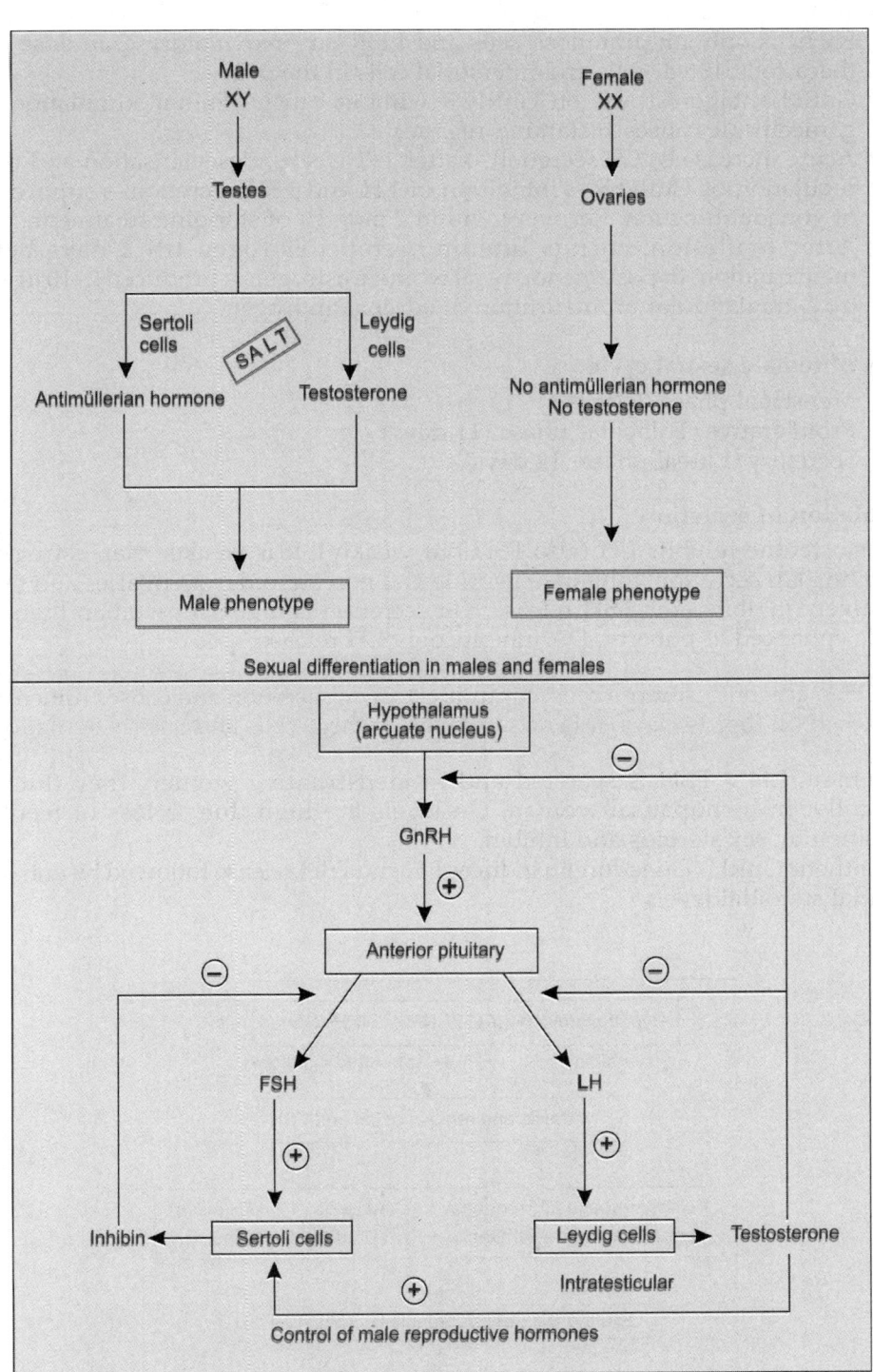

3. FSHR is only on granulosa cells and LHR on preovulatory granulosa cells, theca cells, luteal cells and interstitial cells in the ovary.
4. GnRH antagonist acts on GnRH R without causing initial stimulation, e.g. **ganirelix** (it causes histamine release).
5. Acute increase of Gn secretion → after 1–2 weeks, desensitisation and down regulation of GnRH R → inhibition of LH and FSH secretion → suppression of gonadal function. Recovery within 2 months of stopping treatment.
6. After ovulation, corpus luteum secretes estrogen till 2 days before menstruation. In post-menopausal women, estrogen is produced 2–10 µg/day by extraglandular aromatisation of adrenal androgen.

Days of female sexual cycle
1. Menstrual phase (5 days).
2. ProliFerative/Follicular phase (11 days).
3. Secretory/Luteal phase (12 days).

Regulation of secretion

Testosterone inhibits LH (also FSH but weakly). It is weaker than estrogen in inhibiting **Gn** secretion. Inhibin (a peptide and non-steroid from ovaries and testes) selectively inhibits only FSH release. **Gn** secretion is higher in woman than man and is enhanced at puberty. DA inhibits only LH release.

> FSH acts on granulosa cells, controls estrogen secretion and causes follicular growth (in first 14 days). LH acts on ovarian theca cells and causes ovulation.

In man, LH > FSH is secreted and in menstruating women, they fluctuate cyclically. In menopausal woman, Gn levels are high due to loss of feedback inhibition by sex steroids and inhibin.

Synthetic GnRH/Gonadorelin induces LH and FSH release followed by enhanced gonadal steroidal levels.

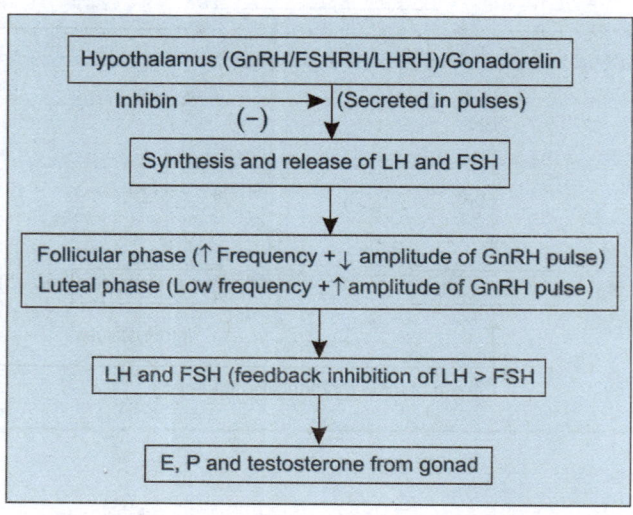

PK: t½ of Gn—4 hrs due to high affinity and resistance to enzymatic hydrolysis. t½ of gonadorelin—6 min, partly metabolised, mainly exerted unchanged in urine. All Gn is given intramuscularly.

Preparation

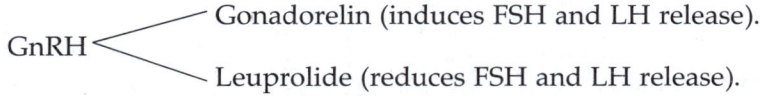

GnRH
- Gonadorelin (induces FSH and LH release).
- Leuprolide (reduces FSH and LH release).

> **Leuprolide Lessens LH and FSH**

Superactive GnRH are
- Buserelin
- Goserelin
- Histrelin
- Nafarelin
- Leuprolide

ADR: GnRH (superactive)
- **H**ot flushes
- **O**steoporosis
- **L**oss of libido   **HOLED**
- **E**motional liability
- Vaginal **D**ryness

U
1. OC in male and female
2. CA prostate and breast
3. Precocious puberty
4. Polycystic ovarian disease
5. Fibroid
6. Infertility from endometriosis (leuprolide)
7. To test pituitary-gonadal-axis in male (gonadorelin)
8. Female hypogonadism (gonadorelin)
9. *In vitro* fertilisation: Menotropin (LH + FSH) obtained from urine of menopausal women
10. Induction of ovulation in women with polycystic ovarian disease. Menotropin/urofollitropin (pure FSH) is used *in vitro* fertilization

> Maternal serum alpha fetoprotein and hCG are reduced in Down's syndrome.
> **Autosomal anomalies**
> 1. Down's syndrome (trisomy 21)—Drinking age 21 (commonest chromosomal disease).
> 2. Edward's syndrome (Trisomy 18)—Election age 18 (2nd commonest chromosomal disease).
> 3. Patau's syndrome (Trisomy 13)—Puberty age 13

Chorionic gonadotropin (CG)

Obtained from urine of pregnant women.
Foetal placenta secretes CG which passes through maternal circulation.

CG is glycoprotein with

- 33% sugar
- MW 38000
- 237 amino acid in 2 chains

Mech

1. Foetal placental CG maintains corpus luteum →excreted by mother in urine.
2. CG binds to LHR.

ADR

1. Mood change, allergy, precocious puberty.
2. Ovarian hyperstimulation (pain, bleeding, polycystic ovary)

U: Commercially available.

1. **Amenorrhoea and infertility:** Menotropin (10 days) followed by CG next day (ovulation in 75%).
2. **Hypogonadotropic hypogonadism in males:** CG IM 3 times/week then menotropin after 3 months.
3. **Cryptorchidism (undescended testes):** CG/serum Gn-LH before the age of 7 yrs in the absence of anatomical obstruction.

Androgens: Gonad produces steroidal hormones having estrogenic, androgenic and progestational activities. Testes of an adult male produce 3–12 mg/day testosterone. Adrenal cortex produces weak androgens (dehydroepiandrosterone and androstenedione) →partial conversion to testosterone by peripheral tissues. In ovary, testosterone is produced (this together with testosterone of adrenal = 0.25–0.50 mg/day).

Plasma level of testosterone in adult male →0.3–1 µg/dl and adult female → 20–60 ng/dl.

Synthetic androgen (orally active)

1. Methyltestosterone
2. Fluoxymesterone

Both are 17-alkyl substituted derivative of testosterone, and are orally active due to resistance to first pass metabolism.

5 α-reductase: 2 isoforms

1. 5α-reductase-1 (present in urogenital tract of male, genital skin).
2. 5α-reductase-2 (present widely in genital and non-genital skin).

Mech: A part of testosterone (prohormone) in extraglandular tissue.

Dihydrotestosterone R complex is more active than testosterone R complex in combining with DNA. But testosterone is active in foetal genital rudiments, pituitary and hypothalamus site involved in feedback inhibition, and in spermatogenic cells of testes.

Sex hormone binding globulin binds to estradiol and testosterone.

Finasteride inhibits 5α-reductase-1 strongly and 5α-reductase-2 weakly.

Genetic deficiency of 5 α-reductase-1 causes male **pseudohermaphroditism** due to inability of male genitalia to produce active form (dihydrotestosterone) from circulating testosterone.

Physiological function
1. Causes all the changes occurring in a boy at puberty (growth of hair and genitals, deepening of voice, penile erection, skin thickening, increased sebaceous gland, loss of subcutaneous fat and prominent veins). Androgens cause **more RBC** production.
2. Causes intrauterine development of male phenotype (produced by foetal testes itself), spermatogenesis and maturation of spermatozoa.
3. Causes pubertal spurt of growth in boys and to a smaller extent in girls (rapid bone growth both in thickness and length, muscle building, enhanced appetite, enhanced haem synthesis, increased nitrogen, water and minerals—Na, P, S, K, Ca).
4. Mediates feedback inhibition of pituitary LH.

Genital ducts
1. Paramesonephric duct forms female genital tract.
2. Mesonephric (Wolffian) duct forms **M**ale genital tract (develops into **S**eminal vesicle, **E**pididymis, **E**jaculatory duct, **D**uctus deferens). **SEED M = Man = not Woman**

PK: Inactive orally due to high first pass metabolism. Hydrolysed to active free form. 98% bound to globulin and albumin. Metabolites (androsterone and Etiocholanolone) excreted in urine, mostly by conjugation with glucuronic acid and sulfate.

Plasma t½ →10–20 min.

A little estradiol is produced from testosterone by aromatization of a ring in extraglandular tissue. Synthetic androgens are metabolised slowly having longer duration of action.

LH stimulates Leydig cell to produce testosterone. GnRH stimulates FSH secretion which enhances sperm production, and stimulates Sertoli cells of male testes to produce inhibin (it inhibits FSH secretion). FSH **S**timulates **S**permatogenesis by acting on **S**ertoli cells of **S**eminiferous tubules.

ADR
- Edema
- Masculinization
- Priapism
- Acne
- Virilization and menstrual irregularities in women
- Sustained painful erections
- Oligozoospermia
- Precocious puberty and **S**hortening of stature due to early closure of epiphysis

- Reversible **C**holestatic jaundice specially with synthetic androgens
- Hepatic **CA**
- **G**ynaecomastia due to peripheral conversion of testosterone to estrogens.

OCP Grows MASSIVE Carcinoma

CI

- CA prostate and male breast
- Liver and kidney disease
- Pregnancy due to musculinization of female foetus.

U

1. Hypo**G**onadism (increased fertility, potency and growth)
2. Hypo**P**ituitarism.
3. **T**esticular failure (which results in delayed puberty).
4. **C**A breast.
5. **C**A prostate (leuprolide).
6. Menopausal **S**yndrome: Androgen+ estrogen in HRT.
7. Hereditary **A**ngioneurotic edema: Mainly synthetic androgen therapy which enhances synthesis of complement (C_1)—esterase inhibitor.

PG ACTS

Anabolic steroids: These are synthetic androgens with higher anabolic and lower androgenic ratio (Anabolic: Catabolic ratio →>1).

This ratio of testosterone is 1. Mostly ratio is between 1 to 3. Anabolic and androgenic effects are mediated through the same R.

Anabolic steroids are

- **S**tanozolol
- **E**thyl Estrenol
- **M**ethandienone
- **O**xandrolone
- **O**xymetholone
- **N**androlone

SEE MOON

The ratio is measured by injecting the drug into castrated rats and measuring the increase in weight of levator ani muscle to that of ventral prostate.

ADR and CI: Same as testosterone.

U

1. To hasten recovery after **I**njury.
2. **C**atabalic state: To reduce nitrogen loss.
3. **A**nemia (haemolytic, hypoplastic, renal failure and malignancy associated): Drugs enhance RBC count and Hb%.
4. **R**enal insufficiency: Drugs decrease urea production.
5. **E**dema and HTN.
6. **S**uboptimal growth in children.
7. **O**steoporosis.
8. To enhance the physical activity in atheletes. Drugs are included in the list of "Dope Test".

I CARE SO

Impeded androgens/antiandrogens: Estrogens reduce testosterone production by preventing Gn secretion. Estrogens act as antiandrogen up to some extent. The **most** potent inhibitors of gonadal function are superactive GnRH agonists.

KTZ reduces testosterone production. Progesterone has weak but true antiandrogenic action, whereas cimetidine and spironolactone have only weak antiandrogenic actions.

Antiandrogens are
- **D**anazol
- **L**euprolide
- **C**yproterone acetate   **DLC Film**
- **F**lutamide
- Finasteride

Leuprolide

Leuprolide is antiandrogen.

Mech: GnRH analogue with agonistic properties when used in pulsatile fashion and antagonistic properties when used in continuous fashion (continuous fashion causes initial burst of LH and FSH).

ADR: Antiandrogenic action
     Nausea and vomiting
U: 1. Infertility
     2. CA prostate

Finasteride

Finasteride is a competitive inhibitor of 5α-reductase.

Mech: Selectively and competitively inhibits 5α-reductase-2 isoenzyme (inhibits 5α-reductase-1 strongly and 5α-reductase-2 weakly).

PK: Effective orally, extensively metabolized in liver, excreted in urine and faeces, plasma t½ – 4–8 hrs (elderly: 6–15 hrs).

ADR: Decreased **L**ibido
     Impotence
     Decreased volume of **E**jaculate   **LIES = Rumour**
     Swelling of lips
     Rashes
U: 1. BPH: It reduces prostate size and enhances peak urinary flow rate in 50% patient. 6 months for maximum relief (dose: 5 mg OD).
   2. **A**cne   **ABC**
   3. Male pattern **B**aldness
   4. **C**A prostate

Cyproterone acetate: It is a potent antiandrogen, potent antiestrogen and related to progesterone.

Mech: Competes with dihydrotestosterone for the intracellular androgen receptors and inhibits its binding.

Large doses (1) produce castration like effect (failure of pubertal changes in the immature, and loss of libido + androgenic anabolism in adults).

(2) Inhibit Leydig cell function, spermatogenesis and Gn secretion.

ADR: 1. Gynaecomastia in males
2. Hirsutism
3. Virilisation

U: Tested for but not yet marketed.
1. Male pattern baldness
2. Acne
3. CA prostate

Flutamide: It is non-steroidal drug having specific androgenic activity.

Mech: Its active metabolite **"2-hydroxy flutamide"** competitively blocks androgen action on accessory sex organ and on pituitary (it enhances LH secretion by blocking feedback inhibition →enhances plasma testosterone level in males and overcomes antiandrogenic effect of flutamide partially). **Bicalutamide** has same actions.

ADR

1. Gynaecomastia
2. Breast tenderness
3. Liver damage

U

1. **CA prostate:** Flutamide + GnRH agonist to suppress LH and testosterone secretion or flutamide after castration.
2. **Female hirsutism:** Flutamide + oral contraceptive.
3. **Precocious puberty:** Spironolactone and flutamide have antiandrogen activity, hence are used in all of the above.

Danazol

Danazol is orally active **ethisterone** and has mild anabolic androgenic and progestational activity.

Mech: Most prominent action is **"Suppression of Gn secretion"** from pituitary in both male and female leading to inhibition of testicular/ovarian function and suppression of gonadal function. Inhibits cleaving enzyme (CYP450) dehydrogenase, hydroxylase but not aromatase leading to ↑ estrogen and ↑ clearance of progesterone: Partial agonist.

ADR

1. Muscle **C**ramp   **CLASH**
2. **L**oss of Libido in men
3. **A**ndrogenic effects (weight gain, acne, hirsutism, deepening of voice)
4. Night **S**weats
5. **H**ot flushes in women
6. Complete amenorrhoea
7. GIT upset

U

1. Gynaecomastia
2. **Infertility:** Withdrawal of danazol after 3 months of treatment results in rebound fertility in women.
3. **Menorrhoea** (drug reduces menstrual blood loss)
4. **Precocious puberty in boys**

5. Fibrocystic **B**reast disease (chronic cystic mastitis)
6. Hereditary **A**ngioneurotic edema
7. Endometriosis—(DOC) improvement in up to 90% cases.

> **Gynaecomastia Is Mainly Produced By Antiandrogenic Effects**

Estrogens: (a) Source: Testes, ovary (estradiol), placenta (estriol) and blood (aromatization). (b) Potency: Estradiol > estrone > estriol.

Types: 1. Natural
         2. Synthetic

Natural estrogens: "Estradiol" is the major estrogen secreted by ovary and synthesized in graafian follicle, corpus luteum and placenta from cholesterol. Placenta starts secreting estrogen and progesterone from 2nd trimester term.

Synthetic estrogens: Sterically resemble natural estrogens, have transconfiguration. 2 types:

a. **Steroidal**
   - Ethinyl estradiol
   - Mestranol
   - Tibolone

b. **Non-steroidal**
   - Oral-diethylstilbestrol (stilbestrol)
   - Topical-dienesterol, hexesterol.

Actions of estrogen

1. Estrogen enhances progesterone R protein whereas progesterone represses estrogen R and induces degradation of estradiol.
2. Enhances cholesterol secretion and reduces bile salt secretion leading to **lithogenicity**.
3. Levels of sex steroidal, thyroxine and cortisol binding globulins are elevated.
4. Reduces plasma LDL cholesterol and enhances HDL + triglycerides. Raised HDL: LDL ratio → atherosclerosis in premenopausal women.
5. Estrogens are anabolic similar to but weaker than testosterone, promote positive Ca^{++} balance, partly by inducing renal **hydroxylase** enzyme which generates active form of vitamin D_3.
6. Causes pubertal changes (growth of uterus and fallopian tubes, vaginal epithelia cornified, endometrial proliferation, breast growth, feminine body contours, fusion of epiphyses).
7. Induces (a) watery secretion from cervix for sperm penetration, (b) progesterone to bring about secretory changes, (c) increased rhythmic contraction of uterus and fallopian tubes.
8. Estrogen withdrawal alone produces menstruation in the absence of progesterone (anovulatory cycle). Menstruation is not inhibited by high dose of estrogen.
9. Progesterone causes scanty, viscid, cellular cervical secretion hostile to **sperm penetration**.

Mech: Same as other steroid (binds to cytoplasmic R causing proteins synthesis via nucleus). Estogen R is present in female sex organ, breast, vessels, heart, CNS, pituitary and liver.

PK: Natural estrogen:
1. Inactive orally
2. Short duration of action due to rapid hepatic metabolism.

Estradiol ester (IM)—slowly absorbed (prolonged action). Bound to globulin and albumin.

Synthetic estrogens: Well absorbed orally and transdermally, metabolized slowly.

Estradiol $\underset{}{\overset{Liver}{\rightleftharpoons}}$ Estrone → Estriol

Estradiol, estriol and estrone are conjugated with glucuronic acid and sulfate. Excreted in bile and ultimately in urine (**mostly**).

Enterohepatic circulation due to deconjugation in intestines is present.

All estrogen preparations have similar action and their equivalent parenteral doses are:

(Diethylstilbestrol **10** mg) = (Estriol Succinate **16** mg)
= (Conjugated estrogen **10** mg)
= (Mestranol **0.15** mg) = (Estradiol **0.1** mg)
= (Ethinyl estradiol **0.1** mg)

> **CD** = 10,10
> **EE** = 0.1,0.1
> **MS** = 0.15, 16

But oral potencies are different due to different first pass metabolism.
Estradiol is inactive orally.
Oral and parenteral doses are same in:
- Mestranol
- Ethinylestradiol
- Diethylstilbestrol

Preferred route of estrogen is oral.

ADR of estrogen and OC
1. **Acne, Adult** stature reduced when estrogen given to children.
2. **Bleeding: BP** raised by both estrogen and progesterone due to elevated angiotensin level and rennin activity which induce salt and water retention.
   Benificial effect: Estrogen elevates HDL/LDL ratio but progesterone nullifies this benefit.
3. **Coronary and Cerebral** thrombosis resulting in MI/stroke (due to elevated platelet aggregation and clotting factors and reduced antithrombin III and plasminogen activator in **endothelium**).

Chloasma is pigmentation of forehead, cheeks, and nose in pregnancy.

CA produced are
Endometrial
Genital
Breast, and
Hepatomas (benign)

Genital CA is specially in female offspring of pregnant mother. In postmenopausal women, estrogen enhances and progestin reduces endometrial CA. Breast cancer is with estrogen.

4. – DM
   – DVT
   – Thrombophlebitis
   – Leg vein and pulmonary thrombosis mainly in women >35 yrs age, diabetic, smokers and hypertensive.
5. Elevated biliary cholesterol Excretion by Estrogen (increased HDL/LDL ratio) →Gallstone (higher with OC) formation is doubled on chronic use.
6. Feminization and loss of libido with estrogen in males.
7. Gynecomastia
8. Hair of the body is increased   **ABCDEFGHI**
9. Increased weight gain
U: Two **commonest** uses of estrogens
   a. Contraceptive
   b. HRT in postmenopausal women.
1. HRT (hormonal replacement therapy): Manopaused women are in hormone deficient state causing physical and emotional disturbances such as
   – Osteoporosis (loss of Ca^{2+} and osteoid)
   – Dermatological changes.
   – Urogenital atrophy
   – Vasomotor disturbances (hot flushes, chilly sensation, aches, faintness, sweating).
   – Psychological disturbances (depressed mood, loss of self-confidence).
   – CVS disease (stroke, MI)

Estrogen HRT suppresses the menopausal syndrome by restoring Ca^{2+} balance, raising **HDL : LDL ratio**, preventing hyperinsulinemia and LDL oxidation and increasing PGI_2 production.

Doses of estrogen in HRT is lower than that of OC.

Typically conjugated estrogen is used 1 mg/day.

Estrogen Enhances the risk of Endometrial CA due to continuous estrogenic stimulation of endometrium but progestin reduces the risk hence used with estrogen. Estrogen is palliative in CA breast in late postmenopausal women.

Estrogen →Endometrial CA

2. **Hirsutism:** By inhibiting LH production →↓ ovarian androgen production →reduced body hair.
3. **Dysmenorrhoea:** Estrogen inhibits PG synthesis in endometrium and ovulation (DOC—PG synthesis inhibitor).
4. **Senile vaginitis:** Suppression of lactation by inhibiting prolactin release (DOC: Bromocriptine).
5. **Acne:** Estrogen inhibits Gn release from pituitary leading to ↓ ovarian androgen production (hence not used in a boy).
6. **Dysfunctional uterine Bleeding:** Estrogen- adjuvant.
7. **CA prostate:** Estrogen suppresses androgen production. GnRH agonist preferred.
8. **Delayed puberty in girls** is due to ovarian agenesis (Turner's syndrome)/ Hypopituitarism.

RHDs ABCD

Tibolone

Tibolone is 19-nonsteroid having estrogenic, progestational and weak androgenic activity.

Mech: Suppresses raised Gn level and menopausal symptoms.

CI

1. Undiagnosed vaginal **B**leeding
2. Hormone dependent **C**ancer
3. **M**igraine
4. **E**pilepsy
5. **L**iver disease
6. **T**hromboembolic disease

> Barium Carbonate (BaCO$_3$) **MELT**

ADR

1. Increased facial hair
2. Weight gain

U

1. **U**rogenital **A**trophy
2. **P**sychological **S**ymptoms
3. **O**steoporosis
4. **L**oss of libido

> **ASO Level**

Antiestrogens

Antiestrogens are non-steroidal compounds:
1. Clomiphene citrate
2. Tamoxifen citrate, aromatase inhibitors (anastrozole, letrozole)
3. Chlormadinone acetate
4. Raloxifene, ormeloxifene.

Chlormadinone acetate has anti-estrogenic and progestational action.

Antiestrogen/SERM (selective estrogen receptor modulator) has estrogenic and antiestrogenic effect. First SERM: Tamoxifen.

Clomiphene citrate: It is antiestrogen that reduces feedback inhibition of estrogen on pituitary gland and hypothalamus.

Mech: Binds to intracellular estrogenic R and produces antagonistic, agonistic or partial agonistic actions.

Increased Gn secretion by blocking estrogenic feedback inhibition of pituitary gland →↑ LH/FSH at each secretory pulse → ovulation.

Agonistic and antagonistic actions are due to activation of estrogen responsive genes by clomiphene-estrogen R complex.

PK: Well absorbed orally, deposited in tissues, t½ → 6 days.
Largely metabolized and excreted in bile.

ADR

1. Gastric upset
2. Polycystic ovaries and multiple pregnancy
3. Hot flushes due to peripheral antagonistic action of estrogen.

4. Vertigo
5. Allergic dermatitis

Gastric pH—Very Acidic

U
1. **Sterility** (50 mg OD for 5 days starting from 5th day of cycle per month).
2. *In vitro* **fertilization** (clomiphene + Gn).
3. **Oligozoospermia/male infertility** (25 mg OD for 24 days plus 6 days rest for up to 6 months).
   ↑ Gn →spermatogenesis and testosterone secretion.
   Higher doses cause estrogenic action.

Tamoxifen citrate: It is mainly antiestrogen.
It is the first SERM.

Mech: Binds to intracellular estrogen R and produces antagonistic, agonistic or partial agonistic actions. Agonist > antagonist on bone.

ADR
1. Hot flushes
2. Vomiting
3. Vaginal bleeding and menstrual irregularities.

PK
Effective orally
Biphasic plasma t½ = 10 hrs and 7 days
Excreted in bile

U
1. **Male infertility:** Due to weaker estrogenic action, it is preferred over clomiphene.
2. **CA breast:** (DOC) and less toxic than other anticancer drugs.

Raloxifene is second generation SERM. Ehances women's bone density without increasing risk of endometrial cancer.

Mech
1. Acts on estrogen R →estrogenic and antiestrogenic effects.
2. No effect on endometrium. Enhances risk of thromboembolism.
3. Lowers cholesterol and LDL in serum (no effect on HDL and TG).
4. Reduces bone resorption and overall bone turnover.

PK
Readily absorbed orally.
Converted to glucuronide conjugates through first pass metabolism.
>95% bound to plasma protein, enterohepatic circulation, excreted in bile to faeces.

IA
1. Absent, but raloxifene + cholestyramine reduce raloxifene absorption by 60%.
2. Warfarin + raloxifene →10% drop in PT.

ADR: 1. DVT
        2. Pulmonary embolism
        3. Retinal vein thrombosis.
CI: 1. Pregnancy

2. DVT
3. Raloxifene + cholestyramines

U: Osteoporosis in postmenopausal women.

Ormeloxifene: It is SERM.

Mech: Estrogen antagonist in uterus and breast. Suppression of endometrial proliferation by regulating ER. Normalized uterine bleeding with anovulatory cycle near menopause. Contraceptive property present.

ADR: HTN, weight gain, fluid retention, headache, prolonged MC.

U: Dysfunctional uterine bleeding.

Progestin

Progestin means favouring pregnancy. 2 types: (1) Natural progestin, (2) Synthetic progestin.

Natural progestin is progesterone derived from cholesterol. It is 21 C steroid, secreted by corpus luteum (10–20 mg/day) in the later half of the cycle.

After fertilisation, hCG sustains corpus luteum. 1–5 mg/day progesterone from adrenal and testes is secreted in men.

Synthetic progestin

A. 19-Nortestosterone derivatives (18 C)
- Norethindrone (norethisterone)
- Norethynodrel
- Ethynodiol diacetate
- Lynestrenol (ethinyl estrenol)
- Allylestrenol
- Norgestrel (Gonane)
- Newer compounds (desogestrel and norgestimate are prodrugs, gestodene).

B. Progesterone derivatives (21 C)
- Megesterol acetate
- Medroxyprogesterone acetate
- Chlormadinone acetate
- Hydroxyprogesterone caproate
- Dydrogesterone
- Newer compounds (norgestrel acetate)

C. Antiprogestin: Mifepristone

Progesterone derivatives are pure progesterone (except chlormadinone) with weaker antiovulatory action and used as adjuvant to estrogen in HRT.

Older 19-nortestosterone derivative is weak androgenic, weak estrogenic with potent antiovulatory and used as contraceptives. Levoisomer (levonorgestrel) of norgestrel is more potent.

Newer 19-nortestosterone derivative is potent progestins with strong antiovulatory action, used in women with hyperandrogenemia.

Norgestrel is antiandrogenic but less antiovulatory and effects endometrium.

Mech: Progesterone R is in female genital tract, breast, pituitary and CNS.

Binding to R → translocation of complex to nucleus → DNA mediated RNA transcription → protein synthesis.

Estrogen enhances progesterone R protein but progesterone suppresses estrogen R and degrades estradiol.

Actions of progesterone

1. It is for preparation of uterus for implantation and maintenance of pregnancy due to reduced uterine motility and inhibits immunological rejection of foetus by reducing CMI and T cell function, otherwise mucosal shedding in uterus during menstruation takes place.
2. Enhances secretion and suppresses epithelial proliferation. After pregnancy stroma enlarges, glands atrophy and sensitivity of myometrium to oxytocin reduces due to progesterone.
3. Converts watery cervical secretion into viscid, scanty and cellular secretion for sperm penetration.
4. Induces leukocyte infiltration into cornified epithelium.
5. Causes acini proliferation in mammary glands. Estrogen + progesterone prepare breast for lactation and their withdrawal after delivery cause prolactin release from pituitary for milk secretion.
6. Has sedative affects, causes 0.5°C rise in body temperature by resetting hypothalamic thermostat and enhancing heat production.
7. Stimulates respiration, lowers serum HDL levels, enhances amount of LH secreted/pulse but reduces frequency of LH pulses by action on hypothalamic pulse generator.
8. Gonane 19-nortestosterone is potent antiovulatory.

PK: Progesterone: Inactive orally due to high first pass metabolism in liver. Completely degraded in liver into pregnanediol which is excreted in urine as sulfate and glucuronide conjugates.

Synthetic progestins: Orally active, slow metabolism, plasma t½ → 8–24 hrs.

ADR

1. **A**therogenesis is due to lower plasma HDL levels (19-Nortestosterone derivative causes atherogenesis).
2. **D**M: Potent agent (levonorgestrel, etc.) raises blood sugar to cause DM.
3. **A**menorrhoea
4. **M**asculinisation of female foetus and other congenital abnormalities when progestin given in early pregnancy
5. **P**ain on IM progesterone.
6. **S**winging of mood
7. **E**dema, engorgement of breast
8. **A**cne
9. **T**emperature of body elevated

A DAMP SEAT

CI: For diagnosis of pregnancy.

U

1. As **C**ontraceptive (**commonest** use).
2. HRT: Progesterone derivative without androgenic activity + estrogen in endometrial CA in postmenopausal women.

3. Endometrial CA
4. **A**bortion (habitual/threatened): No progesterone deficiency in most patient is present.
5. Premenstrual **T**ension (headache, fluid retention, irritability) is released by suppressing ovulation by estrogen + progesterone treatment.
6. Endometriosis: It is due to the presence of ectopic endometrium. It presents dysmenorrhoea, infertility and painful pelvic swelling.
   Progestin prevents bleeding in ectopic sites by suppressing menstruation. Danazol—alternative.
7. **D**ysfunctional uterine bleeding: It is often associated with anovular bleeding.

CREATED

Mifepristone: It is 19-Nonsteroid with potent competitive antiprogestational and significant antiglucocorticoid activity (but not in normal individual due to inhibition by negative feedback at hypothalamic-pituitary level → ACTH release → cortisol increase).

Mech: In follicular phase, it reduces Gn surge from pituitary → no ovulation. Antagonist of progesterone and glucocorticoid.

In luteal phase, it prevents secretory changes. Later in the cycle, it inhibits progesterone support to endometrium, stimulates uterine contraction and induces menstruation. After implantation, it inhibits decidualisation, hCG production and progesterone secretion.

Due to its partial agonistic action, it has weak progestational activity in the absence of progesterone (anovulatory cycles after menopause).

Antiprogestin mifepristone also acts as glucocorticoid receptor antagonist. It also blocks the preparation of uterus for pregnancy.

PK: Orally active, t½—30 hrs, bioavailability—25%.

Excreted in bile. Metabolised in liver (enterohepatic circulation present).

ADR: 1. Bleeding
2. Anorexia
3. Abdominal discomfort.

U:1. **Cushing's syndrome** (for inoperable cases).
2. **Induction of labour** (in foetal death and abnormal foetus) by blocking **relaxant action** of progesterone on uterus of late pregnancy.
3. **Termination of pregnancy:** Up to 9 weeks, it causes complete abortion in 60–85% cases on taking 600 mg single dose orally.
   Mifepristone + PG analogue in first trimester of pregnancy.
4. **As contragestational drug:** Causes menstruation and dislodges embryo and ova (fertilized or not). **Dose:** once a month on expected date of menses. When taken within 72 hours of intercourse as single dose, it acts as postcoital contraceptive.

Hormonal Contraceptives

Hormonal contraceptives are hormonal preparation used for reversible **suppression of pregnancy.**

Contraceptive reduces the incidence of **fibrocystic breast disease, ovarian cysts, endometrial and ovarian CA, blood loss and anemia: Cycle becomes** regular from irregular, **PID and endometriosis** are improved.

Female contraceptives: Fertility is suppressed at will with 100% confidence and complete return on discontinuation. These should be safe, convenient, efficacious and of low cost.

Two types
 1. Oral
 2. Injectable

Oral contraceptive (OC)

1. **Phased regimen:** It is to reduce total steroid dose → E + P. Estrogen (E) **constant** + Progestin (P) increases **gradually.**
2. **Minipill (luteal supplements):** Only low doses progestin (P) has **96–98%** efficacy. It reduces implantation of fertilized ovum.
3. **Postcoital (morning after) pills: (E/E + P).** High dose estrogen for a few days →discontinued → bleeding→dislodge implanted blastocyst.
   Estrogen (stilbestrol 25 mg/ethinyl estradiol 2.5 mg BD for 5 days) or ethinylestradiol 0.1 mg + levonorgestrel 1 mg BD starting within 3 days of intercourse.
   Efficacy→90–95%
   Used in rape, etc.
4. **Combined pill:** Most efficaceous **(98–99.9%)** and most popular.
   Estrogen (ethinylestradiol/mestranol) + **Progestin (**19-nortestosterone—has potent antiovulatory action).
   Both inhibit ovulation by decreasing LH and FSH release by negative feedback inhibition of estrogen on pituitary. Progestin causes bleeding at the end of the cycle and reduces the risk of endometrial CA due to estrogen.
   Starting on 5th day of menstruation, one tablet is taken OD for next 20 days with a gap of one week in which bleeding occurs.

Pharmacology Review

Oral Contraceptive Pills **OCPS** (1) **4 types:** Only progestin pill (minipill), Combined pill, Phasic pill and Post-coital pill, Sequential pill. (2) **Mechanism of action:** Ovulation inhibition, Cervical mucus thickening, Prevention of implantation, Suppression of contraction.

OC preparations

	Progestin	+	Estrogen
Postcoital pill	1. Levonorgestrel 2.	+	Elhinylestradiol Diethylstilbestrol
Minipill	3. Norethindrone 4. Norgestrel		
Phased pill	5. Norethindrone 6. Levonorgestrel	+ +	Ethinylestradiol Ethinylestradiol
Combined pill	7. Ethynodiol diacetate 8. Lynestrenol 9. Norgestrel 10. Levonorgestrel 11. Desogestrel	+ + + + +	Mestranol Ethinylestradiol " " "

ADR of OC: Venous Thromboembolism due to estrogen. **HATS**
Arterial phenomena due to estrogen + progestin.
HTN due to estrogen + progestin.
Gallstone due to estrogen.
Permanent sterility in some women when injectable pills are given IM as oily solution.

ADR of oral CONTRACEPTIVES: **C**holestatic jaundice, **O**edema of cornea, **N**asal congestion, **T**hyroid dysfunction, **R**aised BP, **A**nemia/**A**cne/**A**lopecia, **C**erebrovascular disease, **E**levated blood sugar, **P**orphyria/**P**igmentation, **P**ancreatitis, **T**hromboembolism, **I**CP raised, **V**omiting (progesterone only), **E**rythema nodosum, **S**ystems involved are CVS/CNS (extrapyramidal effect).

Injectable contraceptives: These are given IM as oily solution. The patients do not need for daily ingestion of pills. 2 types (i) combined (E+P), (ii) P only.

Limitations: Risk of cancer (ovarian, cervical and hepatic) is not enhanced, but risk of breast CA in women (<53 years) is increased.

Amenorrhoea and menstrual irregularities are common. **6–30 months** after discontinuation, return of fertility takes place.

DMPA (Depot Medroxy Progesterone Aectate) is long-acting progestin injected once in 3–6 months and causes complete disruption of menstrual bleeding pattern and total amenorrhoea (most important undesirable property).

NEE (Norethindrone/Norethisterone Ananthate) is long-acting and injected once in 2–3 months, has failure rates. Long-acting progestin and estrogen are injected once a month and allow reasonable menstrual bleeding pattern in most cases.

Mech: Inhibition of Gn release from pituitary through normal feedback inhibition. Progestin reduces LH and estrogen reduces FSH secretion. Both synergise to inhibit midcycle of LH surge. Hence, follicles fail to develop and fail to rupture causing **no ovulation.**

Thick cervical mucus secretion evoked by progestin (except postcoital pill) blocks sperm penetration.

Due to minipills and postcoital pills, endometrium becomes hyperproliferative/hypersecretory/atrophic and hence inhibits blastocyst implantation, these pills also disfavour fertilization.

Practical considerations

Discontinuation of all OCs results in full return of fertility within 1–2 months with a rebound increase in fertility (multiple pregnancy if conception occurs within 2–3 weeks).

But injectable contraceptive may cause permanent infertility.

On missing one tablet when woman is on combined pills, 2 tablets are taken on the next day to continue usual doses.

But on missing >2 tablets, alternative method is used to start the next course on the 5th day of bleeding.

Pregnancy occurring during contraceptive use is terminated by suction—aspiration to avoid genital CA in **female** offspring, undescended testes in **male** offspring and risk of malformation.

The obese needs higher dose (50 µg ethinylestradiol but **most women** need 30 µg ethinyl estradiol). Pills containing higher **estrogen** dose are used if **breakthrough bleeding** occurs. Progestin is used if estrogen is **contraindicated.**

More estrogenic preparation is **preferred** in women with acne and hirsutism while **more progestin** in women with excessive menstrual loss, though **most OCs** are balanced.

Women developing weight gain, raised LDL cholesterol and acne due to androgenic action of older 19-nortestosterone progestin, "**newer progestin, desogestrel lacking androgenic action**" is preferred.

CI

1. **CVS disease** (HTN, hyperlipidemia, coronary thromboembolism).
2. **Surgery** due to postoperative thromboembolism.
3. **Acute liver disease**
   Hepatoma
   Jaundice
   Porphyria
4. **Relative CI:** DM, smoking, obesity, vaginal bleeding, fibroid, gallbladder disease, migraine, mild HTN, age >35 years, mentally ill.

Absolute CI of OC: **A**bnormal, undiagnosed vaginal bleeding, **B**enign and malignant hepatic tumour, **C**A breast, **D**isease of coronary and cerebral artery, **E**strogen dependent tumour, **F**requent thromboembolism and **G**estation.

ABCDEFG

IA

1. Phenytoin, phenobarbitone, primidone, CBZ and rifampin **increase** metabolism of contraceptives and cause their **failures.**

2. Suppression of intestinal **microflora** (tetracycline, ampicillin, etc.)→ estrogen conjugation excreted in **bile** →interruption of enterohepatic circulation→ **fall in blood level.**

Centchroman/Centron/Saheli

It is an **anti-implant agent and** acts by inducing **embryo-uterine asynchrony, accelerated tubal transport,** and **suppression of decidualization.** It is a **nonsteroidal estrogen antagonist** developed at **CDRI** (India) introduced in the **NFWP,** as an OC. It prevents conception with 97–99% success and with return of fertility on withdrawal.

PK: t½ = 1 week.

Dose: 30 mg twice weekly for 12 weeks followed by once a week.

Male contraceptive: The aim is to inhibit spermatogenesis which takes 64 days and is not achievable because practically men do not get pregnant (**most important**).
1. **Complete suppression** of spermatogenesis is difficult because millions of spermatozoa are released at each ejaculation in comparison to single ovulation in women/month.
2. **Gn suppression** inhibits testosterone secretion resulting in loss of libido and impotence.

Drugs are

1. Androgen and antiandrogen
2. Estrogen and progestin suppress Gn (feminization occurs).
3. Superactive GnRH analogues (inhibit Gn release and testosterone secretion).
4. Cytotoxic drugs (cadmium, indoles, nitrofurans) suppress spermatogenesis but toxic and also cause irreversible action.
5. **Gossypol:** It is a non-steroidal compound obtained from cotton seed (China) and has no hormonal/antihormonal activity.

Mech of gossypol suppresses spermatogenesis in 99.9% men and reduces sperm motility developing infertility after a couple of months (mechanism uncertain). Fertility is reported after discontinuation with 10% oligozoospermic men. Destroys seminiferous cells.

ADR (gossypol):
1. Breathlessness
2. Paralysis
3. Hypokalemia due to renal loss of K⁺ (**most important**)
4. Edema
5. Neuritis
6. Diarrhoea

BPH END

Nonoxynol-9 acts as **spermicide.**

Causes of **GYNAECOMASTIA: G**enetic (XXY), **Y**oung age, **N**eonatal, **A**ntifungal (KTZ), **E**strogen, **C**CB/cimetidine, **O**ld age, **M**arijuana, **A**lcohol, **S**pironolactone, **T**esticular and adrenal tumour, **I**NH and inhibition of testosterone, **A**lkylating agent.

Rules of 4 in male and female: These happen when **4** eyes see together in the same direction as **4** eyes are better than 2:

Best semen collection = **4** days after abstinence.
Total volume = **4** ml per ejaculation (semen).
Total count = **4**00 million (sperm).
Infertility = <**4**0 million/ml.
Azoospermia = **A**bsent of sperm.
pH of vagina = **4**, gestation period = **4**0 weeks.
Oocytes released = **4**00 (menarche to menopause).
Oocytes present at puberty = **4**00,000.
MTP: **P**assed by **P**arliament in 1971 and applied
M2P in 1972. **P**ermitted up to 20 weeks.
Mala **D** = **D**-norgestrel (0.3 mg) + 0.03 mg ethinyloestradiol.
Mala **N** = **N**orgestrel (0.3 mg) + 0.03 mg ethinyloestradiol.
Amniocentesis: ALPHA-FETOPROTEIN = **16** letters = measured at **16** weeks.
CHORIONIC = **9** letters = CVS measured at **9** weeks.

25 Drugs for Uterus

1. **Uterine relaxants (tocolytics):** Delay/postpone labour (if cervical dilatation is <4 cm), arrest threatened abortion and control dysmenorrhea.
2. **Uterine stimulant (abortifacients/ecbolics/oxytocics):** Drugs acting on uterus effect endometrium (estrogen and progestin—most important) and myometrium. TocoLytics (reduce uterine motility): **Tone LYTICS**

   1. **P**rogesterone
   2. **A**drenergic agonist
   3. **A**lcohol ($CH_3 CH_2 OH$)
   4. **C**CB
   5. **M**gSO$_4$
   6. **P**G synthesis inhibitors, ritodrine

   Progesterone **A**nd **A**bortion **C**ure **M**adam's **P**ain

Uterine relaxants/stimulants

1. **Hormones:** Oxytocin (pitocin and syntocinon are synthetic oxytocin).
2. **PGs:** PGE$_2$, PGF$_2\alpha$, misoprostol, 15-methyl PGF$_2\alpha$.
3. **Ergot alkaloids:** Methylergometrine, ergometrine (ergonovine).
4. **Others:** Quinine, ethacridine.

Oxytocin

Oxytocin (**P**arturition most important role) and ADH are synthesized within the nerve cell bodies in **P**araventricular nuclei and supraoptic nuclei of hypothalamus respectively, transported down the axon and stored in the nerve endings within neurohypophysis in the separate neurones as complex with their specific binding proteins—**neurophysins**. Both are octapeptides having **6 common amino acid residues** and released by appropriate stimuli.

Milk ejection reflex is initiated by suckling so that it can be easily sucked by infant. Oxytocin contracts myoepithelium of mammary glands and forces milk into bigger sinusoids. Milk ejection reflex is absent in hypophysectomised patients.

Action of oxytocin

1. Causes ADH like action at high doses in kidney.
2. Causes vasodilatation by direct action resulting in fall in BP, flushing and reflex tachycardia.

3. Contracts myoepithelium of mammary alveoli and forces milk into bigger milk sinusoids initiating milk ejection reflex by suckling. Myoepithelial cells are more sensitive than myometrium to oxytocin. **Oxytocin Oozes** (releases) and **PROlactin PROduces** milk.
4. Enhances force and frequency of uterine contractions restricted to fundus and body.
   At low doses, full relaxation occurs in between contraction.
   At high doses, basal tone increases.

Mech: Action on myometrium is independent of innervation. Number of oxytocin R is enhanced markedly during later part of pregnancy (at term) → increased sensitivity to oxytocin. It acts by depolarization of muscle fibres and influx of Ca^{2+} ions through IP_3 generation. Nonpregnant uterus and uterus during early pregnancy are resistant to oxytocin. It also enhances PG synthesis and release by endometrium.

Oxytocin is also released during labour and complementary to it is PG and PAF.

IA: **Estrogen enhances and progestin reduces oxytocin effect on uterus.**

PK

Route (IV/IM), inactive orally due to being peptide, rapidly degraded in liver and kidney with plasma t½ = 10 min.

Pregnant uterus and placenta have **oxytocinase** (a specific aminopeptidase) and can be detected in maternal plasma.

ADR

1. **Water intoxication** is due to ADH like action of large doses given along with IV fluids specifically in toxemia of pregnancy and renal insufficiency.
2. Insidious use during labour causes **strong uterine contractions** forcing presenting part to pass through incompletely dilated birth canal causing rupture of uterus, foetal injury, asphyxia and death.

U

1. **Abortion:** As nasal spray to stimulate milk letdown.
2. **Breast engorgement** which occurs due to inefficient milk ejection reflex.
3. **Caesarean section.**
4. **Oxytocin challenge test** is to determine uteroplacental adequacy in high-risk pregnancy by infusing IV fluid at very low concentration till uterine contraction is elicited every 3–4 minutes.
   Marked increase in foetus HR indicates uteroplacental inadequacy.
5. **Induction of labour and uterine inertia:** Total dose = 2–4 IU.
   Low dose causes ↑ rythmic contraction.
   High dose causes sustained uterine contraction.

   Oxytocin is preferred over ergometrine (methergin) because:
   a. It is short-acting (short t½)
   b. Intensity of action is controllable and quickly terminated.
   c. Fetal oxygenation is maintained due to normal relaxation in between contraction at low concentration.
   d. Foetal descent is not compromised.

Magnesium sulfate

MgSO₄ controls convulsions, reduces BP in toxemia of pregnancy and suppresses uterine contraction effectively.

ADR
1. Cardiac arrhythmia
2. Muscular paralysis
3. CNS and respiratory depression

U: 1. **PRE**eclampsia (**P**roteinuria, **R**aised BP and **E**dema).
    2. Used when beta agonist is contraindicated.
    3. Toxemia of pregnancy (reduces BP and ovulation).

Ritodrine

Ritodrine suppresses premature labour and delays delivery.
    Mech: Selective β₂ agonist.
    ADR: CVS (hypotension, edema, arrhythmia), metabolic (hyperglycaemia, hyperinsulinemia, hypokalcemia), anxiety, headache.
    CI: DM, CHD, with β blocker/steroid
    U: Premature labour/delivery; 50 μg/min IV.

    CCB: It reduces tone of myometrium, opposes contractions and postpones labour.
    Ethyl alcohol: Stops labour.
    ADR: foetal hypoxia, maternal CNS depression.
    Nitrites, GA, diazoxide, atropine (anticholinergic) and phenothiazine reduce uterine contraction but have poor efficacy. PG synthesis inhibitors (aspirin, indomethacin) delay labour when used before it has started.

26
Drugs Acting on Thyroid Gland

Thyroid gland was discovered by Wharton. Isolation and crystallisation of T_4 was done by Kendall. Chemical structure of T_4 was determined by Barger and Harrington.

Normal weight of thyroid gland—**25 gm.** Normal I_2 needed/day is 14 mg. Amino acid needed for thyroxine production is **tyrosine**.

TSH/Thyrotropin is formed from
1. 210 amino acids
2. 2 chain glycoprotein (22% sugar)
3. MW 30,000.

Physiological functions
1. TSH stimulates gland to synthesize and secrete T_3 and T_4.
2. Induces hyperplasia and hypertrophy of thyroid follicles and enhances blood supply to gland. Tumoricidal and iodine uptake.
3. Promotes iodide trapping by the gland, its organification and incorporation into T_3 and T_4 by enhancing peroxide activity.
4. Enhances endocytotic uptake of thyroid colloid by follicular cells and proteolysis of thyroglobulin to release T_3 and T_4.
5. TH enhances rates of most chemical reaction in all cells.

Mech

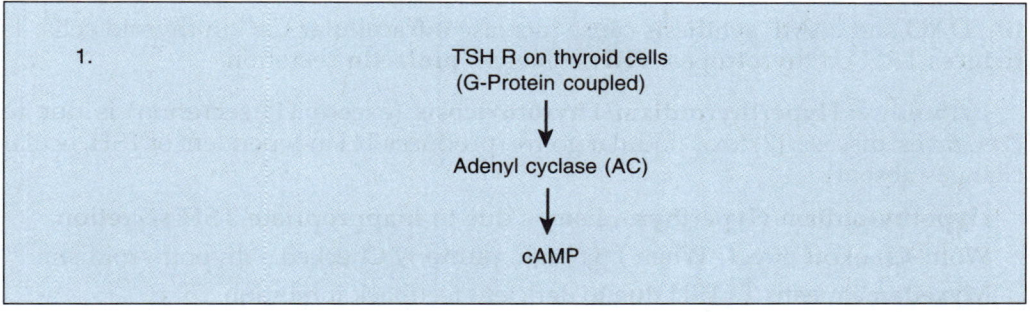

Regulation of secretion

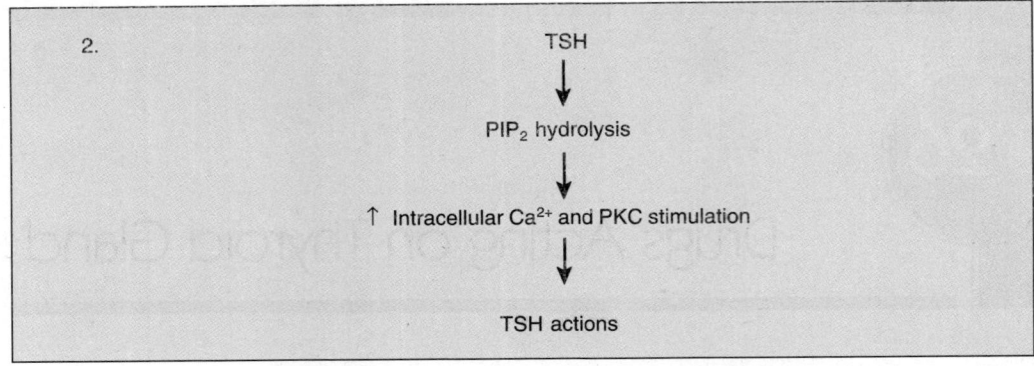

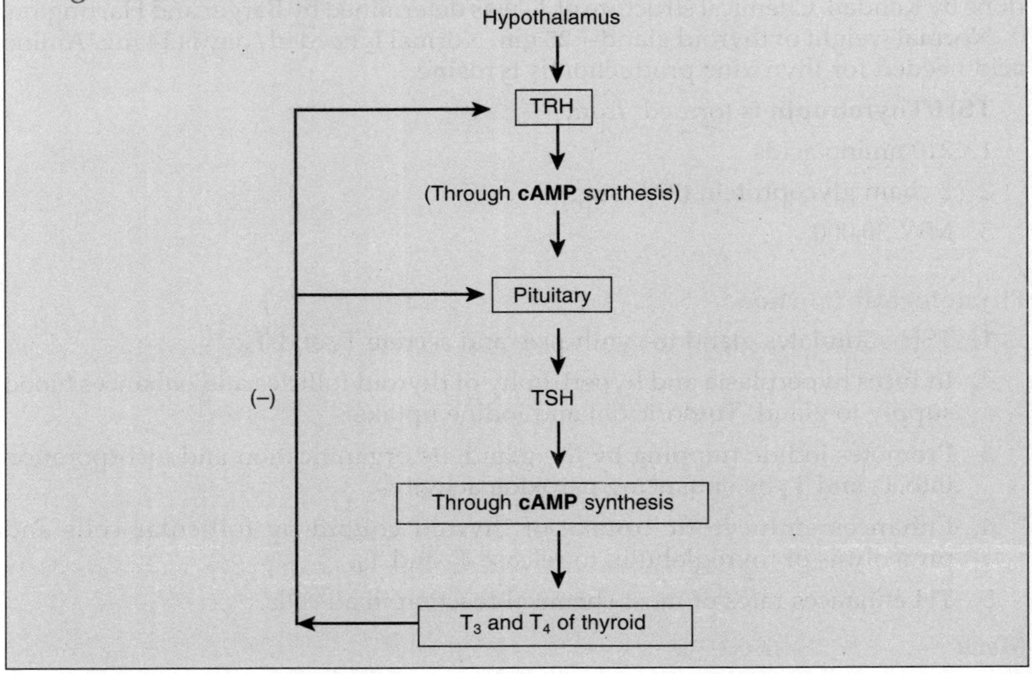

IP_3/DAG and cAMP synthesis cause increase intracellular Ca^{2+} in thyroid cells. T_3 reduces TRH on thyrotropes. **TRH** enhances **prolactin** secretion.

Pathology: Hyperthyroidism/Thyrotoxicosis (excess TH secretion) is due to (1) Graves' disease, (2) toxic nodular goitre (produces TH independent of TSH, ocular changes absent).

Hypothyroidism/Hyperthyroidism is due to **inappropriate TSH secretion.**

Wolff-Chaikoff effect: When I^- is high, pump is Checked →hypothyroidism.

Myxedema means ↑ TSH due to deficient feedback inhibition.

Graves' disease: It is due to IgG **attachment to TSH R** of thyroid cells and their stimulation in the same way as TSH. Due to feedback inhibition, TSH level is low. Hence, IgG is called **LATS (Long-Acting Thyroid Stimulator).** IgG fraction is Ab to TSHR stimulating ↑ T_3/T_4 in Graves' disease.

Autoimmune inflammation of periorbital tissues causes **exophthalmos** (TSH is not the cause of exophthalmos in Graves' disease).

Hypothyroidism 1. Infant (cretinism)
2. Adult (myxoedema)

Graves' disease

Symptoms | GOITRE |

Goitre

Ophthalmic symptoms

Irritability

Tremor

Restlessness

Excitability

Causes:

Autoimmune, Stress, Sex female, EPS (exophthalmos producing substance), Age young, Familial, Emotional, LATS, TSI. | AS SEA FELT |

HyperTHYROIDISM (features):

Tremor, Heart rate increased, Yawning (fatigability), Restlessness, Oligomenorrhea, Intolerance to heat, Diarrhoea, Irritability, Sweating, Muscle wasting with weight loss.

Thyroid hormone (TH): Secreted by thyroid gland.
    3 Types
    1. T_3
    2. T_4
    3. Calcitonin from interfollicular **C cells.**

T_4 (thyroxine) was the first hormone to be synthesized in the laboratory.

T_3 and T_4 are iodine containing derivatives of thyronine (a condensation product of 2 molecules of amino acid tyrosine). The hormones are synthesized and stored in the follicles as a part of TG (thyroglobulin) molecules (a glycoprotein with 10% sugar synthesized by thyroid cells).

I^- uptake occurs by active transport to thyroid cells (1/5th = **8 mg** of total body content of I_2).

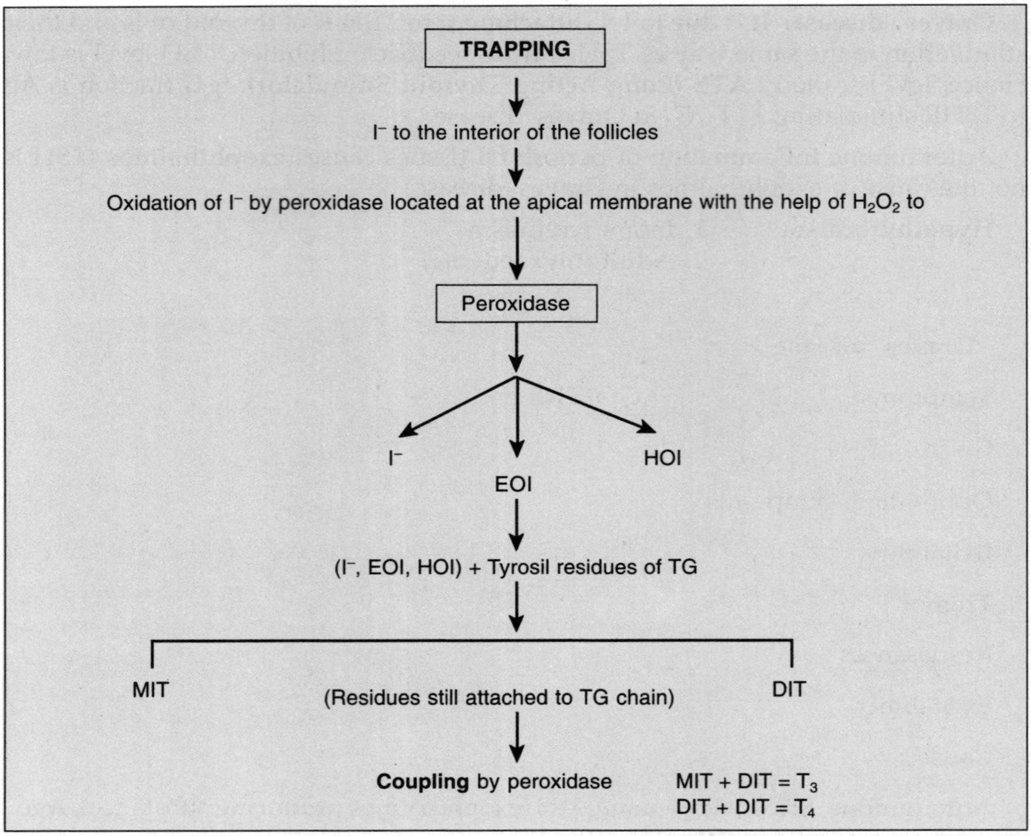

TRAPPING
I⁻ to the interior of the follicles
Oxidation of I⁻ by peroxidase located at the apical membrane with the help of H_2O_2 to
Peroxidase
I⁻
EOI
HOI
(I⁻, EOI, HOI) + Tyrosil residues of TG
MIT
(Residues still attached to TG chain)
DIT
Coupling by peroxidase
MIT + DIT = T_3
DIT + DIT = T_4

During I_2 deficiency, more MIT is available and more T_3 is formed (**more active form** is generated with less amount of I_2). **Normally more T_4 is formed. TG containing iodinated tyrosil and thyronil** residues transported to **interior of follicles** remains stored as **thyroid colloid** till taken back into the cells by **endocytosis and** broken down by **lysosomal protease.**

ENDOCYTOSIS
In the cells
Proteolysis by protease
DIT, MIT
Deiodination
I⁻ to be reutilised
T_4 (90–95%), T_3
Secretion
Circulation
Deiodination of 1/3 T_4 in liver and kidney

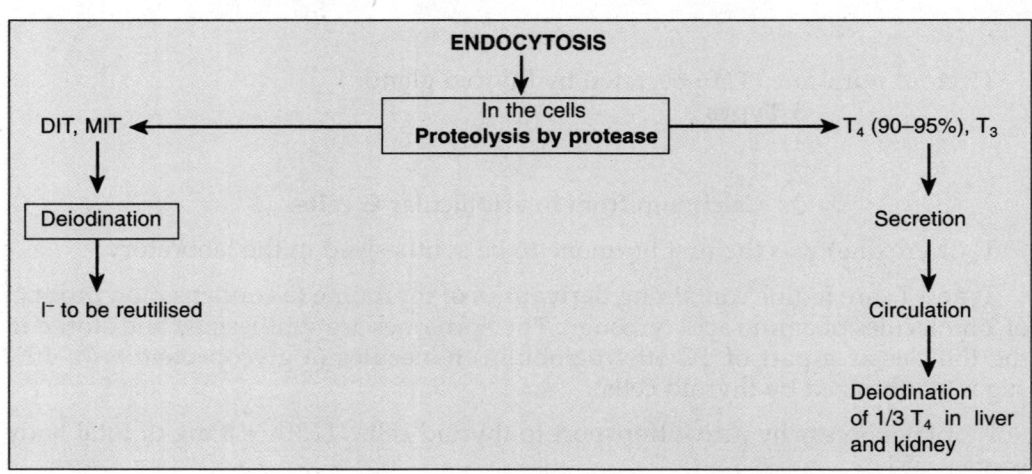

Active form "T_3" from circulation to target tissues (except brain and pituitary which themselves convert T_4 to T_3).

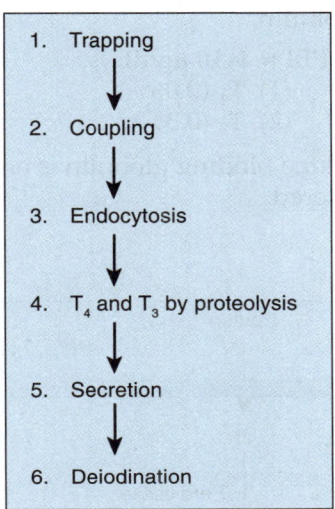

A. **Liver, Kidney, salivary Glands** are the primary site for inactivation of T_4 and T_3.
LKG
B. **TSH stimulates 1, 2, 3, 4, 5** steps.
C. **Ionic inhibitors** block **step 1**.
D. **Excess iodide** interferes with **steps 1, 2, 3, 5**.
E. **Propylthiouracil** inhibits steps **2 and 6**.
F. **Carbimazole** inhibits **step 2**.

Glucocorticoids, **A**miodarone, **P**ropranolol and **P**ropylthiouracil inhibit peripheral conversion of T_4 to T_3 (**except** in brain and pituitary).
GAP

Major source of TH to **developing foetus** is **foetal thyroid**. From **11th week** of pregnancy, foetal thyroid starts producing **thyroxine**. FNAC is for definitive diagnosis of all CA except follicular CA. Calcitonin is the **tumour marker** of medullary CA.

Quiscent gland →Follicles distended with colloid cells are flat/cubical.
TSH stimulated gland →colloid absent and cells columnar.

Normal thyroid secretion 〈 T_4 **80 µg/day** / T_3 **20 µg/day**

1. T_4 = **3, 5, 3, 5-Tetraiodothyronine**.
2. T_3 = **3, 5, 3'-Triiodothyronine (normal T_3: Active)** and **3, 3, 5'-Triiodothyronine (reverse T_3: Inactive)**. **Equal amount** of both is formed in the periphery. **More potent T_3** was discovered in **1952**.

All protein bound iodine (**PBI**) in plasma is in TH. **3 plasma proteins** bound to TH are:

1. Albumin
2. Transthyretin (thyroxine binding prealbumin)
3. Thyroxine binding globulin.

Normal concentration of PBI = **4–10 µg/dl**.
Free form (active form):   (1) T_4 (0.06%)
                                   (2) T_3 (0.3%)

During pregnancy, thyroxine binding globulin is enhanced but concentration of free hormones remain unaltered.

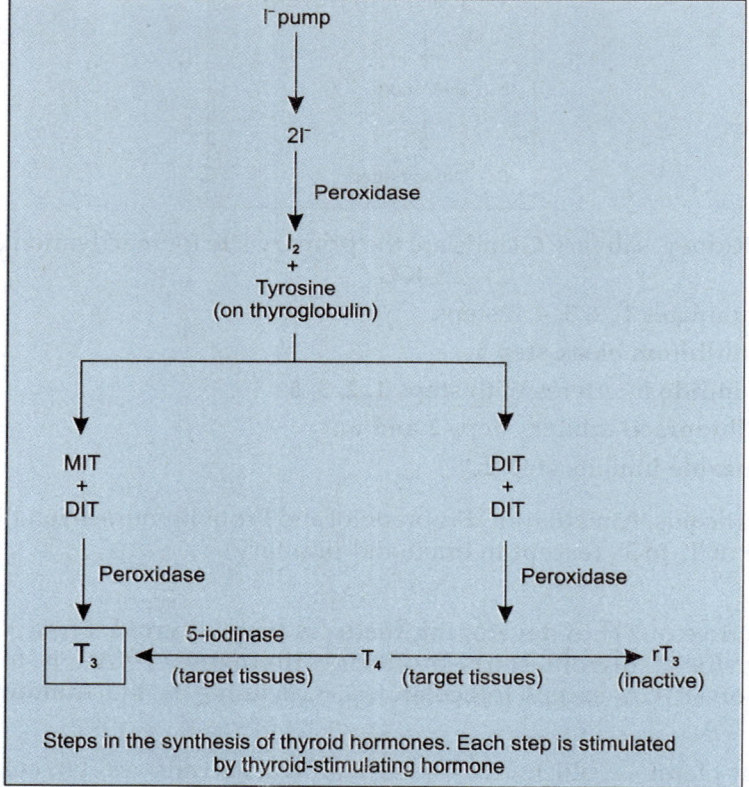

Steps in the synthesis of thyroid hormones. Each step is stimulated by thyroid-stimulating hormone

Normal human thyroid **secretes 70–90 µg of T_4 and 10–30 µg of T_3 daily**. All protein bound I_2 in plasma is TH (**90–95% T_4 and rest T_3**).

$T_4 > T_3$ is secreted by the gland. T_4 is **15 times** more tightly bound to plasma protein. Hence, T_4 is major circulating hormone (but 1/3 of T_4 is converted to T_3 in the periphery). Low potency and delayed action of T_4 are due to low concentration of its free form and its lower affinity for nuclear receptors. T_4 (prohormone of T_3)

is **5 times** less potent than T_3 and acts faster. Peak effect of T_4 comes in 6–8 days and that of T_3 in 1–2 days. Levothyroxine (T_4) is synthetic.

Actions are similar of both T_3 and T_4.
1. Overall effect of T_4 is catabolic → enhanced amount of protein being used as energy source (though protein synthesis is also enhanced). Hence, weight loss in hypothyroidism is present. Hypothyroidism inhibits mucoprotein synthesis which characteristically accumulates in myxoedema.
2. Congenital deficiency of T_3 and T_4 results in cretinism → nervous system is the **most** effected part of the body, which is the result of paucity of axonal and dendritic ramification, synapse formation and impaired myelination.

Hyperthyroidism causes tremors, hyper-reflexia, nervousness and excitability. The flabby and weak muscle with sluggishness is present in myxoedema. Constipation is in hypothyroidism and diarrhoea in hyperthyroidism.

> **Constipation = Hypo = Less, Diarrhoea = Hyper = More**

Thyrotoxic patient has enhanced muscle tone, weakness due to myopathy and tremor. Hypothyroidism causes:
A. Anemia (treated by T_4)
B. Impaired fertility
C. Oligomenorrhoea in women.
3. **Hyperthyroidism** causes **hyperglycaemia** due to glycogenolysis and gluconeogenesis in liver and faster glucose absorption from intestine (though glucose utilization is also enhanced).
Hyperglycaemic and diabetic like state occur in hyperthyroidism.
Diarrhoea occurs in hyperthyroidism.
Constipation occurs hypothyroidism.
4. **BMR** is increased due to stimulation of cellular metabolism by T_3/T_4
5. > **T_3/T_4 suppresses PDE**
   ↓
   ↑ cAMP
   ↓
   ↑ Lipolysis (lipolysis is also due to potentiation of CA action)
   ↓
   ↑ Plasma FFA.

Cholesterol metabolism and its conversion to **bile acids** are enhanced, hence LDL level is reduced → **hypocholesterolemia** (a characteristic of hyperthyroidism).
Weight Loss is also present.
6. **T_4 enhances HR, CO, and contractility.**
T_3/T_4 stimulates beta **receptor and Ca^{2+} ATPase** of heart muscle → hperdynamic state and HTN. It may precipitate **CHF** and angina.

Mech

T_4 Functions **4B**
Brain maturation
Bone growth
Beta-adrenergic effects
BMR↑

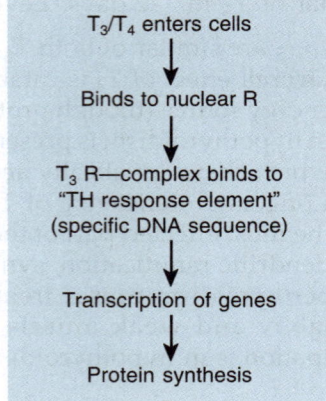

T_3/T_4 enters cells
↓
Binds to nuclear R
↓
T_3 R—complex binds to "TH response element" (specific DNA sequence)
↓
Transcription of genes
↓
Protein synthesis

ADR of TH replacement (due to ↑ BMR)

1. Flushing
2. Weight Loss
3. ↑ Appetite   **AFLAT**
4. Tachycardia
5. Angina

PK: Free T_3 and T_4 are inactivated by **deiodination, glucuronide/sulfate** conjugation in the liver, kidney and salivary gland. Conjugates are exerted in **bile.**
Deconjugated (intestine) and reabsorbed (enterohepatic circulation) forms are excreted in **bile.**
Plasma t½ → 6 days for T_4 and 1–2 days for T_3.
Shortened t½ → in hyperthyroidism due to faster metabolism.
Prolonged t½ → in **hypothyroidism** due to slower metabolism.

U: HRT—**commonest** use in TH deficient patient.
1. Cretinism (↓ TH)
Characteristics X-ray finding → epiphyseal dysgenesis. It is congenital absence of T_3 and T_4. **The greatest** sufferer is the nervous system.

Two types (A) **Sporadic** cretinism: Developmental failure/synthetic defect.
(B) **Endemic** cretinism: Iodine deficiency.

Treatment: Thyroxine 7 µg/kg.
In hypothyroid newborn → treatment within **one month** is needed to avoid cretinism. After 3–4 months of untreated hypothyroidism of newborn, brain dysfunction occurs.

2. Non-toxic **goitre**

Two types (A) **Endemic** (↓ iodine)
(B) **Sporadic** (defect in synthesis)
Both have **deficient** production of TH → excess TSH → enlarged thyroid gland → more efficient trapping of iodide and ↑ T_3 formation → hence treatment **with T_4.**
(Ca^{2+} in water, goitrogen/thiocynates in food/milk cause **endemic** goitre).
Treatment of endemic goitre and cretinism due to iodide deficiency in pregnant mother = 150–200 µg iodine/day **best in the form of edible salt.**

3. **Papillary CA of thyroid (commonest** CA of thyroid**):** It has Orphan–Annie-eyed nuclei.
   Treated by T_4 which suppresses TSH production.
4. **Adult hypOthyroidism:**
   Treatment with T_4 is **most gratifying,** because it avoids CVS symptoms. **L-isomer** is **30 times** more potent than D-isomer. Hence, **L-thyroxine** is used, dose (50 µg/day starting gradually, increasing up to **200 µg/day maximum**).
5. **Myxoedema coma:**
   Liothyronine (triiodothyronine) 100 µg IV followed by 25 µg QID. Alternate is thyroxine.

   Cretinism Never COME

6. **Empirical use:** T_4 in   **AMU Court**
   A. Refractory Anemia
   B. Mental disorder
   C. Chronic/non-healing Ulcer
   D. Constipation

Classification

Thyroid inhibitors/antithyroid drugs
(They lower the functional capacity of hyperactive glands)

1. **Goitrogens**
   a. **Ionic inhibitors/Iodide trapping inhibitors**
      Thiocyanates (SCN^-)
      Perchlorates (ClO_4^-)
      Nitrates (NO_3^-)
   b. **Synthesis inhibitors/thioamide/antithyroid drugs by convention**
      Propylthiouracil
      Carbimazole
      Methimazole (active metabolite of carbimazole)
2. **TH release inhibitors**
   NaI, KI, I_2, organic iodide.
3. **Thyroid tissue destroyer**
   Radioactive iodide (^{123}I, ^{125}I, ^{131}I)

Other drugs
   a. Li →inhibits TH release.
   b. Amiodarone →inhibits peripheral conversion from T_4 to T_3.
   c. Sulfonamide and para-aminosalicylic acid inhibit T_4 iodination and coupling reaction.
   d. CBZ, rifampin, phenytoin and phenobarbitone induce metabolic degradation of TH.

TH synthesis inhibitors
Act due to **peroxidase** binding by drugs.

PropylThioUracil (PTU) inhibits **P**eroxidase/**P**eripheral deiodination, **T**yrosine iodination and **U**nion (coupling).

Mech

1. Inhibit **oxidation** of iodide/iodotyrosyl residues.
2. Inhibit iodination of tyrosin residues in TG (the most important).
3. Inhibit coupling of iodotyrosine residues to form TH by binding **peroxidase**.
4. Propylthiouracil also inhibits peripheral conversion of T_4 to T_3 (methimazole and carbimazole may antagonise this action of propylthiouracil).

ADR

1. **Goitre** is due to enhanced TSH release as a consequence of reduction in feedback inhibition (hypothyroidism due to over treatment but reversible on stopping).

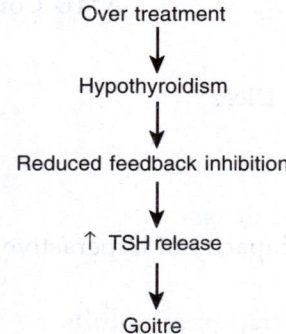

2. Skin rashes:
   Maculopapular pruritic rash (**commonest** ADR).
3. **GIT intolerance.**
4. Joint pain.
5. Rarely fever, liver damage, hair defect and agranulocytosis (**the most severe** ADR).

PK

Absorbed orally, widely disributed in the body (cross placenta, enter milk), hepatic metabolism, renal excretion, effect foetus by crossing placenta. All are concentrated in thyroid with longer intrathyroid t½.

Plasma t½ of **propylthiouracil = 1–2 hrs** and **carbimazole = 8 hrs**. Carbimazole acts 12–24 hrs (single dose per day is given).

Single daily dose of propylthiouracil acts for 4–8 hrs, hence BD/TDS is given.

Propylthiouracil is highly plasma protein bound whereas carbimazole is less plasma protein bound.

U:

1. **Thyrotoxicosis (Graves' disease and toxic nodular goitre)**

   Graves' disease = 50% cure after 1–2 yrs of treatment.
   Toxic nodular goitre = In frail elderly patient, drugs are used (permanent therapy). Remission is rare, hence **surgery** (or ^{131}I) is preferred.
2. **Preoperatively in partial thyroidectomy:** Reduce size and vascularity.
3. **Thyroid storm** (acute hyperthyroid crisis) is treated with **propranolol and antithyroid** drugs. Propranolol reduces heart stimulation due to enhanced TH.

4. **TH synthesis inhibitor + ^{131}I**
   Advantages: a. No surgical risk
                     b. Reversible hypothyroidism
                     c. Used in children
   Disadvantages: a. Lifelong treatment due to relapse
                     b. ADR
                     c. Not used in non-cooperative patient.

Antithyroid drugs are preferred over surgery because:
a. Injury to nerve/tissue is absent
b. Hypothyroid is reversible
c. Useful in children and young adults.

CI
1. ^{131}I and thyroidectomy in pregnancy.
2. **Foetal hypothyroidism and goitre** (CI = antithyroid drugs). But propylthiouracil in pregnancy and nursing mother is given due to its greater protein binding capacity and hence less transfer to the foetus.

Ionic inhibitors
Relative inhibitory potency: ClO_4 (10): SCN (1): NO_3 (1/30).
Mech: Monovalent anions inhibit ion trapping by thyroid because of similar ionic size. Inhibit iodide concentrating mechanism in thyroid.

ADR:
1. NO_3^- causes vasodilatation and methemoglobinemia.
2. SCN^- causes liver, kidney and brain toxicity and bone marrow depression.
3. ClO_4^- causes fever, rashes, aplastic anemia and agranulocytosis.

TH release inhibitors
I_2 is the **fastest** acting thyroid inhibitor and is reduced to iodide in the intestine. Both I_2 and I^- have similar response and cause enlarged gland to shrink, as well as to make firm and less vascular.

Mech: "Thyroid constipation" (TH release inhibition) is the **most** important action. Endocytosis of colloid and proteolysis of TG are stopped. Excess I^- inhibits its own transport in thyroid cells.

U
1. Preoperative preparation for **thyroidectomy** to make the gland firm and less vascular.
2. **Thyroid storm:** NaI/KI
3. **Expectorant**
4. **Antiseptic:** Tincture iodine
5. **Prophylaxis** of endemic goitre

ADR

A. Acute reactions
1. **Swelling** of lips and eyelids
2. **Angioedema** of larynx
3. **Fever, joint pain, petechial haemorrhage**
4. **Lymphadenopathy and thrombocytopenia**

B. Chronic reactions (iodism)
1. **Swelling** of eyelids.
2. **Inflammation** of mucous membrane and burning sensation in the mouth.
3. **Salivation** and **lacrimation.**
4. **Sneezing and rhinorrhoea.**
5. **Hypothyroidism and goitre** even in foetus when given to a nursing mother.

Radioactive iodine: Fastest acting thyroid inhibitor is iodine.
- A. Stable isotope—^{127}I.
- B. Radioactive isotopes
    1. ^{125}I—physical t½ = 60 days.
    2. ^{123}I—physical t½ = 13 hrs.
    3. ^{131}I—physical t½ = 8 days (**commonest** used isotope, 20–40% patient needs >1 dose).

Mech: They emit X-rays and β-particles. X-rays are used for tracer studies. β-particles are used for destruction of thyroid cells. β-particles penetrate 0.5–2 mm of tissues and cause (pyknosis + necrosis + fibrosis). **Most** important action of iodine is inhibition of hormone release.

ADR
1. Thyroid constipation
2. Hypothyroidism (50%) → constipation

U
1. Thyroid **scanning** (^{123}I).
2. Tracer **studies** (X-rays).
3. Thyroid cells **destruction** (Beta-particles).
4. As Na salt of ^{131}I **dissolved** in water and taken orally:
    a. Diagnostic: 25–100 µ curie.
    b. Therapeutic: ^{131}I **(DOC)** after 35 yrs of age.

Hyperthyroidism due to Graves' disease or toxic nodular goitre (**commonest** indication):
Dose = 5 µ curie.
Once hyperthyroidism is controlled, cure is **permanent**.
Peak effects are in **10–15** days with daily iodine administration, after that **thyroid escape** occurs and **thyrotoxicosis returns.**

Advantages
a. Simple treatment
b. Permanent cure
c. No surgical risk

Disadvantages
a. Hypothyroidism
b. Long latent period of response
c. Not suitable for young patients
d. **Contraindicated** during pregnancy
5. **Metastatic CA of thyroid.**
6. **Thyrotoxicosis** (for 14 days preoperatively).

CI
1. Pregnancy
2. Age < 35 yrs

Thyrotoxicosis with
1. Enhanced radioiodine uptake = **Graves' disease.**
2. Enhanced radioiodine uptake and normal T_4 (serum)–T_3 **toxicosis.**
3. Reduced radioiodine uptake:
   - De Quervain's thyroiditis
   - Thyrotoxicosis factitia
   - Jod Basedow thyrotoxicosis.

Drugs causing **ALOPECIA: A**ntithyroid, **L**ithium, **O**C withdrawal, **P**henytoin, **E**thionamide, **C**ytotoxics, **I**nterferon, **A**nticoagulants and albendazole.

Lugol's solution is iodine plus KI. Ipodate reduces T_3 in thyrotoxicosis.

27. Drugs Affecting Calcium Metabolism

Drugs are
a. **Bisphosphonates**
b. **Hormones**
   1. Parathormone (PTH)
   2. Calcitonin
   3. Calcitriol (active form of vitamin D)

Calcium

Ca^{2+}/Ca^{++}/calcium ion is the **5th most abundant** body constituent after H, C, O and N, 2% (1–1.5 kg) of body weight and 99% of it is stored in bones.

Normal plasma Ca^{2+} is 10 mg/dl. 40% is bound to albumin and 50% is ionised (acidosis favours it).

Actions

1. Controls **excitability** of nerves and muscles.
2. Regulates **permeability** and **integrity** of membranes and cell adhesion.
3. Causes **coagulation** of blood, excitation–contraction **coupling of all muscles,** excitation–secretion **coupling of all glands** (both exocrine and endocrine) and **transmitter** release from nerve endings.
4. Acts as **intracellular messenger** of transmitter, hormones and autacoids.
5. Generates **impulse** in heart.

Regulation of plasma Ca^{2+} level

a. **Decrease resorption is due to:**
   - Mithramycin   **MEAT Grows Bone**
   - Estrogen
   - Androgen
   - Thiazide
   - GH and Gallium nitrate
   - Bisphosphonate
b. **Increase resorption is due to**
   - Corticosteroid   **CAPITAL**
   - Alcohol
   - PGE_2
   - IL 1 and 6

- TH
- PArathormone
- Loop diuretic

Three hormones (PTH, calcitriol and calcitonin) regulate plasma Ca^{2+} level which is normally **10 mg/dl** (40% bound to plasma protein chiefly **albumin, 50%** is in **ionised** form). **Acidosis** favours and **alkalosis** disfavours ionisation of Ca^{2+}. Daily excretion is **300 mg** (150 mg in urine and 150 mg in faeces). About one-third is absorbed from GIT, hence daily dose in diet should be about **1 gm**, to maintain Ca^{2+} balance. Ca^{2+} deficiency causes **tetany** and **laryngospasm**.

Tetracycline, Oxalate, Phosphate and Phytate reduce Ca^{2+} absorption by forming **insoluble** complex.

Glucocorticoid and phenytoin also reduce Ca^{2+} absorption.

TOP

ADR: GIT:
    Bloating   BCG
    Constipation
    Gas

U

1. Supplement: SEAT
    Usual dose = 1 gm
    Pregnancy and lactation = 1.5 gm
2. Empirically (weakness, etc.)
    Benefit is psychological.
3. Antacid
4. Tetany

Parathormone

PTH/Parathormone is a single chain 24 amino acid polypeptide with MW 9500.

Decrease Ca^{2+} induces PTH release by increasing cAMP.

Increase Ca^{2+} inhibits PTH release by decreasing cAMP.

Prolonged hypocalcaemia also causes hypertrophy and hyperplasia of parathyroid. Calcitriol inhibits PTH gene expression.

There is no trophic hormone for it.

Actions

1. The **most** important action is increase in resorption of Ca^{2+} from bone.
2. Enhances Ca^{2+} reabsorption from DCT and promotes PO_4^{3-} excretion.
3. Reduces Ca^{2+} level in milk, saliva and ocular lens (cause of cataract).
4. Inhibits 1α-hydroxylase and enhances Ca^{2+} reabsorption.
5. Enhances serum Ca^{2+}, reduces serum PO_4^{3-}, enhances urine PO_4^{3-}, stimulates both osteoclasts and osteoblasts.

    PTH = Phosphate Trashing Hormone

Mech: ↑ cAMP → ↑ intracellular Ca^{2+} in target cells (osteoblasts).
Osteoclast has no receptor for PTH, but is indirectly activated by it.
Calcitonin inhibits osteoclastic activity and enhances osteoblastic activity.

Hypoparathyroidism causes Low plasma Ca^{2+}, Paresthesias, Tetany, Cataract, Psychiatric changes and Laryngospasm.

Pharmacology Review

Low Plasma Ca^{2+} Level Produces Tetany

Pseudo-hypothyroidism is due to reduced sensitivity of target cells to PTH caused by mutant G protein.

Hyperparathyroidism is **mostly** due to parathyroid tumour, causes decalcification of bone, renal stone and muscle weakness.

PK: Degraded in liver and kidney with plasma t½ = 4 minutes.

U

1. **Diagnosis:** To differentiate pseudo—from true hypoparathyroidism. On injection (200 U teriparatide IV), plasma Ca^{2+} level fails to rise in pseudoparathyroidism.
2. Not used therapeutically because PTH is given **P**arenterally while vitamin D is given orally and is cheap (hence vitamin D is used).

Calcitonin: It is 32 amino acid single chain polypeptide with MW 3600 produced by parafollicular 'C' cells of thyroid.

Increased Ca^{2+} increases and decreased Ca^{2+} decreases calcitonin release.
CALCItonin of **C** cells reduces **CALCI**um and **P**TH reduces **P**hosphate from plasma.

Actions

Action is opposite to PTH, inhibits bone resorption by osteoclasts and Ca^{2+} + PO$_4^{3-}$ reabsorption from PCT.

Pathology: Hypercalcemic states are hyperparathyroidism, hyper-vitaminosis D and osteolytic bony metastasis.

Mech: Acts by increasing cAMP formation.

ADR

1. Tingling of fingers
2. Bad taste   **TAB**let
3. Allergic reaction

PK: Plasma t½ = 10 min.

U

1. Paget's disease
2. Hypercalcemic states
3. Postmenopausal osteoporosis, but causes epistaxis, rhinitis and nasal ulcer.

Bisphosphonates

Bisphosphonates are analogues of pyrophosphate.

They are

a. Pamidronate sodium
b. Etidronate sodium
c. Alendronate
   PEA
d. Gasidronate, Ibandronate, Risedronate, **GIRLS ~ GIRTZ**
   Tiludronate, Zolendronate

Mech: Inhibit bone resorption without effecting bone growth and mineralization by slowing hydroxyapatite crystals activity in mineralised bone matrix and by inhibiting osteoclast.

PK: Given orally/intravenously, excreted unchanged in urine, patient should be hydrated.

ADR
1. Hypocalcemia
2. Osteomalacia by chronic use of etidronate. But alendronate lacks this effect.
3. Thrombophlebitis on IV injection.
4. Leucopenia initially and Pyrexia.
5. Gastric Irritation on oral intake.   **HOT LIP**

U
1. Hypercalcemia of malignancy
2. Paget's disease: They decrease pain and arrest osteolytic lesions.
3. Osteoporosis
4. Osteolytic bone metastasis   **HPO$_2$**
   (Bisphosphonate + calcitriol) are given.

> OsteoBlast Builds bone
> OsteoClast Consumes bone

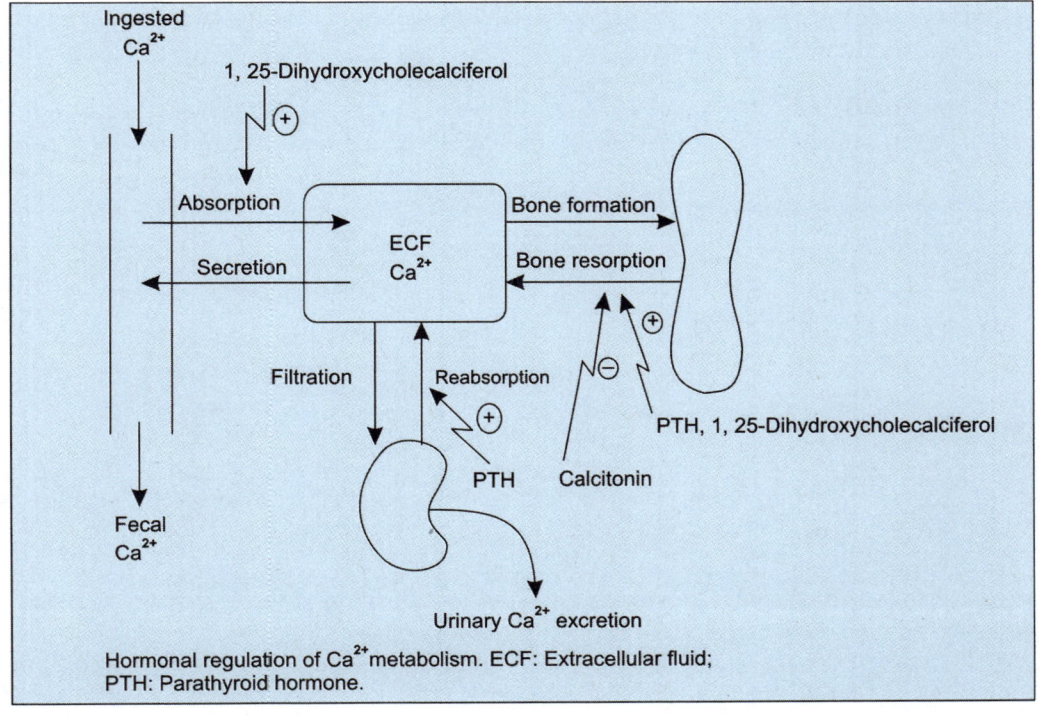

Hormonal regulation of Ca^{2+} metabolism. ECF: Extracellular fluid; PTH: Parathyroid hormone.

Summary of hormones that regulate Ca^{2+}			
	PTH	*Vitamin D*	*Calcitonin*
Stimulus for secretion	↓ serum $[Ca^{2+}]$	↓ serum $[Ca^{2+}]$ ↑ PTH ↓ serum [phosphate]	↑ serum $[Ca^{2+}]$
Action on			
Bone	↑ resorption	↑ resorption	↓ resorption
Kidney	↓ P reabsorption (↑ urinary cAMP) ↑ Ca^{2+} reabsorption	↑ P reabsorption	
Intestine	↑ Ca^{2+} absorption (via activation of vitamin D)	↑ Ca^{2+} absorption (vitamin D-dependent Ca^{2+}-binding protein ↑ P absorption	
Overall effect on			
Serum $[Ca^{2+}]$	↑	↑	↓
Serum [phosphate]	↓	↑	

28. Corticoids or Corticosteroids

Corticoids or corticosteroids are drugs with one of the **broadest** spectrum of clinical utility, have glucocorticoid, mineralocorticoid and weakly androgenic activities.

They include natural glucocorticoid, mineralocorticoid and their synthetic analogues.

Steroid nucleus

Corticoids (both glucocorticoid and mineralocorticoid) are 21 C compounds having *cyclopentanoperhydrophenanthrene* (steroid) nucleus.

> Adrenal cortex is essential for survival.
> **Adrenal cortex layers are:**
> 1. **Zona glomerulosa** (outermost) secretes **aldosterone (mineralocorticoid).**
> 2. **Zona fasciculata** (middle) secretes glucocorticoid.
> 3. **Zona reticularis** (inner) secretes androgen (dehydroepiendrosterone).

Classification

A. Glucocorticoids (**most** potent anti-inflammatory drug)

1. Short-acting (biological t½ <12 hrs)
   - Cortisone
   - Hydrocortisone (cortisol)

   Dose 20 mg

2. Intermediate acting (biological t½ 12–24 hrs)
   - Prednisone
   - Prednisolone
   - Methylprednisolone
   - Triamcinolone

   Dose 4 mg

3. Long-acting (biological t½ >24 hrs)
   - Paramethasone
   - Dexamethasone
   - Betamethasone (highest glucocorticoid activity)

   Dose 1–2 mg

B. Mineralocorticoids
($\downarrow H^+ \downarrow K^+ \uparrow Na^+$)
— Aldosterone (not used clinically).
— Fludrocortisone (dose: 0.2 mg).
— Desoxycorticosterone acetate (DOCA, dose: 2.5 mg).

Actions

1. They maintain **functional status** of skeletal muscle and nervous system, cardiovascular and energy substrate homeostasis along with fluid electrolyte and prepare the body to withstand effects of all kinds of noxious stimuli and stress.
   They have both direct and indirect (permissive) actions.
2. Mineralocorticoids enhance **Na^+, HCO_3^- and H_2O reabsorption** and cause **K^+ plus H^+ excretion** in tubules.

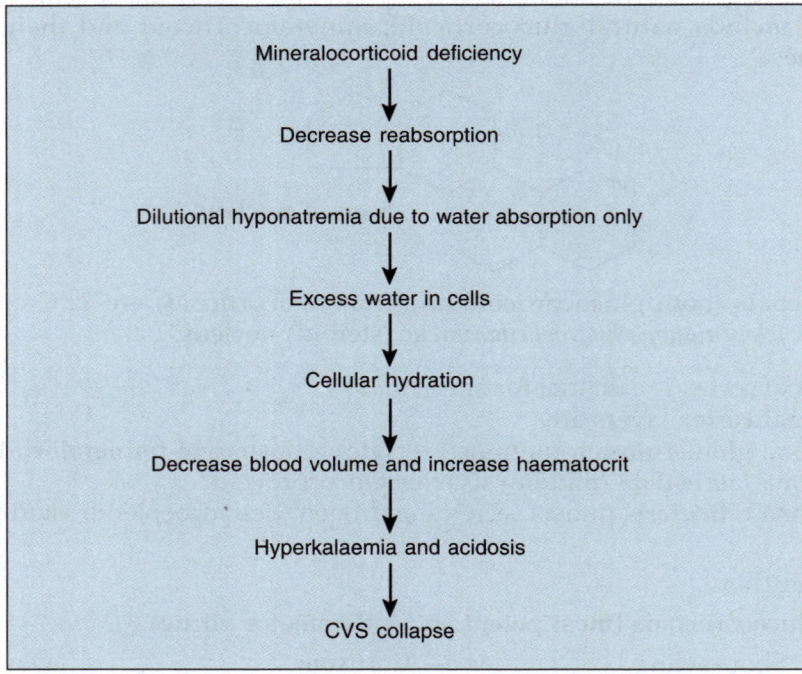

Mech. of mineralocorticoid: Action is due to gene mediated increase in RNA transcription in renal tubular cells which direct synthesis of AIP (aldosterone induced protein).

$Na^+ K^+$ ATPase of tubular basolateral membrane is the major AIP which generates gradients for movements of cations in the cells.

Synthesis of β-subunit of amiloride sensitive Na^+ channel is also induced.

ADR of mineralocorticoid

1. HTN
2. Fluid retention
3. Alkalosis and hypokalaemia due to elevated aldosterone.

Normal secretion of cortisol = 15–30 mg/day.
Normal secretion of aldosterone = 0.125 mg/day.
Source of urinary 17-ketosteroid in male is adrenal and the test to estimate it is **Zimmerman reaction.**

Glucocorticoids

Glucocorticoids are the **first** hormone to be replaced in hypopituitarism. Transcortin/CBG (corticosteroid binding globulin) binds 75% cortisol in circulation. Bound hormone is inactive. Estrogen and TH increase CBG. **Androgen** decreases CBG.

Actions (glucocorticoids)

1. Favour **of gluconeogenesis** by both increasing amino acid uptake by liver and kidney and elevating activities of **gluconeogenic enzymes** (glycogen synthetase, etc.).
2. Stimulate protein catabolism (except in liver) and lipolysis, thereby providing building blocks and energy needed for glucose synthesis.
3. Inhibit glucose utilization by peripheral tissues.
4. Increase lipolysis is due to GH, TH, glucagon and adrenaline. cAMP induced breakdown of triglyceride is enhanced. Subcutaneous tissue over extremities loses fat which gets deposited over shoulder, neck and face causing:
   - **Moon face**
   - **Fish mouth**
   - **Buffalo hump**
5. Inhibit intestinal absorption and increase renal excretion of Ca^{2+} →plasma Ca^{2+} level decreases.
   Negative Ca^{2+} balance results in spongy bones (ribs and vertebrae more sensitive).
6. Increase water secretory activity of renal tubules.
7. Cause euphoria. They cause depression and apathy in **Addison's disease.**
8. Restrict capillary permeability, maintain tone of arterioles and myocardial contractility and have permissive effect on pressor action of adrenaline and angiotensin resulting in HTN.
   Adrenal insufficiency causes CVS collapse.
9. Maintain normal muscular activity. Both hypo- and hypercorticism cause weakness. **Hypocorticism** causes weakness due to hypodynamic circulation. Hypercorticism causes weakness due to hypokalemia, myopathy and muscle wasting.
10. **Enhance gastric secretion.**
11. Increase rate of destruction of lymphoid cells (T cells > B cells) hence used in lymphomas. Enhance number of **RBC, platelets, and neutrophils** in circulation and reduce **eosinophil, basophil, monocyte,** and **lymphocyte.** After 24 hrs, blood counts come back to normal. Steroids reduce all leukocytes except neutrophils. Suppress the inflammatory response which is the basis of **most** of their clinical uses. This action is non-specific and covers all stages and components of inflammation (reduction of capillary permeability, cell infiltration, collagen deposition, scar formation and all cardinal signs—heat, redness, swelling, pain).

The most important overall mechanism is to limit the recruitment of inflammatory cells at the local site. But they do not remove the cause. They favour the spread of infection.

Corticoids are only **palliative** (do not remove the cause of inflammation, the underlying disease continues to progress while manifestations are dampened).

They suppress **all types** of allergic phenomena and hypersensitization due to suppression of recruitment of leukocyte at the site of contact with Ag and of inflammatory response to immunological injury.

Basis of use in autoimmune disease and organ transplantation is suppression of CMI and natural killer cells, inhibition of IL-1 release and IL-2 formation. Reduce the production of **IL-1,2,3,6, TNFα, GM-CSF and γ-interferon.** Broad action is due to interruption of communication between cells involved in the immune process by interfering with production or action of lymphokines.

Steroid/thyroid hormone mech

Hormone→binds to R of nucleus/cytoplasm→DNA-binding domain exposed →mRNA synthesis → response by protein synthesis.

Mech of glucocorticoids

1. Glucocorticoid receptors are present **in all cells.**
2. Cytoplasmic receptors → translocate into nucleus to bind on specific site of chromatin → mRNA transcription → protein synthesis inhibition (catabolic effect) in many tissues. Steroids diffuse across cell membrane and bind to steroid receptor in cytoplasm. Steroid-R-complex migrates to nucleus and acts on DNA to transcript mRNA and to regulate protein synthesis.
3. They reduce POMC gene expression in pituitary corticotropes to reduce ACTH production.
4. They induce lipocortin to inhibit **phospholipase A_2 (↓PG, ↓LT, ↓PAF).**
5. They reduce ELAM-1 and ICAM-1 production in endothelial cell to interfere with adhesion and localization of leukocytes.

PK of glucocorticoids

All natural and synthetic corticoids are effective by oral route except DOCA (this is the only steroid having no glucocorticoid activity).

All are orally active.

Water soluble → given IV/IM.

Hydrocortisone is 90% plasma protein bound, t½ of hydrocortisone = 1.5 hr. Acetonide to C-17 of steroid ring causes greater surface activity.

Most steroid is bound to a specific corticosteroid binding protein (albumin and transcortin).

Transcortin level is increased during pregnancy and treatment with OC. Steroids are metabolised primarily by hepatic microsomal enzymes → conjugated with sulfate/glucuronide through oxidation/reduction pathways. (Cortisol is metabolised by MFO/mixed function oxidase.)

Excreted in urine.

IA of glucocorticoids

Drugs inhibiting adrenal cortical function are:
1. Aminoglutethimide inhibits **desmolase** and reduces the production of all adrenal steroids.
2. KTZ reduces cortisol synthesis and release.
3. Spironolactone inhibits aldosterone receptor.

Prednisone

Mech: Higher apoptosis

ADR
1. Immunosuppression
2. Cushing-like symptoms

U: Commonest glucocorticoid used in cancer—prednisone.
1. CLL
2. Asthma
3. RA
4. Hodgkin's lymphoma

Prednisone is least expensive steroid preparation.

Prednisolone

4 times more potent than cortisol. Dose: 60 mg OD (maximum).
Also given IM/topically/intra-articularly.
Cortisol concentration is **highest** at 6 am.
ACTH concentration is **highest** at 4 am.
Aldosterone is the **most** potent mineralocorticoid but not used clinically due to low oral bioavailability and difficulty in regulating the dose.
Triamcinolone and long-acting steroid have no mineralocorticoid activity. Betamethasone has **highest** glucocorticoid activity. Dexamethasone is the **most** selective for glucocorticoid activity (maximum glucocorticoid activity).
Fludrocortisone is the **most** selective for mineralocorticoid activity (**maximum mineralocorticoid activity**).
Cortisone is glucocorticoid with **least** glucocorticoid activity.
Glucocorticoid having mineralocorticoid activity is cortisone, hydrocortisone, prednisone and prednisolone.
Hydrocortisone is the glucocorticoid with **highest** mineralocorticoid activity.

Cushing's syndrome (↑ glucocorticoid)
Commonest cause—iatrogenic
Next common cause—pituitary dependent Cushing's disease
Commonest symptom—weight gain
Most frequent sign—obesity
Lemon on tooth picks feature—present
Commonest bone involved—vertebra (osteoporosis)
Commonest site of vertebral collapse—T_{12} L_{1-2}
Commonest symptom of osteoporosis—backache
Treatment of choice = Trans-sphenoidal surgery

> **Nelson's syndrome (pituitary dependent Cushing's disease)**
> Treatment of choice—proton beam therapy
>
> **Conn's syndrome (primary hyperaldosteronism)**
> DOC—spironolactone (aldosterone antagonist).
>   Most important differentiating feature in primary and secondary forms = edema is present in secondary hyperaldosteronism.
>
> **Bar Her's syndrome (↑ PGE_2 and I_2)**
> DOC—indomethacin.

ADR of glucocorticoids

1. **Cushing's habitus:** Round face/moon face, narrow mouth/fish mouth, thin limb, buffalo hump/supraclavicular hump/truncal obesity.
   For diagnosis of Cushing's syndrome, dexamethasone is used.
2. **Fragile skin** (typically on thigh and lower abdomen): Hirsutism, thin skin.
3. **Hyperglycaemia/glycosuria**
4. **Infection**
5. **Delayed healing**
6. **Peptic Ulcer:** Silent perforation may occur
7. **Muscular weakness/wasting (myopathy)**
8. **Glaucoma and cataract (posterior subcapsular)**
9. **Osteoporosis:** Its radiological evidence is indication for withdrawal of corticoid therapy.
10. **Psychosis**
11. **Suppression of HPA axis** (hypothalamopituitary–adrenal axis):
    Withdrawal syndrome (joint and muscle pain, fever, malaise, reactivation of disease) precipitates after stoppage of steroid or due to adrenal cortex atrophy (ACTH suppression).
    Commonest cause of adrenal crisis is sudden withdrawal of steroids. **Commonest** cause of adrenal insufficiency is autoimmune adrenalitis. **Most** sensitive test of primary adrenal failure is simultaneous measurement of plasma cortisol and ACTH. HPA axis suppression is minimised by the use of **lowest** dose of shorter acting drugs for **shortest** period of time with single day therapy in the morning or alternate day therapy, preferably with local use.
    ADR of long-term therapy is minimised by using alternate day therapy (doubling dose on one day and using only NSAID on the next day). Adrenocortical steroid used for chronic therapy is the last resort.
12. **Hypokalemic alkalosis.**

> **Adverse effects of GLUCOCORTICOID**
>   Glucose level increase—diabetes mellitus may prepcipitate, Long time to heal, Ulcer—peptic, Cushing's syndrome, Osteoporosis and myopathy, CNS disorders—insomnia, psychosis, Ocular diseases—cataract, glaucoma, Retardation of growth, Thin fragile skin, Immunosuppression—infection predisposition, CHF, Oedema, Increased BP, Depression of hypothalamic–pituitary–adrenal axis.

U of corticoid/corticosteroid

A. HRT
1. **Acute adrenal insufficiency**
   Hydrocortisone/dexamethasone IV
2. **Chronic adrenal insufficiency (Addison's disease)**
   Commonest clinical finding is hyperpigmentation.
   Commonest used drug is hydrocortisone (DOC) given orally with saline.
   (Busulfan—a cytotoxic drug produces Addisonian like feature).
3. **Adrenogenital syndrome (congenital adrenal hyperplasia)** is due to genetic deficiency of steroidogenic enzymes (21-Hydroxylase → **commonest**). Compensatory increase in ACTH secretion is due to adrenal hypertrophy.
   Treatment: Hydrocortisone 0.6 mg/kg/day.

B. Non-endocrine disease
1. **Arthritides**
   a. **Rheumatoid arthritis:** Corticoid is the last resort.
      Treatment: Corticoid + NSAID
   b. **Rheumatic fever**
      Aspirin + corticosteroid
   c. **Osteoarthritis**
      Steroid + NSAID
   d. **Acute gouty arthritis** (but not in chronic gout)
2. **Sarcoidosis:** Prednisone 1 mg/kg/day for 6 weeks

Sarcoidosis is associated with (lung most commonly involved):
— **Granuloma**
— **Rheumatoid arthritis**
— **Uveitis**
— **Erythema nodosum**   **GRUELING**
— **Lymphadenopathy**
— **Interstitial fibrosis**
— **Negative TB test**
— **Gammaglobulinemia**

---

3. **Collagen disease** (SLE, NS, dermatomyositis, polyarteritis nodosa): Steroid is lifesaving.
4. **Autoimmune disease** (active chronic hepatitis, autoimmune hemolytic anemia, thrombocytopenia).
5. **Bronchial asthma:** Status asthmaticus, severe chronic asthma → bronchodilator plus steroid.
6. **Lung disease:** Pneumonia, pulmonary edema, foetal respiratory distress syndrome (ARDS of foetus).
7. **Severe allergic reaction:** Anaphylaxis, angioneurotic edema, urticaria, serum sickness.
   Acts in **1–2 hrs**, hence adrenaline is essential which acts immediately in anaphylactic shock and angioedema of larynx (and other types of shock). DOC—adrenaline.

8. **Eye disease (inflammatory ocular disease)**
   Anterior chamber (topically).
   Posterior segment affliction (systemic therapy).
   CI: Herpes simplex keratitis and ocular injury.
9. **Intestinal disease**
   Acute phase is the indication of steroids.
10. **Skin disease**
    Topical →eczematous skin disease.
    Systemic therapy → severe afflictions (pemphigus vulgaris, exfoliative dermatitis, Stevens-Johnson syndrome).

> **Epidermis layers** (from base to surface):
> Stratum **G**erminativum
> Stratum **S**pinosum
> Stratum **G**ranulosum
> Stratum **L**ucidum
> Stratum **C**orneum
>
> **Gentle Skin Gets Lavish Care**

11. **Cerebral edema:** It is due to tumour and TBM.
    Treatment: Dexamethasone/betamethasone due to absence of Na^+ retaining activity.
12. **Leukemia/malignancy** (ALL, lymphomas due to lympholytic activity):
    Drug for CA breast → due to suppression of adrenal–pituitary axis → ↓androgen →↓estrogen formation from androgen.
13. **NEphrotic syndrome**
    NEgative charge is lost (plasma protein is lost).
14. **To test adrenal pituitary axis**
    Dexamethasone suppresses the axis (hence steroid metabolites in urine are absent).
15. **Tissue rejection** (skin allograft and organ transplantation).
    Treatment: Steroid + immunosuppressant.
16. **To minimise hypothalamopituitary axis suppression:** Shorter acting steroid at the **lowest** doses is given.

> **Uses of steroids**
> **B**ronchial asthma   **BE A CLASSICAL Actor**
> **E**ye disease
> **A**utoimmune disease
> **C**ollagen disease
> **L**ung disease
> **A**llergic reaction
> **S**arcoidosis and shock
> **S**kin disease
> **I**ntestinal disease
> **C**erebral edema

Corticoids or Corticosteroids

Allograft and arthritides
Leukemia
Axis (hypothalamopituitary and adrenal pituitary axis)

CI of corticosteroids
1. Peptic ulcer
2. Pregnancy
3. Psychosis
4. Herpes simplex keratitis
5. Enhanced BP
6. Epilepsy
7. DM
8. CHF
9. Osteoporosis
10. Renal failure
11. TB

Please Precautionly **PHEED (feed) CORT**

Glucocorticoid antagonists
1. **Mitotane**
2. **Amphenone B:** It inhibits 11-, 17-, and 21-hydroxylase.
3. **Metyrapone:** It inhibits 11-hyroxylase. It is the common drug in assessing adrenal function.
4. **Aminoglutethimide**
5. **Mifepristone/Ru-486:** It is glucocorticoid receptor antagonist, and mifepristone is antiprogestin.
6. **Ketoconazole:** Inhibits 11β- and 17-hydroxylase (steroidogenic enzyme).

Metyrapone: It is glucocorticoid antagonist.

Mech: It inhibits 11β-hydroxylase in the cortex and inhibits hydrocortisone synthesis →↑ ACTH release →↑ urinary excretion of 11-desoxycortisol.

U
1. Cushing's syndrome due to adrenal tumour.
2. To test responsiveness of pituitary and its ACTH producing capacity.
3. To assess adrenal function.

Drugs for Glucose Metabolism

Diabetes Mellitus

DM (Diabetes Mellitus) is a **metabolic disorder** (increase glucose, hyperlipidemia, glycosuria, negative nitrogen balance) with thickening of capillary basement membrane, increase in vessel wall matrix and cellular proliferation resulting in vascular complications (lumen narrowing, atherosclerosis, sclerosis of glomerular capillaries, retinopathy, neuropathy and PVD). These are due to increase nonenzymatic glycosylation of tissue protein due to persistent exposure to more glucose and accumulation of sorbitol (a reduced form of glucose). An index of protein glycosylation is concentration of **glycosylated Hb (HbA$_{1c}$)** which reflects the glycaemia over preceding 2–3 months.

Pancreas

1. **Weight**—80 gm.
2. **Main pancreatic duct**—duct of Wirsung.
3. **Accessory pancreatic duct**—duct of Santorini.
4. Pancreatic secretion/day—**one litre and pH 8.4** (acinar cells synthesize and secrete enzymes).
5. Duct cells synthesize—**HCO$_3^-$** (secretin increases it).
6. Most sensitive method of assessing pancreatic exocrine function: **Secretin pancreozymin** stimulation test. Pancreozymin hormone increases pancreatic enzyme secretion.
7. **Serum amylase** (starch splitting enzyme) measurement is **most** widely used test of pancreatic damage. Amylase is also produced in salivary gland, lactating breast, liver, bile duct and fallopian tube.
8. **Serum lipase** is most specific enzyme study in pancreatitis. **Investigation of choice** in acute pancreatitis beyond 5 days is serum lipase.
9. Normal glucose requirement of brain is **120 gm/day.** 56 gm glucose per 100 gm protein is produced in the body.
10. The only type of DM with definite pattern of inheritance is **MODY.**
11. **Best indicator** of DM control over a period of 3 months is glycosylated Hb.
12. **Somogyi phenomenon** is corrected by reducing insulin and Dawn phenomenon is corrected by increasing insulin.
13. **Commonest cause of lactic acidosis** is shock.
14. **Commonest** cause of **hyperkalemia** and chronic metabolic acidosis is renal failure.

15. **Trypsin** (a proteolytic enzyme) is the **most** abundant enzyme present in pancreatic juice.

Two types of DM
1. **Type I/IDDM:** Juvenile onset, autoimmune disorder and viral etiology. **Antibodies** → β cells destruction → low or absent insulin → prone to ketosis. Islet cell Ab is the **earliest** feature and **next earliest** feature is abnormal plasma free fatty acid level.
Honeymoon period is seen.
Ketoacidosis is **most** commonly seen.
2. **Type II/NIDDM:** Maturity onset, genetic predisposition. Post-middle age is more prone.
Insulin is normal/high.

Causes
I. Abnormal gluco-receptor of β cells
II. Reduced insulin receptor
III. Insulin resistance
IV. Excess of hyperglycaemic hormone such as glucagon, etc.
    A. Normal postprandial blood sugar level is <140 mg%.
    B. Normal fasting sugar level of blood—80 mg%.
    C. Normal random sugar level of blood — <120 mg%.
    D. Commonly used method of blood sugar estimation in clinical practice is Folin-Wu method.
    E. Confusion, seizure and coma occur in glucose level <40 mg%.

Insulin
First discovered by **Best and Banting** and chemical structure first discovered by **Sanger**.
It is 2 chain polypeptide (A and B) having 51 amino acid (aa) with MW 6000.
Chain A = 21 amino acid
Chain B = 30 amino acid
Both A and B are held together by 2 disulfide bonds.
Insulin is synthesized in β cells as single polypeptide chain of 110 amino acid (preproinsulin).
Proinsulin = 110 aa – 24 aa = 86 aa.

$$86\ aa \xrightarrow[\text{[86 aa – 35 aa (connecting/C-peptide)]}]{\text{Proteolysis in Golgi apparatus}} 15\ aa$$

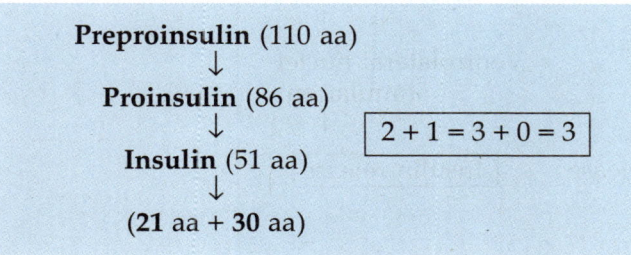

Preproinsulin (110 aa)
↓
Proinsulin (86 aa)
↓   2 + 1 = 3 + 0 = 3
Insulin (51 aa)
↓
(21 aa + 30 aa)

Normal daily secretion of insulin in pancreas—50 U/day.
Amount of insulin present in pancreas—200 U (8 mg).
Insulin is bioassayed by its potency to induce hypoglycemic convulsion in mice/ by measuring blood glucose depression in rabbits.
1 mg of international standard of insulin = 24 units.

Regulation of insulin secretion

1. **Hormonal regulation**
   I. **α cells** secrete proglucagon (20%) and glucogon (20%).
      (**A**lpha causes **A**ccess β and δ stimulation)
   II. **β cells** secrete (75%) proinsulin, insulin and C-peptide (**B**eta **B**locks α action)
   III. **δ cells** secrete (4%) somatostatin which inhibits release of
        (**D**elta **D**ecreases α and β actions)

   4G TIP
   - Gastrin
   - GH
   - Glucagon
   - Gastric acid
   - TSH
   - Insulin
   - Pancreatic enzymes

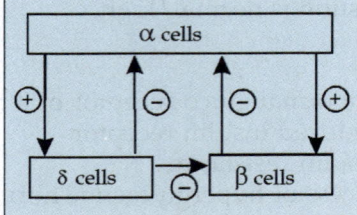

   IV. **PP cells** secrete (<2%) pancreatic polypeptide (PP).
       Streptozocin damages β cells.
       One unit insulin is secreted per hour and more after every meal.
       β cells are the **most** abundant cells of islets.
       PGE inhibits insulin release.

> **Ket**ONE bodies are seen in type **ONE** DM.
>
> **R**BC, **B**rain and **C**ells of liver (hepatocyte) take up glucose independent of insulin.   **RBC**
> **IN**sulin moves glucose **IN**to cells. **GLUC**a**GON** = **GLUC**ose is **GON**e out of cells

2. **Neural regulation:** Islets are supplied by vagal and sympathetic nerves.
   a. $α_2$ stimulates insulin release by inhibiting adenyl cyclase of β cell. $β_2$ stimulation enhances insulin release by stimulating adenyl cyclase of β cells.
   b. **Vagal stimulation/N_M stimulation by ACh** → IP_3/DAG stimulation → ↑ intracellular Ca^{2+} in β cells → insulin secretion.

WBC and medullary cells are independent of insulin. Insulin has insulin sparing effect.

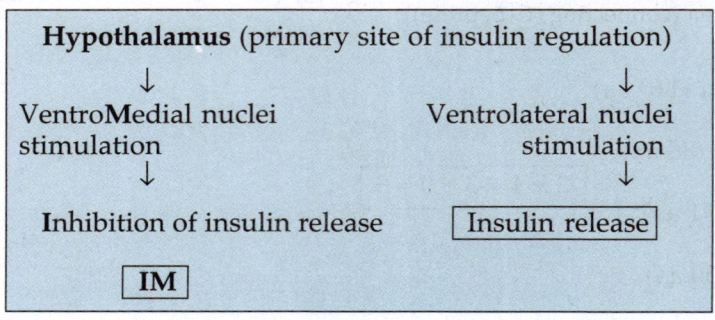

3. **Chemical regulation**
   Oral glucose → incretin release → glucose sensing mechanism of **β cells** (depends on glucose entry and its phosphorylation by glucokinase) → ↑ **intracellular Ca^{2+}** (↓efflux, ↑ influx and release from intracellular stores) → exocytotic release of insulin.
   Oral glucose → incretin release (VIP, GIP, gastrin, secretin, glucagon).
   Glucagon → ↑ cAMP in β cell →insulin release.

Actions of insulin

Site of action →cell membrane. It has short, intermediate and long-term action. Favours storage of fuel.

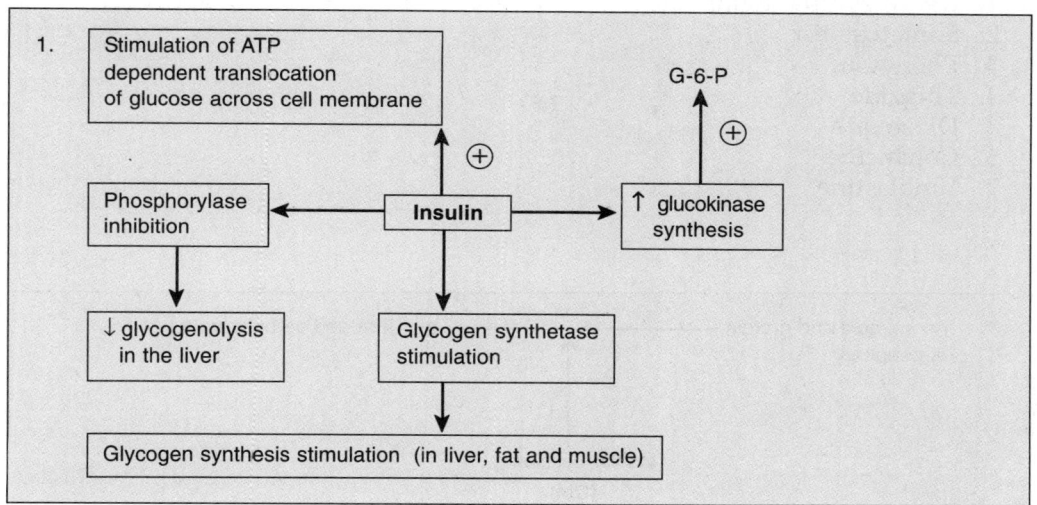

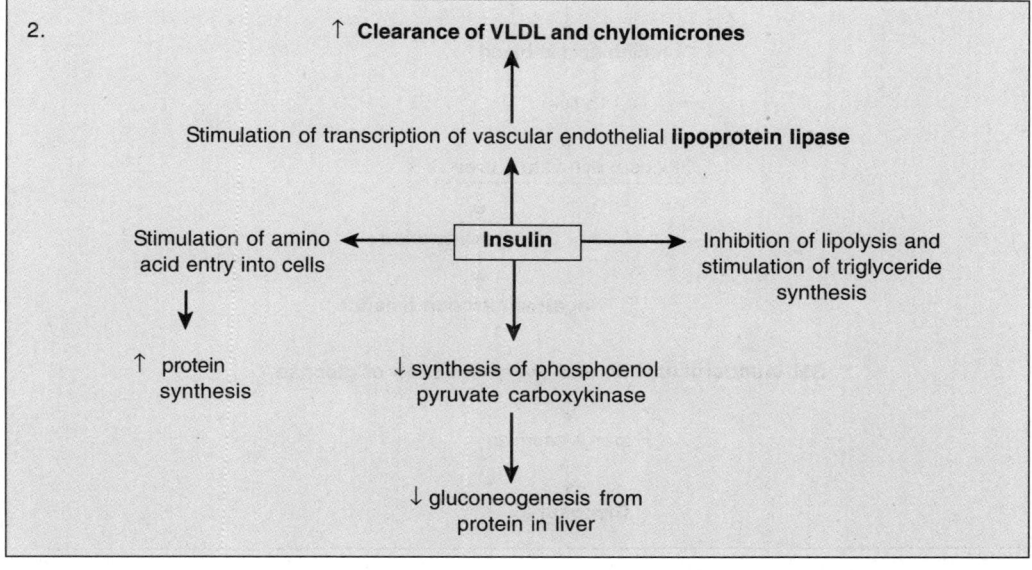

Overall effects of insulin
Insulin reduces plasma glucose level by:
- Increasing glucose transport across cell membrane
- Increasing glucose conversion to glycogen
- Inhibiting FFA release from adipose tissue
- Inhibiting lypolysis + glycogenolysis.

Stimulant of insulin release
1. Glucose—most potent stimulus for synthesis and release
2. Leucine
3. Vagal stimulation and sulfonylureas.

Inhibitor of insulin release
1. CA (α-sympathomimetic)
2. Somatostatin
3. Phenytoin
4. Thiazide
5. Diazoxide
6. Colchicine
7. Vinblastine

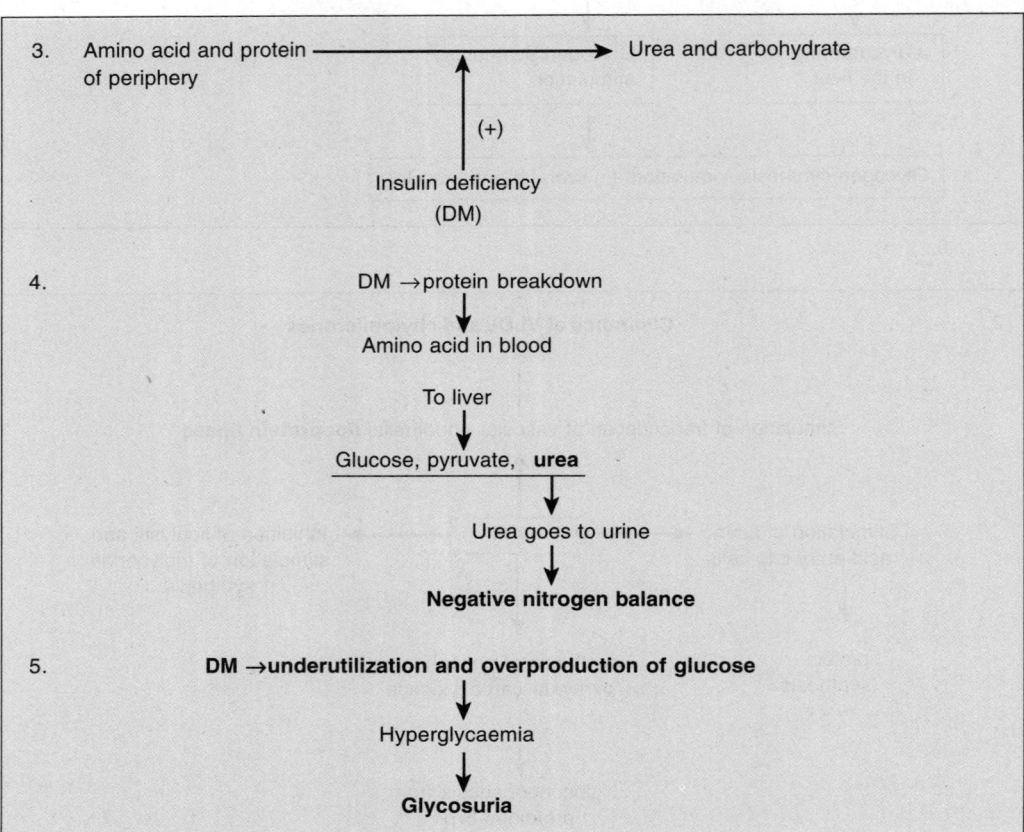

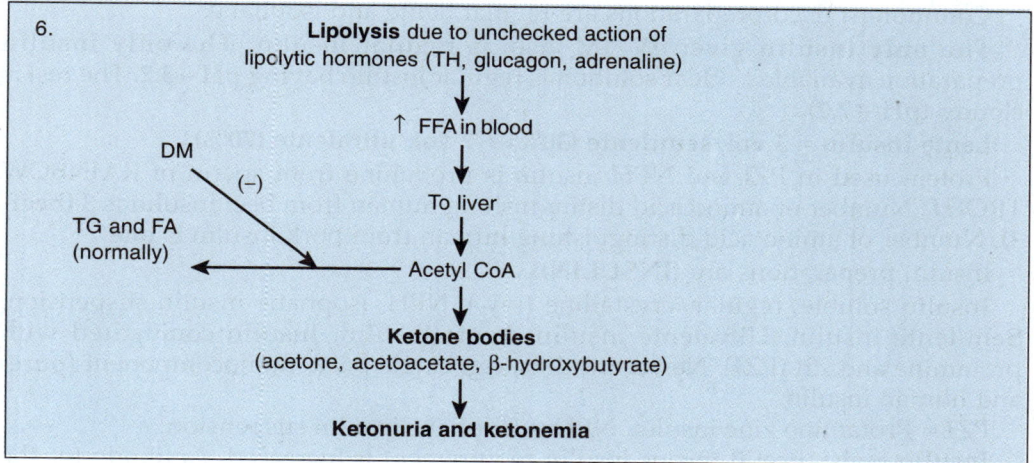

Amplifiers of glucose induced insulin release
1. β receptor stimulation
2. Arginine
3. Xanthine drug
4. Enteric hormones:
   – CCK
   – Gastrin
   – Gastric inhibitory polypeptide
   – Secretin

Mech: Insulin receptor is heterotetrameric glycoprotein formed of **2α** (located outside the membrane for binding insulin) and **2β** subunits (located inside the membrane for tyrosine protein kinase activity) linked together by disulfide bonds.

Insulin + α subunits (binding site) → stimulation of tyrosine protein kinase → autophosphorylation of tyrosine residues of β-subunits to phosphorylate tyrosine residues of other substrate protein.

PK: Plasma t½—7 min, distributed only extracellularly, oral → degraded in GIT because it is peptide, parenteral → hepatic metabolism only, also metabolized in muscle and kidney, degraded in **most target** cells.

Insulin **(biotransformation)** → A and B chains separate → amino acid formation. All preparations contain zinc.

Usual route: Subcutaneously (for all insulin preparations **except** regular insulin which is given IV/IM also).

Standard (conventional) insulin preparation
Derived from beef and pork pancreas and modified by adding Zn/another protein (protamine) to yield slowly absorbable and lower acting preparations, all are cloudy in appearance available in 40 U or 80 U/ml strength and given subcutaneously **except** regular insulin which is clear in appearance, given IV/IM also and available in **100 U or 500 U/ml** strength.

Pharmacology Review

Commonest used preparations are regular, lente and isophane.

The only insulin given IV/IM also, is regular insulin. **The only insulin** preparation available as clear solution is regular insulin having **pH – 3.2**. The rest is cloudy **(pH – 7.2)**.

Lente insulin = 3 vol, semilente (30%) + 7 vol, ultralente (70%).

Protein used in PZI and NPH insulin is protamine from sperm of RAINBOW TROUT. Number of amino acid distinguishing human from beef insulin is **3 (beef-3)**. Number of amino acid distinguishing human from pork insulin is **one**

Insulin preparations are **(INSULIN):**

Insulin soluble/regular/crystalline (ivy.), NPH/isophane insulin suspension, Semilente insulin, Ultralente insulin, Lente insulin, Insulin conjugated with protamine and Zn (PZI), Newer insulins, e.g. single peak, monocomponent (pure) and human insulin.

PZI = Protamine zinc insulin. NPH = Isophane insulin suspension.

Insulin resistance: It means insulin requirement is increased. Antibody for the resistance is **IgG. Commonest** cause of resistance is:

Insulin preparation	Average value			
	Onset of action (hr)	Peak effect (hr)	Duration of action (hr)	Can be mixed with
Short-acting Regular Semilente	<1	2–6	4–12	Regular Lente
Intermediate-acting NPH Lente	1–4	6–16	12–24	Regular Semilente
Long-acting PZI Ultralente	>4	16–24	24–36	Regular Semilente

1. **Obesity** (DOC in resistance—prednisolone).
2. Pregnancy and oral contraceptive.

The risk of antibody formulation is:

Bovine > Porcine > Purified porcine > Human.

Types of resistance are **two:**
1. **Physiological:** Requirement >100 U/day.
2. **Conventional:** Requirement >200 U/day.

Grades of resistance are

1. **Acute:** Causes are infection, stress, trauma and increase hyperglycaemic hormone.
2. **Chronic:** Due to chronic treatment by conventional preparation of beef and pork insulin, **Ab** is produced which binds to insulin. Commonly seen in **NIDDM. Pregnancy, HTN and OC** induce **low grade and reversible** insulin resistance.

Treatment: **More purified insulin** preparation. After few weeks, dose comes to 60 U/day.

More purified insulin preparations

Insulin preparation has **1% other proteins** which are **antigenic. Pork** insulin is **less immunogenic** because it is **more homologous to human insulin than beef insulin.** Pork and beef insulin are modified like conventional preparation into **longer acting forms** (lente, ultralente, isophane). On the basis of **purification method,** preparation is divided into:

A. **Single peak insulin (50–200 ppm pro-insulin)**
Purified by **gel filtration** and **repeated crystallization. All in 10 ml** vial are marketed in India.

B. **MC (monocomponent) insulin (proinsulin <20 ppm)**
Purified by **gel filtration** then **ion exchange chromatography**.

Immunogenicity of pork insulin is similar to that of human insulin.

Advantages:
  i. Less allergic
  ii. Less resistance
  iii. Less lipodystrophy
  iv. Greater stability

Human insulin: In 1980, it was prepared by **recombinant DNA technology, in**:
  i. E. coli (**P**roinsulin **r**ecombinant **b**acteria/**Prb**)
  ii. Yeast (**P**recursor **y**east **r**ecombinant/**Pyr**)
  iii. By **e**nzymatic **m**odification of **p**orcine insulin (**emp**).

β-cell transplant and incorporation of insulin gene in non β-cell lines are likely to provide a long lasting endogenous source of insulin to diabetic patient.

Indication of purer/human insulin (costly, hence used in developed countries, e.g. **PARIS**): **P**regnancy, **A**llergy to conventional preparations, **R**esistance of insulin specially of chronic type, **I**njection site lipodystrophy, **S**hort-term use. **PARIS**

Lispro insulin: It is synthesized by **recombinant DNA** technology from non-pathogenic E. coli. Differs from regular insulin in that **lysine and proline** at position **28 and 29 in chain B** is reversed, hence more absorption (SC)→**rapid action. Used 15 min prior to meal**. Peak level 30–90 min after injection, as compared to 50–120 min for regular insulin. Always used with long-acting insulin to assure proper glucose control. **Most important ADR** is hypoglycaemia. Insulin aspart is its analogue.

Glargine insulin: Supplied at pH 4 and neutralised at ↑ pH (at SC site). Onset of action 4 hrs (peakless). Duration of action 24 hrs. Uniform basal action.

ADR of insulin HEAL

1. **Hypoglycaemia (the most frequent and the most serious)**. Seen commonly when insulin requirement fluctuates unpredictably (i.e. "LABILE" DM).

Symptoms

A. Due to counter-regulatory sympathetic stimulation:
Palpitation, **A**nxiety, **S**weating, **T**remor. **PAST**

B. Neuroglucopenic symptoms (decrease glucose to brain):
Headache, **H**unger, **H**ypotension, **V**isual disturbance, **M**uscular incoordination.   Human Mosaic Virus = HMV

Diabetic neuropathy abolishes ANS symptoms. Confusion, coma and seizures occur when glucose falls **<40 mg%** and irreversible **neurological deficit** occurs due to prolonged hypoglycaemia. Treatment: **glucose orally/IV rapidly.**

Alternatively—**glucagons** 0.5–1 mg IV or adrenaline 0.2 mg SC

2. **Edema**
3. **Allergy** (urticaria, angioedema and anaphylactic condition)
4. **Local reaction** (erythema, stinging and lypodystrophy)

CI: Intensive insulin therapy in young children due to hypoglycemic brain damage and in elderly (more prone to hypoglycaemia and its serious consequences).

IA:
1. β-blockers prolong hypoglycaemia by inhibiting compensated mechanism.
   Hypertension due to adrenaline release occurs.
2. Acute alcohol intake precipitates hypoglycaemia by depleting hepatic glycogen.
3. Salicylates, theophylline and lithium cause hypoglycaemia by increasing insulin secretion and peripheral glucose utilization.
4. Diuretics (loop and thiazide), corticosteroid, oral contraceptive, CCB and salbutamol reduce insulin effect and enhance blood glucose.

Uses of insulin: The chief drawback of insulin use is—it must be given by injection.

A. **Diabetic uses**
  1. **DM**
  2. **Diabetic coma (diabetic ketoacidosis)**
  3. **Hyperosmolar coma (non-ketotic hyperglycaemic coma).**
B. **Non-diabetic uses**
  1. **To test for completeness of vagotomy:** If vagotomy is complete then gastric secretion is absent.
  2. **Schizophrenia**
  3. **Cyclic vomiting: Insulin + IV fluid.**

1. **DM:** Insulin is given in all forms of DM but is a must for IDDM.
   It is preferred in NIDDM in patient with reduced renal plus hepatic function, gestational DM, persistent hyperglycaemia and CVS risks. Effective treatment reduces hyperglycaemia, hypoglycaemia, glycosuria, ketoacidosis and complications (neuropathy, retinopathy, nephropathy and CVS disease). Insulin therapy is started with regular insulin (SC) before each major meal after testing urine/blood by spot test and glucose oxidase impregnated sticks for instant measurement to determine requirement.

Dose: 0.4–0.8 U/kg/day in IDDM.
0.2–1.6 U/kg/day in NIDDM.

Long-term complication of DM is due to glycaemic control, hence the objective is to attain round the clock **euglycaemia**.

2. **Diabetic coma:** Generally occurs in IDDM and the **commonest** cause is infection, others are stress, trauma, inadequate doses of insulin, etc. Typical symptoms are dehydration, hyperventilation and impaired consciousness.

Drugs for Glucose Metabolism

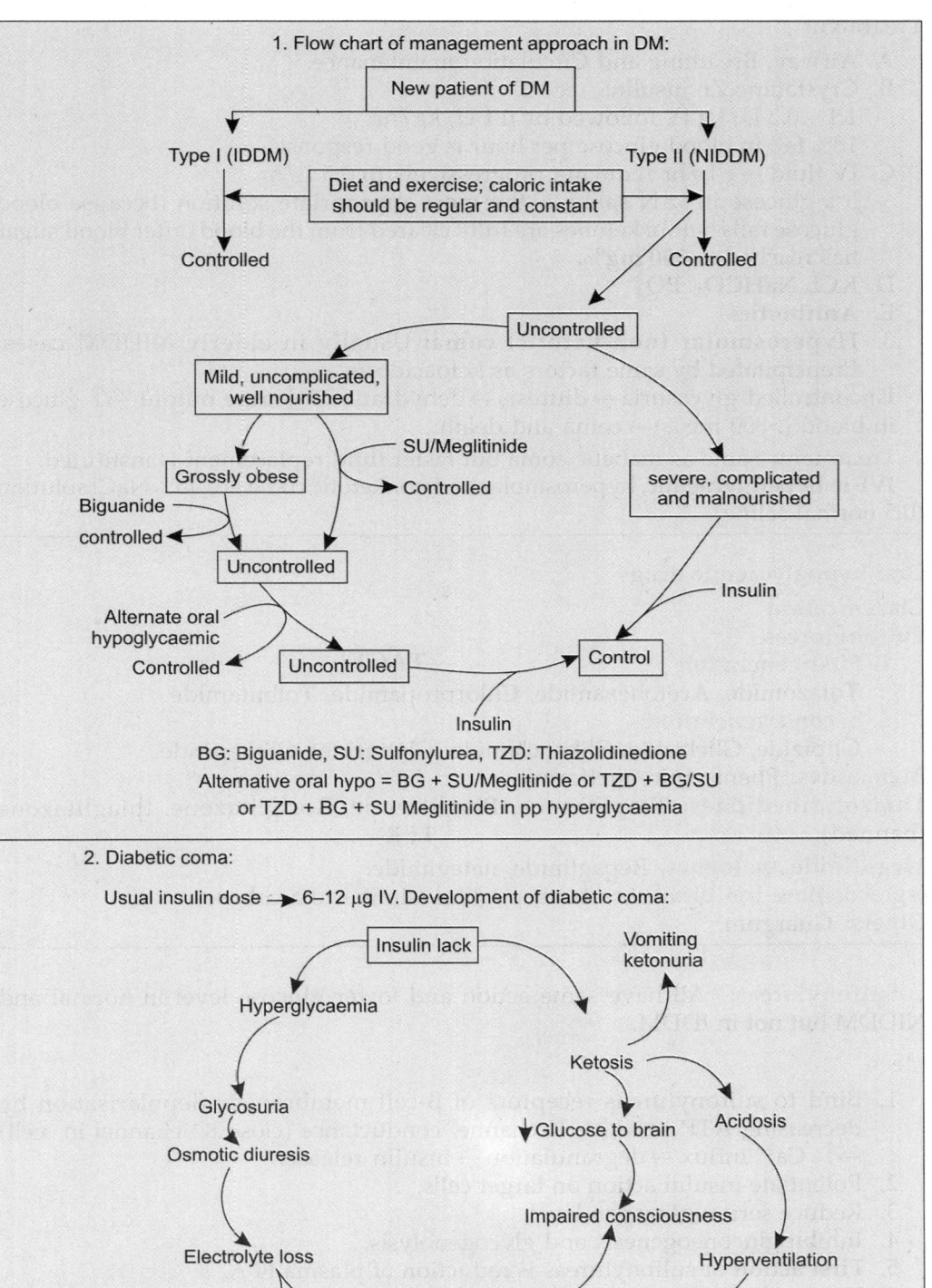

Treatment

A. **A**irway, **B**reathing and **C**irculation maintenance.
B. Crystalline Zn insulin:
   1.1 – 0.2 U/kg IV followed by 0.1 U/kg/hr.
   10% fall in blood glucose per hour is good response.
C. IV fluid →1 L/hr reducing progressively to 0.5 L/hr.
   5% glucose in ½ N saline is the **most appropriate** solution (because blood glucose falls before ketones are fully cleared from the blood) after blood sugar has reached to **300 mg%**.
D. **KCl, NaHCO$_3$, PO$_4^{3-}$**
E. **Antibiotics**

3. **Hyperosmolar (non-ketotic) coma:** Usually in elderly NIDDM cases. Prepcipitated by same factors as ketoacidosis.
   Uncontrolled glycosuria → diuresis → dehydration →↓urine output →↑ glucose in blood (>800 mg%)→ coma and death.
   Treatment: Same as diabetic coma but faster fluid replacement is instituted.
   IVF in hyperglycaemic, hyperosmolar and nonketotic coma is 0.45% NaCl solution (0.5 normal saline).

Oral hypoglycaemic drugs
Classification
Sulfonylureas
1. First generation   **TACT**
   Tolazomide, Acetohexamide, Chlorpropamide, Tolbutamide.
2. Second generation:
   Glipizide, Gliclazide, Glibenclamide (Glyburide), Glimepiride.

Biguanides: Phenformin, metformin.
Thiazolidinediones: Troglitazone, Pioglitazone, Rosiglitazone, thiaglitazone (banned).   **TPR**
Meglitinide analogues: Repaglinide, nateglinide.
α-glucosidase inhibitor: Acarbose, miglitol (similar to acarbose).
Others: Guargum

Sulfonylureas: All have same action and lower glucose level in normal and NIDDM but not in IDDM.

Mech
1. Bind to sulfonylureas receptors of β-cell membrane → depolarisation by decreasing ATP sensitive K$^+$channel conductance (close K$^+$ channel in cell) →↑ Ca^{2+} influx → degranulation → insulin release.
2. Potentiate insulin action on target cells.
3. Reduce serum glucagon level.
4. Inhibit gluconeogenesis and glycogenolysis.
5. **First action** of sulfonylureas is reduction of plasma FFA.
6. Diazoxide inhibits insulin release, acts on ATP sensitive K$^+$ channel opposite to that of sulfonylurea and reduces peripheral use of glucose and CA release.
7. Due to chronic use, insulinemic action of sulfonylureas declines.

PK: All are orally absorbed, **90%** bound to plasma protein, excreted in urine. plasma t½ →8 hrs (**maximum**), **except** chlorpropamide (t½—32 hrs) of first generation, all have plasma t½—8 hrs (**maximum**). Tolbutamide is the **mildest and the safest** sulfonylurea and its action lasts 10 hrs.

Chlorpropamide—action lasts 60 hrs.
Glibenclamide—action lasts 24 hrs.
Glimepiride eliminated in urine and faeces (**first** sulfonylurea used with insulin).

IA:
1. Diuretics (thiazide and loop), diazoxide, corticosteroid and OC inhibit action.
2. Phenobarbitone, phenytoin, rifampicin and chronic alcoholism induce metabolism (reduce their actions).
3. Propranolol, salicylate, lithium, theophylline and sympathetic antihypertensives synergise actions (enhance action).
4. Sulfinpyrazone inhibits excretion of tolbutamide.
5. Phenylbutazone, sulfinpyrazone, sulfonamide, cimetidine, warfarin, phenytoin, acute alcoholism and chloramphenicol inhibit metabolism and synergise action (enhance action).
6. Phenylbutazone, sulfinpyrazone, sulfonamide, PAS, salicylates, clofibrate displace them from protein binding sites (enhance actions).

ADR:
1. **Hypoglycaemia:** The **commonest** ADR. Chlorpropamide has **highest risk**. Tolbutamide has **lowest** risk and it is the **mildest and the safest** sulfonylurea. Hence, tolbutamide is the oral hypoglycaemic of **choice** in renal failure. Hypoglycaemia is treated by glucose.
Tolbutamide = Tolerated best.
2. Disulfiram like reaction.
3. **Hypersensitivity**: Rashes, photosensitivity, purpura, transient leucopenia.
4. Chlorpropamide additionally causes intolerance to alcohol (flushing and disulfiram like reaction), dilutional hyponatremia (due to sensitizing kidney to ADH action) and cholestatic jaundice.
5. Tolbutamide reduces iodine uptake by thyroid but hypothyroidism does not occur.
6. GIT: Diarrhoea/constipation, flatulence, weight gain, nausea and vomiting.

U:
1. NIDDM (mild, uncomplicated and well nourished).
2. **Diagnosis of insulinoma**
Tolbutamide 1 gm IV causes reduced blood sugar in patient with insulin secreting tumour. Hypoglycaemia in insulinoma is treated by diazoxide.
3. **DI:** Chlorpropamide potentiates ADH action on renal tubules.

Biguanides: **Earliest** oral hypoglycaemic drug used for DM is—**synthalin A**. Unlike sulfonylurea, they have no hypoglycaemic effect in nondiabetic subjects and do not stimulate β-cells (no insulin release). Both members have **similar** actions.

Mech:
1. Suppress hepatic gluconeogenesis and glucose output from liver.
2. Inhibit intestinal absorption of glucose, other hexose, amino acid, and vitamin B_{12}.

3. Enhance insulin binding to its receptor and stimulate insulin mediated glucose disposal.
4. Promote peripheral glucose utilization by increase anaerobic glycolysis.
5. Increase insulin sensitivity.

PK: Adequately absorbed, duration of action → 6–12 hrs, plasma t½ of phenformin (7 hrs) and metformin (2 hrs), excreted in urine, metformin not metabolized at all.

ADR:
1. **Common:** Abdominal pain, anorexia, diarrhea, metallic taste.
2. **Lactic acidosis:** The **most** serious complication—phenformin > metformin. Alcohol precipitates lactic acidosis.
3. **Vitamin B$_{12}$:** Deficiency due to interference with absorption.

CI: It is due to lactic acidosis.
1. CVS problem
2. Hypotension
3. Alcoholism   **CHALK**
4. Lung disease
5. Liver disease
6. Kidney disease

U: Used in uncomplicated NIDDM (type II) when not controlled by diet and exercise.

They are **best** used in patients with: **OK SAIF**
1. **O**besity
2. **K**etoacidosis and even its history
3. **S**ugar (fasting blood sugar <200 mg%)
4. **A**ge >40 yrs at the onset of disease.
5. **I**nsulin requirement <30 U/day.
6. <**F**ive years (duration of disease when starting treatment).

Sulfonylureas are preferred over biguanides which reduce fasting blood glucose and glycosylated Hb, and are used in obese NIDDM. 50% patient treated with oral hypoglycaemic ultimately need insulin.

Drugs causing lactic acidosis   **BSF IS SEEN**

Biguanide, **S**alicylate, **F**ructose, **I**NH, **S**orbitol, **S**treptozocin, **E**pinephrine, **E**thanol and methanol, **N**itroprusside.

Acarbose

Acarbose is a mild hypoglycaemic and a complex oligosaccharide.

Mech:
1. Inhibits α-glucosidase (the **final** enzyme in carbohydrate digestion in brush border of small intestinal mucosa).
2. It reduces polysaccharide digestion and absorption, Hb A$_{1c}$, body weight and serum triglyceride.

ADR: Flatulence and loose stool in 50% patient due to formation of unabsorbed carbohydrates.

U:
1. **DM:** 50–100 mg TDS taken at the beginning of each measure meal.
2. As adjuvant to diet in obese patient.

Guargum: It is dietary fibre (polysaccharide) from Indian cluster beans (**Guar**) which forms vicious gel on contact with water.

    Mech: Slows gastric emptying, intestinal transit and cholesterol plus carbohydrate absorption.

    ADR: Flatulence, feeling of fullness, diarrhoea, loss of appetite.

    U:
1. As a hypocholesterolemic
2. To supplement diet
3. To lower sulfonylurea dose.

Repaglinide

Repaglinide is not sulfonylurea. Causes hypoglycaemia lower than sulfonylurea. First member, normalises meal time glucose excursions.

    Mech: Binds to sulfonylurea and other receptors→ATP dependent K⁺ channel closure → depolarisation → insulin release.

    Binds to ATP—sensitive K⁺ channel of β-cells causing insulin release.

    PK: Well absorbed orally, taken TDS before meals, $t½$—1 hr, hepatic metabolism to inactive product, biliary excretion.

    ADR: **W**eightgain, **AR**thralgia, **D**yspepsia. **WARD**

    U: Glycemic control (metformin + repaglinide).

Meglitinide analogues cause quick insulin release (short-acting).

    CI: Liver disease

    U:
1. Type 2 DM (alternative to sulfonylurea)
2. To supplement long-acting insulin and metformin
3. Post-prandial hyerglycaemia

Nateglinide

Stimulates 1st phase insulin secretion leading to rapid onset and shorter duration of hypoglycaemic action than repaglinide.

    U: Postprandial hyperglycaemic in type 2 DM.

    ADR: Dizziness, flu-like symptoms, joint pain.

Troglitazone

First thiazolidinedione for type 2 DM in insulin resistance cases.

    Mech:
1. Troglitazone is insulin sensitizer in liver and skeletal muscle.
2. It **reduces** increased hepatic output of glucose. Promotes insulin dependent glucose utilization in skeletal muscle. Hyperglycaemia, hyperinsulinemia, hypertriglyceridemia and elevated HbA_{1c} levels are improved.
3. It counteracts insulin resistance.
4. Not promote insulin release from β-cells, hence no hyperinsulinemia.

    PK: Increased oral absorption when taken with food, extensively bound to serum albumin, plasma $t½$ of troglitazone is 16–34 hrs, metabolized to **inactive** metabolites, induce cytochrome P450, excreted in faeces.

    CI: Breastfeeding women.

    ADR:
1. Hepatotoxicity (rosiglitazone less hepatotoxic)
2. Upper RTI
3. Headache

4. Anemia
5. Edema
6. Weight gain

IA: 1. Increases metabolism of OC→ovulation and pregnancy occur (hence **contraindicated**).
2. Cyclosporin (metabolized by cytochrome P450) is effected.

U: Type 2 DM in insulin resistance cases (used with insulin→insulin dose is reduced).

Pioglitazone and rosiglitazone

Mech: Selective agonists for nuclear PPARγ (peroxisome proliferator-activated receptor γ) that increases insulin gene transcription. They reverse resistance of insulin by stimulating GLUT4 expression and translocation leading to improved entry of glucose into fat and muscle. Suppression of hepatic gluconeogenesis. Lowering of circulating insulin level in type 2 DM due to improved glycaemic control. Lower serum triglyceride and raised HDL level by pioglitazone.

ADR: Myalgia, plasma volume expansion, CVS dysfunction.

CI: Liver disease and CHF.

PK: Rosiglitazone metabolised by CYP2C8 and pioglitazone by CYP2C8 and CYP3A4.

IA: KTZ inhibits pioglitazone metabolism.

Thiaglitazone has been withdrawn due to hepatotoxicity.

Insulin availability is improved by sulfonylurea and meglitinide and its resistance is overcome by biguanide, α-glucosidase inhibitors and thiazolidinedione.

Glucagon

Glucagon is a single chain polypeptide containing 29 amino acids (MW 3500) secreted by **α-cells** of islets. Beef and pork glucagon are **similar** to human glucagon.

Regulation

1. Increase glucose level inhibits glucagon secrection.
   Incretins evoke insulin release and inhibit glucagon secretion.
2. Ketone bodies and FFA inhibit glucagon release.
3. Amino acid induces both insulin and glucagon secretion.
4. Insulin and somatostatin inhibit glucagon secretion.
5. Sympathetic and parasympathetic stimulation evoke glucagon release.

Actions: These are opposite to that of insulin and are "**the hormone of fuel mobilization**" by mobilizing stored fat plus carbohydrate and by promoting gluconeogenesis in liver during fasting (increasing glycogenolysis and gluconeogenesis). Effect is lost when glycogen stores are depleted. Glucagon secretion is enhanced in **all forms** of severe tissue injuries to supply glucose to injured tissue. It increases force and rate of cardiac contraction and this is not **antagonized by β blockers**. It relaxes gut and inhibits gastric secretion. Diazoxide reduces insulin release.

Mech: Stimulates adenyl cyclase →increase cAMP in liver, fat cells and heart, etc.

U: Orally inactive
1. Hypoglycaemia: Glucagon is secondary to glucose.
2. Cardiogenic shock.
3. Diagnosis of pheochromocytoma: 1 mg IV causes CA release from tumours →↑ BP (treatment is phentolamine to counter BP).

Fungal infection characteristically seen in diabetic ketoacidosis is mucormycosis which leads to **"bone destruction with moth-eaten appearance"**. Infection is the **commonest** cause of death in adult and cerebral edema in children in diabetic ketoacidosis. Diabetic retinopathy is **commonest long-term complication of DM and its earliest sign is micro-aneurysm. Commonest** lesion in diabetic nephropathy is diffuse glomerulosclerosis and **most** specific lesion is nodular glomerulosclerosis. Sorbitol is responsible for manifestation of diabetic neuropathy.

A. DOC
1. Potent once a day drug—glibenclamide.
2. Elderly and those prone to hypoglycaemic—tolbutamide.
3. Potent, faster, short-acting drug—glipizide
4. In patient prone to weight gain—gliclazide

B. Hormones enhancing glucose concentration are
Glucagon, glucocorticoid, GH, epinephrine, estrogen, progestin, TH.

Unit 4
Drugs Acting on CVS

30
An Overview of CVS

CHD (congenital heart disease)
  A. **Right to left shunt (early cyanosis)** →"Blue babies"   **5Ts**
    1. **T**etralogy of Fallot (commonest cause of early cyanosis)
    2. **T**ransposition of great vessels
    3. **T**runcus arteriosus
    4. **T**ricuspid atresia
    5. **T**otal anomalous pulmonary return.
       Tetra(4)-logy of Fallot: **ROADS**
       – **R**VH
       – **O**verriding **A**orta
       – V**S**D
       – Pulmonary Stenosis
  B. **Left to right shunts (late cyanosis)** →"Blue kids"
    1. VSD (commonest)
    2. ASD
    3. PDA
    Frequency: VSD > ASD > PDA.

IHD (insufficient O_2 supply to myocardium)

Manifestations
1. **Angina pectoris (commonest form of IHD): Reversible episodic** O_2 insufficiency.
2. **Acute MI:** Prolonged O_2 deprivation resulting in irreversible tissue necrosis.
3. **Sudden death syndrome:** Episodic recurrences of ventricular **fibrillation (the most organised arrhythmia)**, resuscitation and sudden death.

Etiology
1. **Reduced blood flow** (atherosclerosis, coronary artery spasm, embolism, trauma)

2. **Enhanced O₂ demand**
   (exertion, emotional stress)
   ↓
   Sympathetic stimulation
   ↓
   ↑HR

Enhanced O₂ demand occurs in
   — Contractile (ionotropic) state of heart
   — Enhanced systolic wall tension
   — Lengthening of ejection time
   — Change in HR

3. **Reduced blood oxygenation**
   Risk factor for IHD
   — Hyperlipidemia (↑ LDL/HDL)
   — HTN
   — DM
   — Smoking
   — OC use
   — Obesity
   — Gout
   — Age and sex (risk increases with age and more risk occurs in men)
   — Chronic stress/Type A personality, i.e. aggressive, competitive, ambitious, chronically impatient.

	Factors effecting myocardial O₂ demand				
Factors	HR	BP	Ejection time	Ventricular volume	Ionotropic effect
Excercise	↑	↑	↓	↑↓	↑
Smoking	↑	↑	↑	—	↑
Cold	↑	↑	—	—	—
Beta blocker	↓	↓	↑	↑	↓
Nitroglycerine	↑	↓	↓	↓	↑

Angina pectoris

First described by William Heberden. Transient chest discomfort due to insufficient myocardial O₂.

Types

1. **Stable/Classical angina (predictable):** The **commonest** form due to fixed obstruction in coronary artery. The discomfort builds up to a peak **radiating** to jaw, neck, shoulder and arms, then subsides. End diastolic LV pressure rises from 5 to 25 mm Hg and produces "subendothelial crunch". Relieved by rest.
2. **Unstable angina: New onset,** pattern changes.
3. **Nocturnal angina (angina decubitus):** Occurs in the **recumbent** position.
4. **Prinzmetal's/vasospastic/variant angina:** Due to coronary artery spasm occurring at **rest** and has transient **ST-segment** elevation. Unpredictable. **Most effective drug** is CCB.
   Therapeutic agents for angina pectoris: Nitrates, β blocker, CCB.

> Patient with angina develops ST segment **elevation or depression** on EKG during myocardial hypoxia. This can be induced diagnostically by:
> 1. Tread mill stress testing.
> 2. Dobutamine (↑ HR and ↑ contractility)
> 3. Ergonovine induces coronary vasospasm
>
> ECG is normal in **50–70%** at rest (ST depressed in all **except** variant).

MI: Severe and prolonged restriction of oxygenated blood to heart muscle resulting in cellular **ischaemia**, tissue **injury**, and tissue **necrosis**. The **foremost** symptom is persistent, severe chest pain or pressure likened to having an **elephant sitting on chest**, pain **radiates** to left arm, neck, jaw, teeth and abdomen.

Sensation lasts >30 minute and heart attacks without pain (**silent MI**) occurring in **up to 30%**.
1. **CK/CPK** (MB isoenzyme) elevation present.
2. **SGOT/AST** elevation present (peak in 1–2 days).
3. $LDH_1 > LDH_2$ present.
4. **WBC** 12000–15000 per microlitre indicates necrosis.

Therapeutic agents for MI
1. O_2
2. Lidocaine
3. Thrombolytic agent
4. β blocker
5. Nitrates
6. **Morphine (DOC):** It causes venous pooling, reduces preload, cardiac workload and O_2 consumption.

Systemic HTN: The commonest cardiovascular disorder.
Definition: **Systolic** BP   ≥ 140 mm Hg
                  Diastolic BP   ≥ 90 mm Hg
(HTN means BP ≥160/90 mm Hg—**WHO 1978**).

It is the **commonest** health problem in developed countries (the **commonest** health problem in India is **pulmonary TB**).

Classification
A. Based on BP range (mmHg)

Category			Systolic	Diastolic
HTN	Stage	1 (mild)	140–159	90–99
"	"	2 (moderate)	160–179	100–109
"	"	3 (severe)	180–209	110–119
"	"	4 (very severe)	>210	>120
Normal			<130	<85
High normal		130–139	95-89	

> **Isolated systolic HTN:** Systolic BP >160 mm Hg with diastolic BP <90 mm Hg.

B. **Based on incidence**
1. **Primary/essential HTN:** Causes **unknown in 90% of all** systemic HTN (commonest). Average age of onset is **35 years**.
2. **Secondary HTN: 10% of all** systemic HTN.

Causes of secondary HTN
a. Renal artery stenosis (**commonest** cause of treatable HTN), usually develops **before 35 years** or **after 55 years**.
b. Hypersecretion of aldosterone (pheochromocytoma).

> **Malignant HTN** means HTN with papilloedema. **Accelerated HTN** means HTN with exudate plus haemorrhage.
> **Best screening test** for renovascular HTN is IVP.
> **Commonest** cause of death in HTN is heart disease.
> In **hypertensive retinopathy, silver wire** appearance of retinal vessel is in Grade III and **copper wire** appearance is in Grade II.
> **Rules of Halves:** In 100% population → 50% general population aware of HTN → 25% treated → 12½% adequately treated.
> **Tracking of BP:** Low BP tends to remain low and high BP tends to remain high as individuals grow older. It identifies individuals of developing HTN at future date.

Physiological regulation of BP
1. **Sympathetic nervous system:** Baroreceptor (pressure receptor) is stimulated by hypotension resulting in
    — ↑ HR
    — ↑ CO
    — ↑ force of contraction
2. **Renin-angiotensin-aldosterone system:** It is stimulated by reduced renal perfusion pressure in afferent arteriole resulting in renin release from JG cells.
3. **Fluid volume regulation**
    BP = CO × Peripheral Resistance
    CO = HR × Stroke Volume

CO is regulated by
1. **Cardiac factors:** HR and contractility
2. **Blood volume**
    — Mineralocorticoid
    — Atriopeptin
    — Sodium

Peripheral resistance is regulated by
1. **Local factors:** Autoregulation and ionic (Ph, hypoxia)
2. **Neural factors:** Dilator (β agonist) and constrictor (α agonist)
3. **Humoral factors**
a. **Dilators:** PG, kinins, nitric oxide and EDRF (endothelial derived growth factor)
b. **Constrictors:** Angiotensin II, CA, thromboxane, LT and endothelin.

Therapeutic agents
1. Diuretic (thiazide and loop)
2. K⁺ sparing diuretic
3. Sympatholytic (β blocker, α blocker, centrally acting α agonist—clonidine and methyldopa).
4. Vasodilator (nitrate and ACE inhibitor) and CCB.
5. Reserpine, guanethidine, guanadrel.

CHF (Congestive heart failure)

Abnormality in myocardial function results in the inability of the ventricles to deliver adequate quantities of blood to the metabolising tissues during **normal activity or at rest**. Congestion is due to edematous state commonly produced by fluid back up resulting from **poor pump function**. 5-year survival after initial diagnosis is 50%.

All types of common congenital heart disease cause CHF **except** tetralogy of Fallot. **Most important intrinsic compensatory mechanism** in heart failure is **myocardial hypertrophy**.

Forms of heart failure
1. **Low output failure (commonest types):** Metabolic demand is **normal** but the heart is unable to meet the demand.
2. **High output failure:** Metabolic demand is **more** and heart is unable to meet the demand.
3. **Left-sided failure:** Blood is not adequately pumped from the left ventricle to the peripheral circulation and accumulates within left ventricle. Hence, this ventricle is unable to accept blood from the left atrium and lung.

    Fluid portion of the blood backs up into the pulmonary alveoli producing **pulmonary** edema. **Dyspnoea** and **dry cough** are also present. Preload needed to cause pulmonary congestion is >25 mm Hg.
4. **Right-sided failure:** Blood is not pumped from right ventricle into the lungs and accumulates within right ventricle. Fluid portion of blood backs up throughout the body producing **systemic edema.**

> **Symptoms:** My **skin** feels too tight. My **ring** is too tight.

Cardiac disease commonly underlying CHF

Age range (years)	Common underlying cause
20–40	Rheumatic fever, RHD
40–50	MI, HTN, pulmonary disease
>50	Calcific aortic stenosis

Substances exacerbating CHF
1. **Promote Na retention**

Medicine GLASSED

— Methyldopa
— Estrogen
— Diazoxide
— Guanethidine

2. **Produce osmotic effects**

SUGAr
- Saline
- Urea
- Glucose
- Albumin
- Mannitol

— Li$_2$CO$_3$
— Androgen
— Salicylate
— Steroid (corticosteroid)

3. **Reduce contractility**

ABCD
— β blocker and CCB
— Antiarrhythmic drugs
— Doxorubicin

Cardiac arrhythmia (deviation from normal pattern of heart beat) is due to **abnormal impulse formation** and **disturbed conduction**.

Sinus Brady-cardia	Normal	Sinus tachycardia	AV nodal tachycardia	A. flutter	A. fibrillation
60	100	180	250	350	600 beats/min.

SA node (in the wall of right atrium)

Contains cells that spontaneously initiate AP. This pacemaker normally initiates **60–100 beats/min.**

Four tracts of SA node (internodal tract)
1. **Anterior** tract
2. **Middle** tract (Wenckebach's bundle)
3. **Posterior** tract (Thorel's bundle)
4. **Anterior** interatrial tract (Bachmann's bundle)

Impluse goes through

SA node
↓
AV node (in the lower interatrial septum), impulse delays briefly to complete atrial contraction before ventricular contraction begins.
↓
Bundle of His (left and right) on either side of interventricular septum.
↓
Purkinje fibres

Types of cardiac arrhythmias

Bradyarrhythmia
- Sinus bradycardia
- Sick sinus syndrome
- Different degree of block

Tachyarrhythmia
- Narrow QRS tachycardia **(SV origin)** — • Benign
- Wide QRS tachycardia; **ventricular origin** (also SV origin) — • Lethal • Potentially lethal

Types of arrhythmia (by origin)
1. **Supraventricular arrhythmia:** Due to enhanced **automaticity** of pacemaker/from **re-entry** conduction.
2. **Ventricular arrhythmia:** When an ectopic (abnormal) pacemaker triggers a ventricular contraction before SA node **fires**.

Two types of myocardial fibres (electrophysiologically)
1. **Non-automatic (ordinary):** It cannot generate an impulse of their own.
2. **Automatic (SA and AV nodal fibres)**
   Most characteristic feature of automatic fibres is slow diastolic depolarization. Generate impulse, are present in **SA node, AV node, His-Purkinje system** (i.e. specialised conducting system).
   In addition, patches of automatic fibres, are present in **interatrial septum, AV ring,** around **opening of great vein.**
   Slow diastolic depolarisation means **"after repolarisation to maximum value, the membrane potential decays spontaneously (i.e. phas 4)"**. SA node has the **steepest** phase 4 depolarisation, undergoes **self-excitation** and propagates the impulse to the **rest of** the heart (i.e. normally acts as **pacemaker**).
   Other fibres undergo phase 4 depolarisation but at a slower rate, receive a propagated impulse before reacting the threshold and remain as **latent pacemaker**.

> SA node has the **steepest** phase 4 depolarisation hence acts as the pacemaker.

Two types of AP in automatic muscle are
1. **Fast** channel AP
2. **Slow** channel AP (not has clear cut phase 1–3 of AP).

Latent pacemaker: AV junction, bundle of His and Purkinje fibres contain cells capable of **generating impulses** but have **slower firing rate** than SA node. Hence, SA node predominates **except** when it is depressed" or injured which is called **"Overdrive Suppression"**.

Action potential (AP) of heart has 5 phases
1. **Phase 0 (rapid depolarisation):** Na^+ **influx** through **fast** channel. Charge changes from **negative to positive (+ 30 mV).** Resting membrane potential of myocardial cell is **90 mV**.
2. **Phase 1 (early rapid repolarisation)**
   As **fast Na^+ channel** closes, K^+ **channel** leaves the cell. The cell rapidly repolarises (i.e. return to resting potential).

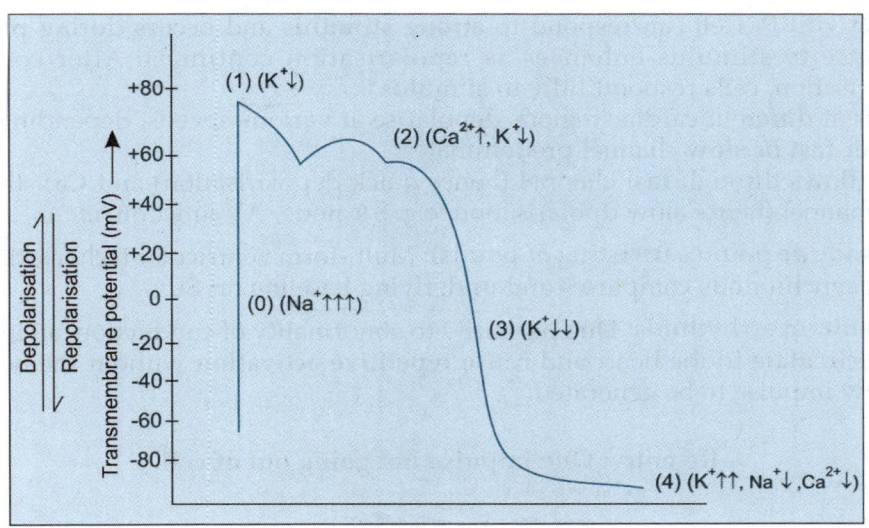

Within the cell	$Na^+\uparrow\uparrow\uparrow$	$K^+\downarrow$	$Ca^{2+}\uparrow, K^+\downarrow$	$K^+\downarrow\downarrow$	$K^+\uparrow\uparrow, Na^+\downarrow, Ca^{2+}\downarrow$
Phase	0	1	2	3	4 (Resting State)

3. **Phase 2 (plateau):** Ca^{2+} **influx** through slow channel while K^+ **exit (efflux).** **Membrane's electrical activity** temporarily stabilises, AP reaches a plateau.
4. **Phase 3 (final rapid repolarisation):** K^+ is pumped out of the cell as the cell rapidly completed repolarisation and returns its intial activity.
5. **Phase 4 (slow depolarisation):** Cell returns to its resting state with K^+ ion inside and ($Na^+ + Ca^{2+}$) ions outside the cell.

Two types of AP in autonomic muscle are

1. **Fast channel AP:** Present in atria, ventricle, Purkinje fibres with Na^+ mainly at the speed of **0.5–5 m/sec** and inhibited by **LA (ERP < APD),** i.e. ERP/APD is <1. It is initiated at **higher threshold.**
2. **Slow channel AP:** Present in SA node, AV node, around AV ring, coronary sinus opening with Ca^{2+} mainly at the speed of **0.01–0.1 m/sec** and is inhibited by **CCB (ERP > APD),** i.e. ERP/APD is >1.

Normally, Purkinje fibres have the **highest** conduction velocity (4000 mm/sec) except near their junction with ventricular fibres gate region or if they change over from fast channel to slow channel response. Most antiarrhythmic drugs enhance ERP/APD ratio.

Initiation of AP varies during both **depolarisation** and **repolarisation.**

Absolute refractory period: Cells cannot respond to any stimulus beginning during phase 1 and ending at the start of phase 3.

ERP: Minimum interval between two propagating action potential **(most important).**

Relative RP: Cell can respond to **strong stimulus** and occurs during **phase 3**. Response to stimulus enhances as repolarisation continues. After complete repolarisation, cells respond fully to stimulus.

Cells at different cardiac regions depolarise at various speeds, depending upon whether **fast or slow** channel predominates.

Na^+ flows through **fast** channel (hence quick depolarisation) and Ca^{2+} through **slow** channel (hence slow dpolarisation, e.g. SA node, AV junction, etc.).

Torsade de pointes (twisting of points): Multi-form ventricular tachycardia with rapid asynchronous complexes and underlying baseline on ECG.

Re-entrant arrhythmia: Due primarily to abnormality of conduction, an impulse may **recirculate** in the heart and cause **repetitive activation** without the need for any new impulse to be generated.

> Re-entry: One impulse not going out of cell.

Re-entry circuit is due to abnormal conduction within heart and may be due to circus movement, e.g. PSVT. For en-entry to happen, the pre-requisite is that the **path length** of the circuit should be **greater than the wavelength** of the impulse. **Fractionation** of impulses is preceded by **premature depolarisation** and is **self-sustaining** due to inhomogenous nature of the ERP generally under the influence of **vagal** overactivity. Impulse passes rapidly through fibres with **short effective RP**, slowly through fibres with **long effective RP** and **not at all through the fibres still refractory**, e.g. auricular fibres of MS.

Normal ECG waveform

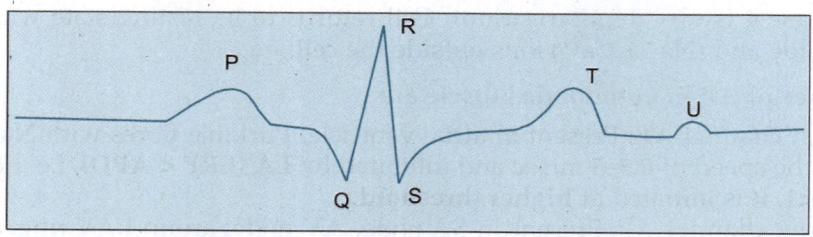

1. P wave reflects **atrial depolarisation.**
2. PR interval represents impulse spread from atria through Purkinje fibre.
3. QRS complex represents **ventricular depolarisation.**
4. **ST segment** represents phase 2 of AP → **absolute** RP (part of ventricular repolarisation).
5. **T wave** shows phase of AP →ventricular repolarisation.
6. PR interval   =   0.83 sec
   PR/PQ interval =   0.12–0.2 sec
   QRS complex   =   0.04–0.10 sec
   QT interval   =   0.35–0.42 sec
7. **U** wave is caused by hyp**O**kalemia.   **U and O are vowels**

Pressure presents in the chamber and the vessels

Structure	BP (mmHg)
Right atrium	0 (mean pressure)
Right ventricle	25/0–1
Left atrium	2 (mean pressure)
Left ventricle	120/0
Aorta	120/80
Pulmonary artery	25/10

> **Ionotropic** means force of contraction
> **Chronotropic** means **C**ardiac Rate (HR)
> **Dromotropic** means con**D**uctivity
> **Lusiotropic** means re**L**axation (**L**oose)

Effects of stimulation on heart functions

Heart function	Parasympathetic stimulation (ACh)	Sympathetic stimulation (Adr)
1. Automaticity (SA node)	Bradycardia	Tachycardia
2. RP:		
Atria	Decreased	Decreased
Conducting tissue	Increased	Decreased
3. Conductivity	Decreased	Increased
4. Contractility	Decreased	Increased

On **parasympathetic stimulation, all** parameters **decrease except** ERP of conducting tissues.

ACh (parasympathetic) causes bradycardia, atrial RP shortened with reduced contractility and conductivity.

Adrenaline (sympathetic) causes ↑ HR, ↓RP with increased contractility and conductivity.

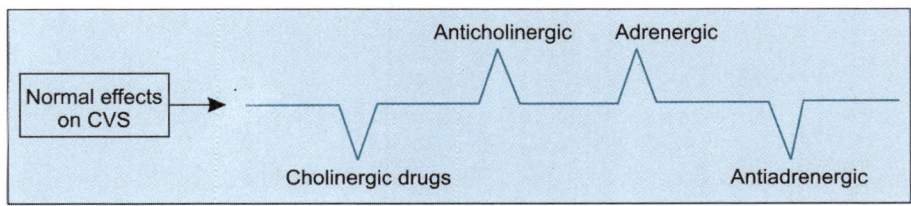

Overall effects of above drugs on CVS.

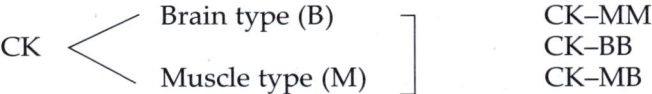

LDL ⟨ Heart type (H)
      Muscle type (M) ⟩ H_4
                        H_3M (highest)
                        H_2M_2
                        HM_3
                        M_4

Sequence of elevated enzymes in MI

CK–MB (first), **AST** (second), LDH (third) and ESR (fourth)   **CASTLE**

Heart murmurs

AS and MR = Systolic   **ARMS~Defence**
AR and MS = Diastolic

31. Cardiac Glycosides/Digitalis

Cardiac glycosides = Sugar + Genin
Genin (aglycone) = Steroid + Unsaturated lactone ring.

Sugar is **glucose/digitoxose**.
Steroid is **cyclopentanoperhydrophenanthrene**. Pharmacological action is due to **glycone**. **Sugar moieties** give solubility and cell permeability.

Digitalis glycosides are called **cardiotonic**. They are **natural steroidal glycoside** and mainstay of **CHF treatment**.

Digoxin is the **most versatile** and widely used cardiac glycosides first described by **William Withering**. They are derived from **Foxglove (digitalis) plant**. This steroid is the longest word in medical science.

Important digitalis	Source
1. Digitoxin	→ Digitalis purpurea (leaf)
2. Digoxin	→ D. lanata (leaf)
3. Gitoxin	→ D. lanata and D. purpurea (leaf)
4. Quabain (strophanthin-G)	→ Strophanthus gratus (seed)
5. Strophanthin-K	→ Strophanthus kombe (seed)
6. Lanatoside-C	→ Semisynthetic

Action of digitalis: Most marked action in AV node and bundle of His

1. Rate of 0 phase depolarisation is reduced in AV node and bundle of His. **Amplitude** is reduced. **AP duration of phase 2** is reduced.
2. **RMP** is reduced. At high doses, RMP shows acceleration at phase 4.
3. In **Purkinje** fibres, the ectopic automaticity is enhanced. It reduces **ERP of atria** and enhances **EPR of AV node** and **bundle of His. Conduction** is delayed. **Effective RP** in atrium is reduced by **vagal action** and enhanced by **direct action**.
4. **Positive ionotropic effects** provide **most of the benefits**
   a. It enhances **contractility** and **CO** in hypodynamic heart without increase in O_2 use. It increases **force of contraction.**
   b. It reduces **cardiac filling pressure, venous plus capillary pressure, heart size, fluid volume, edema**, etc.

c. It enhances **renal blood flow** and deactivates **reinin-angiotensin-aldosterone compensation** promoting **diuresis**.
d. Excitability is enhanced at **low doses** and reduced at **high doses**.
e. It slows the **heart–vagal actions** (↓HR), does not enhance HR but has **prolonged** action (↓HR in CHF, improved circulation due to +ve ionotropic action restores reduced vagal tone and abolishes **sympathetic** overactivity). It enhances **vagal tone of SA node**.
f. **Systole** is **shortened** and **diastole** is **prolonged** (↑ systolic BP and pulse pressure, ↓diastolic BP).

5. It reduces **CNS sympathetic flow** from **enhanced carotid sinus baroreceptor sensitivity. Vagus** reduces **HR** by vagal centre stimulation in brain, enhanced sensitivity of SA node to **ACh** and through **baroreceptors.** These actions can be inhibited by **atropine** but actions on SA node/AV node are not inhibited by atropine.
6. It causes **vasoconstriction (systemic)**

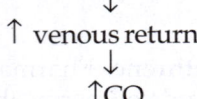
↑ venous return
↓
↑CO

7. It stimulates **CTZ** →nausea and vomiting.
8. **Heart stimulants** (adrenaline, theophylline) reduce myocardial efficiency by reducing HR and having short duration of action.
   Cardiotonics have prolonged duration of actions and do not enhance HR.
9. **Digitalis** causes the failing heart to react more forcefully in the face of increased resistance. **Force of contraction of normal heart** is also enhanced. The failing heart is unable to do so on its own.
10. **Negative ionotropic effect** occurs at SA node at higher doses **(17 μg/kg)**.
11. ECG changes: T wave inversion, ↑ PR interval, ↓QT interval, depressed ST segment.
12. **Effect of digoxin**

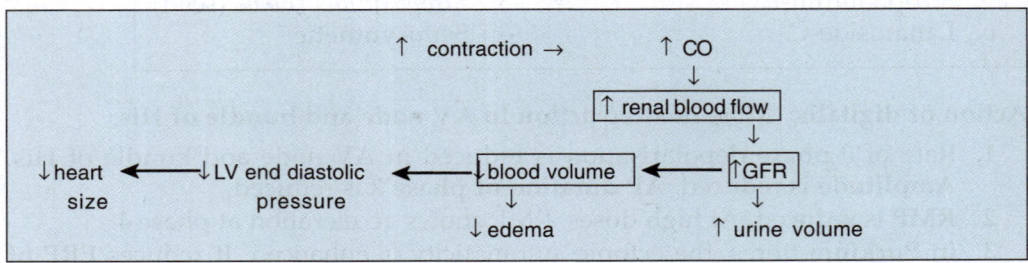

Mech: Cardiac glycoside inhibits **Na^+-K^+ ATPase** of cell membrane causing **enhanced intracellular Ca^{2+}. Na^+-Ca^{2+} antiport** does not function as efficiently causing enhanced intracellular Ca^{2+} and leads to **positive ionotropy** (enhanced Ca^{2+} influx/mobilisation from SR).

Systolic contraction velocity is enhanced due to inhibition of Na^+ and K^+ activated ATPase.

Cardiac Glycosides/Digitalis

Electrolytes of intracellular compartment are K^+, Mg^{2+} and PO_4^{3-}.
Electrolytes of extracellular compartment are Na^+, Cl^-, Ca^{2+} and HCO_3^-
Normally Na^+K^+ ATPase pumps $3Na^+$ out of cell and $2K^+$ into the cell
$Na^+ \rightarrow N, a, + = 3$
$K^+ \rightarrow K, + = 2$

Purkinje fibre is the most sensitive to react to digitalis.
At high doses →intracellular K^+ depletion and alternate after contraction and after depolarisation.
Digitalis selectively binds extracellular face of K^+ binding site of the membrane associated **Na^+K^+ ATPase** of myocardial fibres to inhibit the enzyme. It leads to
inhibition of cation pump
↓
↑ **intracellular Na^+**
(inhibits Na^+ influx hence inhibits Ca^{2+} efflux)
↓
↑ **intracellular Ca^{2+}**
(Ca^{2+} influx but not efflux during depolarization through voltage-gated Ca^{2+} channel).
Small percentage increase in Na^+ concentration causes **large percentage increase in Ca^{2+} concentration (1 Na/3 Ca exchange)**
↓
Excitation–contraction coupling.

Digitalis causes ↑ $[Ca^{2+}]$ within myocardial cell and causes contractility.

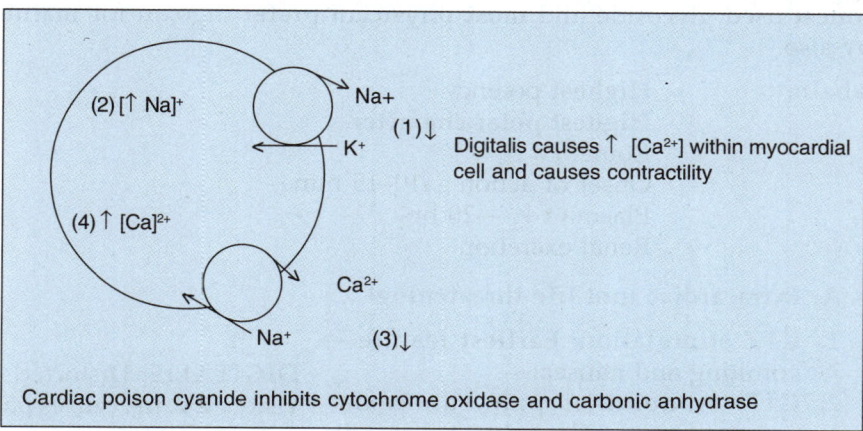

Cardiac poison cyanide inhibits cytochrome oxidase and carbonic anhydrase

Drugs causing cardiac poisons
Tobacco, HCN, Oleander, Digitalis, Aconite and Quinine

> **THODA** Quinine is cardiotoxic

Digitalis inhibits **Na^+K^+ ATPase** of cell membrane which reduces active Na^+/K^+ transport causing increased intracellular Na^+ and Ca^{2+}. $Na^+ - Ca^{2+}$ antiport does not function as efficiently causing increased intracellular Ca^{2+} and leads to **positive ionotropy.**

PK: All are irritants, have the **same safety margin** and concentrated in heart **(20 times more than plasma)** and other body parts.

A. **Digitoxin: Most lipid soluble** and **least potent.**
   90–100% oral absorption **(oral route). 95%** plasma protein bound.
   Hepatic metabolism **(enterohepatic** recycling, no need to reduce dose of digitoxin in renal failure), plasma t½ = 7 days
   Biliary excretion: Onset of action = ½–2 hrs

   Digitoxin $\xrightarrow{\text{Liver}}$ Digoxin.

B. **Digoxin: 60–80%** oral absorption.
   Route: **Oral/IV**
   Plasma therapeutic concentration → 0.8–2 ng/ml.
   Volume of distribution → 6 L/kg due to accumulation in tissues but **not in fat**
   Onset of action → 15–30 min
   Peak action → 4 hrs
   Duration of action → 4 days
   Time for digitalization → 5–7 days
   25% plasma protein bound.
   Plasma t½ →40 hrs (that means steady state serum drug concentration is not achieved for 6–8 days without loading dose).
   Elimination → **35% daily**

Unchanged renal excretion: Rate of excretion is directly proportional to **rate of creatinine clearance.** Steady state level is attained after **4 t½** of digoxin. Digoxin is **commonest** used glycoside and **most physician prefer** digoxin for **maintenance therapy** also.

   Quabain: **Highest** potency
                   Highest polar character
                   Route: IV
                   Onset of action →10–15 min
                   Plasma t ½ →20 hrs
                   Renal excretion

ADR: A. **Extracardiac (not life-threatening)**

1. **CTZ stimulation: Earliest** feature → vomiting and nausea.
2. **GIT:** Abdominal pain, anorexia, nausea appear **first** due to gastric irritation. Diarrhoea, mesenteric vasoconstriction.
3. **Last CNS ADR:** Distorted colour vision. Others are—psychosis and disorientation.

> **DIGITALIS: Distorted colour vision, I.V. inj. causes pain and necrosis, Gastric irritation, Imbalanced orientation, Tachycardia, AV block, Loss of body K⁺, Increased Ca²⁺, Severe bradycardia.**

4. **All glycosides:** Cause pain and necrosis on **IV injection.**

B. **Cardiac (life-threatening):** In **67%** cases with digitalis toxicity, the **first** symptom is **extracardiac** symptom.
   In the **33%** cases, **cardiac arrhythmia** is the **first** symptom.

Cardiac Glycosides/Digitalis

1. **Commonest** cardiac manifestations of glycoside toxicity.
   — Premature ventricular depolarisation
   — AV junctional rhythm.
2. Tachycardia, AF/AFl and severe **arrhythmia.** Severe bradycardia and partial/complete AV block.
3. **Hypokalemia (commonest)**
   Hypomagnesemia
   Hypercalcaemia
   Hypothyroidism
   Age, ischaemia, hypokalaemia and hypercalcaemia enhance toxicity.
   Toxic plasma concentration of digoxin is >2 ng/ml.

Treatment
   a. Tachyarrhythmia
   (chronic use of digitalis and diuretic → K^+ depletion).
   KCl (K^+ antagonises digitalis induced enhanced **automaticity** and reduces glycoside binding to **Na^+K^+ ATPase**).

CI: In higher degree of AV block → may precipitate **complete AV block.**
   b. **Ventricular arrhythmia: Lignocaine (IV–DOC)** suppresses excessive automaticity. Quinidine and procainamide are **contraindicated.**
   c. **Supraventricular arrhythmia:** Propranolol.
   d. **AV block and bradycardia due to vagal stimulation:** Atropine.

   Cordioversion by DC shock is **contraindicated** due to conduction defect.

4. **ECG changes**
   Early: ↑ PR interval, ↓HR, flattened T wave.
   Later: Inverted T wave, ST depression, and changed QT interval.
   Late: ↑ automaticity, delayed after depolarization, PVC and **Bigeminy.**
   In **Wolf-Parkinson-White syndrome,** QRS complex is widened on digitalis administration because conduction through aberrant path is not reduced.
5. **Digoxin toxicities** (>2 ng/ml is toxic plasma concentration).
   Digoxin Ab is **Fab fragment (Digibind)** and is **nonimmune** because it has **no Fc fragment.**
   Digoxin–Fab complex is rapidly excreted by **kidney.**
   Digoxin toxicities are **enhanced** by:
   — **Renal failure** (↓excretion)
   — **hydrochlorthiazide** (via hypokalemia)
   — **Quinidine** (↓ digoxin clearance, displaces digoxin from tissue binding sites).

Treatment of toxicity
   a. **Treatment of choice** →**Fab–Ab** (anti-digitalis Fab fragments)
   b. **Other measures (antidotes)**
   Slowly normalise K^+
   Cardiac pacer
   Lidocaine
   Atropine

Toxicity: Acute (↑ K^+) and chronic (↓K^+). K^+ competes with digitalis for Na pump →↑K^+ of ECF dephos-phoryly-ses enzymes →↓digitalis binding affinity→↓ K^+ (due to ↑ renal blood flow and inhibited renal Na^+ transport by Na pump also) and ↓toxicity (↑ toxicity at ↑ dose).

Precautions and contraindications
1. **Contraindications**
   a. **Wolf-Parkinson-White syndrome.**
   b. **Partial AV block** (may cause complete AV block)
   c. **Ventricular tachycardia** (may cause ventricular fibrillation)
   d. **Hypokalemia:** Enhances digitalis toxicity by enhancing its binding to Na^+K^+ ATPase.
   e. **Liver disease: Digitoxin** must not be given.
2. **Elderly**
3. **Renal disease:** Digoxin excreted unchanged in urine.
4. **Thyrotoxicosis:** Causes arrhythmia.
5. **Myxoedema:** Patients eliminate digoxin more slowly.
6. **Acute myocarditis.**
7. **MI:** Digitalis is used **after MI** only when heart failure is accompanied with AF and rapid ventricular rate.

IA:
1. Quinidine, CCB and hypothyroidism due to reduced renal clearance **enhance** toxicity. Quinidine **reduces** digoxin binding to tissue protein.
2. Diuretics cause **hypokalemia.**
3. Ca^{2+} **synergises** with digitalis.
4. Amiodarone, ACE inhibitor and CCB **enhance** plasma concentration of digoxin.
5. K^+ sparing diuretics **reduce** renal excretion of digoxin.
6. Adrenergic drugs **enhance** ectopic automaticity. β blocker and CCB **oppose** positive ionotropic action.
7. Succinylcholine causes **arrhythmia** in digitalised patient.
8. Phenobarbitone and other **enzyme inducers** enhance digitoxin metabolism.
9. Antacids, metoclopramide, sucralfate, sulfasalazine and neomycin **reduce** digoxin absorption.
   TCA and atropinic drugs enhance absorption.
10. Tetracycline, erythromycin and omeprazole **enhance** digoxin bioavailability.

Plasma drug concentration should be monitored in:
Aminoglycosides
Lithium therapy   **A LEAD Type**
Epileptic treatment
Antiarrhythmic treatment
Digoxin
Theophylline

U: For **rapid onset of action**, use a **divided loading dose** to avoid toxicity.
1. **CHF**
2. Control of ventricular rate in auricular flutter or fibrillation **(cardiac arrhythmia).**
3. **Cardiomyopathy:** Digitalis in **all cardiomyopathy** (**except** hypertropic cardiomyopathy where **DOC** is CCB/β blocker).

Treatment of cardiac arrhythmia: Digoxin **depresses** AV nodal conduction (enhanced myocardial contraction and long duration of action of digoxin are **unusual** for antiarrhythmia).
  a. **AF (atrial fibrillation): DOC–Digoxin.** Digitalis reduces ventricular rate in AF by **reducing number of impulse** that is able to pass down the AV node and bundle of His. It enhances **ERP of AV node** by antiadrenergic, vagomimetic and direct actions and establishes AV block in AF. Digitalis **reduces** average atrial ERP and average ventricular rate.
  b. **AFl (atrial flutter):** Atrial rate is less than that in AF **(200–350 b/min).** Digitalis **enhances** this AV block, reduces ventricular rate and inhibits sudden shift of AV block to a lower degree. AFl may be converted to AF by reducing atrial ERP. Control of ventricular rate is **easier** in AF (graded response occurs) than in AFl (AV block shifts in steps).
  c. **Arrhythmia with CHF.**
  d. **PSVT** (paroxysmal supraventricular tachycardia →HR = 150–200 b/min) is **mostly** due to re-entry involving **SA/AV node.**
  Glycoside (IV) enhances vagal tone, **depresses** the path through SA/AV node or ectopic focus and **terminates** arrhythmia **(success 34%). Verapamil** is more effective, less toxic and acts faster. **Digitalis** is used now in recurrences.

> **Drugs for CHF treatment**
> 1. **6Ds** (Digitalis, Diuretic, VasoDailator, DA, Dobutamine, PDE inhibitors).
> 2. **Bipyridines (PDE III inhibitor):** Amrinone, milrinone. PDE inhibitors: Bipyridine, dipyridamole, methylxanthine.

Treatment of CHF: CO is insufficient to meet the demand of tissue perfusion. **Ventricle** is dilated and its wall is **thickened.**
  I. **Digitalis:** Enhances contractility and shifts the curve towards normal→ (↑ CO). Improved tissue perfusion inhibits sympathetic overactivity→↓ HR and ↓**central venous pressure** → inactivation of compensatory mechanism retaining Na^+ and H_2O → diuresis → edema is cleared. Liver regresses and pulmonary congestion is reduced → dyspnoea abates and cyanosis absent.

To generate the same ejection pressure, a dilated ventricle has to develop higher wall tension, according to **Laplace equation.**

> **Wall tension = Intraventricular pressure × ventricular radius.**

Dose: Mild to moderate CHF = 0.25 mg/day
A. **Slow digitalisation:** Drug is stopped if heart rate is **< 60 b/min (bradycardia)**
B. **Rapid oral digitalisation**
   0.5–1 mg stat →1.25 mg QID.
Usual dose of digoxin: 0.25 mg/day for 1 week →0.375 mg/day for 1 week → 0.5 mg/day for 1 week.

Digitalis is still **the most effective drug** in **all patients for dilated heart and low ejection fraction if** ACE inhibitor and diuretic have failed.

Continued digitalis therapy is the **best course** in CHF patient with auricular fibrillation.

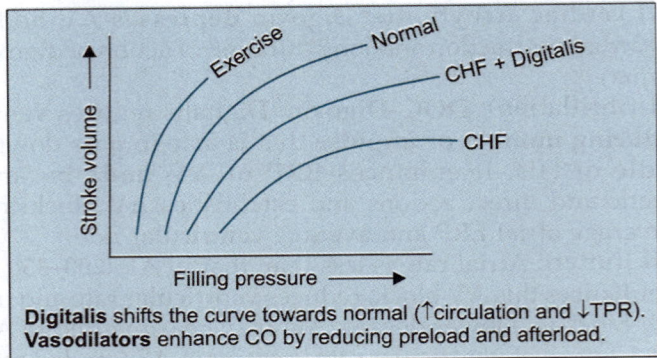

Digitalis shifts the curve towards normal (↑circulation and ↓TPR).
Vasodilators enhance CO by reducing preload and afterload.

In **high output** heart failure (anemia and thyrotoxicosis), response to digitalis is poor. In **low output** heart failure (HTN, CHD, RHD), digoxin is used (**best response** in normal myocardium of these conditions).

II. **Diuretics:** Loop diuretics—DOC (reduce peripheral edema and pulmonary congestion)

III. **Vasodilators:** Reduce preload and afterload. **Mainstay of anti-CHF measures.**

Given orally (given IV in acute heart failure of MI and shock).

Venodilator is for pulmonary congestion with breathlessness and CVP >25 mm Hg.

Arteriolar dilator is used in low cardiac index (minute output/body surface area)

Nonselective vasodilator is for enhanced CVP and low cardiac index.

(ACE inhibitor + Digoxin + Diuretic + Hydralazine) have extra benefit than (ACE inhibitor + Diuretic + Hydralazine).

Cardiac stimulants (β agonist and dopaminergic agonist) have positive ionotropic and vasodilator properties.

Dopamine (3–10 µg/kg/min IV) is used in **cardiogenic shock** due to MI.

Vasodilators
1. **Arteriolar dilators (↓ afterload)**
   A. Hydralazine
   B. CCB
   C. K⁺ channel openers:
      — Minoxidil
      — Nicorandil
      — Diazoxide
2. **Venodilators (↓ preload)**
   Nitrates (GTN, isosorbide dinitrate)
3. **Mixed dilators/arteriovenous dilators**
   (↓ preload and ↓ afterload)
   A. ACE inhibitors
   B. α_1 blockers
   C. Nitroprusside (sodium nitroprusside)

D. AT II antagonist (losartan)
E. K⁺ channel openers:
— Pinacidil
— Cromakalim

PDE III inhibitors: These are amrinone and milrinone.
Mech

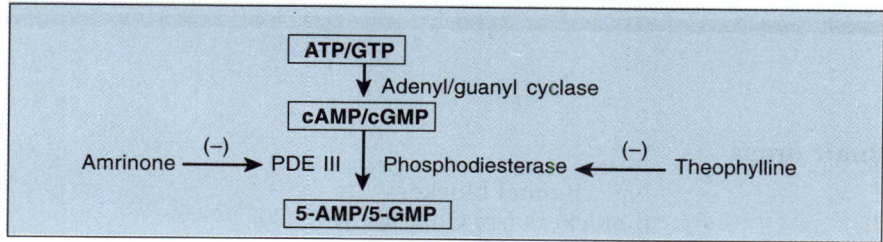

Amrinone is **selective PDE III inhibitor** (specific for intracellular degranulation of cAMP in heart, blood vessels, and bronchial smooth muscles). It enhances myocardial **cAMP** and **transmembrane influx of Ca^{2+}**, rate of development of tension in myocardial fibres and peak tension. **Systemic vascular resistance is reduced.**

Two **most important actions of amrinone**
1. **Positive ionotropy.**
2. Direct vasodilatation hence it is called **inodilator.**

ADR: 1. **Thrombocytopenia (most prominent, mostly transient and asymptomatic)**
2. **Liver damage and fever**
3. **Arrhythmia**
4. **Abdominal pain and diarrhoea.**

U: 1. **CHF:** Short-term IV use in **severe** and **refractory CHF** (10 mg/kg/day max.) Amrinone (IV) acts in 5 min and lasts 2–3 hrs.
2. **DOC in CHF:** ACE inhibitors, diuretic, vasodilators. Second line: Digoxin.
3. **CHF with auricular fibrillation:** Digitalis.

Milrinone: It is **similar** to amrinone and **10 times** more potent.

Drugs used in CHF are   **6Ds**
1. **D**igitalis group of drugs, e.g. digitoxin, digoxin.
2. **D**opamine and **D**obutamine (sympathomimetics).
3. **D**iesterase (phosphodiesterase) inhibitors, e.g. amrinone, milrinone.
4. **D**ilators of both arterioles and venules (decrease CHF mortality also)
   • ACE inhibitors, e.g. captopril, enalapril
   • Dihydralazine + Isosorbide dinitrate
5. **D**iuretics like loop diuretics, thiazides and potassium sparing diuretics.

32. Antiarrhythmic, Antianginal and Antihypertensive Drugs

Antiarrhythmic drugs

1. Class I   : Na^+ channel blockers
2. Class II   : β blockers (*see* Chapter 8)
3. Class III   : K^+ channel blockers
4. Class IVA   : Ca^{2+} channel blockers (CCBs)
   Class IVB   : K^+ channel openers
                  — ATP
                  — Adenosine
5. Others   : Digoxin
                  Atropine
                  Isoprenaline
                  Mg^{2+} and K^+

Antianginal drugs

1. β blockers
2. CCB
3. Nitrates
4. K^+ channel openers
5. Others: Dipyridamole
   Lidoflazine
   Oxyphedrine

Antihypertensive drugs   ABCD

1. **A**CE inhibitors
2. **A**ngiotensin I (AT I) antagonist (losartan)
3. α blockers
4. β blockers
5. α + β blocker (labetalol)
6. **C**CB
7. Central sympatholytic:
   — Clonidine
   — Methyldopa
8. **D**iuretics
9. Vaso**D**ilator
10. Ganglionic blocker:
    — Pentolinium
    — Trimethaphan

11. 5-HT antagonist (ketanserin)
12. Adrenergic neurone blockers:
    — Reserpine
    — Guanethidine

A. Class I: Na⁺ channel blockers (membrane stabilising agents)

1. **Class IA:** Disopyramide
   Moricizine
   Procainamide
   Quinidine — Queen Pe Dil Mera

2. **Class IB:** Lidocaine — Lo Phir Mein Tera
   Mexiletine
   Tocainide
   Phenytoin

3. **Class IC:** Propafenone
   Flecainide
   Encainide
   Moricizine
   Indecainide

B. Class III: K⁺ channel blockers

(Agents widening AP/prolonging repolarisation and ERP)
1. Amiodarone
2. Bretylium
3. Sotalol

C. CCB:

1. Phenyl alkylamine : Verapamil (hydrophilic)
2. Benzothiazepine : Diltiazem (hydrophilic)
3. Dihydopyridine (DHP)—lipophilic:
   Felodipine
   Amlodipine
   Isradipine
   Lacidipine — FAIL
   Nicardipine — NNNN
   Nemodipine
   Nitrendipine
   Nifedipine

D. K⁺ channel openers

Nicorandil — NAD
Pinacidil — cAMP
Minoxidil
Cromakalim
Diazoxide
Adenosine
ATP

E. ACE inhibitors

Captopril
Enalapril
Ramipril

Perindopril
Benazepril
Lisinopril

F. Nitrates

1. **Short-acting**
   Glyceryl trinitrate (GTN, nitroglycerine), isosorbide dinitrate (sublingually).
2. **Long-acting**
   Isosorbide mononitrate
   Isosorbide dinitrate
   Erythrityl tetranitrate
   Penta erythritol tetranitrate

Class	Channel effects
IA	— Na^+ channel inhibition + Dissociation time constant from channel (10 sec) + ↑ AP.
IB	— Na^+ channel inhibition + Dissociation time constant from channel (0.5 sec) + ↓ AP.
IC	— Na^+ channel inhibition + Dissociation time constant (20 sec) + slow conduction in His-Purkinje tissue
II	— Suppress phase 4 depolarisation.
III	— Repolarise K^+ current + ↑ ERP by increasing AP
IVA	— Ca^{2+} channel inhibition.
IVB	— K^+ channel open (hyperpolarisation)

Quinidine

Quinidine is an **alkaloid** obtained from **cinchona bark**. Dextroisomer of quinine is quiniDine

Actions

1. Has **class IA + class III + antivagal** action and reduces **automaticity** in PF and other ectopic foci. Membrane response is reduced.
2. Enhances **threshold** for excitation. ERP is prolonged more than APD (**ERP/APD is enhanced**)—tissues remain refractory even after full repolarisation (**class III property**). **Repolarisation** is prolonged.
3. **Antivagal actions** terminate AF, AFl and PSVT. **Direct** action of drug enhances and its antivagal action reduces AV nodal ERP (overall effect is **inconsistent**). It reduces **contractility**.
4. Reduces BP due to α blockade.
5. Reduces contractility of **skeletal muscle. Uterine contraction** and **antimalarial action** is present. In GIT, diarrhoea and vomiting are due to its **bitter** and **irritant** nature.

Mechanism of Class IA: Slows **phase 0 depolarisation.** It is **open state Na^+ channel inhibitor** with moderate delay in channel recovery **(1–10 sec)**. Suppresses AV conduction and prolongs PR, QRS, QT and APD. APD prolongation is due to

K⁺ channel blockade. ERP/APD is increased.

At high doses, it inhibits **L type Ca²⁺ channel**.

Drugs of class I limit the conductance of **Na⁺** and **K⁺** across cell membrane (a local **anaesthetic action**). Prolongation of repolarisation and refractoriness is present.

Mechanism of action of quinidine

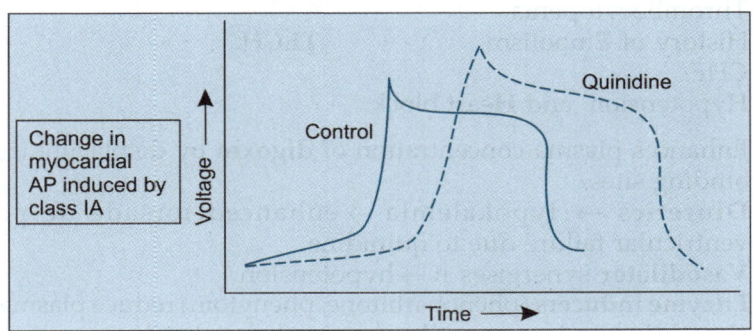

1. **Phase 4** (slow diastolic depolarisation →↓ automaticity)
2. **Phase 0** (slow rate of rise of AP) →↓ excitability and ↓ conduction velocity.

Change in myocardial cell properties due to **direct** (Na⁺ channel blockade) and **indirect** (vagal blockade) actions of class IA antiarrhythmics.

Na⁺ channel blockade	Vagal block (CA and AV node)
↓ Automaticity	↑ Automaticity
↓ Excitability	↑ Excitability
↑ ERP	↓ ERP

Sum total of effects
1. At SA and AV node →variable effects.
2. At atria and ventricular muscle →direct effects.

PK: 75% absorbed and 80–90% plasma protein bound. **Hepatic metabolism** by **hydroxylation**. Completely excreted in **urine** in 24 hrs (20% in unchanged form). t½—**6 hrs**. Single dose effect lasts—**7 hrs**. The plasma concentration = 2–5 µg/ml.

Route and dose:
1. **Orally 200–400 mg TDS** (prophylaxis and maintenance)
2. **IV** — rarely
3. **IM** — never (causes **pain** and **local necrosis**)

ADR:
1. **Sudden death:** May be due to **cardiac arrest/ventricular failure**.
2. **GIT intolerance (commonest): Dose limiting**—nausea, vomiting and diarrhoea.
3. **Cinchonism:** Ringing in ear, deafness, vertigo, loss of vision, delirium.
4. **Idiosyncrasy and hypersensitivity:** Fever, angioedema, asthma, CV collapse. Hypotension and syncope on **IV** due to α blocking action.
5. **Arrhythmia at high dose:** Prolonged QRS complex and QT interval.
6. **Paradoxical tachycardia** (paradoxical effect due to cardiac depressant action of drug):

↓ atrial rate ──────→ ↓ impulse to AV node.

Antivagal action → ↑ impulse to ventricle → paradoxical tachycardia (treated by digitalis)

Precaution: Can precipitate **heart failure** in patient with low cardiac reserve (reduce the dose of quinidine if QRS is broadened beyond **25%** of its normal limit).

CI:
1. Thrombocytopenia
2. History of Embolism
3. CHF
4. Hypotension and Heart block.

TECH

IA:
1. Enhances plasma concentration of **digoxin** by displacing it from tissue binding sites.
2. **Diuretics** → Hypokalemia → enhanced torsade de pointes and ventricular failure due to quinidine.
3. **Vasodilator** synergises it → hypotension.
4. **Enzyme inducers** (phenobarbitone, phenytoin) reduce plasma level while **cimetidine** and **verapamil** enhance plasma level.
5. **Codeine** ──────────→ morphine
   CYP2D6
   (−)↑
   Quinidine
6. **β blocker** and **K⁺ salt** → synergistic cardiac depression with quinidine.

U: **Tachyarrhythmia** is treated by **antiarrhythmics** which depress electrical activity of myocardial cells → ↓ ectopic **automaticity** and → ↓ conduction to reduce **re-entry**.
Bradyarrhythmia is treated with **atropine/β agonists**.
Class IA drugs are often combined with **cardiac glycosides**.
1. Prophylaxis of re-entrant arrhythmia.
2. Atrial and ventricular arrhythmia.
3. Recurrences of ventricular tachycardia.
4. To maintain sinus rhythm after atrial fibrillation/atrial flutter (AF/AFl).
5. Tachyarrhythmia.

Procainamide

Procainamide is **amide** derivative of **LA procaine**.

Actions: Same as quinidine

Difference is:
1. It is dose-to-dose **less potent**.
2. It causes **less depression of contractility** and **AV conduction**.
3. At high dose, hypotension is due to ganglionic blockade **(no α blockade)**.

Mech: Does not block Na⁺ channel but **blocks K⁺ channel** and prolongs repolarisation (**APD** is lengthened).

PK: Orally active
Oral bioavailability   −   **75%**
Peak plasma concentration   −   **1 hr**
Plasma protein binding is **minimal** but **distribution** is wide.
Hepatic metabolism primarily by **acetylation** to **NAPA** (N-acetyl procainamide).

Like isoniazid, **fast** and **slow acetylator** for procainamide is present.
>50% excreted **unchanged in urine.** Plasma t½ →**3–4 hrs.**
Dose: 1. **0.5–1 gm** oral/IM followed by **0.5 gm** every 2 hrs. OR
       2. **Loading dose:** 25 mg/min IV for 20 min followed by 2 mg/kg/hr.
IA: It reduces **sulfonamide** effects.
ADR: 1. **CNS:** Flushing and hypotension on IV, hallucination and mental confusion.
       2. Hypersensitivity (rash, fever, angioedema).
       3. **CVS:** Cardiac toxicity, torsade de pointes, paradoxical tachycardia.
       4. 20% SLE, >50% antinuclear Ab.
U: 1. **VES** and **VT**
    2. Persistent ventricular ectopic (DOC).
    3. **No chronic therapy** due to incidence of SLE and frequent administration.
    4. Alternative to quinidine due to safer and faster actions.

Disopyramide

Disopyramide is **oral antiarrhythmic** and **most potent antimuscarinic.**
  Mech: **Quinidine like cardiac depressant and anticholinergic action.**
No α-blocking property.
No effect on sinus rate due to opposing direct depressant and antivagal action. QRS broadening and PR interval prolongation are less marked.
  PK: Bioavailability—**80%.**
Partial hepatic metabolism by **dealkylation, 50%** unchanged urinary excretion, plasma t½—**7 hrs** (average 6–8 hrs), t½ **increases** in MI and renal insufficiency. The plasma concentration range → **2–5 µg/ml.**
  Dose: 2 mg/kg/day QID oral/IV
  ADR: 1. Cardiac decompensation, greater cardiac **depression,** hypotension.
        2. **Anticholinergic ADR (most important):** Dry mouth, constipation, urinary retention, blurred vision.
  CI: BPH, Sick sinus, Cardiac failure   **BSc**
  U: Recurrent ventricular arrhythmia **(DOC)**

Moricizine

Moricizine has **class IA** and **IC** actions.
  Mech: Less marked CNS effects and cardiodepressant effects.
  ADR: Increased mortality in **post MI patient.**

Some common ADR to class IA antiarrhythmics	
Ventricular arrhythmia	→ Syncope
AV block	→ ↑ PR interval
	↑ QRS complex
	↑ QT interval
↓ contractility	→ Heart failure
Vasodilatation	→ Hypotension

Mexiletine

Mexiletine is **LA** and active **antiarrhythmic** by oral route. Chemically and pharmacologically **similar** to lidocaine.

Mech: Reduces **automaticity** in PF both by decreasing phase 4 slope and by increasing **threshold voltage**.

> **Mech of IB:** Blocks Na^+ channel in both activated and inactivated state. Channel recovery time is <1 sec. Blocks **inactive** Na^+ **channel** in ischaemic area. Minimum **phase 0 depression** and **slow conduction**. Shortens **phase 3 repolarisation** and APD plus refractoriness. ERP/APD is enhanced.

PK: Completely absorbed **orally**.
90% hepatic metabolism.
Renal excretion.
Plasma t½—**10 hrs** (range 9–12 hrs).
Therapeutic plasma conc →0.75–2 μg/ml.

IA: 1. **Phenytoin** and **rifampin** induce its metabolism.
2. **Morphine** reduces its oral absorption.

ADR: 1. Block (AV block)
2. Ocular manifestation.   **BOND**
3. Neurological (nausea, vomiting, tremor, dizziness, confusion, ataxia, blurred vision)
4. Decrease BP and HR.

U: 1. **Post-infarction ventricular arrhythmia** as alternative to lidocaine in resistance cases.
2. Orally in **VES** and **VT** suppression over long-term.

Tocainide

Tocainide is lidocaine analogue

PK: Bioavailability: **90%**.
Excreted **unchanged in urine.**
Plasma level: **6–15 μg/ml**

ADR: 1. Pulmonary fibrosis
2. Paresthesia
3. Agranulocytosis   **PACT**
4. Convulsion
5. Thrombocytopenia

U: Ventricular arrhythmia (it is rarely used due to ADR)

> **Mech. of class IC**
>
> 1. Class IC is **the most potent Na^+ channel blocker** with prominent action on open state and **longest** recovery time (>10 sec). Propafenone is the **most important** Na^+ channel blocker.
> 2. Suppresses **ectopic activity,** slows **conduction,** enhances **PR** and **QRS,** retards **antegrade** and **retrograde conduction** in WPW syndrome.
> 3. Slows **phase 0 depolarisation (maximum phase 0 depression)** and **conduction,** prolongs PR interval, broadens QRS with variable effect on APD. Little effect on repolarisation.

Flecainide
Flecainide: No effect on APD.

Mech: Suppresses **VES, VT, WPW tachycardia** and prevents recurrence of **AF** and **PSVT**. Induces marked reductions of change in **Na⁺ permeability**.

ADR:
1. Mortality in patient recovering from **MI**.
2. **Proarrhythmia**
3. **CNS stimulations**

U:
1. Reserved for resistant cases of recurrent **AF**, supraventricular arrhythmia and **WPW** rhythms without associated CHF.
2. **Ventricular tachycardia → VF.**

> **ADR of class IC**
> 1. High proarrhythmic potential (sudden death)
> 2. Neurological
> 3. Gastrointestinal
> 4. Visual disturbance

Propafenone
Mech: Blocks **Na⁺ channel** and depresses **conduction**. Has **β blocking** property.

ADR:
1. **Precipitate CHF** and **bronchospasm**
2. **SA block.**

U: Resevered for **ventricular arrhythmia** and for maintenance of **sinus rhythm** in AF.

> **Mech of class 3**
> Prolongation of repolarisation of phase 3
> ↓
> Widened AP and ↑ ERP
> (**The most characteristic** function of this class)
> **Refractory tissue** even after full repolarisation.
> **Re-entrant arrhythmia** is terminated.

Amiodarone: It is **unique wide spectrum** antiarrhythmic agent (chiefly **class III** but **class IA + II + IV** activity are also present). It is **unusual iodine containing highly lipophilic long-acting antiarrhythmic.**

> **AMIODARONE** is the drug with prominent actions:
> Antiarrhythmic
> Multiple actions, i.e. block K^+, Na^+, Ca^{++} channel and beta receptors.
> Iodine containing (so may interfere with thyroid functions)
> Orally used mainly
> Duration of action is very long (t½ 3–8 weeks)
> APD and ERP increased (so conduction decreased and depress ectopics).
> **Resistant AF, VT** and **Recurrent VF** are the only clinical uses because of its toxicity.
> On IV injection, myocardial depression and blood pressure decrease. On prolonged use, pulmonary fibrosis and alveolitis.
> Neuropathy may occur
> Eye: Corneal microdeposits may occur

It acts at **all sites** in myocardium which is **unusual for antiarrhythmic**. It effectively reduces almost **any arrhythmia**.

Mech: Prolongs **ERP** by prolonging APD in **all cardiac tissues** and prolongs repolarisation by blocking **K⁺ channel**. Inhibits inactivated **Na⁺ channel** at high stimulation frequency (**class I activity**). Non-competitively blocks α and β **receptors** to cause coronary and peripheral **vasodilatation**. Blocks **Ca²⁺ channel** to cause **bradycardia** and **AV nodal inhibition** (**class IV activity**). APD and ERP are prolonged, conduction slowed and **ectopic automaticity** depressed.

PK: IV causes **myocardial depression** and **hypotension**. Duration of action → **3–8 weeks**. Variable absorption from GIT → 30–50%. Elimination t½ → 20– 60 days.

Lipid soluble with high tissue distribution. Converted to **desethylamiodarone** by hepatic metabolism. Protein binding—**95%**.

Therapeutic plasma concentration → 1–2.5 µg/ml.

Dose: Oral — **8 mg/kg/day** for a few weeks.
— **2 mg/kg/day** maintenance therapy.
IV — 5 mg/kg/hr for 1 hr.

ADR:
1. **Most serious toxicities** (rare if dose is <200 mg):
   Pneumonitis
   Alveolitis
   Pulmonary fibrosis
2. **Torsade de pointes**
   SA and **AV nodal block**
   Hypotension
3. **Peripheral neuropathy** (weakness of shoulder and pelvic muscle)
4. **Hypo- and hyperthyroidism:** No conversion of T_4 to T_3.
5. **Photosensitisation and skin pigment (10%)**
6. **Corneal microdeposits (but no blindness)**
7. **Hepatic damage and nausea.**

ADR of amiodarone — **ABCDEFGHI**

Anorexia, **B**ilateral optic neuropathy, **C**orneal deposits, **D**amage to heart and liver, **E**xcess photosensitivity, **F**ibrosis of lung, **G**irdle weakness due to peripheral neuropathy, **H**ypothyroidism, **I**nteraction with warfarin and digoxin.

Drugs causing corneal opacities
Vit **D**
Mepacrine
Chloroquine — **D and MCI**
Indomethacin

CI:
1. Sinus bradycardia
2. Syncope
3. Heart block
4. Hypersensitization
5. Not administer with drugs prolonging QT interval.

IA: 1. Additive AV block with **β blocker** and **CCB**.
2. Enhances **digoxin** and **warfarin** level by reducing their renal clearance.

U: 1. **Prophylaxis** of ventricular tachycardia
2. **Post MI**
3. **WPW** arrhythmia
4. **PSVT**
5. Recurrent paroxysmal **AF/AFl**.

Bretylium: It is **β blocker** and has **complex electrophysiological effects.**

Mech: 1. Causes **initial NA release** in heart, later **blockade of NA release (↓CA release).**
2. Prolongation of **APD** and **ERP** due to K⁺ channel blockade. Na⁺ **channel blockade** is absent.

PK: **Polar** compound, **erratic** oral absorption, excreted **unchanged in urine,** plasma t½ → **6–10 hrs.**

U: 1. **Ventricular failure** refractory to electrical defibrillation.
2. **Post-MI** resistant ventricular arrhythmia.
Dose: 5 mg/kg 6–8 hously IM/IV.

CCB

Ca²⁺ **channel** is important for **AP generation** in SA node and AV node.

Three types

1. **Voltage sensitive** channel (membrane potential ≤ −40 mV).
2. **Receptor operated** channel (activated by adrenaline and other agonist)
3. **Leak channel:** Ca²⁺ leaks into resting cell and is pumped out by **Ca²⁺ ATPase.**
   Voltage sensitive Ca²⁺ channel: It is **hetrogeneous, membrane spanning funnel-shaped glycoprotein** acting as ion selective valve. Composed of α (α₁, α₂), β, γ, δ subunits. All subunits are modulatory **except** α₁ which encloses channel. 3 types of this channel:

A. L-type (long-lasting current)

a. **Slow inactivation** of cardiac and smooth muscle → excitation–contraction coupling.
b. **SA** and **AV node** → conductivity
c. **Endocrine** → hormone release
d. **Nerve** → transmitter release
L-type has subunit in multiple isoforms and **only this is blocked by CCB,** which binds to α₁ subunit, all restricting Ca²⁺ entry. L-type has **protein kinase activity also.**

B. N-type (neuronal)

Medium action. SA node → pacemaker activitiy. **T current** and **repetitive spike in thalamus.**
Artery → constriction
Endocrine → hormone release

C. T-type (transient)
Fast action on neurone in CNS, sympathetic and myenteric plexus → transmitter release.

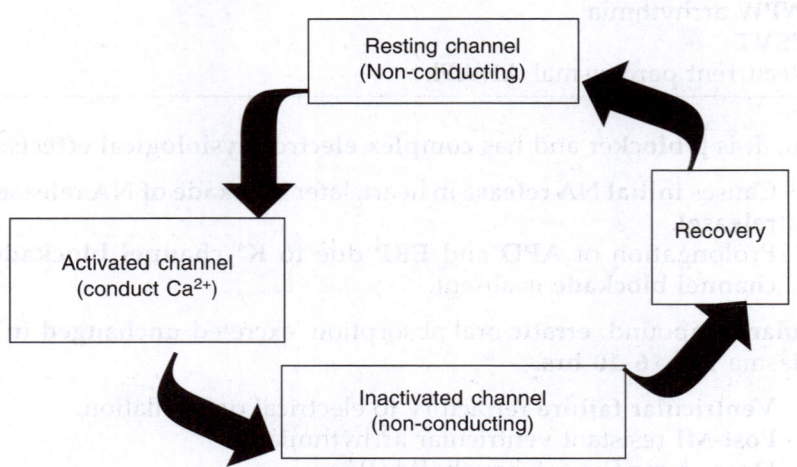

Recovery process is delayed by **verapamil more than diltiazem** but **not by DHP** due to no negative chronotropic/dromotropic action resulting in **depression** of pacemaker activity and conduction.

Dihydropyridine (DHP): All DHPs have pharmacodynamic profile **similar** to nifedipine but vary in PK.

DHPs specially nifedipine are the **most potent Ca^{2+} channel blockers.**

Actions: (A) 2 most important actions of CCB
1. **Negative chronotropic** (HR), **dromotropic** (conductivity) and **ionotropic** action on muscle of heart.
2. **Smooth muscle** (specially vascular) relaxation.

Other actions are

3. **CCB → artery effected more than veins. Extravascular smooth muscle** (uterine, vesical, intestine, biliary, bronchial) is also relaxed.
4. **Channel blocking potency**
   Nifedipine > Verapamil > Diltiazem.
5. **Heart (frequency dependent channel blockade)**
   Verapamil > Diltiazem > Nifedipine (independent).
6. **Vascular smooth muscle relaxation:**
   Nifedipine > DHP > Verapamil.
7. HR + AV conduction + contractility are decreased by **Verapamil + Diltiazem.**
8. Nifedipine reduces RR interval. Diltiazem enhances PR interval but reduces/enhances RR interval.

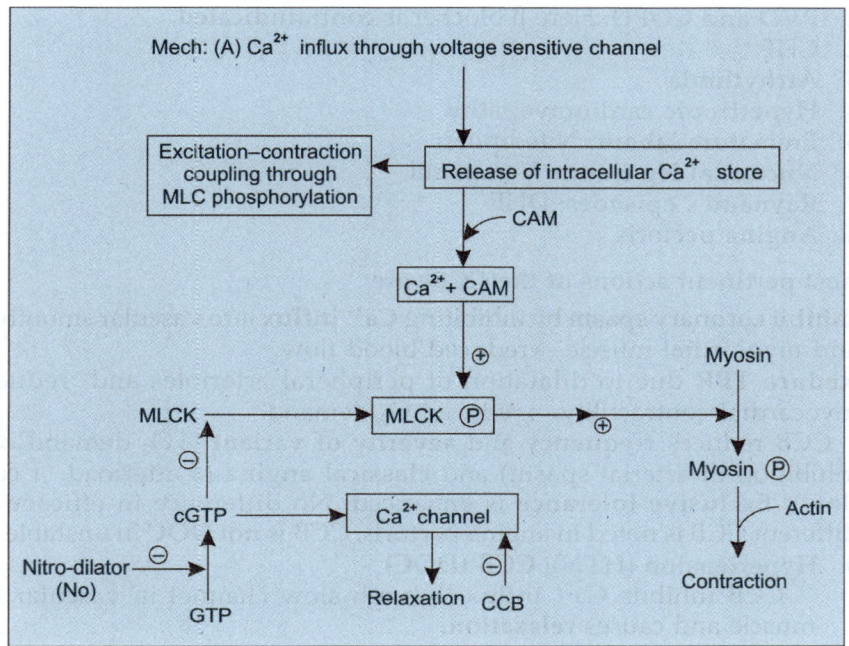

(B) DHP inhibits cyclic nucleotide PDE →↑ cAMP in smooth muscle causing relaxation.

(C)
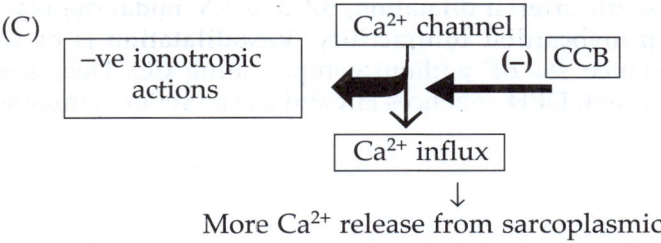

More Ca^{2+} release from sarcoplasmic reticulum
↓
Contraction through binding to troponin (myosin–actin interaction) in heart.
(D) L-type Ca^{2+} channel activates and inactivates at slow rate.
↓
Ca^{2+} depolarising cells (SA and AV node) have less steep 0 phase and longer refractory period.
(E) CCBs are **mistakenly called Ca^{2+} antagonist** as they do not block action of Ca^{2+}. Effects of CCB on myocardium are antagonised by **CA, Ca^{2+}** and **digoxin**.

PK of CCB: All are 90–100% orally absorbed, peak **1–3 hrs except** amlodipine (peak 6–9 hrs).
Oral bioavailability of CCB is **incomplete** and **variable** due to high first pass metabolism. **All are** highly plasma protein bound. **>90% hepatic metabolism.**
Renal excretion for all.
Elimination t½→**2–6 hrs except** amlodipine (elimination t½—40 hrs) and **felodipine** (elimination t½—12–18 hrs).

U:
1. **PVD and COPD:** Here β blocker is **contraindicated**.
2. **CHF**
3. **Arrhythmia**
4. **Hypertropic cardiomyopathy**
5. **Premature labour:** Nifedipine
6. **Nucturnal leg cramp:** Verapamil
7. **Raynaud's episodes:** DHP
8. **Angina pectoris**

Two most pertinent actions of the CCBs are
A. **Inhibit coronary spasm** by inhibiting **Ca^{2+} influx** into vascular smooth muscle and myocardial muscle →reduced blood flow.
B. **Reduce TPR** due to dilatation of peripheral arterioles and reduction in myocardial contractility →reduced O_2 demand.
  CCB reduces **frequency** and **severity of variant** (↓O_2 demand of heart, inhibition of arterial spasm) and **classical angina** (↓ afterload, ↑ coronary flow). **Exclusive tolerance** is enhanced. No difference in efficacy among different CCB is noted in angina pectoris. CCB is **not DOC** in unstable angina.
9. **Hypertension (HTN): CCB (DOC)**
  CCB inhibits Ca^{2+} influx through slow channel in vascular smooth muscle and causes **relaxation**.
  Low renin hypertensive patient, blacks and elderly respond well. **All 3 subgroups** have **equal efficacy as antihypertensives**. **All CCBs** share a **similar** mechansim of action, each agent produces **different degrees of coronary** and **systemic arterial dilatation, SA and AV nodal depression** and **a decrease in myocardial contractility. Vasodilatation** is present. ↓peripheral resistance →↓ BP without compensating CO. Decrease in venous return is absent. **DPH** enhances HR and CO by reflex sympathetic stimulation.

Advantages
A. Action is **quick**.
B. **Most agents** are administered once or at the most twice a day (**monotherapy** effective in **50%** hypertensives and actions independent of patient's renin status).
C. Do not compromise **haemodynamics** hence no physical work capacity impairment is present.
D. **CNS** side effects absent.
E. Not impair **renal** perfusion. Not effect **male sexual** function, plasma **lipid profile, electrolyte balance, uric** acid level and **quality of life**.
F. Can be given in **pregnancy, asthma, angina** and **PVD**.

Disadvantages
A. Worsening of **unstable angina**. Worsening of **CHF** due to absence of reduced venous return (negative ionotropic/dromotropic action of verapamil/ diltiazem).
B. **DHP** enhances **HR+ CO** by reflex sympathetic stimulation.
C. Enhanced mortality of CHD patient due to repeated surge of **adrenergic discharge** and marked swing of BP attending each dose of rapidly acting DHP.

Antiarrhythmic, Antianginal and Antihypertensive Drugs

D. **Ankle edema** due to enhanced hypostatic pressure across capillaries of dependent parts as a result of **reflex vasoconstriction** of postcapillaries in these vascular beds.

E. Nifedipine reduces **insulin release** →DM is accentuated. (Carbohydrate tolerance is not impaired.)

CCB specially nifedipine accentuates **bladder voiding difficulty** in elderly males and **gastroesophageal reflex**.

Nifedipine

Nifedipine is **CCB** with **antiplatelet** activity and **least effect on AV conduction**.

Mech:
1. Causes **arteriolar dilatation** →↓TPR → **hypotension**.
2. Not depressed SA/AV nodal conduction. (AV nodal ERP increases/decreases).
3. **RR interval** is reduced.
4. **Reflex sympathetic stimulation** of heart predominates.
↓
Tachycardia, ↑ CO, ↑ contractility but no decrease in venous return. **Coronary flow** is **enhanced**.

PK: Bioavailability—**100%** as it bypasses liver metabolism.
Volume distribution—**10 L/kg**.
Clearance—**1 L/hr/kg**.
Elimination t½ →**12–18 hrs**.
Dose: **5–20 mg BD—TDS** oral.
Highly **lipid soluble**

CI: Non-β-blockade patient.

ADR
1. Palpitation
2. Flushing
3. Ankle edema
4. Hypotension
5. Headache
6. Drowsiness and nausea
7. Relaxant effect on bladder→difficult urine voiding in elderly males.
8. Reduced **insulin release** →hampering DM control.
9. Increased angina due to **"coronary steal" phenomena**.
10. CCB causing **gum hypertrophy** and **peripheral edema** is nifedipine.

U:
1. CHF
2. Angina
3. HTN
4. Premature labour and bronchial asthma due to **relaxant action**.

Nicardipine: Greater smooth muscle selectivity (direct cardiodepression is absent). **More coronary dilatation** is present.
Dose: 20–40 mg TDS.

Felodipine: Greater **vascular selectivity, large tissue distribution** and **longer t½** present.
- **PK:** Plasma protein binding → **99% (maximum)**
  Bioavailability → **15–25%**
  Volume of distribution—**10 L/kg**
  Clearance—**1 L/hr/kg**
  Elimination t½ → **12–18 hrs**

Amlodipine: **The most distinct DHP. Complete but slow oral absorption** present (peak after **8 hrs**). Oral bioavailability is higher and consistent due to **less variable** and less **consistent first pass metabolism.**
- **PK:** Bioavailability—**60%.**
  Volume of distribution—**21 L/kg**
  Clearance—**0.42 L/hr/kg.**
  Elimination t½ (longest)—**40 hrs**
- **U:** **Alternative to DHP as retard preparation due to slow absorption.**

Nitrendipine: Vaso-selective, no cardio-depressant, not depress AV conduction.
- **U:** **Angina prectoris**
  HTN

Lacidipine: **Vasoselective,** higher concentration in **vascular smooth muscle membrane.**
U: HTN

Nimodipine: Short acting. Crosses BBB (blood–brain barrier). **Cereberal vascular relaxation** present.
- **U:** Prevention and treatment of **neurological deficit** due to cerebral vasospasm following subarachnoid haemorrhage of ruptured congenital intracranial aneurysm.

Diltiazem: Direct cardiac actions of diltiazem are **similar** to those of verapamil. **Less potent** vasodilator than nifedipine and verapamil and has **modest direct negative chronotropic, dromotropic** and **ionotropic action** but direct **depression of SA node** is **similar** to verapamil. **Dilates** coronary vessels.
  PR interval increases
  RR interval increases/decreases
  AV nodal ERP increases
- **ADR** (**similar** to verapamil):
  1. **Dose:** Hypotension and bradycardia
  2. **Overdose/IV:** ↓ TPR
- **CI:** Pre-existing sinus, AV nodal or myocardial disease.
- **PK:** Bioavailability **40–60%**
  Elimination t½ → **5–6 hrs**
  Dose: 30–60 mg TDS/QID oral
  Clearance—**0.7 L/hr/kg**
  Volume of distribution—**3 L/kg**
  Plasma protein binding—**80%**

IA: 1. Enhances plasma **digoxin** like verapamil.
2. Low dose should be given with **β blocker**.

U: 1. **Angina**
2. **HTN**
3. **MI**
4. **Arrhythmia**
5. **β blocker contraindicated patient of COPD/PVD.**

Verapamil

Verapamil is a **phenylalkylamine hydrophilic papaverine congener** and has **most prominent cardiac electrophysiological action.**

Actions

A. Antiarrhythmic actions

Mainly reduces **heart rate** and slows **conduction** through AV node. Blocks **L-type Ca^{2+} channels** and delays their recovery.

Reduces SA nodal and ventricular **automaticity** plus reduced **depolarisation** rate. Prolongs **AP** and **ERP**.

RR and **PR** intervals are enhanced. Depresses Ca^{2+} mediated depolarisation → suppresses **automaticity or re-entry.** Phase 4 depolarisation in SA node and PF is reduced →**bradycardia** and **extension** of latent pacemaker.

The most consistent action is prolongation of AV nodal ERP →slow AV conduction + termination of re-entry.

Negative ionotropic action is present due to interference with Ca^{2+} mediated excitation–contraction coupling.

B. Antianginal actions

Has **a blocking activity** and **dilates arterioles** (↓TPR and ↓BP).

Direct **cardiodepression** (reduced contractility).

HR is reduced. **AV conduction** is slowed but CO is maintained by **reflex sympathetic stimulation** and **decrease in aortic impedence.** Coronary flow is enhanced due to **vasodilatation. Dilates peripheral arterioles.**

PK: On **chronic use,** verapamil reduces its own metabolism (bioavailability is **doubled** and **t½** is prolonged).
Bioavailability—**15–30%**
Volume of distribution—**5 L/kg**
Clearance—**0.9 L/hr/kg**
Elimination t½—**4–6 hrs**

ADR: 1. **Bradycardia, AV block, hypotension.**
2. **Cardiac arrest** on IV and in **sick sinus.**
3. **Constipation,** nausea, **flushing, headache, ankle edema.** (**alternative treatment**—amlodipine which has slow absorption).

CI: 1. CCB absolutely **contraindicated** in heart failure—verapamil.
2. **PSVT** with CHF/hypotension
3. **VT** →VF
4. **Digitalis toxicity** → AV block
5. Partial **heart block** and **sick sinus**

IA:
6. **Conduction defects** accentuation. Hence, contraindicated in 2nd and 3rd degree block.
7. **HTN with CHF**/conduction defects.
1. Not given with β blocker → causes **additive sinus depression, conduction defects** and **asystole**.
2. Reduces **digoxin excretion** → ↑ plasma digoxin level → digoxin toxicity
3. Not used with other cardiac depressant (quinidine, disopyramide).

Phenylephrine enhances BP, reflexly reduces HR and PSVT.
Edrophonium enhances vagal tone to heart → ↓ HR and ↓ PSVT.

U:
1. **PSVT: DOC** (5–10 mg IV in 2–5 min → effective in **80%**).
2. **Recurrence of PSVT**
3. **AF/AFl**
4. **Re-entrant supraventricular** and **nodal arrhythmia** (WPW) but risky due to **reflex sympathetic stimulation** and **ERP reduction**.
5. **Variant angina—DOC**
6. **Arrhythmia**
7. Suppresses **nocturnal leg cramp, mania and psychosis.**
8. HTN: **CCB–DOC.** Effective in **50%** patients. Used in **pregnancy/asthma/angina** also. Action **independent** of renin status.
   Improves **arterial** compliance
   Retards **atherogenesis**
   Reduces **LVH**

Drugs for AV block
Atropine abbreviates AV nodal ERP and enhances conduction velocity in bundle of His.
Adrenaline facilitates AV conduction, shortens ERP of conduction tissue, enhances automaticity of ventricular pacemaker and is used in partial/complete heart block.

Adenosine
Adenosine is **endogenous** chemical and is **end product of ATP.**

Mech
1. Reduces **automaticity** in SA node and conduction velocity, enhances K^+ efflux leading to **hyperpolarisation.**
2. Activates **ACh sensitive K^+ channel** and causes membrane hyperpolarisation through interaction with A_1 **type G protein coupled adenosine receptor** on SA node (pacemaker depression → ↓HR), AV node (ERP prolongation → slow conduction) and atrium (shortening of AP and reduced excitability).
3. It reduces Ca^{2+} **current** in AV node (depression of re-entrant circuit through AV node → termination of PSVT + transient coronary dilatation).

Antiarrhythmic, Antianginal and Antihypertensive Drugs

4. Slows **sinus rate** and enhances **AV nodal refractoriness** leading to **hyperpolarisation**.

PK:
1. Within **30 sec >90%** episodes of PSVT termination involving AV node on IV **(as free base/ATP)**.
   6–12 mg IV injected **as fast as possible**.
2. Plasma t½—**10 sec** due to uptake into **RBC** and **endothelial cell** (adenosine → inosine + 5-AMP). Complete elimination through **coronary circulation.** Injected ATP is rapidly converted to adenosine.

IA:
1. **Dipyridamole** inhibits its uptake and potentiates its action.
2. **Methylxanthine** blocks adenosine receptors and antagonises its action.

ADR
1. **Commonest ADR** (in 30–60%): **Dyspnoea** due to bronchoconstriction, **flushing** due to vasodilatation, **chest pain**.
2. **VF**
3. **Ventricular stand still** for a few seconds.
4. **Bronchospasm** in asthma.

Advantages
1. **Efficacy better** than verapamil
2. Actions last **<1 minute**
3. Given in hypotension, CHF or with β blocker where verapamil is **contraindicated**.
4. **Safe** in wide QRS tachycardia with WPW syndrome (**unsafe** is verapamil).
5. Sensitive in **verapamil resistant** cases.

Disadvantages
1. **Not for recurrence**
2. **Expensive** and not freely available.

U:
1. Used by **most cardiologist** in PSVT.
   In recurrent cases—**verapamil** or **β blocker** or **digoxin**.
   Adenosine acts by **hyperpolarising** supraventricular muscle membrane.
2. **DOC** in abolishing AV nodal arrhythmia.
3. To produce controlled **hypotension** during surgery.
4. To **diagnose** tachycardia dependent on AV node.
5. To induce brief coronary **vasodilatation**.

> K^+ depresses ectopic pacemaker specially in digoxin toxicity.
> Mg^{2+} effective in torsade de pointes and digoxin toxicity.

Choice of antiarrhythmics (empirical)
Indications
1. Sustained VT
2. Arrhythmia causing hypotension/cardiac failure
3. Marked palpitation
4. Waring arrhythmia (after MI)

Choice depends on
1. ECG diagnosis
2. Mechansim of arrhythmia
3. Mechanism and range of drug and its PK profile
4. Haemodynamic effect of drug.

Aim: To improve cardiovascular function by restoring sinus rhythm or controlling ventricular rate or conversion to desirable pattern of electrical and mechanical activity.

DOC in arrhythmia

1. **Digitalis induced:** — Phenytoin
   — Lidocaine
   — Propranolol

2. **Ventricular arrhythmia**
   Ventricular extrasystole (VES)   **— Acute**   —Lidocaine
                                    — Chronic — Quinidine
                                                   — Amiodarone

   VT   **— Acute**   — Lidocaine and cardioversion
            — Chronic   — Procainamide (most effective)
                                — Dysopyramide
                                — Quinidine

   VF   **— Acute**   — Essential defibrillation
            — Chronic   — Amiodarone
                                — Quinidine

3. **Supraventricular arrhythmia**
   Sinus bradycardia   — Atropine 0.5 mg IV
   Sinus tachycardia   — Sedative, IV propranolol
   Atrial extrasystole (AES)   — Quinidine
   PSVT   **— Acute**   — Verapamil/Adenosine IV
              — Chronic   — Verapamil (prophylaxis also)
                                    — Digoxin
                                    — Propranolol
   AV block   — Atropine/isoprenaline.
   WPW syndrome:
               — Acute   — Flecainide, encainide and cardioversion
               — Chronic   — Amiodarone, propranolol
   AFl and AF   **— Acute**   — Verapamil, cardioversion
                   — Chronic   — Amiodarone, digitalis, quinidine

---

Nitrates: All organic nitrates are **similar** in actions but **differ** only in time course and cause direct non-specific smooth muscle relaxation.

GTN and **isosorbide** dinitrate terminate **attack** and **all other** (antianginal) drugs are used for **chronic prophylaxis.**

Actions

1. **Preload reduction**

   Vasodilatation (most prominent)
   ↓
   (Veins much more than artery)
   ↓
   Peripheral pooling of blood
   ↓
   Decreased venous return
   (preload decreased)
   ↓
   End diastolic pressure and size reduced
   ↓
   Abolished subendothelial crunch
   and decreased cardiac work
   ↓
   Decreased cardiac work
   ↓
   (Laplace relationship
   Wall tension = Intraventricular pressure × Ventricular radius)
   ↓
   Means ↓ radius
   ↓
   ↓ tension
   ↓
   ↓ O_2 demand

2. **Afterload reduction**

   Arteriolar dilatation
   ↓
   ↓TPR
   ↓
   ↓ afterload on heart
   ↓
   Hypotension
   (systolic > diastolic)
   "Reflex sympathetic activity maintains diastolic BP"
   ↓
   Cardiac work is reduced
   (which is **directly proportional to** aortic impedence)

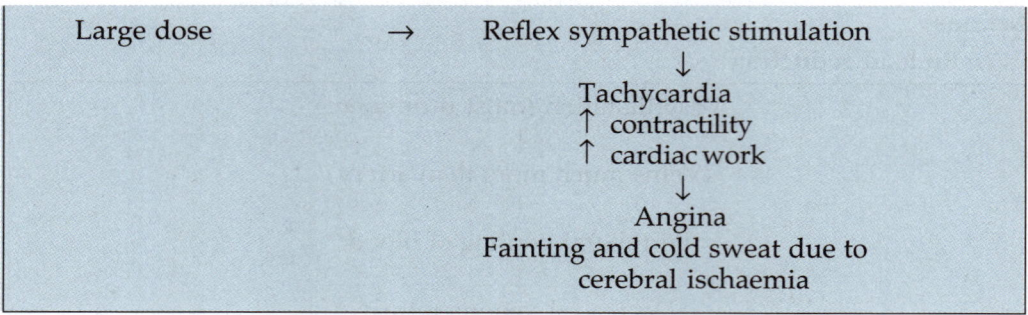

3. **Coronary flow distribution**

   Larger coronary artery dilatation
   (in preference to arterioles/resistance vessel)
   ↓

   Favourable blood redistribution to ischaemic area in angina. But in non-ischaemic area, resistance vessels maintain their tone, hence blood flow is not increased.

   In variant angina, drugs counteract vasospasm. In classical angina, drugs reduce cardiac work by peripheral vasodilatation.

   Exercise tolerance is enhanced due to lesser augmentation of cardiac work by same amount of exercise.

4. Dilates cutaneous (specially on neck and face →flushing) and meningeal vessels (causing headache).

   Splanchnic and **renal blood flow** are reduced to compensate for vasodilatation in other areas and lungs are decongested by shifting blood to systemic circulation.

   Bronchi, biliary tract and **oesophagus are relaxed.**

Antianginal therapy: Goal is to reduce myocardial O_2 consumption (MVO_2) by reducing determinants (end diastolic volume, BP, HR, contractility and ejection time)			
Components	*Nitrates*	*β blocker*	*Nitrates + β blocker*
End diastolic volume	↓	↑	↓/no effect
BP	↓	↓	↓
Contractility	↑ (reflex response) ↓	↓	No effect
HR	↑ (reflex response)	↓	↓
Ejection time	↓	↑	No effect
MVO_2	↓	↓	↓↓
Nifedipine is similar to Nitrates in effect N = N			
Verapamil is similar to β blocker in effect V = B			

Mech

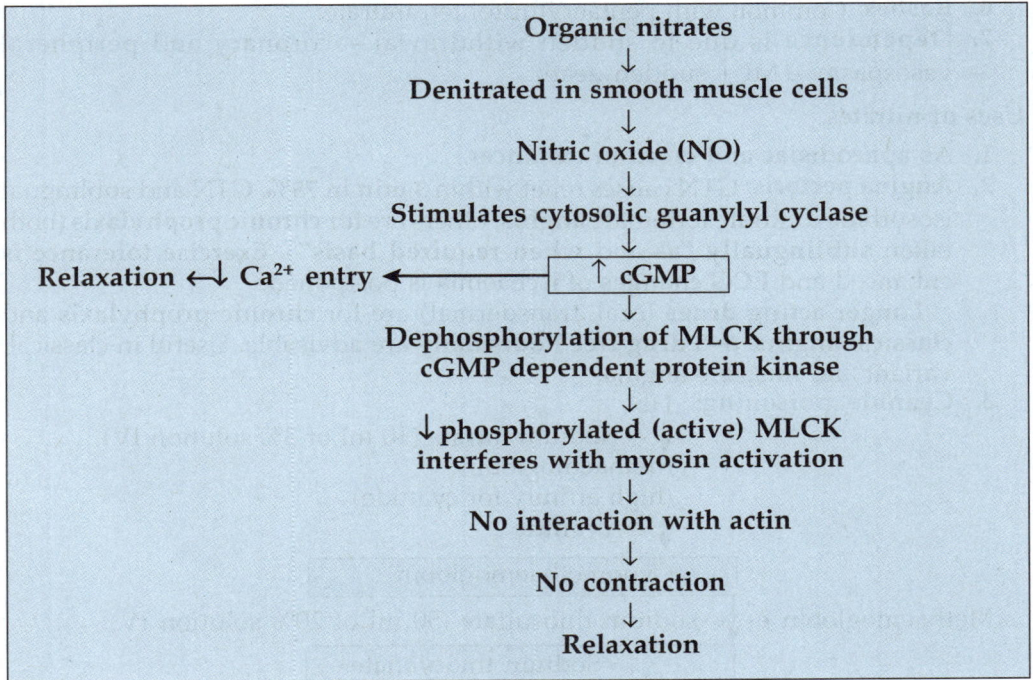

PK: Lipid soluble
Well absorbed from buccal mucosa, intestine and skin.

All undergo extensive and variable **first pass hepatic metabolism except** isosorbide mononitrate. Rapidly denitrated by **glutathione reductase.**

Rate of absorption from administration site and metabolism govern the duration of action (short-and long-acting). **GTN** and **isosorbide dinitrate** are short-acting from sublingual and long-acting from oral route.

ADR (mostly due to vasodilation)
1. **Fullness in head**

    Alternating development of **tolerance** during the **work week** and **loss of tolerance** over the **weekened** for the vasodilating action resulting in tachycardia, dizziness, headache **every Monday.**

    Flushing, weakness, fainting, sweating, dizziness and palpitation are reduced by **lying down** and enhanced by **erect posture plus alcohol.**

    Tolerance with high doses. **Cross tolerance** among **all nitrates.** Agents used to reverse tolerance caused by nitrates →**dithiothreitol or sulfhydryl regenerating agent.**

2. **Throbbing headache (commonest ADR of GTN).**

    Nitroglycerine is used in the manufacture of dynamite, hence "**Monday morning headache**"/**Monday disease** is seen in person working in dynamite factories.

3. **Syncope** (due to postural hypotension).
4. **Methemoglobinemia** is reversed by methylene blue.

5. Reflex tachycardia
6. **Rashes:** Common with pentaerythritol tetranitrate.
7. **Dependence** is due to sudden withdrawal →coronary and peripheral vasospasm →MI + sudden death.

Uses of nitrates

1. As aphrodisiac and erection enhancer.
2. **Angina pectoris:** GTN causes relief within **3 min in 75%**. GTN and sublingual isosorbide dinitrate terminate **angina,** others are for **chronic prophylaxis** (both taken **sublingually "as and when required basis"**). **Exercise tolerance** is enhanced and **ECG changes** of ischaemia is postponed.

    Longer acting drugs (oral, transdermal) are for **chronic prophylaxis** and **classical angina. 6–8 drug free hours daily** are advisable. Useful in classical, variant and unstable angina.
3. **Cyanide poisoning:** Hb
   ↓ ← sodium nitrate (10 ml of 3% solution IV).
   Methaemoglobin
   (high affinity for cyanide)
   ↓ ← cyanide

   Cynomethaemoglobin

   Methaemoglobin ←↓← sodium thiosulfate (50 ml of 20% solution IV).

   Sodium thiocyanate
   ↓
   Excreted in urine

    Thus, oxidative enzymes are protected from cyanide.
4. Esophageal spasm.
5. **Biliary colic** due to disease/morphine: Sublingual GTN/isosorbide dinitrate.
6. **CHF and LVF**

    Nitrates → venous pooling of blood (aided by sitting posture in acute LVF and chronic CHF) →↓ venous return (preload)→↓ end diastolic volume→ improved LV function by Laplace law and regression of pulmonary congestion.

    GTN (DOC) IV: Rate of IV infusion is guided by continuous haemodynamic monitoring.
7. **MI and international cardiac procedure** (coronary angioplasty, thrombolytic therapy of acute MI).

    ### GTN (glyceryl trinitrate/nitroglycerine)

    Volatile liquid absorbed on inert matrix of tablet and rendered **non-explosive,** stored in **closed glass** (no plastic).

Route: **Sublingual** route.

In **oral** route, tablet is crushed over teeth and spread over buccal mucosa.

Mech: **Same** as nitrates (i.e. through NO).

PK: Acts in **1–2 min** due to direct absorption in systemic circulation.

Hepatic metabolism 90%, plasma t½ 2 min.
Duration of action depends on availability of the drug on buccal mucosa.
Oral dose → 5–15 mg.
Rapidly absorbed from **skin** also.
Sustained release capsule for **chronic prophylaxis, IV line** of drug provides rapid, steady, titratable plasma concentration for as long as possible.

U:
1. **Unstable angina:** Sublingual GTN is the **most frequently** used agent for the treatment of angina.
2. **LVF**
3. **Coronary vasospasm**
4. **MI**
5. **HTN** during surgery

Isosorbide mononitrate/dinitrate

Active metabolite of isosorbide dinitrate is isosorbide mononitrate. Isosorbide dinitrate is **solid** and **similar** to GTN in property.

PK: **Sublingually** given in **attack**.
Orally given in **chronic prophylaxis**.

| t½ | — | I. mononitrate | → | 4–6 hrs |
| | — | I. dinitrate | → | 40 min |

Longer acting nitrates are used for **chronic prophylaxis**.

K⁺ channel openers

Intracellular K⁺ concentration — 150 mM
Extracellular K⁺ concentration — 5 mM

Types of K⁺ channels
- Voltage dependent
- Na⁺ activated
- Ca²⁺ activated
- Cell volume sensitive
- ATP sensitive
- Receptor operated

Actions
1. **Most prominent** action of K⁺ channel openers is visceral and vascular smooth muscle **relaxation**.
2. Diazoxide, etc. reduces **insulin** secretion.

Sulfonylurea enhances **insulin** secretion by blocking K⁺ channel leading to **hypoglycaemia**.

Mech: Channel open → K⁺ ion outflow → hyperpolarisation

U: K⁺ channel openers: **ABCDEFGHI-LM**
1. Angina pectoris
2. Bronchial asthma
3. CHF
4. PVD (Raynaud's disease, cerebrovascular disease)

5. Erection disorder of penis
6. Fall of hair/alopecia
7. AntihypoGlycaemic (insulinoma)
8. HTN
9. Urinary urge Incontinence
10. Premature Labour
11. Myocardial salvage in MI.

Nicorandil

Mech: Activates ATP sensitive K^+ channel
↓
Hyperpolarises vascular smooth muscle
↓
Vasodilatation
(antagonised by glibenclamide)

$$\text{Drug} \rightarrow NO \rightarrow \uparrow cGMP \rightarrow \text{vasodilatation}$$

ADR
1. Flushing
2. Palpitation
3. Weakness
4. Headache and dizziness
5. Nausea and vomiting

Oxyphedrine:	Improves myocardial metabolism and sustains **hypoxia** better.
Mech:	Adrenergic effect on heart improving contractility and AV conduction. Reduction in vascular resistance.
U:	Angina and MI.
Cyclandelate:	It is **papaverine like** general smooth muscle relaxant → ↑ cutaneous, skeletal and cranial blood flow in normal person.
ADR:	Palpitation
	Flushing
	Headache
U:	**Placebo for PVD**
	Drugs for PVD are: β agonist
	α blocker
	CCB
	Antioxidant
	(no vasodilator can overcome organic obstruction).

Pentoxiphylline (Oxypentifylline)

It is a **theophylline analogue** and PDE inhibitor.

Mech: Enhanced blood flow in **ischaemic areas** by reducing whole blood viscosity and by improving RBC flexibility.

This **rheological action** (study of property of flow) rather than vasodilatation improves blood flow through microcirculation **(no steal phenomenon)**.

ADR:
1. Dyspepsia
2. Nausea and vomiting
3. Bloating (reduced by taking drug after meal)

U:
1. Non-haemorrhagic **S**troke   **MOST UGC**
2. Chronic cerebrovascular insufficiency
3. **T**ransient ischaemic attack
4. Intermittent **C**laudication (due to diabetic arteriosclerotic and inflammatory vascular disease) →walking distance is enhanced.
5. Trophic leg **U**lcer and **G**angrene.
6. **O**cclusive circulation of retina and cochlea.
7. To improve sperm **M**otility.

Drug therapy in MI

1. Continuous haemodynamic parameter and ECG monitoring
2. Opioid and BZD
3. O_2, IVF (saline/LMW dextran)
4. $NaHCO_3$ for lactic acidosis
5. β blocker (reduces infarct size = myocardial salvage) for arrhythmia
6. Lidocaine (procainamide for tachyarrhythmia)
7. Atropine/electrical pacing for tachyarrhythmia
8. Furosemide (reduces preload), vasodilator, ionotropic agent (to enhance pumping of heart) for pump failure
9. Heparin and oral anticoagulant for thrombus
10. Fibrinolytic agents for thrombolysis
11. ACE inhibitor for remodeling and subsequent CHF
12. Aspirin and hyperlipidemia control for inhibition of future attack

Rational drug combination for angina

1. β blocker + (long-acting Nitrate/slow acting DHP)
   (**verapamil and diltiazem** are SA/AV nodal depressant with β blocker, hence they are **contraindicated**).
   Tachycardia due to nitrate is blocked by **β blocker**. Reduced total coronary flow and ventricular dilatation due to β blocker are **counteracted** by nitrate.
2. Nitrate (↓ preload) + CCB (↓ afterload).
   Used in severe variant angina.
3. Nitrate (↓ preload) + β blocker (↓ cardiac work) + CCB (↓ afterload + ↑ coronary flow) used in severe and resistant cases of classical angina.

B	+	C	+	N
		C	+	N
B	+	D	/	N

Hydralazine

Hydralazine and dihydralazine are direct artery dilators (little action on vein).
  Mech

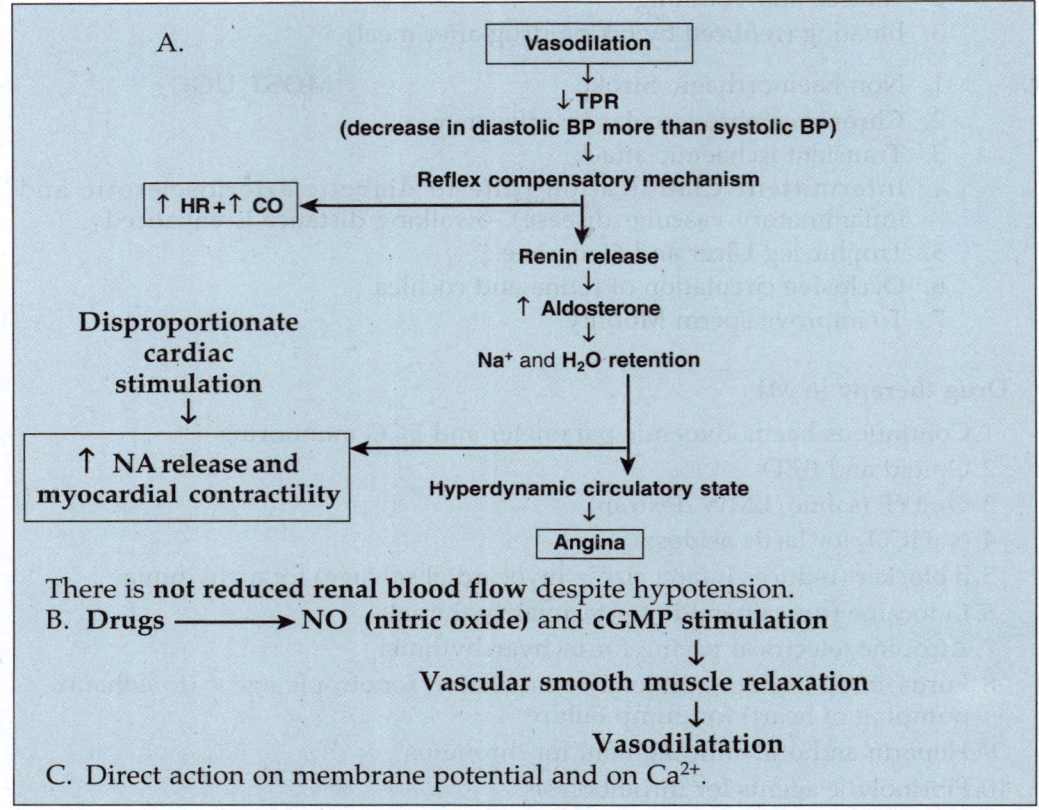

A. Vasodilation → ↓TPR (decrease in diastolic BP more than systolic BP) → Reflex compensatory mechanism → ↑HR + ↑CO; Renin release → ↑Aldosterone → Na$^+$ and H$_2$O retention → Hyperdynamic circulatory state → Angina. Disproportionate cardiac stimulation → ↑NA release and myocardial contractility.

There is **not reduced renal blood flow** despite hypotension.
B. Drugs → NO (nitric oxide) and cGMP stimulation → Vascular smooth muscle relaxation → Vasodilatation
C. Direct action on membrane potential and on Ca^{2+}.

PK: Well absorbed orally (peak 1–2 hrs). Hepatic metabolism through **acetylation** (**slow** and **fast** acetylators).
  Higher bioavailability in **slow** acetylators causing **lupus syndrome**.
  Completely metabolised in liver and plasma → renal excretion.
  t½ → 1–2 hrs
  Dose: **Oral** — 40 mg
       IV/IM — 20 mg

Drugs causing RPGN	
Hydralazine	
Allopurinol	
Rifampicin	
Penicillamine (commonest)	sHARP

ADR (due to vasodilatation)
  1. RPGN
  2. **Longer hypotensive** effect due to its persistence in vessel wall.
  3. Salt rentention, edema

4. Facial flushing, throbbing headache
   5. Nasal stuffiness, dizziness
   6. Angina, MI, palpitation
   7. Peripheral neuritis
   8. Paresthesias, muscle cramp, tremor
   9. **Lupus erythematosus** and **RA like symptoms** develop on prolonged use **(>100 mg/day)** commonly in women and slow acetylator. Slowly reversible on stopping treatment.

CI:
1. Older patient
2. IHD
3. Acute aortic dissecting aneurysm.

U: Not used alone/Large doses not for long period.
1. Moderate to severe **HTN** with diuretic/β blocker.
2. **DOC in HTN during pregnancy.**
3. CHF
4. **Hypertensive emergency.**

Minoxidil

Minoxidil is a vasodilator and action is **similar** to hydralazine (direct artery dilator + little venous dilator). It is a **prodrug.**

Mech:

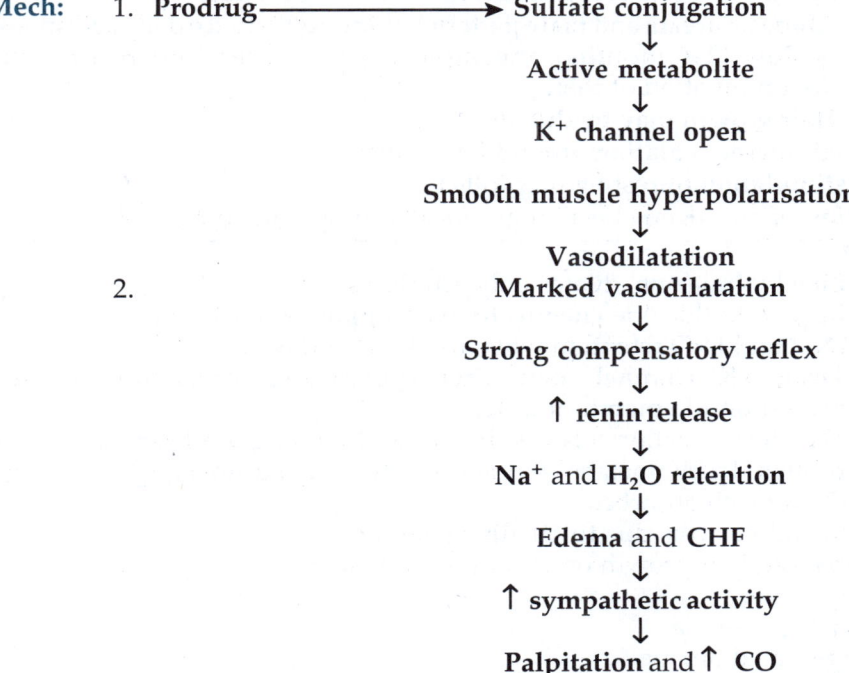

3. Vasodilators (minoxidil, hydralazine) are **alternative to CCB, β blocker, α blocker** and **ACE inhibitor** and are **direct peripheral vasodilator, not used alone due to increase plasma renin activity + CO + HR.**

Actions:
1. Vasodilation
2. Tachycardia

	3. Reduced peripheral resistance
	4. Enhanced CO
	5. Enhanced renin secretion
PK:	Well absorbed **orally**
	Hepatic metabolism and **renal** excretion
	Plasma t½ → 3–4 hrs.
	Duration of action—24 hrs (accumulates in vessel wall).

ADR:
1. **Hair growth** on face, back and arm due to enhanced **cutaneous blood flow.**
   — **Hirsutism**
   — **Hypertrichosis** (so not given in female)
2. **Salt** and **water** retention
3. Local irritation, itching, burning
4. Pericardial effusion with tamponade
5. Angina, tachycardia, MI
6. Headache, dizziness, palpitation and skin reaction in **1–3%**.

CI:
1. Pheochromocytoma
2. Female due to hypertrichosis.

U: Always used with **loop diuretic** and **β blocker**.
1. Life-threatening **HTN** (associated with renal failure).
2. **Alopecia areata** and **male pattern baldness** (2% twice daily). Response is slow (2–6 months), incomplete, 60% success but recurs after discontinuation of therapy.

Hair growth may be due to
A. Enhanced **microcirculation** around hair follicle.
B. **Direct stimulation** of resting hair follicle.
C. **Alteration** of androgen effect on genetically programmed hair follicle.

Diazoxide: Like hydralazine, dilates only **arterioles.**
Related to thiazide **chemically** with **opposite** renal action (Na^+ and H_2O retention when used for >2 days).

Mech: Drug → K^+ channel open → hyperpolarization of smooth muscle → relaxation of smooth muscle.

PK: Duration of action >24 hrs due to tight binding to plasma and tissue protein. Partly metabolised and partly excreted **unchanged in urine.** Orally well absorbed.

ADR:
1. Pain and necrosis due to **alkaline** solution.
2. Enhanced hair growth on chronic oral therapy.
3. Palpitation
4. Hyperglycaemia
5. Aggravated angina

Disadvantage of long-term therapy
1. Na^+ and H_2O **retention** → plasma volume expansion.
2. **Inhibits insulin** secretion from β cells of pancreas → **hyperglycaemia** and DM.
3. Inhibits **uric acid** excretion → hyperpolarisation → gout.

Route: Orally effective in HTN, but causes DM, gout in long-term.
   A. **IV** →antihypertensive.
   B. **Orally** →decreased insulin release from pancreas (hence ineffective to treat if insulin has induced hypoglycaemia).

U:
1. Hypertensive emergency (IV 50–100 mg/10 min)
2. **Alopecia**
3. **Uterine relaxant** to arrest premature labour.
4. **Insulinoma** (antihypoglycaemic): To treat hypoglycaemia from hyperinsulinoma.

> **Trimethaphan:** Rapidly acting ganglionic blocker →reduces sympathetic tone to blood vessel.

Na nitroprusside: It is rapidly and consistently acting **vasodilator**.
   Duration of action→**2–5 min**

Mech
1. **Relaxes** both capacitance and resistance vessels →reduced venous return →↓**TPR** and ↓**CO**
2. Decreased myocardial work but no ischaemia.
3. Increased plasma **renin**.
4. **Drug** $\xrightarrow{\text{RBC, Endothelial cell}}$ **NO** →Relaxation of vascular smooth muscle.

PK:
A. Decomposes on **alkaline pH** and **light**. (hence bottle is covered with **black paper**).
B. **Drug** $\xrightarrow{\text{Liver}}$ **Thiocyanate** →Excreted
   ↓
   Accumulated (if excess)
   ↓
   Toxicity and **psychosis**

ADR:
1. Enzyme for NO production is different from that of GTN (hence **different pattern of vasodilatation** and **no tolerance**).
2. **Cyanide toxicity** (releases CN).
3. **Nervousness, disorientation, perspiration, palpitation, weakness, vomiting.**

U:
1. **Acute hypertensive crisis/hypertensive emergency**
   Acts on both **artery** and **vein**. Used only in **short-term emergency** treatment of acute hypertensive crisis. Onset of action is **instantaneous** and is maximal in **1–2 min**.
2. Refractory CHF, pump failure with MI and acute MR →↓**pre-** and **afterload**.

Dofetilide: Pure class III antiarrhythmic (no autonomic/peripheral action).

Mech: Prolongs APD and ERP by selectively blocking K^+ current only.

U: AF/AFI converted to sinus rhythm in 30% on maintenance).

ADR: Torsade de pointes.

Trimetazidine: Reduces frequency and enhances exercise capacity by non-haemodynamic mechanisms.

Mech: Unknown but improved cellular tolerance to ischaemia is achieved by
 (a) Inhibiting mitochondrial 3-KAT → ↓FA and ↑ glucose metabolism in heart.
 (b) Protecting membrane from free radical (oxygen atom) and limiting intracellular acidosis plus Ca^{2+}, Na^+ accumulation during ischaemia.

PK: Oral absorption, partly metabolised and excreted unchanged in urine, half-life = 6 hours.

ADR: Dizziness, tiredness, muscle cramp, gastric burning sensation.

U: As adjuvant in angina and post MI.

Reserpine: It is an **alkaloid** from roots of *Rauwolfia serpentina* **(Sarpgandha). Pure alkaloid** was isolated in **1955.**

Mech
1. Causes **CA and 5-HT depletion.**
2. Acts at membranes of **intraneural granules storing monoamines** (NA, DA, 5-HT) and **irreversibly** inhibits active amine transport → monoamines depleted and MAO degraded.
   Effects last after drug is eliminated **(hit and run drug)** because tissue CA stores are restored only gradually.

ADR **HEAP**
1. Postural Hypotension and bradycardia (take **2–3 weeks for full effect).**
2. Higher doses → depletion of **CA** and **5-HT in brain also** → sedation and mental depression.
3. Antipsychotic effects + Extrapyramidal symptoms due to DA depletion.
4. Parasympathetic overactivity:
   Bradycardia, diarrhoea, enhanced gastric acid, miosis, postural hypotension, nasal stuffiness, impotence, weight gain, **suicidal** tendency.

CI: 1. Pregnancy 2. Peptic ulcer
 3. Epilepsy 4. Depressive illness

U: As mild antihypertensive: Dose: **0.25 mg/day.**
Acts centrally and peripherally by depleting **CA stores** in the brain and periphery. **Postganglionic adrenergic neurone blockers** are given in patients unresponsive to **all other medications** due to poor tolerance by **most patient (best to avoid)**

Guanethidine: It is a **polar guanidine** compound taken up into adrenergic nerve ending by **active amine transport.**

Mech of actions
1. Decreases NA from storage granules →**NA depletion**.
2. Blocks NA uptake mechanism at axonal membrane → **NA depletion**.
3. Inhibits nerve impulse coupled NA release→**hypotension** and **bradycardia**.
4. **Triphasic action of guanethidine on BP.**

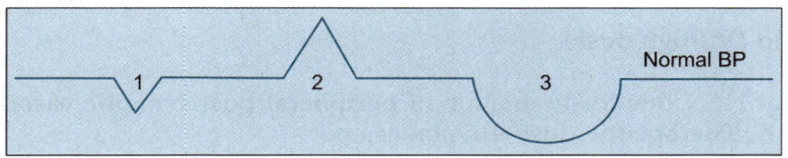

Phase 1 — Direct vasodilatation so hypotension.
Phase 2 — Initial release of NA so HTN
Phase 3 — NA depletion so gradual hypotension

5. Causes **sympathetic blockade** in peripheral neurones. With chronic administration, its **cumulative effect** reduces tissue concentration of NE. This lasts several days after **discontinuation** of drug.

ADR
1. Postural (orthostatic) and excercise **hypotension**.
2. Weakness and **sexual dysfunction**.
3. **Diarrhoea** due to parasympathetic overactivity.
4. **Frank edema** and **CHF** due to Na and H_2O retention.
5. Inhibition of **ejaculation** and impotence in males.

U: HTN: Guanethidine
Guanadrel does not cross to CNS and reduces adrenergic neural activity like guanethidine.

Clonidine: It is a moderately potent **antihypertensive** and is an **imidazoline derivative,** related to:

Nephazoline (α agonist)
Tolazoline (α antagonist)   All these 3 properties are present in clonidine
Antazoline (H_1 antagonist)

Imidazole preferring receptor (IPR) is present in **brain** and **periphery** and is activated by clonidine but not by NA.

Clonidine and methyldopa are central sympatholytics.

Mech: Sympathomimetic (periphery) and ↓sympathetic outflow (CNS).
1. **Selective $α_2$ agonist activity**
   ↓
   Stimulation of central $α_2$ receptor
   ↓
   Sedation and **analgesia**.

   Stimulates presynaptic outflow →↑ vagal tone (↓HR) and ↓ sympathetic derive.

2. Acts as **α-methyl NE** in medulla
3. Reduces NA release from peripheral adrenergic nerve endings (release inhibitory $α_2$ action), by stimulation of presynaptic $α_2$ R.

4. **Stimulates α_2 R in medulla (vasomotor centre) leading to**
   ↓ **sympathetic outflow**
   ↓

   > ↓ vasomotor tone (↓ BP) and ↓ HR
   > (also due to ↑ vagal tone).
   >   Plasma NA declines.

5. **Rapid IV (high dose)**
   ↓

   Transient HTN due to stimulation of **peripheral post-synaptic vasoconstrictor** α_1 and α_2 R. Therapeutic dose → hypotension.

   On **chronic** use → more hypotension is due to reduced CO rather than reduced TPR.

6. Reduces **sympathetic flow** to kidney → reduced **renin** release.
7. Reduces **CNS sympathetic** output.

PK: Well absorbed **orally, 60%** excreted unchanged in urine, plasma t½—**8–12 hrs,** effect last **6–24 hrs.**

Dose: **300 microgram (maximum)** TDS orally/IM

IA: TCA and CPZ block α R and abolish antihypertensive activity.

ADR
1. Acute **withdrawal** HTN.
2. Sedation, mental depression, dry mouth, dry nose, dry eyes (**reduced secretion** by central action).
3. **Impotence, salt** and **water** retention.
4. **Bradycardia** due to reduced sympathetic tone.
5. Postural **hypotension.** Decreases plasma NA concentration and its renal excretion.
6. **Severe rebound HTN,** tachycardia, restlessness, anxiety, sweating, headache, nausea, vomiting on **1–2 missed doses.**
   (**Syndrome** same as in **pheochromocytoma**)

   Increased CA is due to:
   A. Sudden **removal of central sympathetic stimulation** → stored CA release.
   B. **Supersensitivity** of peripheral adrenergic nerve to CA developing due to **chronic reduction of sympathetic tone** during clonidine therapy. **Rigid schedule** prevents withdrawal **syndrome.** Syndrome is treated by **labetalol.**

U:
1. **Moderate HTN** (clonidine + diuretic).
2. **Hypertensive emergency.**
3. **Before surgery:** Reduces dose of GA/LA/analgesia → less CVS depression.
4. **Intrathecal clonidine** (substituted for morphine).
5. **Smoking cessation. Alcohol withdrawal. Opioid withdrawal** (opioid and clonidine stimulate G_i regulatory protein and reduce sympathetic overactivity of opioid withdrawal syndrome).
6. **As analgesia** (substitutes morphine for intrathecal/epidural surgical and postoperative analgesia).
7. Alternates **vasomotor symptoms of menopausal syndrome.**
8. **Diarrhoea** due to diabetic neuropathy (α_2 mediated increased salt absorption in gut mucosa).

9. **Clonidine suppression test for pheochromocytoma** (reduces plasma NA to <0.25 ηg/ml in essential HTN but not in pheochromocytoma).

Methyldopa: It is a **moderate efficacy antihypertensive** and **α methyl analogue of dopa**. It is **precursor of DA** and **NA**.
Mech
1. Reduces **CNS sympathetic outflow** (α_2 action).
2. Methyldopa ⟶ ↓ TPR > ↓HR/↓CO

α-methyl DA ⟵ (Brain)
↓
α-methyl NA (selective α_2 agonist)
↓
Acts on central α_2 R
↓
↓ efferent sympathetic activity from medulla
(nucleus tractus solitarius)
↓
Decreased circulating NA and renin

3. **Large doses** → Inhibits **dopamine decarboxylase** in brain and periphery.
↓
↓NA synthesis and false transmitter
(methyl NA) formation in periphery

PK: Transported actively by amino acid carrier, <33% absorbed orally, **partly metabolised** and **partly excreted unchanged in urine,** effects develop over **6 hrs** and last over **24 hrs.**

ADR
1. **Common:** Sedation, lethargy and reduced mental capacity.
2. **Hypotension**
3. **Cognitive impairment**
4. **Dryness** of mouth, nasal stuffiness, headache
5. **Fluid retention,** weight gain.
6. **Impotence**
7. **Hypersensitivity:** Postive Coombs' test in **17%**, haemolytic anemia, thrombocytopenia, lupus syndrome, flu-like illness, hepatitis, fever, rash.
8. **Rebound HTN** on sudden withdrawal.

ADR of METHYLDOPA
Mental retardation
Electrolyte imbalance
Tolerance
Headache and hepatotoxicity
Yesness/nodding due to parkinsonism
Lactation (in female)
Dry mouth
Oedema
Psychological upset
Anemia (hemolytic)

IA: 1. **TCA** blocks its active transport to adrenergic neurons and reverses its action.
2. **Haloperidol** and **reserpine** enhance CNS symptoms.
U: 1. **Moderate HTN:** Methyldopa + diuretic
2. **LVH** is reversed.
3. **Diastolic dysfunction** is improved.

Treatment of HTN: Treatment is initiated if diastolic BP is >90–95 mm Hg and the **goal** is to reduce the incidence of:
— Heart failure and renal failure.
— Stroke, MI, coronary artery disease.

DOC for HTN — ACE inhibitor
   Beta blocker
   ABCD   CCB
   Diuretic

But "**individual care approach**" is adopted for the selection of initial monotherapy (**50–70% success**).

ACE inhibitors

Indications   ACE
1. Active young patient
2. Coexisting angina, post-MI
   Coexisting LV dysfunction (LVH)/**C**HF
3. **E**nhanced renin cases (those on low salt diet)
   Enhanced glucose intolerance
   Enhanced uric acid
   Enhanced PVD and dyslipidemia

Contraindications
1. Pregnancy
2. Single kidney/bilateral renal artery stenosis.

Cautions
1. Diuretic therapy and dry cough
2. More salt intake

β blockers

Indications   PLANT
1. **P**regnancy
2. **L**ow cost therapy/**L**ow salt diet (high renin cases).
3. **A**ngina/post-MI and coexisting **A**nxiety.
4. **N**on-obese.
5. **T**achycardia and **T**ence young patient

Not indicated in   ABCDEFG
1. **A**sthma, **A**bnormal lipid profile.
   Requirement of optimum physical and mental **A**ctivities.
2. **B**orderline glucose tolerance and **B**radycardia.
3. **C**HF and **C**onduction defects.
4. **D**M and PVD

5. Elderly
6. LV Failure

CCB

Indications   PACES
1. **P**regnancy and **P**VD
2. **A**sthma, **A**ctive patient
3. **C**OPD
4. **E**lderly
5. Isolated **S**ystolic HTN

Not indicated in
1. CHF, conduction defect ⎤
2. Receiving β blocker   ⎥ Verapamil
3. Sick sinus, myocardial inadequacy ⎦ and diltiazem given
4. IHD, LVH
5. BPH
6. Gastroesophageal reflux

Diuretics

Indications   ROLES
1. **R**enal disease with Na^+ retention
2. **O**bese with volume overload
3. **L**ow renin HTN and **L**ow cost therapy
4. **E**lderly
5. Isolated **S**ystolic HTN

Not indicated in   A GDP
1. **A**bnormal lipid profile, **A**ctive young hypertensive.
2. **G**out
3. **D**M
4. **P**IH

Combination therapy for HTN
1. (ACE inhibitor, CCB, vasodilator, diuretic) **enhance plasma renin activity** and (β blocker, methyldopa, clonidine) **reduce plasma renin activity.**
2. **All sympathetic inhibitors** (except β blocker) and **vasodilators** (cause fluid retention and are tolerance dependent) + **diuretics** (inhibit fluid retention and are tolerance dependent).
3. **ACE inhibitor + diuretics** for CHF and LVH.
4. **Hydralazine** and **DHP** (tachycardia by both and ↓TPR by vasodilator) + **β blocker** (↓tachycardia, ↑ TPR by non-selective β blocker).
5. **ACE inhibitor + β blocker/CCB/clonidine or methyldopa.**
   DHP (long-acting) + **clonidine/methyldopa.**
   Prazosin + β blocker.

3 drugs combination for HTN
(i) ACE inhibitor + CCB + diuretic
(ii) ACE inhibitor + β blocker + diuretic
(iii) β blocker + CCB + diuretic   ABC → AC, AB, BC

Combination (i) is for malignant HTN.

Combination to be avoided
1. α/β blocker + clonidine (antagonism).
2. Hydralazine + DHP/prazosin (same haemodynamic action).
3. Diuretic + DHP (no additional antihypertensive action of diuretic).
4. Verapamil/diltiazem + β blocker (AV block and bradycardia).
5. Clonidine + methyldopa or any 2 drugs of same class.
6. Reserpine + β blocker (bradycardia/syncope).

HTN in pregnancy
BP >135/85 mm Hg is dangerous for pregnancy.

Antihypertensives to be avoided in pregnancy
1. ACE inhibitor, losartan → foetal damage and growth retardation.
2. Diuretic → ↓ blood volume → ↑ uteroplacental perfusion deficit.
3. Na nitroprusside → **contraindicated** in eclampsia.
4. Non-selective β blocker → LBW, hypoglycaemia, neonatal bradycardia, decreased placental size.
5. Reserpine: Suicidal depression in mother, nasal obstruction, deranged respiration and temperature control in newborn.

Safer antihypertensive in pregnancy
1. **H**ydralazine
2. **M**ethyldopa
3. **P**razosin and **C**lonidine
4. Cardioselective **β** blocker
5. **D**HP (but weaken uterine contraction during labour).

> HMP and BDC

Hypertensive emergency and urgency
Hypertensive emergency is a severe elevation of BP **(>200/140 mm Hg)** that demands either immediate (within minute/emergency) or prompt (within hours) reductions of BP.

Conditions requiring immediate reduction
— Acute LVF with pulmonary edema
— Dissecting aortic aneurysm
— Acute MI with HTN
— Intracranial haemorrhage
— Hypertensive encephalopathy
— Cheese reaction, clonidine withdrawal

Conditions requiring prompt reduction
— Malignant/accelerated HTN.

Treatment: Reduction in BP must be gradual in prompt reduction **(15 mm Hg decrease in mean arterial pressure over first hour).** Diuretic is avoided initially due to hypovolemia and vasoconstriction induction, unless intravascular fluid overload has been demonstrated.

Combination in urgency (within 2–4 hrs)
1. Nifedipine   + **furosemide**
2. Clonidine   + **furosemide**
3. Captopril   + **furosemide**
4. Hydralazine + **furosemide**

Drugs in emergency (within minute)
1. Na Nitroprusside IV (eclampsia is **contraindicated**).
2. Nitroglycerine IV (in LVF, MI, unstable angina).
3. Diazoxide (aortic aneurysm is **contraindicated**).
   Dose: 20 mg/minute.
   Onset of action → 1–2 min
   Duration of action → 17 hrs

In hyperadrenergic states (pheochromocytoma, cheese reaction, clonidine withdrawal):
DOC—phentolamine/phenoxybenzamine/prazosin (IV).

In aortic dissection:
A. Trimethaphan IV **(most suitable)**
B. β blocker + Na nitroprusside

> **Hypertensive crisis,** is due to **secondary mechanism** →CA is enhanced.
> **Phentolamine test is diagnostic** (phentolamine rapidly **reduces BP** elevated due to **pheochromocytoma, MAO inhibitors, clonidine withdrawal, sympathomimetics/cocaine**).
> Measurement of **urinary CA** is also diagnostic.
> **Treatment:**   α blockers
>   β blockers
>   α + β blockers
>   **Metyrosine** (tyrosine hydroxylase inhibitors)

Unit 5
Drugs for Kidney

33 An Overview of Kidney

180 L of fluid is filtered everyday. **Thick ascending LH** (thick ascending loop of Henle) is **impermeable** to water. Kidney comprises only **0.5% of body weight** but receives **25% of CO**. All Na^+ entered are pumped out into **renal interstitium at basolateral membrane by Na^+, K^+-ATPase energised Na^+-K^+ antiporter.** Basolateral membrane = Blood side.

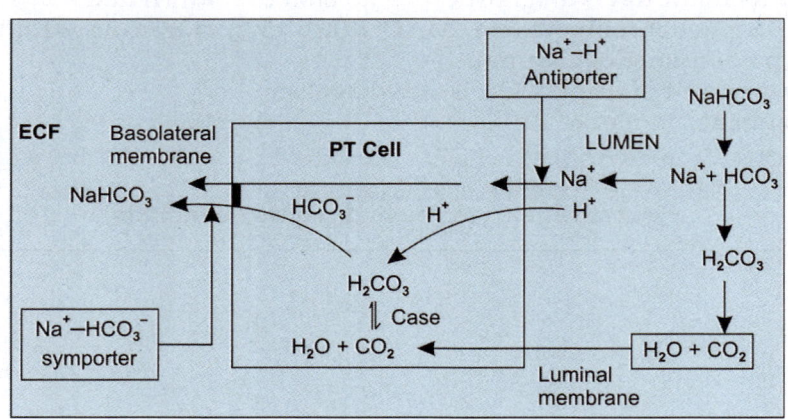

Thick ascending LH has 2 distinct portions
1. Medullary (cuboidal cell)
2. Cortical (flattened cell)

Cuboidal cell
↓
(Na^+-K^+-2 Cl^- cotransport to ECF by Na^+, K^+ ATPase at basolateral membrane plus Na^+-Cl^- symporter moves Cl^- down its electrochemical gradient to ECF and carries Na^+ along)
↓

Hypotonic fluid in tubule
↓
Hypertonic fluid by NaCl accumulated in medullary interstitium (osmotic gradient)
↓
Draws water from descending LH

4 times higher osmolarity of medullary tip **(papilla)** is maintained by **hairpin structure of LH** (acting as passive current multiplier) and **vasa recti** with shunts. Hence, renal papilla is prone to **necrosis**.

Na^+ is reabsorbed at different sites

PT	→	65–70%
Ascending LH	→	20–25%
DT	→	8–9%
CD	→	1–2%

80% nephrons lie in outer cortex with short LH and low Na^+ reabsorption. **20%** nephrons are **juxtamedullary**, have long LH and create **corticomedullary osmotic gradient**. Redistribution of blood flow between these 2 types of nephrons alters **salt and H_2O excretion**.

Sympathetic stimulation of kidney causes **renin release. Adrenergic** drugs enhance **Na^+ and H_2O reabsorption. PG** produced in kidney acts modulator of renal circulation and renin release. **PGE_2** inhibits ADH action. Natriuretic hormone of atrium **ANP** (atrial natriuretic peptide) induces natriuresis in response to salt and volume overload.

Renin-angiotensin-aldosterone system has distal tubular reabsorption of Na^+ and secretion of K^+/H^+.

Site of action of diuretics

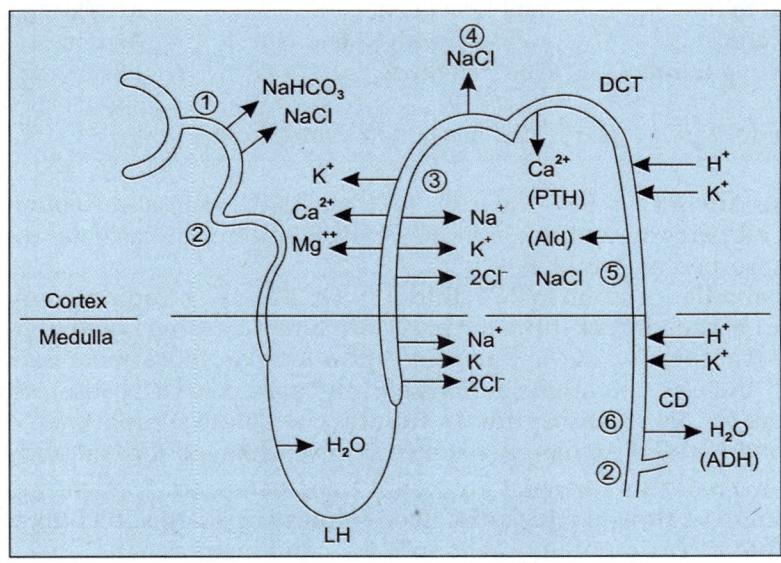

1. Acetazolamide (inhibits Na⁺/H⁺ exchange)
2. Osmotic agent (mannitol)
3. Loop agents (inhibit Na⁺-K⁺-2Cl⁻ cotransport)
4. Thiazides (inhibit Na⁺-Cl⁻ cotransport)
5. Aldosterone antagonist (inhibits Na⁺/K⁺ exchange)
6. ADH antagonist

Site of action of diuretics

Loop diuretics	—	Thick ascending Limb of LH
ThiaziDes	—	DCT
Case inhibitor	—	PCT
K⁺ sparing	—	Cortical collecting tubule
ADH blocker	—	Collecting tubule (CT)
Osmotic diuretic	—	PCT, descending limb of LH, CT

	Sites	Mechanism	Drugs
1.	**PCT**	Osmotic diuretic and C. anhydrase inhibitor	Acetazolamide, mannitol
2.	**Ascending LH**	↓Na⁺ reabsorption with loss of K⁺ at distal tubule → ↓ medullary hypertonicity	**Loop diuretics** Furosemide Bumetanide Piretanide Ethacrynic acid
3.	**Cortical diluting segment**	↓Na⁺ reabsorption with loss of K⁺ at distal tubule	**Thiazides** Chlorthalidone Xipamide Metolazone Mefruside Clopamide
4.	**Distal tubule and cortical collecting tubule**	Inhibition of Na⁺ exchange with K⁺ and H⁺ → K⁺ retention	**K⁺ sparing diuretics** Amiloride Triamterene Spironolactone

(Mefruside is non-thiazide but has action similar to it).

Reabsorption in PCT: 80% NaHCO₃, 40% NaCl, 60% H₂O, and all filtered organic solutes. In all parts of nephron, Na⁺, K⁺-ATPase (pump) in basolateral membrane pumps reabsorbed Na⁺ to ECF.

Cuboidal cells are found in PCT, thick LH, DCT and CD. Sodium pump (Na⁺, K⁺-ATPase) of LH causes back diffusion of K⁺ into lumen causing positivity→electrical potential→reabsorption of Mg²⁺ and Ca²⁺ (thus loop diuretics enhance excretion of NaCl, Mg²⁺ and Ca²⁺). Xanthine inhibits Na⁺ and passively Cl⁻ reabsorptions. **Three mechanisms for Na⁺ reabsorption in tubule:** Na⁺ solute symport, Cl⁻ driven Na⁺ transport and Na⁺/H⁺ exchange (secreted H⁺ is exchanged for Na⁺ and HCO₃⁻).

Seven mechanisms for renal epithelial transmembrane transport of solutes
1. **Connective flow** in which dissolved solutes are dragged by bulk water flow.
2. **Simple diffusion** of lipophilic solutes across membrane.

3. **Channel mediated** diffusion (diffusion of solute through pore).
4. **Carrier mediated** (facilitated) diffusion/uniport:
   Solute transport by carrier protein down electrochemical gradient.
5. **Primary active transport** (ATP mediated): Solute transport by carrier protein against electrochemical gradient using ATP.
6. **Secondary active transport** (ATP mediated)→free energy of electrochemical gradient: (a) **Symport** (cotransport of solute in same direction): Transport of one solute coupled to that of another, both being transported across a membrane in the same direction. (b) **Antiport** (countertransport of solute in opposite direction): Two solutes are exchanged across a membrane. Symport and antiport respectively, of solutes with one solute travelling "uphill" against electrochemical gradient and the other solute travelling down electrochemical gradient.

CD: Principal cells cause Na^+, K^+ and H_2O transport. Intercalated cells cause H^+ secretion. Aldosterone in CD causes Na^+ reabsorption via conductive channel and H^+ plus K^+ secretion (CD has apical membrane channel and basolateral membrane sodium pump).

Distal nephrons reabsorb Na^+, urea and water and secrete K^+ and H^+, Na^+ reabsorption occurs along with electrochemical gradient followed by active extrusion across basolateral membrane. In **thick ascending LH**, Na^+ reabsorption is coupled to K^+ and $2Cl^-$ (Na^+-K^+-$2Cl$ symport).

34

Diuretics

Diuretics (net loss of Na^+ and water in urine). One of the **most widely** prescribed drugs is diuretic.

Classification
1. **High efficacy diuretics (inhibitors of Na^+-K^+-$2Cl^-$ cotransport)**
   (a) **Sulphamoyl derivatives:** Furosemide, bumetanide, piretanide
   (b) **Phenoxyacetic acid derivative:** Ethacrynic acid
   (c) **Organomercurials:** Mersalyl
2. **Medium efficacy diuretics (inhibitors of Na^+-Cl^- symport)**
   (a) **Benzothiadiazines (thiazides):** Chlorothiazide, hydrochlorothiazide, polythiazide, cyclopenthiazide, benzthiazide, hydroflumethiazide, bendroflumethiazide, clopamide.
   (b) **Thiazide like (related heterocyclics):** Chlorthalidone, metolazone, xipamide, indapamide.
3. **Weak/adjuvant diuretics**
   (a) **Carbonic anhydrase inhibitors:** Acetazolamide, ethoxzolamide topical ($\downarrow$IOP): Brinzolamide, dorzolamide.
   (b) **Potassium sparing diuretics**
      (i) **Aldosterone antagonist:** Spironolactone
      (ii) **Directly acting (inhibitors of renal epithelial Na^+ channel):** Triamterene, amiloride.
   (c) **Xanthines:** Theophylline (renal adenosine α_1 blocker)
   (d) **Osmotic diuretics:** Mannitol, isosorbide, glycerol
   (e) **Acidifying or alkalinizing salts:** Ammonium chloride, potassium citrate, potassium acetate.
   (f) **Action on renin—AT system:** NSAIDs and ACE inhibitors.
   (g) **Uricosuric diuretics:** Tienilic acid, indacrinone.

> Diuretic efficacy: Loop > thiazide > K^+ sparing diuretics.

Furosemide/frusemide (prototype drug): It is **sulfonamide** loop diuretic. It is **stronger** diuretic and **weaker** antihypertensive than thiazides. This **high ceiling (loop)** diuretic inhibits Na^+-K^+-$2Cl^-$ **cotransport**.

Maximum **natriuretic effect** is greater than that of other classes (**10 L/day** urine may be produced). Acts at LH hence called Loop diuretic.

Mech (furosemide)

1. Na^+ and Cl^- **cotransport** is blocked at macula densa.
2. Inhibits Na^+-K^+-$2Cl^-$ **cotransport** at **thick ascending LH (site 3)**.
3. Abolishes **corticomedullary osmotic gradient to block positive and negative free water clearance**. Abolishes **hypertonicity** of medulla inhibiting urine concentration.

> **Loop** diuretics principally act at **ascending LH** where they inhibit cotransport of Na^+ and Cl^- from lumen filtrate. They enhance excretion of Na^+, Cl^- and H_2O and reduce **uric acid** secretion but cause no change in urinary pH. **High efficacy** diuretics mainly act at **thick ascending LH**, **medium efficacy** diuretics act at **cortical diluting segment of LH**. Diuretics are **contraindicated** in toxaemia and pregnancy as blood volume is low despite edema.

4. Enhanced K^+ **excretion** is due to high Na^+ load reaching DT.
5. Furosemide and bumetanide have **weak CAse inhibitory** action and enhance HCO_3 excretion (action independent of acid–base balance of body).
6. Increases Ca^{2+} and Mg^{++} excretion (thiazide reduces Ca^{2+} excretion).
7. Reduces **renal uric acid excretion** (blood uric acid level is enhanced) due to interference with tubular secretion of uric acid and enhanced reabsorption in PT. **Hyperuricemic** and **hyperglycaemic** actions are lower than that with thiazides.

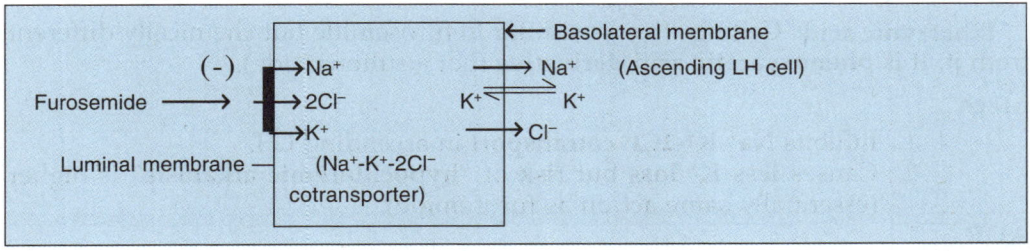

8. **Glycoprotein with 12 membrane spanning domains** acts as Na^+-K^+-$2Cl^-$ cotransporter in epithelia performing secretory or absorbing function including Ascending LH. Furosemide is attached to Cl^- binding site of this protein and inhibits its transport function **(molecular mechanism)**.
9. Furosemide IV causes enhanced systemic venous capacitance and reduced LV filling pressure → quick relief in LVF and pulmonary edema.
10. Causes acute changes in **systemic** and **renal haemodynamics**. After 5 min of IV, renal blood flow is transiently enhanced and there is redistribution of blood flow from outer to mid cortical zone (**GFR unaltered** due to compensatory mechanism).

    Reduced PT reabsorption is due to altered pressure relationship among **vascular, interstitial** and **tubular compartments**. Enhanced local **PG synthesis** causes intrarenal haemodynamic changes.

> Loops Lose Ca^{++}, Mg^{++}, and K^+

PK (Furosemide): **Onset** of action:
- IV → 5 min
- IM → 10–20 min
- Oral → 20–40 min

Duration of action → 3–6 hrs. Rapidly absorbed **orally**.

Bioavailability **60%**. Low **lipid** solubility and highly bound to plasma protein. Partly conjugated with **glucuronic** acid and mainly excreted unchanged by glomerular filtration and proximal tubular secretion. Some excreted in **bile** and directly in intestine.

Competition with transport of uric acid at same site leads to **hyperuricemia**. Plasma t½ → **1–2 hrs** (prolonged in pulmonary edema, renal and hepatic insufficiency).

Usual dose → **20–80 mg** OD in morning.

Piretanide: **3–5 times** more potent than furosemide.

Bumetanide: **Same** as furosemide but **40 times** more potent and induces very rapid diuresis.

PK: More **lipid** soluble, oral bioavailability → **80–100%**, bound to plasma protein, partly metabolised and partly excreted **unchanged in urine**, plasma t½ → **1–1½ hrs**.

Dose: — Oral → 1–5 mg
IV/IM → 2–4 mg (**maximum** 15 mg in renal failure).

U: 1. Pulmonary edema
2. Furosemide resistant cases

Ethacrynic acid: Ceiling effect is **similar** to furosemide but chemically different from it. It is **phenoxyacetic acid derivative** (not a sulfonamide).

Mech
1. Inhibits Na^+-K^+-$2Cl^-$ **cotransport** in ascending LH.
2. Causes **less K^+ loss** but risk of **"hypochloremic alkalosis"** is higher (essentially **same action** as furosemide).

ADR
1. **Similar** to furosemide **except** no hyperuricemia and no sulfa allergy are present.
2. Hearing loss
3. Hepatotoxic

U: Diuresis in patient allergic to sulfa drugs.
(Uricosuric congener of ethacrynic acid in patient with hyperuricemia is **Indacrinone** and **Tricrynafen**).

Uses of loop diuretics
1. Edema (renal and resistant)—**DOC**
2. Acute pulmonary edema (acute LVF with MI)—**DOC**
3. ARF—**DOC** furosemide
4. CHF—**DOC** furosemide
5. **Cerebral edema**
6. **Forced diuresis**
7. **Anemia:** Given with blood transfusion to inhibit vascular overload.

8. **Hypercalcaemia** and **renal Ca²⁺ stone**
   Enhance Ca²⁺ excretion and urine flow → excess salt loss must be replaced. **DOC**—loop diuretic.
9. HTN due to renal failure, fluid retention and CHF: Action is more intense but of shorter duration **(1–4 hrs)** than that of thiazides. Causes decrease in BP due to decrease plasma volume and decrease CO. **Fluid** and **electrolyte imbalance** is caused by loop diuretic. In **HTN due to chronic renal failure, thiazide is ineffective.**
   Loop diuretic is also used in **resistant to combination regimen containing thiazide.**

Advantages of diuretic as antihypertensive
A. Once per day
B. No fluid retention and no tolerance
C. Low incidence of postural hypotension
D. Low cost
E. Less risk of hip fracture in elderly in comparison to hypocalciuric action of thiazide

Thiazides and related diuretics (inhibitor of Na⁺-Cl⁻ symport)

Moderately efficacious diuretics (as 90% glomerular filtrate is reabsorbed before it reaches their site of action). Thiazide reduces **MI by 27–44%** and incidence of stroke by **31–49%**.

Mech of thiazide

1. Inhibits **Na⁺-Cl⁻ symport** at the luminal membrane of cortical diluting segment/early DCT (site 4)→inhibition of NaCl reabsorption in early DCT reducing diluting capacity of nephron and Ca²⁺ excretion.
2. Reduces **+ve free water clearance** (in the absence of ADH) but does not effect –ve free water clearance (in the presence of ADH).
3. Like Na⁺-K⁺-2Cl⁻ cotransport, Na⁺-Cl⁻ symporter is a **glycoprotein with 12 membrane spanning domains** but it does not bind furosemide or any other class of diuretics.
4. Causes **decreased Ca⁺⁺** and **urate excretion** and increased **Mg⁺⁺ excretion** (**Ca⁺⁺** and **Mg⁺⁺** by direct distal tubule action). Increased Na⁺ in tubular fluid holds:
   A. Water in the nephron → **diuresis**.
   B. Enhanced Na⁺/K⁺ exchange →**hypokalemia**.
      Increased Na⁺ is presented to distal nephron and exchanges with K⁺ → urinary K⁺ excretion is enhanced.
5. Reduces blood volume→↓**GFR** (hence not effective in patient with low GFR). Causes slow BP fall.
6. Reduces insulin release → **hyperglycaemia**.
7. **Thiazides in DI**
   A. Drug → state of sustained electrolyte depletion → glomerular filtrate completely reabsorbed **iso-osmotically** in PT.
   B. Drug → ↓**salt absorption** in CD → smaller volume of less dilute urine passed out. (Salt restriction has same effect.)
   C. Drug → ↓**GFR** →↓ tubular fluid load.

8. **90%** glomerular filtrate has been reabsorbed before reaching the site of action of these diuretics, hence they are **medium efficacy diuretic.**

Effects of thiazides

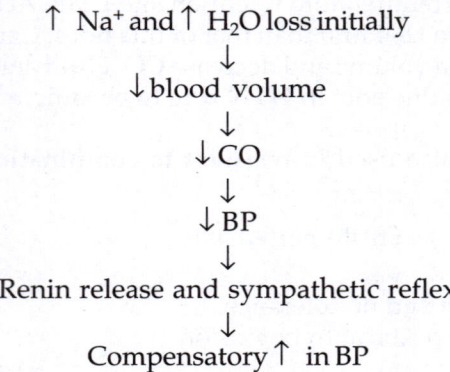

Thiazides later cause **direct vasodilatation** which reduces **peripheral resistance** →↓ **BP.**

PK (thiazides): High salt intake leads to **H_2O retention** which reduces **effectiveness** of thiazides. All are absorbed **orally.**
Onset of action → **one hr**
Duration of action → **varies**
More **lipid** soluble agents have longer volume of distribution, lower rate of renal clearance and are longer acting. **Little hepatic** metabolism. Excreted **unchanged.** Filtrated at glomerulus and secreted in PT. Competition with the transport of **uric acid at the same site** leads to **hyperuricaemia.**

IA of thiazides and loop diuretics

1. Thiazides potentiate **all antihypertensives except DHP** and prevent tolerance by inhibiting plasma volume expansion.
2. Both potentiate **all other antihypertensive** drugs (therapeutically useful).
3. **Hypokalemia** induced by these diuretics enhances **digitalis toxicity** and incidence of **polymorphic ventricular tachycardia** due to quinidine, **potentiates** competitive **neuromuscular** blocker and reduces **sulfonylurea** action.
4. Loop diuretics and aminoglycosides produce additive **toxicity** and **nephrotoxicity** due to their toxic action (hence **not given together**).
5. Loop diuretics enhance nephrotoxicity of **aminoglycosides** and first generation **cephalosporin.**
6. Diuretics and cotrimoxazole cause **thrombocytopenia.**
7. **Most NSAIDs** reduce actions of loop diuretics by inhibiting **PG synthesis** in the kidney.
8. **Probenecid** competitively inhibits tubular secretions of diuretics (reduces their action by reducing the concentration in the tubular fluid through which they reach the site of action).
    Diuretics reduce **uricosuric** action of probenecid.
9. Enhanced **Li^+ reabsorption** in DT due to diuretics enhances serum Li^+ level.

ADR of thiazides and loop diuretics (due to fluid and electrolyte changes)
1. Acute **isotonic saline** depletion (hence Na⁺ and Cl⁻ levels are normal).
2. Dilutional **hyponatremia** of CHF→H₂O retention but salt excretion→diluted ECF→hyponatremia (**but edema persists**).

   Treatment: A. Stop diuretic
   B. Restrict water intake
   C. Glucocorticoid (enhances water excretion)
3. **Mg⁺⁺ depletion.**
4. **Hypokalemia: Most significant ADR, duration of action dependent. Serious complication:** Weakness, fatigue, muscle cramp, cardiac arrhythmia.

   Treatment: A. Increased dietary K⁺ intake.
   B. **KCl 24–72 mEq/day.**
   C. Use of K⁺ sparing diuretic
   D. **Maintain K⁺ >3.5 mEq/L**
   E. Captopril + thiazide (inhibit hypokalemia)

   KCl plus diuretic (combined) are not given due to
   A. Containing insufficient K⁺ (**8–12 mEq only**)
   B. **Gut ulceration** by releasing KCl
   C. **Better K⁺ retention** (after diuresis is over)
5. **Hypocalcaemia with loop diuretics**

   Diuretics Deplete **Na⁺, Mg⁺⁺, K⁺, Ca⁺⁺** and **saline.**

6. HyperGlycaemia is due to inhibition of insulin release →**DM.**
7. HyperLipidaemia: A. ↑ LDL cholesterol
   B. ↑ total cholesterol
   C. ↑ triglyceride
   D. ↓ HDL
8. HyperCalcaemia with thiazides. High ceiling diuretic→Low Ca²⁺

   Thiazide is **the only diuretic** causing hypercalcaemia.
9. HyperUricaemia occurs in **30% cases → 2% develops gout. Thiazide > Furosemide.** hyper, GLUC
10. Hepatic coma due to hypokalemia, alkalosis and enhanced level of NH₃ in blood.
11. **ADR commonest** with Ethacrynic acid is GIT and CNS disturbance.
12. Sulfa Allergy: Rashes and photosensitivity specially in sulfonamide hypersensitive patient.
13. Renal insufficiency due to ↓GFR. Nephritis (interstitial) is also present.
14. Deafness (with loop diuretics specially ethacrynic acid).

    Earliest symptom of ototoxicity is "high pitched tinnitus".

    Deafness is due to increased salt content of **endolymph** and **direct toxic action on hair cells** in internal ear. **Reversible dose related ototoxicity** (both cochlear and vestibular) is present.

15. **ADR of furosemide** **HEARD**
    A. Delayed closure of **patent ductus arteriosus** of infant when given to nursing mother.
    B. Nocturia ⎫
    C. Prostatism ⎬ In elderly patient
    D. Urinary retention ⎭

CI of thiazides and loop diuretics

PIH due to low blood volume despite edema
↓
Further decrease in blood volume and compromised placental circulation
↓
Miscarriage and foetal death

Uses of thiazides

1. **HTN (thiazides DOC): Hydrochlorthalidone 50 mg (maximum antihypertensive action).** Effective in **30%** cases (**mostly** in low grade HTN). Mild antihypertensive (average decrease in mean arterial pressure **10 mm Hg**). Thiazides cause **arteriolar dilatation** directly and reduce **total fluid volume**. They enhance:
   A. Urinary **excretion of Na⁺** and **H₂O** by inhibiting **Na⁺** and **Cl⁻** reabsorption in the distal renal tubules.
   B. Urinary excretion of **K⁺** and **HCO₃⁻**.
   C. The **effectiveness** of other antihypertensive agents by preventing **re-expansion** of extracellular and plasma volume, except CCB but inihibit development of **tolerance** in them.

   Thiazides reduce plasma and ECF volume by 15%
   ↓
   ↓ CO
   ↓
   **Na⁺ balance and CO restoration
   (by compensatory mechanism)**
   ↓
   Hypotension due to ↓TPR

   (**most probably** due to 5% persisting Na⁺ deficit).
   ↓TPR is also produced by salt restriction and antihypertensive action is lost on high salt intake. **Hypotension** develops gradually over 2–4 weeks.

2. **Nephrogenic diabetes insipidus**
   Paradoxically exert **antidiuretic** effect. Reduce urine volume in both **pituitary origin** and **renal DI** (specially in renal origin where ADH is **ineffective**). But urine is never hypertonic.
   Hydrochlorthalidone **250–50** mg TDS with K⁺ supplements is needed.
   Other drugs for **pituitary DI** is **chlorpropamide** and **clofibrate**.

3. **Hypercalciuria: (DOC—thiazides)** with recurrent renal Ca²⁺ stone:
   Thiazides **(DOC)** act by reducing Ca⁺⁺ excretion.

4. **Edema:**   **Better** for maintenance therapy
          Best in cardiac edema
          But powerless in renal failure

Kwashiorkor results from protein deficient **MEAL**:	
M	— Malabsorption
E	— Edema
A	— Anemia
L	— Liver (fatty)

5. **Hypocalcemia: Thiazides**
   (**Hypercalcemia**—furosemide is given).

Chlorthalidone: It is a long-acting agent
- PK: t½   —   40–50 hrs
- U: HTN.

Metolazone: Also inhibits PO_4^{3-} reabsorption.
- PK: Excreted **unchanged in urine.**
- U: Severe renal failure.

Xipamide: Diuretic action **similar** to low doses of furosemide.
- ADR: Hypokalemia (due to longer duration of action)

Indapamide: Highly **lipid** soluble mild diuretic.
Chemically related to **chlorthalidone.**
- Mech: Reduces **TPR** but **CO is unchanged. Reduces BP at doses which cause little diuresis (hence minimal electrolyte imbalance** and **potassium loss).**
- PK: Well absorbed **orally,** extensively **metabolised.**
    - Elimination t½   —   16 hrs
    - Single dose   —   2.5 mg
- ADR (minor)
    1. **Electrolyte disturbance and K^+ loss**
    2. **GIT intolerance and fatigue**
- CI: Liver and kidney disease
- U: HTN

Resistance of loop diuretics: Refractoriness (progressive edema despite diuretic therapy) is more with **thiazides than loop diuretics.**

Causes of resistance
A. **Nephrotic syndrome** (due to diuretic binding to urinary protein)
B. **Cirrhosis of liver** due to abnormal pharmacodynamic
C. **CHF** due to delayed absorption as a result of intestinal congestion
D. **Renal insufficiency** and **advanced age** due to decreased diuretic to its site of action as a result of low GFR and proximal tubular secretion
E. **Distal nephron hypertrophy** due to chronic use of loop diuretic

Carbonic anhydrase inhibitors (CAse inhibitors)
Organs in which CAse is present: Carbonic anhydrase **PER KG**
— CNS
— Pancreas (exocrine)
— Eye
— RBC
— Kidney (PCT in the cortex)
— Gastric mucosa

Pharmacology Review

$$H_2O + CO_2 \xrightleftharpoons{\text{CAse}} H_2CO_3 \rightleftharpoons H^+ + HCO_3^-$$

Functions of CAse: (i) H^+ ion secretion
(ii) CO_2 and HCO_3^- transport

>99% inhibition is needed to produce effects.

Acetazolamide: It is a **sulfonamide** derivative and acts at **PCT**.

Mech:
1. Inhibits **CAse in PCT cell (reversibly** and **non-competitively)** for slow hydration of $CO_2 \rightarrow$ reduces H^+ to exchange with luminal Na^+ through Na^+-H^+ antiporter.
2. Causes **self-limited $NaHCO_3$ diuresis** and decrease in total body HCO_3^- stores.
3. Inhibition of brush border **CAse** retards H_2CO_3 dehydration in tubular fluid so that less CO_2 diffuses back into the cells. **Net effect** is inhibition of HCO_3^- (and accompanying Na^+) reabsorption in PT $\rightarrow$ **alkaline diuresis** ensues.
4. Secretion of H^+ **in DT** and **CD** is inhibited (a subsidiary site of action of carbonic anhydrase inhibitor). CAse mediated reaction generates H^+-**ATPase** which causes H^+ **secretion**.
5. Distal part exchanges Na^+ with K^+ loss.
6. Alkaline urine is produced (rich in HCO_3^-) $\rightarrow HCO_3^-$ depletion $\rightarrow$ **acidosis.**

> **Acetazolamide:** Inhibits both **membrane bound** and **cytoplasmic** forms of CAse $\rightarrow$ complete abolition of Na^+ and HCO_3^- reabsorption. Major site of action is **PT** and **CD**. Inhibition of H^+ secretion, decreased HCO_3^- absorption and decreased net Na^+ reabsorption take place.

7. **Extrarenal actions**
   A. Reduces **IOP in eye** due to reduced **aqueous humour** formation (rich in HCO_3^-).
   B. Reduces **gastric HCl** and **pancreatic $NaHCO_3$** secretion.
   C. Enhances CO_2 **in brain** and reduces pH $\rightarrow$ **sedation** and **seizure** threshold are enhanced.
   D. Alters CO_2 **transport** in lungs and tissues.

PK: Well absorbed **orally**. Excreted **unchanged in urine**.
Duration of action of single dose $\rightarrow$ 8–12 hrs.
Onset of action $\rightarrow$ 1–1½ hrs. Dose $\rightarrow$ 250–1000 mg/day.

ADR
1. **Kaliuresis (most marked** by CAse inhibition among **all diuretics)**.
2. K^+ **depletion**
3. Metabolic **Acidosis** (specially in COPD)

> **ACID**azolamide causes **ACID**osis.

4. **Sulfa Allergy** and NH_3 toxicity
5. **Abdominal** discomfort
6. **Bone marrow depression** (rare but serious)

> Obsoleted CAse inhibitors: Methazolamide, Ethoxzolamide, Dichlorphenamide MED

7. Ca phosphate stone formation due to phosphaturia and hypercalciuria
8. Drowsiness
9. Bicarbonate depletion → hyperchloremic metabolic **alkalosis.**

ABCD

10. **Hypersensitivity** reaction (fever, rashes)
11. Fatigue
12. Paresthesias
13. Neuropathy

CI: Liver disease (hepatic coma)

U: 1. Glaucoma (**commonest** indication)
2. Metabolic **alkalosis** (and to alkalinise urine) because it reduces total body HCO_3^- stores.
3. Epilepsy
4. Acute mountain sickness and periodic paralysis.

Ethoxzolamide: More potent than but similar to acetazolamide.

K^+ sparing diuretics (conserve K^+): These are aldosterone blocker/inhibiting Na^+ channel in **DT** and **CD cells.**

K^+ STAys
Spironolactone
Triamterene and **A**miloride

Spironolactone: It is a **weak diuretic, a mild saluretic** (as more Na^+ is reabsorbed proximal to its site of action) and a **steroid** (chemically related to mineralocorticoid—aldosterone).

Site of action: Cortical collecting tubule. It acts only when **aldosterone** is present.

Mech:
1. Site of action of both aldosterone and drug is **late DT** and **CD cells.**
2. Acts from **interstitial side of tubular cells** and inhibits **AIP** formation. Both drug and aldosterone acts at intracellular **MR** (mineralocorticoid receptor) from interstitial side of tubular cells.

A.
Drug
↓
MR
↓
Competitively inhibition of AIP (aldosterone induced protein) formation
↓
↑ Na^+ and ↓K^+ excretion
(K^+ retaining action develops over 3–4 days)

B.
Aldosterone (Ald)
↓
MR
↓
Complex translocates to nucleus
(mRNA formation)
↓

AIP synthesis
(Na^+, K^+-ATPase and Na^+ channel)
↓
Stimulates Na^+ channel.
Translocates Na^+ channel from cytosolic site to luminal membrane and Na^+, K^+-ATPase to basolateral membrane
Enhances ATP production by mitochondria
↓
Na^+ reabsorption (and K^+ plus H^+ secretion indirectly)

3. **Drugs bind to MR and inhibit aldosterone action.**
4. Enhances Ca^{2+} **excretion** by direct action on renal tubules.

PK: Oral bioavailability—**75%, complete hepatic metabolism.**

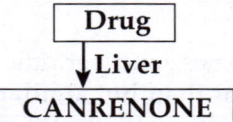

(**Most important** active metabolite 50–70%)
Highly bound to plasma protein

ADR
1. Hyperkalemia **(most serious)**
2. Hyperchloremic metabolic acidosis
3. Hirsutism
4. Impotence
5. Intestinal irregularities and abdominal upset
6. Gynaecomastia
7. Confusion and drowsiness

CI: **Renal failure** (diuretics contraindicated—K^+ sparing diuretics)

IA:
1. Spironolactone and K^+ supplement cause **dangerous hyperkalaemia.**
2. **Aspirin** blocks tubular secretion of canrenone and inhibits action of spironolactone.
3. Enhances plasma **digoxin** concentration.
4. Inhibits **carbenoxolone sodium** induced Na^+ and water retention.

U: (**Spironolactone** and **thiazide** for better action and less K^+ loss)
1. **Hypokalemia** due to loop and thiazide.
2. **Refractory edema** (cirrhotic and nephrotic edema): Drug breaks **resistance** to thiazide developed due to secondary hyperaldosteronism to re-establish the response.
3. **HTN (spironolactone + thiazide):** The most pertinent shared feature of K^+ sparing diuretics is promotion of K^+ retention. They are **less potent** than thiazides and loop diuretics.

Triamterene and amiloride are **nonsteroidal** organic bases with **identical actions.**

Mech
1. **Site of action: CCT** (cortical collecting tubule)/**DT** and **CD cells.** Act directly on **Na^+-K^+ transport** process and are effective even after **adrenalectomy** and **loss of endogenous aldosterone,** then cause **small Na^+ loss and weak diuresis** and reduce K^+ **excretion.** Reduced K^+ excretion is the most important action.

2. Inhibit Na⁺ channel in CCT (DT) thereby causing **diuresis** without risk of K⁺ loss. Amiloride **blocks** Na⁺ channel.
3. Directly acting inhibitor of **renal epithelial Na⁺ channel** generated by **Na⁺, K⁺-ATPase of basolateral membrane**.

$$\downarrow$$

Na⁺ entry causes PD (− 15 mV) = depolarisation

$$\downarrow$$

↑ K⁺ secretion into lumen through K⁺ channel

$$\downarrow$$

Deriving force for K⁺ secretion is increased

$$\downarrow$$

Lumen membrane more depolarised

$$\downarrow$$

↑ Na⁺ delivery to distal nephron
(due to its greater entry through Na⁺ channel)

4. **All diuretics** enhance **K⁺ secretion** but amiloride and triamterene prevent K⁺ excretion by blocking luminal Na⁺ channel.
5. **Intercalated cells** in CD possess **ATP driven H⁺ pump** to secrete H⁺ into the lumen (pump facilitated by **lumen negative potential**).
Amiloride **reduces** lumen negative potential → reduces H⁺ secretion.
6. **Amiloride** is **10 times more potent** than triamterene.
At higher doses, it inhibits **Na⁺** reabsorption in PT. It reduces calcium excretion and enhances **urate** excretion. It blocks **Li⁺ entry** through Na⁺ channel in CD cells and mitigates **Li⁺ induced DI**.

PK

A. **Amiloride:** 1/4th orally absorbed, t½ → 10–20 hrs.
B. **Triamterene:** Incompletely absorbed **orally, hepatic** metabolism → active metabolite, **renal** excretion, plasma t½ → 4 hrs, duration of action → 8 hrs.

ADR

A. **Amiloride:** Muscle cramp, increase urea of blood, impaired GTT and photosensitivity.
B. **Triamterene:** Nausea, diarrhoea and headache.
C. **ADR of both:** Hyperkalemia and antiandrogenic effect **(gynaecomastia)**.

IA

1. Both enhance plasma **digoxin** level.
2. With **ACE inhibitors,** they cause hyperkalemia.

U

A. **Amiloride**
1. **Cystic fibrosis** by increasing fluidity of respiratory secretions.
2. Li⁺ induced nephrogenic **DI** (amiloride—**DOC**).

B. **Uses of both**
1. **Hyperaldosteronism**
2. **Hypokalaemia** (thiazide/loop) + (amiloride/triamterene)
Inhibit hypokalaemia and enhance antihypertensive and natriuretic effects.

> **Diuretics** and **metabolic disorders**
> 1. Acetazolamide →**hypokalaemic hyperchloremic metabolic acidosis.**
> 2. K⁺ sparing diuretic→**hyperkalaemic hyperchloremic metabolic acidosis.**
> 3. Thiazide and loop diuretic →**hypokalaemic metabolic alkalosis.**

Osmotic diuretics

Functional criteria
1. Inert with **limited** metabolism
2. Freely **filtered** at glomerulus
3. Enhanced **renal flow**

Mannitol
Mannitol is a **6 carbon alcohol**, pharmacologically **inert** and **non-electrolyte** of MW-**182**. Site of action: Proximal tubule.

Mech
1. Enhances **urinary** volume with enhanced excretion of **all ions** (cations and anions).
2. **Limits** tubular **water** and **electrolyte** reabsorption in many ways:
   A. Expands ECF volume (increases **GFR**, inhibits **renin** release and reduces **blood viscosity**).
   B. Enhances renal blood flow
   ↓
   Reduces medullary hypertonicity
   (specially to medulla)
   ↓
   Reduces H₂O extraction from descending thin limb
   (Dissipated corticomedullary osmotic gradient)
   ↓
   Reduces passive salt reabsorption in thin ascending LH
3. Retains water **iso-osmotically** in PT (lumen fluid dilution →inhibition of NaCl reabsorption).
4. Inhibits **transport** process in thick ascending LH **(most important)**.
5. Osmotic diuretics are **filtered** by kidney and **not absorbed**.
   ↓
   Thus, **osmotically** hold water in **tubules**.

↑ urine flow
↑ ECF volume
↓
Edema

PK: Not metabolised in the body, freely filtrated at glomerulus and undergoes **limited** reabsorption (hence **exceptionally** suited as osmotic diuretic). Not absorbed orally.

Diuretics

IV (10–20% solution given), t½ →30–90 min.

ADR: Headache, nausea, vomiting and **hypersensitivity** reaction.

CI 　　　　　No CAN HELP
1. As **N**atriuretic
2. Treatment of **C**hronic edema
3. **A**nuria
4. Acute tubular **N**ecrosis
5. Cerebral **H**aemorrhage
6. **E**stablished ARF
7. Acute **L**VF
8. **P**ulmonary edema

U: 1. To maintain **GFR** and **urine flow** in "**impending ARF**" (trauma, cerebrovascular surgery, haemolytic reaction).

Mannitol is **contraindicated** if kidney forms **no urine** (as it expands plasma volume → pulmonary edema and heart failure).

2. **Cerebral edema**
3. **Glaucoma**
4. Forced diuresis in hypnotic and other **poisoning.**
   A. Decreases tubular H₂O reabsorption → decreases poison reabsorption.
   B. Dilution of poison.
5. To counteract **low osmolarity of plasma/ECF** due to rapid haemodialysis/peritoneal dialysis.

Diuretics and electrolyte changes
1. **Urine NaCl** → is enhanced by **all** diuretics (loop, thiazide, CAse inhibitor and K⁺ sparing).
2. **Urine K⁺** → is enhanced by **all** diuretics except K⁺ sparing diuretics.
3. **Blood pH** is reduced by K⁺ sparing diuretics and CAse inhibitors **(acidosis)** and enhanced by loop and thiazide diuretics **(alkalosis)**

　　　　　　　Loop and thiazide Lower H⁺

Diuretics	Renal excretion			
	Na⁺	K⁺	Cl⁻	HCO₃⁻
Furosemide	↑↑↑	↑	↑↑	↑
Ethacrynic acid	↑↑↑	↑	↑↑↑	×
Thiazide	↑↑	↑	↑	↑
Acetazolamide	↑	↑↑	↓↑	↑
Spironolactone	↑	↓	↑	↑
Triamterene	↑	↓	↑	↑
Mannitol	↑↑	↑	↑	↑

NH₄Cl (Ammonium chloride)
Mech

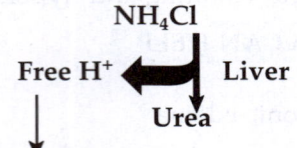

Acidosis (acidifies urine and enhances elimination of weak base)
↓
Enhanced elimination of acid and Cl⁻ (compensatory mechanism of kidney)
↓
Diuresis

PK: Less effective than mannitol as **50%** urea is reabsorbed from tubular fluid, unpleasant taste. **Dose:** 4–8 gm/day.

ADR: 1. Thrombosis and pain   2. Unpleasant taste

CI: Renal insufficiency; **Liver** disease.

U: To acidify urine (30% urea + 10% dextrose IV). Dextrose prevents **haemolysis**.

Pot. citrate/acetate: Alkalinise urine, change pH but are not diuretic.

Uricosuric diuretics (tienilic acid and indacrinone)

Mech: Act at multiple sites in nephron.

U: Not used due to toxic effect.

Ototoxic drugs | BCD, SEP   MAC, VAC |

A. Beta blocker (propranolol, oxprenolol, practolol)
   Cisplatinum
   Diuretic (loop) and quinine
   Salicylate
   Ethosuximide ⎤
   Phenytoin   ⎦ Vestibulotoxic

B. Minocycline
   Ampicillin
   Chloramphenicol
   Capreomycin
   Vancomycin
   Aminoglycoside
      (i) Amikacin and neomycin
          Auditory > vestibular
      (ii) Gentamicin and streptomycin
          Vestibular > auditory

K^+ sparing diuretics:
Spironolactone, Triamterene, Amiloride.
Clinical uses:
1. **Secondary hyperaldosteronism:** As seen in cirrhotic, nephritic and refractory edema.
2. **To** counter K^+ loss due to thiazide and loop diuretics.
3. **Adjuvant** use with other diuretics as in hypertension.

35

Antidiuretics

Antidiuretics (reduce urine volume specially in DI)
1. **ADH/vasopressin, desmopressin, lypressin, terlipressin.**
2. **Thiazide—amiloride.**
3. **Others—clofibrate, carbamazepine, chlorpropramide.**

ADH (Antidiuretic Hormone)

ADH is an **octapeptide** secreted by posterior pituitary **(neurohypophysis)** along with **oxytocin**, synthesized in hypothalamic **(supraoptic** and **paraventricular)** nerve cell bodies as a large cell precursor peptide along with **neurophysin** (its binding protein) and transported down the axon to nerve endings in **median eminence** and **pars nervosa. Osmoreceptors** of hypothalamus and **volume receptors** of left atrium, ventricles and pulmonary veins regulate **rate of ADH release** governed by body hydration. Impulses from **baroreceptors** and higher centres also regulate its synthesis and release. Increase plasma osmolarity and contraction of ECF volume are 2 physiological stimuli for ADH release.

ADH secretion is enhanced by   **PHARMA**
PG
Histamine
ACh
neu**R**opeptide
Morphine
AT II

ADH secretion is inhibited by   **GAP**
GABA
ANP (atrial natriuretic peptide)
Peptide (endogenous opioid peptides)

AVP (8-arginine-vasopressin) is mammalian ADH.
Lypressin (8-lysine-vasopressin) is found in swine.
ADH receptors (G-protein coupled cell membrane receptors) are of **2 types:**
A. V_1 B. V_2

A. V_1 **receptors: Except** in renal CD cells and some **vessels, all receptors** are V_1 types. **2 subtypes (V_1 R).**
   a. V_1a present on smooth muscle, platelet and liver.
   b. V_1b present on anterior pituitary.

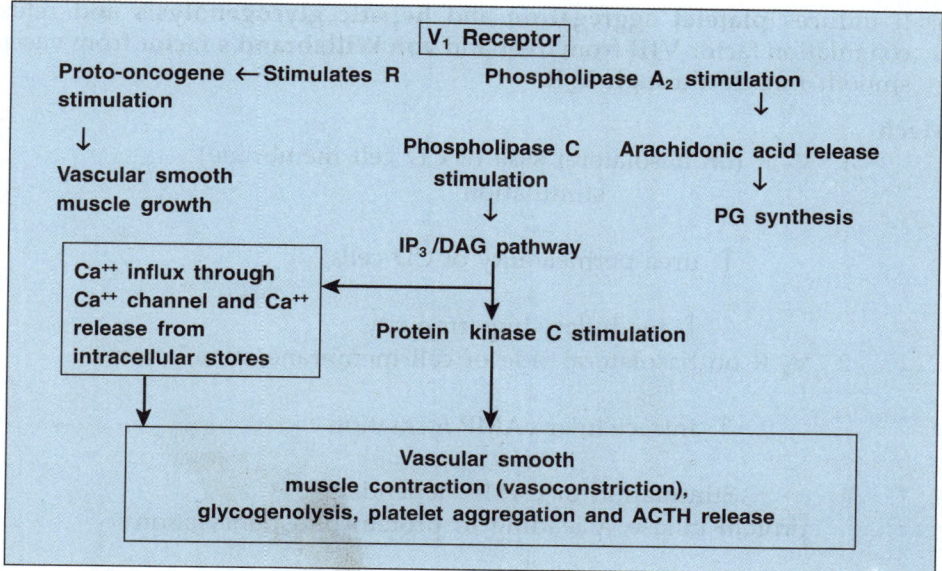

B. **V₂ receptors**: These are present on **renal CD cells** (for water permeability regulation through **cAMP** production) and on blood **vessels** (for vasodilatation). V₂ receptors are **more sensitive to ADH** than V₁ receptors.

Actions

1.
$$\text{ADH acts on CD cells}$$
$$\downarrow$$
$$\uparrow H_2O \text{ permeability}$$
$$\downarrow$$
H₂O from lumen to interstitium
(maximum osmolarity of urine attained
is 4 times higher than plasma)

   Dilute urine is produced in the absence of ADH.

2. **V₁ actions** restrain V₂ mediated water permeability and restrict V₂ effect (when **plasma AVP** level is high)

3. **At high dose**
$$V_1 \text{ Receptor}$$
$$\downarrow$$
$$\text{Vasoconstriction}$$
$$\downarrow$$
$$\uparrow BP \text{ (hence the name vasopressin)}$$

   Cutaneous, mesenteric, thyroid, skeletal muscle, fat depot and coronary beds are **constricted**.

   Chronic AVP use causes **vascular smooth muscle hypertrophy**.

4. **Gut** and **uterus** are contracted. AVP acts on oxytocin receptors. Oxytocin is **equipotent** to AVP in non-pregnant and early pregnancy but at term, its sensitivity is enhanced **selectively**.

5. It does **not cross blood–brain barrier** but in **CNS**, it is a **peptide neurotransmitter** for temperature regulation, circulation, ACTH release and learning of tasks.

6. It induces **platelet aggregation** and **hepatic glycogenolysis** and releases coagulation factor **VIII** from liver and **von Willebrand's factor** from vascular smooth muscle through **V₂R**.

Mech

1. $V_2 R$ (on basolateral side of CD cell membrane) stimulation
   ↓
   ↑ urea permeability of CD cells
   ↓
   ↑ medullary hypertonicity

2. $V_2 R$ on basolateral side of cell membrane stimulation
   ↓
   ↑ intracellular cAMP formation
   ↓
   Stimulation of cAMP dependent protein kinase A leading to protein phosphorylation
   ↓
   Promotes exocytosis of "Aquaporin CD" water channel having vesicles (WCV) through apical membrane
   ↓
   ↑ aqueous channel insertion into apical membrane
   ↓
   ↓ rate of endocytosis and degradation of WCV
   ↓
   ↑ H_2O permeability of CD cells

PK: Exogenous **ADH** does not penetrate blood–brain barrier.
Inactive orally, destroyed by **trypsin.**
Route: parenteral/intranasal.
Plasma t½ → 25 min
Duration of action → **3–4 hrs**

IA:
1. Carbamazepine and chlorpropamide potentiate **AVP.**
2. NSAID (specially indomethacin) enhances **AVP** induced antidiuresis by inhibiting renal PG synthesis.
3. Li⁺ and demeclocycline **antagonise** ADH action, **reduce** urine concentrating ability of kidney and **produce** polyuria plus polydipsia.

ADR
1. **On local use:** Nasal irritation, congestion, ulceration, epistaxis, rhinitis.
2. **Abdominal** cramp, belching, palor, nausea, urge to deficate.
   Backache in female due to uterine contraction.
3. **Bradycardia, angina** due to coronary vasoconstriction, increased afterload, fluid retention, hyponatremia.
4. **Allergy:** Urticaria, etc.

CI: 1. IHD 2. HTN 3. Chronic nephritis

Uses of ADH

1. **DI** of pituitary/neurogenic origin **(most important indication of ADH).**
   Ineffective in renal (nephrogenic) DI. **Lifelong therapy** is needed **except** in neurosurgery due to transient DI → **Desmopressin (DOC)**
   Aqueous ADH differentiates **neurogenic** from **nephrogenic DI**→**5 U ADH** diluted in **1 L** and infused **IV** at the rate of **1 ml/min** →urine volume is reduced and its osmolarity is increased if DI is due to **ADH deficiency**. Desmopressin 2 µg (IM) is DOC for it.
2. **Renal DI:** Indomethacin reduces polyuria, hence it is used.
3. **Bed wetting (nocturia)** in children: **Desmopressin 10–20 µg** nasal spray at bedtime (periodic monitoring of BP and body weight to check fluid overload).
   One week withdrawal in every 3 months is needed for **reassessment**.
4. **Renal concentration test:** Maximum **urine** concentration at **5–10 U intramuscularly, given.**
5. **Haemophilia and von Willebrand's disease:** **AVP** inhibits bleeding by releasing coagulation factor **VIII, von Willebrand's** factor and **desmopressin (DOC).**
6. **Esophageal variceal bleeding:** ADH constricts **mesenteric vessel**, allows clot formation and reduces blood flow.
7. To drive out **gases** from bowel before abdominal radiotherapy.

Desmopressin: It is **selective V$_2$ agonist, synthetic analogue, 12 times more potent antidiuretic** than natural AVP and has **no vasoconstrictor action.**
PK: Duration of action → 6–18 hrs.
U: 1. **DI (DOC—Desmopressin):** Lifelong therapy.
   Neurogenic DI: ADH **(IM)**
   Desmopressin and lypressin **(intranasally).**
   Nephrogenic: **Thiazide**
   2. **Bed wetting in children**
   3. **Diagnosis of DI**
         Administer Desmopressin (DOC)

Concentrated urine (↑ **urine osmolarity**) ←┤
       ↓
Cranial origin **(pituitary deficiency).** No effect → Nephrogenic DI

Terlipressin: It is synthetic prodrug of vasopressin.
U: Bleeding esophageal varices.

---

1. **Exudates** = 1.020 and
   TRANSUDATES = 1.011 → | 11 letters |
2. **Spleen** | 1, 3, 5, 7, 9, 11 |
   Size = **1 × 3 × 5** inches
   Weight = **7** ounces
   Position = **9** to **11** ribs

Unit 6
Autacoids and Related Drugs

36 ACE Inhibitors

Autacoid means **self-healing substance/remedy.**

Generally acts **locally,** hence called **local hormone/neuromodulator.** But it differs from hormones because hormones are produced by **specific cells** and are transported through circulation to act on distant target cells/tissues.

Functions: A. Reactions to injury   B. Immunological insult
C. As transmitter   D. Modulator in nervous system.

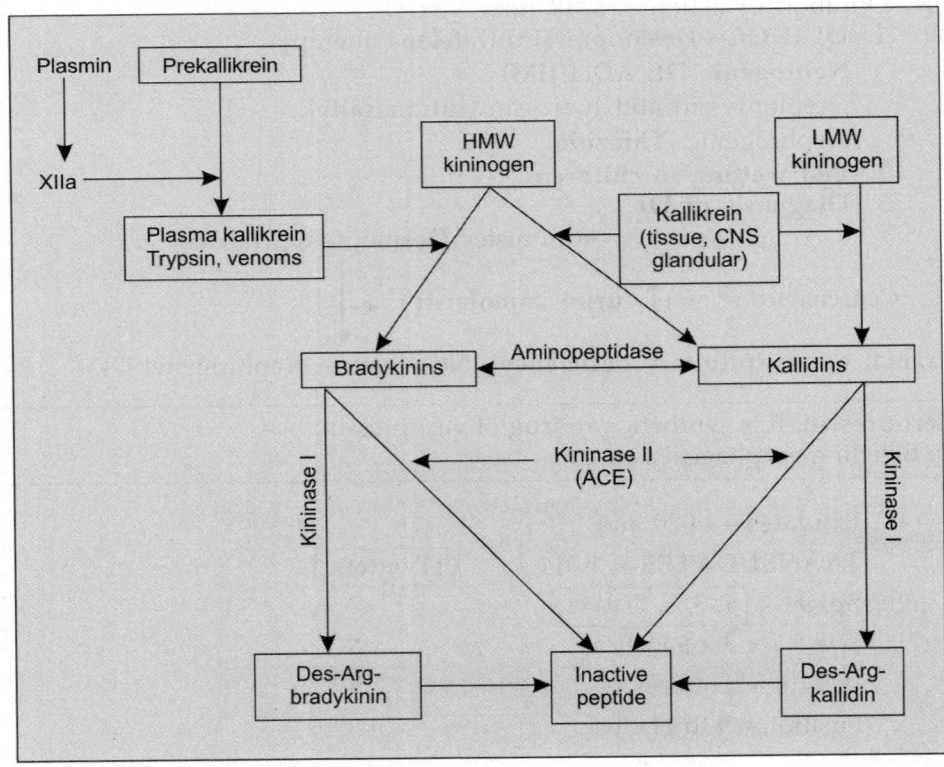

Classical autacoids are

A. Amine autacoids: Histamine, serotonin/5-HT (**5-HydroxyTryptamine**)
B. Peptide autacoids: Angiotensin (AT).
   Plasma kinins such as bradykinin and kallidin.
C. Lipid derived autacoids: PG, LT, PAF.

Generation and metabolism of plasma kinins (see diagram)

1. **Prekallikrein** is activated by **Hegeman factor** and **plasmin**.
2. Plasma and tissue have kininogenase inhibitory factors of which C_1 esterase inhibitor is **the most important**.
3. Kinins are degraded mainly in **lungs by kininase II/ACE** (AT II converting enzyme or dipeptidyl carboxypeptidase) to split off **2** amino acids from carboxy terminal of peptide chain and by kinase I to remove **1** amino acid (arginine) producing selective B_1 agonistic metabolites **(des-arg-bradykinin and kallidin)**.

Actions of plasma kinins

1. Bradykinin **(slow to move)** and kallidin have **same actions**.
2. Direct action on heart is **absent**.
   Hypotension causes reflex stimulation.
   More **vasodilatation (arterioles mainly) than ACh** and **histamine** mediated through **EDRF (NO)** release.
   Flushing, throbbing headache and hypotension on **IV injection. Histamine** is released from mast cells.
   Increased capillary permeability due to **separation of endothelial cells** → exudation and inflammation.
   Wheel and **flare similar to histamine** on intradermal injection.
3. **Most nonvascular smooth muscle** is **contracted**.
   Slow intestinal contraction and bronchoconstriction are present.
4. Stimulate nerve ending that produces pain →**burning sensation**
   Adrenal medulla —Kinin→ CA.
   Brain —Kinin→ ↑ **sympathetic discharge.**
   Increase permeability of blood–brain barrier.
5. Enhance renal blood flow and facilitate **salt + H_2O excretion** by action on tubules. Reduce diuretic effect of **furosemide** by B_2 R antagonist action (by locally generated kinin).
6. **Bronchoconstriction** and **renal vasodilatation** by kinins are attenuated by **aspirin** (PG synthesis inhibitor).

Kinin receptors

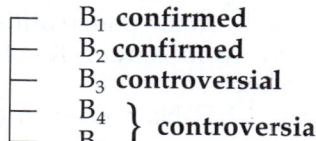

Most kinin actions of non-inflamed tissue are mediated by B_2 **receptors** which are present on:
A. **Visceral smooth muscle:** Contraction of intestine, uterus and airway.
B. **Sensory nerve (pain)**
C. **Vascular endothelium**
EDRF release (vasodilatation) and increased **permeability**.

Mech (A)
$$B_2 R$$
$$\downarrow$$
$$\text{G protein coupled R}$$
$$\downarrow$$
$$\text{Phospholipase C}$$
$$\downarrow$$
$$IP_3/DAG$$
$$\downarrow$$
Intracellular Ca^{2+} mobilization transducer mechanism.

(B) Inflammation induces synthesis of B_1 **receptors** on smooth muscle of large vessels → **vasoconstriction** in normal tissue. Kallidin is **equipotent** on both B_1 and B_2. But **bradykinin** has higher affinity for B_2 than B_1.
Des-Arg metabolites are selective B_1 agonist.

Pathophysiological roles of kinins

1.
$$\text{Tissue injury}$$
$$\downarrow$$
$$\text{Local kinin production}$$
$$\downarrow$$
$$\text{Production of all signs of inflammation}$$
$$\text{(redness, exudates, pain, WBC mobilisation)}$$
$$\downarrow$$
$$\text{Stimulation of } B_1 \text{ R on macrophages}$$
$$\downarrow$$
$$\text{IL-I and TNF-}\alpha \text{ production}$$

2. Stimulate **nerve endings** and enhance **PG production** to act as mediators of pain. B_2 **blockers** block **acute** pain produced by bradykinin but **induced B_1 R** mediate pain of **chronic** inflammation.
3. **Capillary permeability** is enhanced by bradykinin.
4. Regulation of microcirculation specially in **kidney** through local kinin production.
5. **Integration** of kinin with clotting, fibrinolysin and complement systems.
6. **Kinins cause:** Closure of ductus arteriosus, foetal pulmonary artery dilatation and umbilical vessel constriction to adjust from **foetal to neonatal circulation.**
7. **Kinins are involved in**   **SCARFS**
Angioedema, Asthma, ACE inhibitor induced cough, Acute pancreatitis. Carcinoid, Fluid secretion in diarrhoea, Immunological Reaction, Postgastrectomy dumping Syndrome, Rhinitis, Shock.
8. **Aprotinin** is **trypsin** and **kallikrein inhibitor** and has been used in **acute pancreatitis** and **carcinoid.**

RENIN-ANGIOTENSIN SYSTEM

1. $t_{1/2}$—AT II →1 min and renin →15 min.
2. Biological potency of AT I is only 1/100th that of AT II.
3. **ACE is dipeptidyl carboxypeptidase of luminal surface of vascular endothelial cells** (specially in lungs).
4. AT III is the first degradation product, 2–10 times less potent than AT II but in stimulating **aldosterone secretion** it is **equipotent**.
5. **Vessels form AT II within their wall by taking renin and angiotensinogen. Heart, vessels, brain, kidneys and adrenal possess all components of renin-angiotensin system** to generate AT II locally.

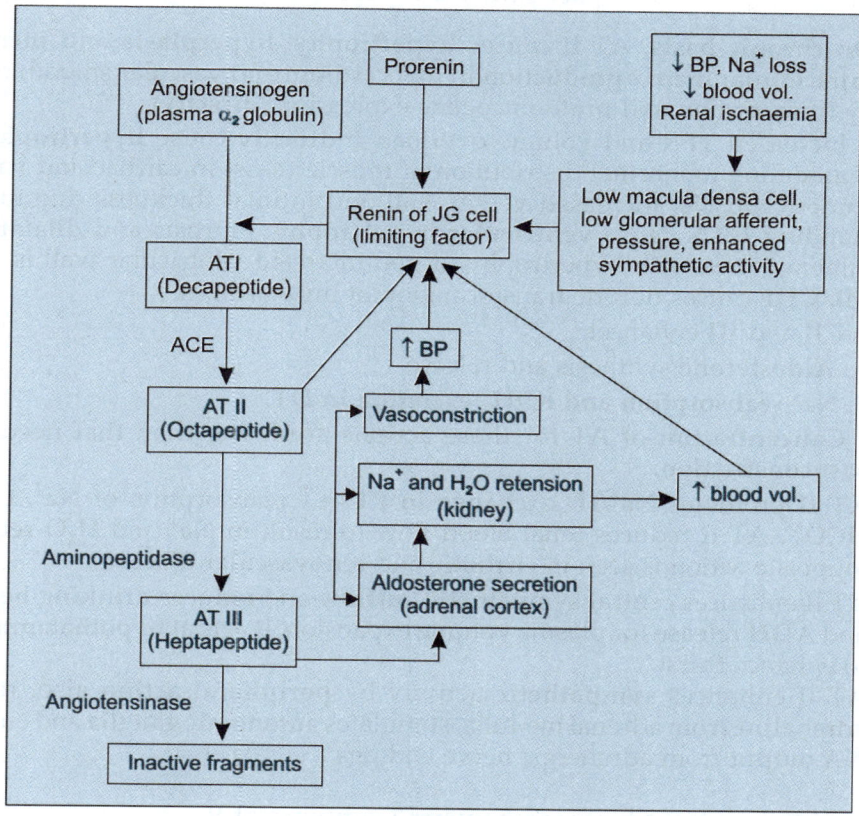

Actions of AT II

1. **Most prominent action** of AT II is **vasoconstriction of all vascular beds** produced directly and by increasing:
   A. **Adr/NA release** from adrenal medulla/adrenergic nerve ending.
   B. **Central sympathetic outflow.**
2. **IP$_3$/DAG constricts** arterioles.
3. AT II induced vasoconstriction causes fluid movement from vascular to **extravascular** compartment. **AT II is more potent than NA.**

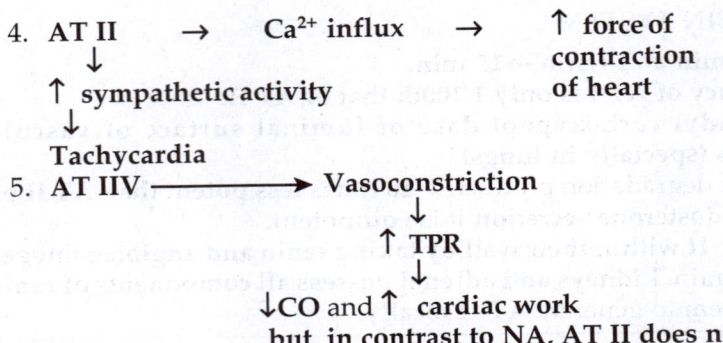

4. AT II → Ca²⁺ influx → ↑ force of contraction of heart
   ↓
   ↑ sympathetic activity
   ↓
   Tachycardia

5. AT II V ──→ Vasoconstriction
   ↓
   ↑ TPR
   ↓
   ↓CO and ↑ cardiac work
   but, in contrast to NA, AT II does not activate latent pacemaker

6. **On chronic basis**, AT II causes **hypertrophy, hyperplasia** and **increased intracellular matrix production** in myocardium and vascular smooth muscle by transcription and proto-oncogene expression **(directly)**.
   Increased TPR and volume overload **indirectly** cause **hypertrophy** and **remodeling** (abnormal distribution of muscle mass) in cardiac and vascular smooth muscle. Increased vessel wall and intimal thickness due to long-standing **HTN** cause **ventricular hypertrophy**. Fibrosis and dilatation of infarcted area with hypertrophy of non-infarcted ventricular wall is due to **MI. CHF** causes fibrotic transformation of myocardium.

7. **AT II and III enhance:**
   A. **Aldosterone** synthesis and release
   B. **Na⁺ reabsorption and K⁺/H⁺ excretion in DT.**
   Concentration of AT for these actions are lower than that needed for **vasoconstriction**.

8. AT II promotes **Na⁺/H⁺ exchange in PT** →↑ reabsorption of **Na⁺, Cl⁻** and **HCO₃⁻**. AT II reduces renal blood flow to result in **Na⁺** and **H₂O** retention (opposite action is seen in **cirrhotic** and **renovascular disease**).

9. AT II enhances **central sympathetic outflow** and induces **drinking behavior** and **ADH release** for plasma volume expansion. It acts at **hypothalamus** level to enhance **thirst**.

10. AT II enhances **sympathetic** activity by **peripheral action** also, releases **adrenaline** from adrenal medulla, stimulates **autonomic ganglia** and enhances **NA output** from adrenergic nerve endings.

AT receptors and transducer mechanism: 2 subtypes of R

A. **AT₁** (selective AT₁ blocker →losartan)
B. **AT₂** (PD 123177 →selective AT₂ blocker)

1. **All known actions** are mediated by **AT₁ R** which is G protein coupled R using different **transducer** mechanism in different tissues.
   Phospholipase C—IP₃/DAG intracellular **Ca²⁺ release** mechanism of vascular and visceral smooth muscle acts by activating **MLCK**.

2. Increased **Ca²⁺ movement** also induces **aldosterone release /synthesis, cardiac ionotropy, depolarisation** of adrenal medullary/autonomic ganglion cell resulting in **CA release/sympathetic discharge**.

ACE Inhibitors

   DAG stimulates **PKc** → phosphorylation of intracellular protein and augments **response + cell growth.**
3. **AT II** inhibits **adenyl cyclase** in **liver** and **kidney.** Intrarenal haemostatic action involves **phospholipase A_2 activation** and **PG/LT production.**
4. **AT_1 R** mediates long-term effects of **AT II** on cell growth in fibroblasts, vascular smooth muscle and myocardium.
5. **AT II** activates **PKc, MAP kinase, tyrosine protein kinase** → increased expression of **proto-oncogenes** and **transcription** of growth factors → ↑ **cell growth** and ↑ **intracellular matrix synthesis.**
6. **AT II** and **III** stimulate **aldosterone** secretion from adrenal cortex and exerts **trophic** influence on **granulosa cells.**

Renin release regulation
1. **Renin is regulated by**
   A. Decreased tension in **afferent** glomerular arterioles (the intrarenal **baroreceptor** pathway).
   B. Decreased **Na^+ concentration** in tubular fluid sensed by **macula densa cells.**
   C. Increased **sympathetic** impulses of **JG cells** by **baroreceptors** and other reflexes, activated through **$β_1$ R.**
2. **AT_1 R stimulation on JG cells** inhibits **renin release.**
3. **ACE inhibitor** and **AT I blockers** enhance renin release.
   Loop diuretics enhance renin production by reducing **Na^+ entry** into macula densa cells.
   Vasodilators and **diuretics** stimulate renin release by reducing BP.
   Central sympatholytics and **β blockers** reduce renin release by depressing **β adrenoceptor** pathway.
   NSAIDs inhibit PG production → ↓ **renin release.**
4. Plasma renin activity is enhanced in **most renovascular HTN.**

ADR of AT II: Myocardial ischaemia.
Uses of AT II: Hypotension during anaesthesia.

Advantages
A. No production of secondary hypotension.
B. No tissue necrosis on extravasation.

Inhibition of renin-angiotensin system
1. Sympathetic blockers (**β blockers, etc.**) reduce renin release.
2. **AT_1 blockers** inhibit AT II action on target cells.
3. **Aldosterone blockers** block mineralocorticoid receptors.
4. **ACE inhibitors** inhibit generation of active AT II.
5. **Renin inhibitory peptides** and **renin specific antibodies** inhibit renin action by interfering with **AT I generation** from **angiotensinogen (rate limiting step).**
6. **Saralasin** is **octapeptide analogue of AT II** which **competitively blocks AT II R.**

Classification
A. **ACE inhibitors:**
   Teprotide (first ACE inhibitor) was synthesized from **BPF** (bradykinin potentiating factor) of **pituitary viper venom.**

- Captopril
- Ramipril
- Perindopril
- Benazepril
- Enalapril
- Lisinopril

Marketed in India
Blood Cell PER Lakh

- Quinapril
- Cilazapril
- Zofenopril
- Fosinopril

Not marketed in India.
Quin-Cilaz-Zofen-Fosin

B. **Angiotensin II antagonist:** Irbesartan, Telmisartan, Candesartan, Zolasartan, Losartan, Olmesartan, Valsartan, Eprosartan

ITCZ LOVE ~ IT'S LOVE

Captopril

Its effects are **class effects common to all ACE inhibitors.** It is **sulfhydryl with dipeptide surrogate of proline** which abolishes **pressor action of AT I only.** Trandolapril and moexipril are also ACE inhibitors.

Mech

1. **ACE inhibitors inhibit ACE**
   ↓
   ↓**AT II** and **inhibition of bradykinin inactivation.**
   ↓
   ↑ renin release due to loss of feedback inhibition.
2. **Most actions** are due to **AT II generation** but **renin** and **AT I** levels are also enhanced.
3. **Blocks AT I pressor action** but **does not block AT II R.**
4. Enhances plasma **kinin** level and potentiates **bradykinin** action.
5. ↑ **Kinin** and ↑ **PG (due to** ↑ **kinin)** cause **cough** induced by ACE inhibitor in susceptible individual.
6. Interferes with degradation of **substance P.**
7. Captopril reduces BP by **reducing TPR** specially in **renovascular, accelerated** and **malignant HTN** and maintains **vascular tone in 80%.** ACE inhibitors prevent bradykinin (vasodilator) inactivation.
   Renin-AT system is overactive in 20%, normal in 60% and hypoactive in 20% cases of essential HTN. Arterioles are dilated, TPR is reduced, **systolic** and **diastolic BP** are decreased but effect on **CO** is **absent.**
8. Captopril does not block **AT II R,** hence **AT II** action is present.
9. **Reflex (postural) changes in plasma aldosterone** are abolished, and basal levels are reduced as a result of loss of their regulation by **AT II** but mineralocorticoid is secreted by **ACTH** and K^+ of plasma (physiologically).
10. **Dilates efferent renal arterioles** which are regulated by AT II.

PK: 70% orally absorbed (bioavailability). Food reduces bioavailability.
Partly metabolised and partly excreted unchanged in urine.
Elimination t½—**2 hrs.**
Duration of action→**6–12 hrs.**

Dose: Daily dose = 25–150 mg
20 mg BD then 50 mg TDS.
In CHF/Diuretic treatment—stat 6.25 mg BD to avoid hypotension. **Take 1 hour before/2 hour after meal.**

ADR: ADR of **all ACE inhibitors** is **same.** Captopril is **well tolerated by most patient** in daily dose <150 mg.

CAPTOPRIL

1. Cough (persistent brassy cough tickling in throat).
   Commonest ADR of ACE inhibitors **(4–16%).** Develops within **1–8 weeks.** Subsides on discontinuation in **4–6 days.** Caused by **inhibition of bradykinin/substance P breakdown in lungs of susceptible individuals → ↑bradykinin.**
2. Angioedema (<1%): Results in sweating of lips, mouth, nose and larynx.
3. Orthostatic hypOtension in diuretic treated or CHF patient.
4. Potassium level raised in patient taking K⁺ sparing **diuretic/NSAID/β blocker.**
5. Proteinuria **and granulocytopenia** in renal disease. **Foetal damage** in later half of Pregnancy.
6. Reversible loss/alteration of Taste sensation (dysguesia).
7. Rashes and urticaria **(1–4%).**
8. Acute Renal failure in bilateral renal artery stenosis due to dilatation of **efferent arterioles and fall in glomerular filtrate pressure.**
9. Headache, dizziness, nausea, bowel upset in 1–4%.
10. Increased renin and Lower AT II.

CI:
1. **Renal failure**
2. **Renal artery stenosis** because dilatation of efferent renal arterioles reduces pressure in the glomerulus.

IA:
1. **NSAIDs** alternate hypotension action.
2. ACE inhibitors + K⁺ sparing diuretic/K⁺ supplement cause **hypokalaemia.**
3. **Antacids** reduce captopril bioavailability.
4. ACE inhibitors reduce **Li⁺ clearance** and predispose to its **toxicity.**

Enalapril: Enalapril **(prodrug)** → **enalaprilat (tripeptide analogue).**

Pharmacological, therapeutic and **adverse effect profile** of captopril and enalapril are same.

Advantages

1. More potent
2. **Not effected** by food.
3. **"Abrupt first dose hypotension"** due to slow onset of action (which is due to the need for conversion to active metabolite) is **less.**
4. Rashes and loss of taste are less.
5. **Longer** duration of action (**most HTN** treated with single or at the most 2 daily doses).

PK: Has **carboxyl** in place of sulfhydryl.

Duration of action	— 24 hrs
Peak duration	— 4–6 hrs
Elimination t½	— **11 hrs**
Renal excretion	
Daily dose	— 2.5–40 mg
Bioavailability	— 40–50%

Bioavailability		
Captopril	—	70%
Enalapril	—	45%
Lisinopril	—	25%
Perindopril	—	20%

Lisinopril: It is a **lysine** derivative of **enalaprilat**. Reduces CO, venous return and contractility. Chemical nature—**carboxyl**.

PK: Slow and incomplete oral absorption uneffected by **food**.
Longer duration of action (single daily dose needed).
Bioavailability	—	25%
Peak action	—	6–8 hrs
Duration of action		>24 hrs
Elimination t½	—	**12 hrs**
Renal excretion		
Daily dose	—	10–40 mg

Perindopril: Restores reduced elastic properties of **artery** and **heart** in HTN. Same efficacy and tolerance as ACE inhibitor.
Chemical nature—**carboxyl**.

PK: 66–95% orally absorbed.
20% perindopril→perindoprilat (active metabolite).
Bioavailability	—	20%
Peak action		6 hrs
Elimination t½	—	**25–30 hrs**
Renal excretion		
Duration of action		>24 hrs
Daily dose	—	2–8 mg

Ramipril: Chemical nature—**carboxyl**
Ramipril is converted into **Ramiprilat** (active metabolite).

PK: **Extensive tissue distribution (distinctive feature** among ACE inhibitors).
Plasma t½	—	8–18 hrs **(ramiprilat)**
Bioavailability 60%		Renal excretion
Duration of action	—	>24 hrs
Daily dose	—	2–10 mg

Benazepril is **nonsulfhydryl** product of ACE inhibitor

PK: Bioavailability—37%   Renal excretion
t½   —   10–12 hrs

U of ACE inhibitors

A. **HTN: DOC**—ACE inhibitors. **Weak vasoconstrictor (AT I)** is converted to **AT II (potent vasoconstrictor)** which is inhibited by **ACE inhibitors** →decreased fluid volume and peripheral vasodilatation.
ACE inhibitors are **DOC in all grades of HTN except** those with bilateral renal artery stenosis. **50–60%** responds to ACE inhibitors.
Majority of rest—ACE inhibitors + diuretic/β blockers.
Antihypertensive of choice in DM is ACE inhibitors.

Advantages

1. **Safe in asthma, DM, PVD and CREST syndrome.**

C	–	Calcinosis
R	–	Raynaud's phenomenon
E	–	Esophageal dysmotility
S	–	Sclerodactyly
T	–	Telangiectasia

2. **Lack of postural hypotension, electrolyte** disturbances, **weakness** and **CNS effects.**
3. **Inhibition of secondary hyperaldosteronism and K^+ loss due to diuretics.**
4. **No hyperuricaemia, no rebound HTN** on withdrawal, no effect on plasma **lipid** profile.
5. Reverse **LV hypertrophy** and enhance **wall-to-lumen ratio** of blood vessels of hypertensive patient.
6. Less worsening of **quality of life parameters.**
7. Reduce **cardiovascular** morbidity and enhance life expectancy of hypertensive patient.
8. **Greater protective potential** than other antihypertensive drugs due to specific effect on myocardial and vascular cell growth/remodeling.
9. Improve **renal blood flow,** retard **diabetic nephropathy** and repress **vascular/ LV hypertrophy.**
10. ACE inhibitors are the **most appropriate** antihypertensive in:

SCALD

MI **S**pecially Post MI, **C**HF, **A**ngina, **L**VH, **D**iabetic nephropathy.

B. MI
C. **Scleroderma crisis:** HTN and renal function deterioration are due to **AT II**.
D. **Diabetic nephropathy:** Inhibit renal disease in **all types of DM**.
Albuminuria (glomerulopathy index) remains stable in treated patient.
E. **CHF (DOC): Drugs** → vasodilatation
↓
↓ preload and afterload
↓
↓ right atrial pressure
↓ pulmonary arterial pressure
↓ systemic vascular resistance
↓ systolic wall stress and systemic BP
↓ PCWP and HR
↓ cardiac work

Stroke volume and **CO** are enhanced.

Salt and H_2O are lost due to **improved renal perfusion.**

Drugs also retard the progression of LV systolic dysfunction and prolong survival of CHF patient of **all grades (I to IV).**

Captopril test is to diagnose **renovascular HTN** and to obviate the need of **renal angiography.**

Basis: Captopril inhibits AT II formation → ↑ TPR (more in renovascular than essential HTN).

Losartan: It is **AT II blocker,** and has **all advantages of ACE inhibitors.**

Mech: 1. **Competitive AT II blocker. Inhibits all actions of AT II** (vasoconstriction, sympathetic stimulation, aldosterone and adrenaline release, salt and H_2O reabsorption, ADH release, growth promoting action on heart and vessels).
2. **Reduces BP in HTN.**
3. Regresses **hypertensive LVH** like ACE inhibitors.
4. **10,000 times more selective for AT_1 R than AT_2R.**

PK: Bioavailability due to first pass metabolism—**33% renal** excretion.
Peak duration of action—3–6 weeks.
Plasma t½—2 hrs (losartan) and 6–9 hrs (E 3174).
Losartan (partially carboxylated in liver) → E 3174.
Active metabolite (E 3174) is **10–30 times more potent non-competitive AT_1 blocker.**
Peak plasma level — Losartan – **1 hr**
— E 3174 – **3–4 hrs**
(Both are **98% plasma protein bound**).
Dose: 50 mg/day in HTN.

ADR: No significant ADR as it does not enhance **kinin** levels. Hence, cough, urticaria, angioedema and taste disturbance are absent.
1. **Hypotension** and **hyperkalaemia.**
2. **Headache, weakness** and **upper GI intolerance.**

CI: Pregnancy due to fetopathic potential
U: HTN: Losartan 50 mg/day
Losartan + 20 mg chlorthiazide enhance **effectiveness.**

Candesartan

Mech: AT_1 antagonist
PK: Duration of action = 24 hours
Hepatic metabolism and renal excretion.
Half-life = 12 hours. Dose = 8 mg OD/BD.

Irbesartan

Mech: AT_1 antagonist
PK: High oral bioavailability
Partial metabolism
Excreted in bile. Half-life = 12 hours
Dose = 4 mg/kg/day OD.

AT II R blockers (ARB) bind to AT_1 R (selectivity: AT_1 10,000 fold > AT_2 R). Affinity order of AT_1 R: candesartan > irbesartan > telmisartan = valsartan = EXP 3174 (active form of losartan) > losartan.

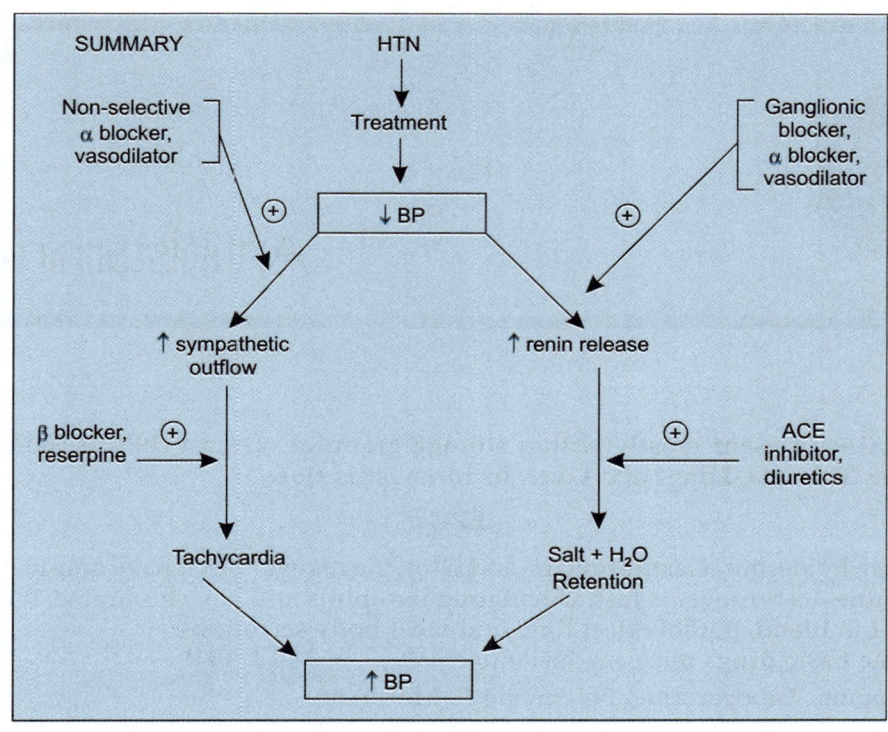

37 Antihistaminics

Histamine: Present **mostly** within **storage granules** of mast cells of Skin, GIT mucosa, Placenta, Lungs and Liver. Its turnover is **slow**.

LPGs

Brain, Epidermis, Gastric mucosa and Growing region $\boxed{\text{BEG}}$ have **non-mast cell histamine**. Its turnover is **fast. Circulating basophils** also have histamine. It is also present in **blood, pathological** fluid and **most body secretions**.

Some basic drugs releasing histamine are: **Most ATP**

Atropine, Tubocurarine, Polymyxin B, Morphine.

Synthesis and degradation of histamine

Histidine
↓
Histamine —Diamine oxidase→ Imidazole acetic acid
↓ N-methyl transferase
N-methyl histamine
    ↓ Oxidase
Methyl imidazole acetic acid

Histamine is **β-imidazolylethylamine** and is **positively charged molecule held** by **acidic protein and heparin (negatively charged)** within intracellular **granules** of mast cells → **exocytosis**

↓
Na^+ in ECF exchanged with histamine
↓
Free histamine (histamine release)
(−) ↑
↑ intracellular cAMP

Inactive orally because liver degrades **all** histamine absorbed from intestines.

Histamine receptors
— H_1
— H_2
— H_3 **(auto-receptor)** → controls histamine release from neurones in brain.

Antihistaminics

Effects of histamine

A. **H_1 R:** Controls **bronchial** and **intestinal** smooth muscle. Acts on **sensory nerve** endings to cause pain and itching.

B. **H_2R:** Enhances **gastric secretion, HR** and **contractility**.

C. **H_1 and H_2 R:** Vasodilatation (arterioles and venules) → **shock.** ↑ capillary permeability → **edema**.

Actions of histamine

1. Causes **vasodilatations (arterioles, capillary venules)**. Flushing, heat, tachycardia and increase CO are produced on **SC injections**. Hypotension on **IV injection with shorter H_1** and **longer H_2 components** is produced. H_1 has higher affinity (at low doses only H_1 component manifests). **Combination of H_1 and H_2 blockers** completely block hypotension due to **large doses**.
   Pulsatile headache is caused by cranial vasodilatation.

2. Histamine ⟶ H_1 R on endothelial cells
   ↓ ↓
   H_2 R on vascular   EDRF mediation
   smooth muscle
   ↓   ↓
   Vasodilatation   Vasodilatation

3. Histamine ⟶ H_1 R on vascular smooth muscle
   ↓ ↓
   H_1 Receptor   Constriction of large artery and vein
   ↓
   Separation of
   endothelial cells
   ↓
   ↑ capillary permeability
   ↓
   Plasma exudation

4. **On intradermal injection, triple response** produced is:

   A. **Flare:** Redness in surrounding area due to **arteriolar dilatation** mediated by axon reflex.

   B. **Red spot:** Due to **capillary dilatation**.

   C. **Wheal:** Due to fluid exudation from capillary and venules (↑ capillary permeability).

5. Histamine ⟶ H_1 R ⟶ negative dromotropic effect
   ↓   (slow AV conduction)
   H_2 R
   ↓
   ↑ HR and ↑ force of contraction

6. Bronchoconstriction and intestinal contraction.

7. Histamine ⟶ H_2 R on parietal cells
   ↓
   ↑ cAMP
   ↓
   Stimulates membrane proton pump
   (H^+, K^+-ATPase)
   ↓
   ↑ gastric secretion
8. Histamine (IV/intracutaneously or more deeply)
   ↓
   Stimulates sensory nerve ending
   ↓
   Pain and itching
9. Histamine ⟶ stimulate autonomic ganglia and adrenal medulla
   ↓
   Adrenaline release
   ↓
   HTN
10. Histamine on intracerebroventricular administration (because it does not cross BBB)
    ↓
    H_1 and H_2 R
    ↓
    HTN, cardiac stimulation, behavioral arousal, ADH release, hypothermia, vomiting

Pathophysiological roles of histamine

1. All stimuli evoking gastric secretion (gastrin, cholinergic drug, feeding, vagal stimulation)
   ↓ ⊕
   Histaminocyte of gastric mucosa
   ↓
   Non-mast cell histamine release
   ↓
   Gastric secretion

   H_2 blockers block acid secretion induced by histamine.

2. **Histamine of mast cells**
   ↓
   H_1 R
   ↓
   Ag-Ab reaction on the surface
   (involving **IgE** type of reaginic Ab)
   ↓
   Urticaria, angioedema, bronchoconstriction and anaphylactic shock.

3. Histamine is **afferent** transmitter initiating sensation of itch and pain at sensory nerve endings. **Non-mast cell histamine** of brain (hypothalamus and

midbrain) maintains **wakefulness** through H_1 R. **H_1 agonists** of brain also suppress **appetite**.

Histamine regulates body temperature, cardiovascular function, thirst and hormone release from anterior pituitary.

4.
$$\text{Histamine} \downarrow$$

Vasodilatation and promotion of WBC adhesion to vascular endothelial cell by expressing adhesion molecule **P-selectin** on the cell surface
$$\downarrow$$
WBC sequestration at inflammatory site.

5. Histamine is needed in **tissue growth** and **repair**.

Uses of histamine (no therapeutic use). Diagnostic uses are
1. **Test of acid secreting capacity of stomach: Pentagastrin** is a **synthetic gastrin analogue** which enhances **gastrin secretion**.
2. **Test for pheochromocytoma** (Dangerous test).
   Histamine →CA release from tumour → HTN.
   Treatment: Phentolamine immediately.
3. **To test bronchial hyperactivity in asthma.**
4. **Test for achlorhydria for diagnosing pernicious anemia.**
   Treatment: **Vitamin B_{12}**

Beta-histamine is H_1 selective histamine analogue.
Indication: Central vertigo in Menier's disease.
CI: **Asthma** and **ulcer**.

Histamine releasers
The **stimuli** (tissue damage, Ag, polymers, drugs and surface acting agent like Tween 80, etc.) release histamine from **mast cells.** Tween mainly releases histamine from mast cells, hence called **"histamine liberators"** and produces **anaphylactoid reactions** (itching, burning sensation, hypotension, urticaria, tachycardia, headache, colic and asthma) which are controlled by H_1 and H_2 blockers.

Classification
A. **H_1 blockers (competitive blockers)**
   a. **First generation**
      1. **Highly sedative**
         Diphenhydramine*
         Dimenhydrinate*
         Hydroxyzine*
         Promethazine
         Doxylamine
      2. **Moderately sedative**
         Meclizine*
         Buclizine

---
*4 drugs are for treatment of motion sickness

Trimeprazine
Pheniramine
Antazoline
Cyproheptadine
3. **Mild sedative**
Chlorpheniramine
Cyclizine
Clemastine
Dimethindene
Methdilazine
Mepyramine (pyrilamine)
Mebhydroline
Triprolidine
  b. **Second generation**
  1. **Antivertigo drug:** Cinnarizine
  2. **Non-sedating antiallergics**
Tarfenadine ⎱ Least
Astemizole ⎰ sedative
Cetirizine
Azelastine
Loratadine, desloratadine, mizolastine, ebastine
B. **H_2 blockers** (first H_2 blocker **burimamide** was developed by **Black** in 1972).
Cimetidine
Ranitidine
Famotidine
Roxatidine
Nizatidine
Loxatidine
C. **H_2 agonist:** Betazole (enhances gastric secretion)
D. **H_3 blocker:** Thioperamide (no clinical use)

CLASSIFICATIONS

Antivertigo drugs

A. **Vasodilator:** Nicotinic acid.
B. **Diuretics:** Loops, thiazide and acetazolamide.
C. **Anxiolytic** and **antidepressant** (modify sensation of vertigo): Diazepam, amitriptyline.
D. **Corticosteroid** (reduces intralabyrinthine edema due to viral infection).
E. **Labyrinthine suppressants** (suppress end organ receptors/inhibit central cholinergic pathway in vestibular nuclei):
  1. **Anticholinergics:** Atropine, hyoscine.
  2. **Antihistaminic with anticholinergic actions:** Cinnarizine, cyclizine, promethazine, dimenhydrinate, diphenhydramine.
  3. **Antiemetic phenothiazines:** Thiethyle perazine.
Prochlorperazine (perenterally, **the most effective** drug for controlling vertigo and vomiting).

H_1 Blockers

Mech: Competitively antagonise histamine actions at H_1 R.

Pharmacological actions

1. **All H_1 blockers** have **similar** actions **(qualitatively)** but have **quantitative** differences specially in **sedative** property.
2. Inhibit histamine induced **bronchoconstriction**, intestinal and smooth muscle **contraction**, and **triple response (itch, flare, wheal)**. Hypotension is blocked by H_1 blocker (and $H_1 + H_2$ inhibition are needed for **complete** blockade). Large vessel constriction is **antagonised.**
3. **Type I** reaction of hypersensitivity is suppressed.
   (LTC_4 and D_4 and **PAF** are mediator for asthma).
4. Cause **direct smooth muscle relaxation** leading to hypotension.
5. **Mepyramine** and **antazoline** have strong membrane stabilizing property (hence **antiarrhythmic** property) but cause irritation.
6. Inhibit **neural uptake of NA** and potentiate it like cocaine.
7. Antagonise **muscarinic** actions of ACh. **High anticholinergic** actions are present in:
   - A. Cyproheptadine
   - B. Dimenhydrinate
   - C. Diphenhydramine
   - D. Pheniramine
   - E. Promethazine
8. Produce **CNS depression** depending on blood–brain barrier penetration and H_1 R. affinity (**no central effect** of histamine is seen on IV injection because it does not cross BBB—blood–brain barrier). **Promethazine** controls **vomiting** of pregnancy, reduces **tremor, rigidity** and **sialorrhoea of parkinsonism**. Some are **antitussives**.

PK: Absorbed **orally** and **parenterally**. **Hepatic** metabolism and **renal** excretion. Widely distributed in the body and enter brain. Duration of action of **most agents** → 4–6 hrs **except** Astemizole, Cetirizine, Clemastine, Loratadine, Meclizine **CALM** which act for → 12–24 hrs.

ADR of H_1 blockers

1. **Commonest:** Sedation, diminished alertness and concentration, light headedness, motor incoordination, fatigue, tendency to fall asleep.
2. **Anticholinergic effects:** Dry mouth, urine hesitancy, blurred vision, altered bowel movement.
3. **Headache and epigastric stress.**
4. **Contact dermatitis** on local application.
5. **Acute overdose:** Tremor and convulsion, flushing and hypotension, central excitation, fever and **features of belladonna poisoning and** death due to CNS and respiratory failure.

Nonsedating antiallergic drugs (second generation compound)

Free of CNS effect, psychomotor performance is absent, **anticholinergic** ADR absent, H_1 **receptor specific.**

Uses: Acute allergy to drugs and foods, atopic eczema, allergic rhinitis and conjunctivitis, dermographism, hay fever, pollinosis, urticaria.

Desloratadine: Active metabolite of loratidine effective at half the dose (5 mg OD) of it. Psychomotor and cardiac safety persent.

Mizolastine: Non-sedative, non-active metabolite, half-life = 10 hrs.

U: Urticaria, allergic rhinitis (10 mg OD).

Ebastine: Converted to carbastine, half-life =10–16 hrs, non-sedating.

U: Nasal and skin allergies.

Terfenadine: It is a **selective H_1 blocker** and produces **active carboxy metabolites** (fexofenadine).

    Mech: 1. Blocks **selectively H_1 R.**
           2. Inhibits **cardiac K^+ channel** in overdose →polymorphic ventricular tachycardia **(torsade de pointes).**

    PK: Onset of action → 1–2 hrs, duration of action → 12–24 hrs.

                Terfenadine
                   ↓   **Cytochrome P450 isoenzyme 3A4**
          Fexofenadine (active carboxymetabolite)

t½ (Fexofenadine):   1. **25 hrs (Reference Katzung)**
                           2. **17 hrs (Reference KDT)**

Excreted **equally in urine** and **faeces.** Dose (fexofenadine)—**60 mg.**

ADR: Cardiotoxicity
IA: Erythromycin   } These are **the most important**
            Clarithromycin   drugs precipitating cardio-
            Ketoconazole   toxicity with terfenadine
            Itraconazole   or astemizole

Terfenadine blocks cardiac K^+ channel → cardiotoxicity. Most common drugs causing this with **Terfenadine** are **KTZ, ITraconazole, Erythromycin KITE** and Clarithromycin → Cardiotoxicity.

U: Atopic and exercise induced **asthma.** Terfenadine is good for **short-term** and **intermittent** use whereas astemizole is good for **maintenance** therapy.

Astemizole

    Mech: **Same** as terfenadine, due to **week anti-5-HT action,** it causes increase appetite, weight gain and flatulence.
    PK: **Onset** of action   → 2–4 hrs
            Duration of action →2–5 days, **97%** plasma protein bound, **t½—20 hrs,** drug → active metabolite with t½ **12–19** days, excreted in **faeces.**
            On daily administration, **steady state** is attained in 1–3 weeks.
    ADR: **Same** as terfenadine
    U: **Perennial rhinitis (better efficacy** than terfenadine or chlorpheniramine)

Loratadine: It is **selective peripheral H_1 blocker. Lacks CNS depressant** effects.
                Acts **faster** than astemizole.
                    Drugs ⟶ **Active metabolite**

Cetirizine: It is **selective peripheral H_1 blocker with no CNS depressant effects (like loratadine).**

Mech
1. **Peripheral H_1 R** action through (H_1 antagonism).
2. Inhibits **histamine release** and release of **cytotoxic mediators** from platelets and eosinophil chemotaxis during secondary phase of **allergic response**.
3. **Hydroxyzine** → cetirizine

PK: $t\frac{1}{2}$ → 8 hrs, dose → 25–100 mg

U:
1. Upper respiratory **allergy**
2. **Pollinosis**
3. **Urticaria**
4. Adjuvant in seasonal **asthma**.

Azelastine

Mech
1. Inhibits **histamine release** and **inflammatory reaction** triggered by LT and PAF.
2. Blocks H_1 R (with good topical activity and bronchodilator property)
3. Down regulates ICAM-I expression (intracellular adhesion molecule 1) on nasal mucosa.

PK: $t\frac{1}{2}$—24 hrs
ADR: Stinging in nose, altered taste perception.
U: As nasal spray for seasonal and perennial allergic rhinitis.

Cinnarizine

Mech
1. Blocks H_1 R
2. **Anticholinergic, sedative, vasodilator** and **anti-5-HT** properties are present.
3. Modulates Ca^{2+} **flux** and attenuates **vasoconstriction**.
4. Inhibits **vestibular sensory nuclei** of inner ear, suppresses **postrotatory labyrinthine reflexes** reducing Ca^{2+} influx from endolymph into vestibular sensory cells.

ADR: Sedation and mild GI upset.
U: (1) Menier's disease; (2) Vertigo and motion sickness.

ADR of H_1 blockers
1. Sedation
2. **Anticholinergic ADR** (dry mouth, constipation, urinary retention).
Second generation H_1 blockers do not have these ADR.

Uses of H_1 antihistaminics (based on sedative, antihistaminic and anticholinergic properties).

1. **Allergic disorders**
   A. **Only palliative:** Not suppress **Ag : Ab reaction**, prevent effects of **released histamine**.
   B. Control **urticaria, hay fever, itching, allergic conjunctivitis** and **angio-edema**.

C. Come **second** in anaphylactic shock. **DOC** is adrenaline, adrenaline is also life-saving in laryngeal edema.
D. $H_1 + H_2$ **blockers** prevent atopic dermatitis, chronic urticaria, and perennial vasomotor rhinitis.
E. **Type I hypersensitivity** reactions to drugs (except asthma and anaphylactic shock) and skin rashes.
F. **Seasonal allergic** rhinitis (H_1 blocker), acute urticaria (H_1 blocker).

Reasons of ineffectivity of older antihistaminic in bronchial asthma
A. LTC_4 and D_4 and PAF are more important mediator than histamine.
B. Insufficient concentration of antihistaminics at the site to block histamine of bronchi.

2. Prevent ADR produced by **histamine liberators** (ivy poisoning, insect bite) and suppress **abnormal dermographism. Prophylaxis** in blood/saline infusion induced **rigor.**
3. **Common cold:** Only **symptomatic** relief by sedative and anticholinergic action (reduce **rhinorrhoea**). Do not effect course of illness.
4. **Pruritides: Antipruritic actions** independent of H_1 antagonism are present (but incomplete relief occurs). **DOC** in idiopathic pruritis.
5. **Motion sickness (prophylaxis)**   **CMDT**
   Cyclizine, **M**eclizine, **D**iphenhydramine and **D**imenhydrinate, Prome-Thazine (taken 1 hr before starting journey).
   Promethazine is also used in: Radiation sickness, morning sickness, vomiting (drug induced and postoperative).
   Meclizine is used in **sea sickness** for 24 hrs. **All antimotion sickness drugs** are more effective when taken **30–60 min before** commencig journey because after journey has started, sickness control is very difficult. **Antihistaminic is teratogenic** so better to avoid in morning sickness.
6. **Vertigo**
7. **Preanaesthetic medication** and **parkinsonism**
   Promethazine due to sedative and anticholinergic actions.
8. **As sedative** and **hypnotic (insomnia, etc.):** Due to **antihistaminic** and **CNS depressant** effects.
9. As **anxiolytic: Hydroxyzine** due to autonomic action.
10. **Acute muscle dystonia: Promethazine** and **hydroxyzine** due to anticholinergic action.

Uses of H_1 blockers   **CAMP and DAMP**
Common cold
Allergic disorder, ADR of histamine liberators.
Motion sickness
Parkinsonism, preanaesthetic medication.
Depressant (sedative and hypnotic)
Anxiolytic
Muscle dystonia (acute)
Pruritides, and prophylaxis

38. Drugs Related to 5-Hydroxytryptamine System

Serotonin/5-HT (5-hydroxytryptamine): Serotonin (vasoconstrictor substance of serum) and **enteramine** (smooth muscle contracting substance of enterochromaffin cells of gut mucosa). 90% 5-HT is present in **intestine, rest** is found in brain and platelets. Also present in wasp, scorpion sting, invertebrates and plants (banana, pear, tomato, pineapple, cow-hage and stinging nettle).

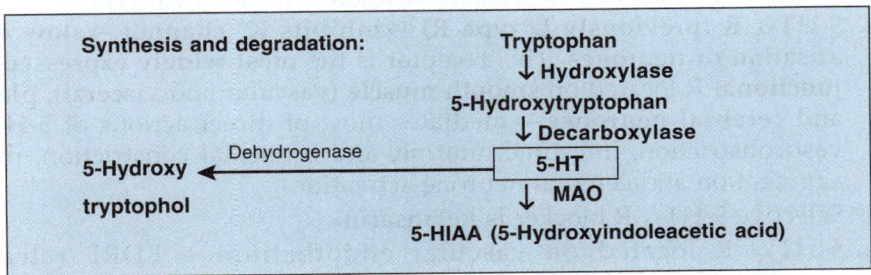

5-HT is **β-amino-ethyl-5-hydroxyindole** and is actively taken up by **amine pump of membrane of platelet** and **serotonergic nerve ending** (like NA uptake) → no free 5-HT in plasma. Both **NA** and **5-HT uptake** are inhibited by TCA. Again like **CA**, 5-HT stored is within storage granules and its uptake at granular membrane is inhibited by **reserpine** → depletion of 5-HT and CAs.

$$DOPA \xrightarrow{Decarboxylase} NA$$

5-HT receptors: 4 families

A. $5-HT_1$
B. $5-HT_2$
C. $5-HT_3$
D. $5-HT_{4-7}$
} **14 receptors subtypes**

Mech: Except $5-HT_3$ all are G-protein coupled R

$5-HT_1$ → ↓ cAMP
$5-HT_2$ → IP_3/DAG generation
$5-HT_4$
$5-HT_6$ } → ↑ cAMP
$5-HT_7$

$5-HT_3$ → **Ligand-gated** cation channel (Na^+ and K^+ channel) stimulation leading to fast depletion.

1. **5-HT$_1$ R (6 subtypes)**
   - 5-HT$_{1A}$ → also prevents Ca^{2+} channel and stimulates K$^+$ channel.
   - 5-HT$_{1B}$
   - 5-HT$_{1C}$ (now designated as 5-HT$_{2C}$)
   - 5-HT$_{1D}$
   - 5-HT$_{1E}$
   - 5-HT$_{1F}$

   A. **All inhibit adenyl cyclase** and act as **autoreceptors** in brain (inhibit firing of 5-HT nerves or release of 5-HT from nerve ending).
   B. **Raphe nuclei** of brainstem and **hippocampus** are **most important** location of 5-HT$_1$ R. **Buspirone** is partial agonist of 5-HT$_{1A}$ R.
   C. 5-HT$_{1D}$ R regulates dopaminergic tone in **substantia nigra–basal ganglia** and causes **cranial vasoconstriction. Sumatriptan** is selective 5-HT$_{1D}$ agonist.
   D. 5-HT$_{1D}$ R → prevents **NA release** from sympathetic nerve ending and inhibits **inflammatory neuropeptide release** from nerve ending in cranial blood vessels.

2. **5-HT$_2$ R:** 3 subtypes, coupled to **phospholipase C**, function through **IP$_3$/DAG generation. α-methyl 5-HT** is selective agonist for **all 3 subtypes**.
   A. **5-HT$_{2A}$ R** (previously D type R) → inhibits K$^+$ channel → slow depolarisation of neurones. This receptor is the **most widely expressed postjunctional R** located on **smooth muscle (vascular and visceral), platelets** and **cerebral neurones** → mediates most of direct actions of 5-HT like vasoconstriction, intestinal, uterine, and bronchial constriction, platelet aggregation and cerebral neurone activation.
   B. Selective 5-HT$_{2A}$ R blocker is **ketanserin**.
   C. 5-HT$_{2C}$ R located on vascular endothelium → EDRF release → **vasodilatation**. 5-HT$_{2C}$ R is also found in **choroid plexus**.

3. **5-HT$_3$ R (previously classified as M type R)**
   Depolarises nerve ending by opening cation channel.
   A. **Mediates indirect** and **reflex effects of 5-HT**
      a. Somatic and autonomic nerve ending → **itch, pain, coronary chemoreflex (↓ BP, ↓ HR, apnoea)**.
      b. Nerve ending in myenteric plexus → ↑ **peristalsis,** ↑ **emetic reflex**.
      c. Area postrema and nucleus tractus solitarius in brainstem → **nausea** and **vomiting**.
   B. **2-methyl 5-HT** is selective 5-HT$_3$ agonist. **Ondansetron** is selective 5-HT$_3$ blocker in gut wall and brainstem and prevents vomiting.

4. **5-HT$_{4-7}$ R: 5-HT$_4$ R:** Present in **mucosa, plexus** and **smooth** muscle of gut → increased peristalsis and intestinal secretion.
   5-HT$_4$ R of hippocampus and **colliculi of brain** → ↓ K$^+$ conductance → **hyperpolarisation. Cisapride** and **renzapride** are selective 5-HT$_4$ agonist.
   5-HT$_{5-7}$ R are closely related to 5-HT$_4$ R located in brain.
   Clozapine has affinity for **5-HT$_{6,7}$ R** and is **5-HT$_{2A/2C}$ blocker**.

Actions of 5-HT: 5-HT is a potent **depolariser of nerve ending** and exerts direct, reflex and indirect effects.

1. Artery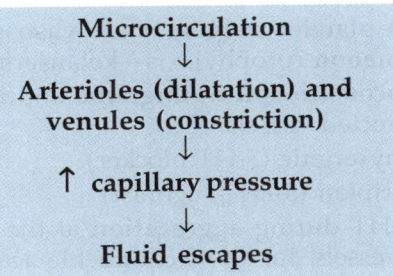
   - Constricted (action on smooth muscle)
   - Dilated (EDRF release).

   Larger vessels are constricted. **Adrenal medulla** →adrenaline is released.

   Microcirculation
   ↓
   Arterioles (dilatation) and venules (constriction)
   ↓
   ↑ capillary pressure
   ↓
   Fluid escapes

2. **Stimulates heart** (both directly and by NA release from nerve ending)
3. **Coronary chemoreflex (Bezold-Jarisch reflex):** Activation through action on **vagal** afferent nerve ending of coronary bed→bradycardia, hypotension and apnoea.
4. **Triphasic response of BP on IV injection**
   A. Early sharp fall in BP due to coronary chemoreflex.
   B. Brief rise in BP due to ↑ CO and vasoconstriction.
   C. Prolonged fall in BP due to arteriolar dilatation and extravasation of fluid.

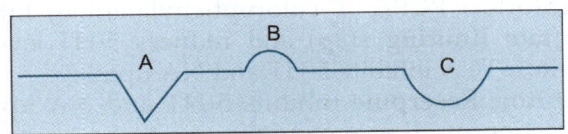

5. 5-HT is a potent stimulator of GIT (direct action and through enteric plexus). ↑ peristalsis → ↑ secretion → ↑ **diarrhoea**.
   Bronchoconstriction (less potent than histamine).
6. Prevents **gastric secretion of acid** and **pepsin** but enhances **mucus** secretion.
7. **Tachyphylaxis** is common with repeated dose of 5-HT.
8. Stimulates **afferent nerve ending** →pain, tingling and pricking sensation.
   Histamine in releasing **CA** from adrenal medulla is more potent than 5-HT.
9. **Visceral afferent depolarisation** elicits respiration and cardiovascular reflexes, nausea and vomiting. **Respiratory stimulation** (mostly from reflex bronchial afferents) and hyperventilation occur.
10. **Partly crosses BBB**, produces **sleepiness**, causes change in **body temperature** and change in **behavior**.
11. 5-HT changes **shape of platelet**, causes **weak aggregation** through **5-HT$_{2A}$ R.**

Pathophysiological roles

1. 5-HT as **neurotransmitter** is found in brain (raphe nuclei of brainstem and substantia nigra), sends axons **rostrally** to (limbic system, cortex, neostriatum) and **caudally** to spinal cord and is involved in sleep, temperature regulation, thought, cognitive function, mood, behavior, vomiting and pain perception.

2. 5-HT is a precursor of **melatonin** in pineal gland, regulates **biological clock** and maintains **circadian rhythm**.
3. **Nausea** and **vomiting** are specially evoked by cytotoxic drugs /RT, mediated by **5-HT release** and its action on 5-HT$_3$ R in gut, area postrema and nucleus tractus solitarius.
4. 5-HT release **from** platelet triggers acute vasospasm of larger arteries → **Raynaud's phenomenon** (prophylaxis—ketanserin).
5. 5-HT initiates **vasoconstriction** in **migraine** and is involved in **neurogenic** inflammation of affected vessels.
   Prophylaxis—methysergide (5-HT blocker)
   Treatment—sumatriptan (5-HT$_{1D}$ agonist)
6. Platelets release 5-HT during **aggregation** at the site of **vessel injury** and accelerate injured vessels due to its contractile action → **haemostasis**.
7. **(5-HT+TXA$_2$)** from platelets cause coronary spasm and variant angina.
8. **HTN** is caused by 5-HT in pre-eclampsia (**ketanserin** is anti-hypertensive).
9. **Enterochromaffin cells** and **5-HT containing neurones** regulate peristalsis and local reflexes.
10. **Carcinoid syndrome** (tumour) → ↑ 5-HT → bowel hypermotility and bronchoconstriction.

Drugs effecting 5-HT system

1. **5-HT precursor:** Tryptophan enhances 5-HT.
2. **Synthesis inhibitor:** PCPA (P-chlorophenylalanine) inhibits tryptophan hydroxylase (**rate limiting step**) and reduces 5-HT level.
3. **Uptake inhibitor:** TCA inhibits 5-HT and NA uptake.
4. **Storage inhibitor:** Reserpine inhibits 5-HT and NA uptake into storage granule → depletion of **all monoamines**.
   Fenfluramine releases 5-HT.
5. **Degradation inhibitor:** MAO inhibitors prevent degradation of 5-HT.
6. **Neuronal degeneration:** 5, 6-dihydroxytryptamine destroys 5-HT neurones.
7. **5-HT R agonists**
   A. **LSD** (potent hallucinogen, non-selective 5-HT agonist) stimulates 5-HT$_{1A}$ on raphe cell body, and 5-HT$_{2A}$, 5-HT$_{2C}$ and 5-HT$_{5-7}$ in brain.
   B. **Azapirones** (non-sedative antianxiety) is partial agonist of 5-HT$_{1A}$ R.
   C. **Sumatriptan**
   D. **Cisapride** and **renzapride** are prokinetic drugs, enhance GIT motility and are 5-HT$_4$ agonist.
   E. **Trazodone** → active metabolite—mCPP (m-chlorophenyl piperazine). mCPP is 5-HT$_{1B}$, 5-HT$_{2A}$/5-HT$_{2C}$ agonist in brain.

5-HT blockers

A. **Nonselective/partial agonist**
   1. **Ergot derivatives:** LSD, L-Bromo LSD, ergotamine, methysergide.
   2. **α blocker:** Phenoxybenzamine
   3. **Antihistaminic:** Cyproheptadine, cinnarizine
   4. **CPZ**
   5. **Morphine**

Drugs Related to 5-Hydroxytryptamine System

B. **Clinically used drugs** **PCM ROCK**
   Pizotifin (pizotyline)
   Cyproheptadine
   Methysergide
   Risperidone
   Granisetron
   Clozapine
   Ketanserin and ritanserin.

Ketanserin: It is **clinically used 5-HT blocker.**
Mech: 1. Weak α_1, H_1 and **dopaminergic blockers.**
2. **5-HT$_2$ inhibition (5-HT$_{2A}$ > 5-HT$_{2C}$)** →antagonises vasoconstriction, platelet aggregation and airway smooth muscle contraction→ **antihypertensive action.**

PK: Oral bioavailability—**50%** due to first pass metabolism, extensively metabolised, t½—24 hrs at **steady rate,** dose →**20–40 mg BD.**

ADR: 1. Dizziness and nausea
2. Tiredness
3. Dry mouth

U: 1. Raynaud's disease

Ritanserin: It is **5-HT$_{2A}$ selective congener of ketanserin.**

Pizotifen: **Mech:** 1. 5-HT$_{2A}$/5-HT$_{2C}$ blockers
2. Antihistaminic
3. Anticholinergic
U: Migraine prophylaxis

Clozapine is a typical antipsychotic.
Mech: 1. Dopaminergic blocker
2. 5-HT$_{2A}$/5-HT$_{2C}$ blockers
U: Resistant schizophrenia

Risperidone is a typical antipsychotic.
Mech: 5-HT$_{2A}$ and **5-HT$_{2D}$ (combined) blockers** (actions **similar** to clozapine).
ADR: Extrapyramidal side effects.
U: **Reduces negative symptoms of schizophrenia.**

Cyproheptadine

Mech: 1. Prevents 5-HT$_{2A}$ R **(primarily)**
2. H_1 antihistaminic
3. Sedative
4. Anticholinergic
5. Cyproheptadine and methysergide block **D type receptor.**

U: 1. Allergy
2. As antipruritic
3. Enhances **appetite** → used in children and poor eaters to promote weight gain.

4. **Carcinoid** and **post-gastrectomy dumping syndrome**.
5. In antagonising **priapism/orgasmic delay** caused by 5-HT uptake inhibitors.
6. **Migraine prophylaxis**.

Ergot alkaloids

Ergot alkaloids are **adrenergic blockers**. **Ergot**, a fungus *Claviceps purpurea*, growing on **grains** (rye, millet), forms a purple hard body (curved) called **Sclerotium**. **Ergotism** (ergot poisoning by contaminated grain consumption) produces **dry gangrene of hand** and **feet of black colour like burn (most important feature)** and results in **miscarriages** in women and **convulsion**. Ergots have **alkaloids, LSD, ACh, histamine, tyramine, sterols**, etc.

1. **Natural ergot alkaloids** are **tetracyclic indole containing compounds** (a derivate of **lysergic acid**). Two types:
    A. **Amine alkaloids**
       a. **Ergometrine (ergonovine)**—oxytoxic
       b. **Methylergometrine**
    B. **Amino acid alkaloids**
       a. **Ergotoxine** (mixture of ergocristine, ergocryptine and ergocornine)
       b. **Ergotamine**
2. **Semisynthetic derivatives**
    a. Dihydroergotamine (DHE)
    b. Dihydroergotoxine (codergocrine)
    c. Bromocryptine (2-bromo-α-ergocryptine).
    d. Methysergide
3. **Synthetic nonlysergic acid derivatives:** Lisuride, pergolide, lergotrile, metergoline.

Ergotamine: It is **amino acid alkaloid of natural type**. Amino acid alkaloids are **α blockers** and **vasoconstrictors**. Natural ergot alkaloids → vasoconstriction → **ergotism** (peripheral vascular insufficiency and gangrene). **Hydrogenation** reduces constriction and enhances α blocking action. Ergot poisoning is known as St. Antony's fire.

Mech

1. Partial agonist and antagonist at **α R** and **all subtypes of 5-HT$_1$ and 5-HT$_2$ R** → sustained **vasoconstriction, visceral smooth muscle contraction, vasomotor centre depression, antagonism** of NA and 5-HT action on smooth muscle.
2. **Emetic** action through CTZ and moderately potent anxiolytic.
3. **Chronic use: Vasoconstriction** → **damage to capillary endothelium** → **thrombosis, vascular stasis** and **gangrene (ergotism)**.
4. **Ergotamine** causes **HTN** and **dihydroergotoxine** causes **hypotension** on **IV injection**.
5. **Amino acid alkaloids** (ergotamine and ergotoxine)→partial agonist—antagonist at α adrenergic, serotonergic and dopaminergic R.
6. **Ergotamine is most potent vasoconstrictor** (unrelated to autonomic receptor action). **Ergotoxine** is the **most potent α blocker**.

7. **Ergotamine in migraine**
   A. Constriction of **dilated cranial vessels**.
   B. Constriction of **AV shunt channel** → reduced shunting of blood flow from carotid artery.
   C. Ergotamine and DHE reduce **neurogenic inflammation and plasma leakage in dura mater** occurring due to **retrograde stimulation** of perivascular afferent nerves (mediated through partial agonism at **5-HT$_{1D/1B}$ R** in and around cranial vessels).

Uses of ergotamine: The **most effective** ergot alkaloid for migraine treatment.
Dose: 1 mg half hourly (fatal **6 mg**).
In **vomiting,** drug per rectum as suppository is given.
Amine alkaloids: Only **amine** alkaloids are used in **obstetrics**.
Ergonovine (ergometrine) is the **most potent oxytocic**.
Methylergometrine and **ergometrine** have **same pharmacological profile**. Both enhance **force, frequency** and **duration** of uterine contraction due to partial agonistic action on **5-HT$_2$** and **α R** (methylergometrine is **1½ times more potent** on uterus than ergometrine). Both are **weaker vasoconstrictor** and enhance **peristalsis** at high doses. Both are **sensitive** on gravid uterus specially at term and in early peurparium. They reduce **milk secretion** (dopaminergic action).

Mech:
1. Ergonovine: **Weak α agonist**.
   Partial 5-HT R agonist in uterus, placenta and umbilical blood vessels. **Potent 5-HT$_2$ blocker** in GIT smooth muscle. **Weak dopaminergic agonist** on pituitary lactotropes and CTZ. **Less emetic,** contraction of myometrium (**most important action**).
2. Methylergometrine is **1½ times** more potent than ergometrine on uterus.

PK:
1. Ergometrine and methylergometrine: Both are **rapidly** and **completely** absorbed from **oral** route.
   Effect of single dose is **3–4 hrs**.
   Onset of uterine action
   Oral — 15 min
   IM — 5 min
   IV — Immediate
   Partly hepatic metabolism and **plasma t½→1–2 hrs, excreted** in urine.
2. **Ergot alkaloids:** Oral bioavailability **<1%** due to slow and incomplete absorption and high first pass metabolism, **hepatic** metabolism, **excreted in bile,** sequestered in tissue (**action longer**), plasma t½— 2 hrs.
   Cross BBB.

ADR:
1. **Amine alkaloids** reduce **milk secretion** at higher doses due to inhibition of prolactin release (**dopaminergic action**).
2. **Ergot alkaloids:** Chest pain and vascular spasm, paresthesias, nausea and vomiting, weakness.

Cautions (amine alkaloid)
1. HTN and vascular disease
2. Toxaemia and sepsis
3. Liver and kidney disease

CI: (1) Ergot alkaloid
   (a) HTN, IHD, PVD
   (b) Pregnancy and sepsis
   (c) Liver and kidney disease
(2) **Amine alkaloid:** (a) Pregnancy, (b) Before 3rd stage of labour.
   CI of **ERGOTS:** **E**clampsia and pre-eclampsia, **R**h –ve mother (fetomaternal microtransfusion) and renal + liver diseases, **G**estation (multiple), **O**bstructive vascular and collagen diseases, **T**oxaemia in pregnancy, **S**epsis.

U: (1) **Amine alkaloids**
   (a) **PPH:** Compress uterine vessel and induce placental expulsion (in **third stage** of labour).
   (b) Instrumental delivery
   (c) To ensure normal involution
   (d) Preferred over oxytocin to stop bleeding (premature labour is reduced by β_2 agonist action).

Dihydroergotoxine

Dihydroergotoxine is a **semisynthetic** ergot alkaloid. **Nicergoline** has **same** action as dihydroergotoxine.

Mech: 1. Potent **α blocker** and weak vasoconstrictor.
2. Partial agonistic/antagonistic action on **5-HT R.**
3. Metabolic and vascular effects and enhanced ACh release in cerebral cortex occur. **ACh released** from cortical slices alters brain metabolism.
4. **Adrenergic blocker**
5. Enhances cerebral blood flow (**selectively**).

ADR: Flushing, hypotension and bowel upset.
U: Dementia.
DHE: It is semisynthetic ergot alkaloid.
Mech: 1. Reduces **serotonergic** and **α-adrenergic** agonistic action and enhances **α blocking** property (less potent vasoconstrictor).
2. **Weak emetic, oxytocic,** and **antidopaminergic** action present.
3. **DHE** and **dihydroergotoxine** are antiadrenergic and cerebroactive substances.

U: Migraine: **Equally** effective to ergotamine. Injected DHE is less hazardous. **Ergotamine + 100 mg caffeine** enhance ergotamine absorption from oral and rectal route and help in cranial vasoconstriction.

Methysergide

Methysergide is **semisynthetic** derivative of ergot alkaloid and is **anti 5-HT.**

Mech: 1. $5\text{-}HT_{2A}/5\text{-}HT_{2C}$ and $5\text{-}HT_1$ **blockers** on smooth muscle.
2. Acts as prophylaxis of migraine due to 5-HT antagonism.

ADR: 1. **CNS effects:** Nervousness, etc.
2. **GIT effects:** Abdominal pain, nausea, diarrhoea.
3. **On chronic use:** Abdominal, pulmonary and endocardial fibrosis. **A gap of one month** is given after **5 months** of treatment.

U: 1. Migraine prophylaxis
2. Cluster headache

3. Carcinoid and post-gastrectomy dumping syndrome.

> **Rule of one-third for carcinoid**
> 1. One-third metastasized
> 2. One-third multiple
> 3. One-third present with second malignancy

Migraine: **Pulsatile headache** usually restricted to **one side** with attacks lasting **4–48 hrs** and associated with **sensitivity** to light, nausea, vomiting, sound, vertigo and loose motions. Familial in **60–80%**, common in **women**, precipitating factor is **stress**.

Types: a. **Classical** (migraine with aura)
b. **Common** (migraine without aura)

Classical migraine shows **neurological** symptoms. Immediate cause of pain in migraine is **pulsatile dilatation** of large cranial vessels. An **initial intracranial vasoconstriction** is followed by **prolonged extracranial** vasodilatation during which headache occurs.

Mech: Unknown. Two theories are
1. **Vascular:** Vasoconstriction/blood shunting through carotid arteriovenous anastomoses produces **cerebral ischaemia** and starts attack.
2. **Neurogenic:** Spreading **depression** of cortical electrical activity and neurogenic inflammation of affected blood vessel wall amplified by retrograde transmission in afferent nerves and release of mediators (5-HT, substance P, neurokinin, NO, and calcitonin gene related peptide-CGRP).

Severity: A. **Mild:** **Fewer than one attack/month** of throbbing but tolerable headache lasting up to **8 hrs**.
B. **Moderate:** **One or more attacks/month**. Throbbing headache more intense, lasting for **6–24 hrs**.
C. **Severe:** **>2–3 attacks/month** of severe throbbing headache lasting **12–48 hrs**, accompanied by vertigo, vomiting, etc.

Treatment of migraine

A. **Mild:** NSAID (± antiemetic)
Antiemetics: Domperidone
Diphenhydramine
Metoclopramide
Promethazine
Prochlorperazine
B. **Moderate:** NSAID/ergot alkaloid/sumatriptan (+ antiemetics).
Prophylaxis: When attack >2–3/month.
C. **Severe:** Ergot alkaloid/sumatriptan (+ antiemetic).
Prophylaxis (≥6 month): β blocker, TCA, CCB, methysergide, cyproheptadine.

Prophylaxis of migraine

1. **Propranolol: Commonest** used drug. Reduces **frequency** and **severity** of attacks in **70% patient**, effects seen in one month.

Dose: 40 mg (starting) to **160 mg (maximum)**.
2. **Amitriptyline: Most extensively** tried.
3. **Flunarizine:** Weak **cerebroselective Ca²⁺ channel blocker** and also inhibits **Na⁺ channel** (reduces frequency and intracellular Ca²⁺ overload due to brain hypoxia).

ADR of flunarizine: Sedation, constipation, dry mouth, hypotension and weight gain. (Methysergide, pizotifen, valproate, verapamil are also used.)

Sumatriptan: Selective 5-HT$_{1D}$ agonist, cerebral vasoconstrictor, most effective treatment of acute attack.

Mech
1. **Novel selective 5-HT$_{1D}$ (also less potent 5-HT$_{1B}$) R agonist and inflammatory neuropeptidase release** around affected vessels (antimigraine action). Neuropeptidase suppresses **neurogenic inflammation** of cranial vessels.
2. **At high doses,** activates 5-HT$_1$R (vasoconstriction by activating 5-HT$_1$ R).
   75% complete relief in 3 hrs.
3. Suppresses nausea and vomiting of migraine.

PK: Oral bioavailability—15%. Absorbed rapidly and completely after **SC injection.** Rapidly metabolised by **MAO-A isoenzyme** and metabolites are excreted in **urine.** Elimination t½— <2 hrs.

IA: Interacts with 5-HT uptake inhibitor and **lithium**.

ADR:
1. Tingling and dizziness
2. Tightness of head and chest
3. Feeling of heat and weakness
4. HTN, bradycardia, risk of MI and vasospasm
5. SC injection → painful
6. Sudden death

CI:
1. IHD, HTN, CAD or prinzmetal angina
2. Epilepsy
3. Pregnancy
4. Hepatic and renal disease
5. Driving
6. Ergotamine and sumatriptan are not administered together within 24 hrs

U: Moderate and severe migraine **(the most effective treatment of acute attack).**

Sublingual drugs: **BUccal Mastication is NICE KNIFE** **BU**prenorphine, **M**ethyltestosterone, **N**itroglycerine; **I**soprenaline, **C**lonidine, **E**rgot, **NIFE**dipine.

39. Platelet Activating Factor, Prostaglandins and Leukotrienes

In the body, **PG, LT** and **TX** are all derived from **eicosa (20 C atoms) tri/tetra/penta enoic acid** and collectively called **Eicosanoids. LT = Leuko-Trienes**.

Leuko = Leukocyte (i.e. first obtained from it) and trienes = 3 conjugated double bonds. PG and LT are derivatives of **polyunsaturated essential fatty acid of 20C atoms**, released from **cell membrane phospholipid** and currently the **most intensely investigated substance**. PG is derivative of **prostanoic acid** (not present in the body) — **5 membered ring** and **2 side chains** projecting in **opposite** directions at **right angle to the plane of the ring**. PG and TX are designated as **A, B .... I** (depending on ring and its substituents). Each series has members with **subscript 1, 2, 3** (i.e. number of double bonds in side chains). LT is designated as **A,B, ... F** with subscript **1, 2, 3, 4**. Fatty acid (FA) released from membrane lipids in **largest** quantity is **arachidonic acid (5, 8, 11,14-eicosa tetraenoic acid)**. 4 double bonds are reduced to 2 double bonds due to saturation in **PG, PGI, TX synthesis** → subscript 2 PG **(most important in man)** → PGE_2, $PGF_{2\alpha}$, PGI_2, TXA_2. In LT synthesis, **no double bond reduction (no cyclization)** occurs → LTB_4, LTC_4, LTD_4. **Most universally distributed autacoids** in the body are **eicosanoids** which are synthesized locally and released as needed (*de novo* synthesis) with duration of action = **1 minute**. Every **cell** synthesizes PG/LT. There is **no preformed stores of PG/LT**.

Stimuli → ↑ intracellular Ca^{2+} → stimulates hydrolases and phospholipases A → PG and LT synthesis (rate is governed by arachidonic acid release from membrane lipid).

Primary PG

A. PGE_2 → partitioned into **ether buffer**.
B. $PGF_{2\alpha}$ → partitioned into **phosphate buffer**. α indicates "OH" group orientation on ring.

PG A, B, C are not found in the body. **Spleen** and **lungs** synthesize **whole range** of COX products. **Platelets** synthesize TXA_2 **(unstable)** → TXB_2. Vessel wall synthesize PGF_2 **(unstable)** → 6-Keto $PGF_{1\alpha}$. COX-1 and 2 catalyse the **same reaction**. COX-1 is **constitutive** enzyme in **most cells** (its activity is unchanged once cell is fully grown). **LOX pathway** occurs in lungs, WBC and platelets → LT **(most important product)**. LTB_4, C_4 and D_4 form **SRS-A** (slow reacting substance of anaphylaxis). LTB_4 is potent **chemotaxis**. Platelets have only **12 LOX**.

LOX →HPETE: (1) LT A_4; (2) Hepoxiline, trioxilin, lipoxiline.

Arachidonic acid $\xrightarrow{CYP450}$ 19 and 20-HETE and epoxyeicosatrienoic acid.

↓ Free radical
Isoprostanes

In brain cells, ethanolamine + arachidonic acid form **anandamide**.

Synthesis inhibition: **Aspirin** acetylates **COX** at serine residue irreversibly, while **other NSIADs** are **competitive** and **reversible** inhibitors of COX **(most non-selectively except miloxicam, nimesulide and nabumetone which are selective for COX-2)**. LT is enhanced due to increased **arachidonic acid** available for LOX pathway. **Glucocorticoids** (inhibit arachidonic acid release from membrane lipid →↓LT, ↓TX, ↓PG) → stimulation of **peptide lipocortin production** → inhibition of phospholipase A_2 → reduction of all eicosanoids (PG, TX, LT).

Degradation: Occurs in **most tissues** but is **fastest** in lungs.

Plasma t½ of most PG, TXA_2 and **prostacyclin** is few second to few minute.

Uptake into cells → side chain oxidised and double bond reduced → inactive metabolites → urine. PGI_2 is catabolised mainly in **kidney.**

Actions

1. **TXA_2** from platelets and **PGI_2** from vessel wall are **local hormone** to control microcirculation.

TXA_2 (platelet)	→	Increased aggregation
	→	Vasoconstriction
PGI_2 (vessel wall)	→	Decreased aggregation
	→	Vasodilatation

    PGI_2 = Platelet Gathering Inhibitor

2. **PGE_2** and **$PGF_{2\alpha}$** are **vasodilator** in most vascular beds (more potent than ACh/histamine). **$PGF_{2\alpha}$** constricts larger veins. **PGI_2** is uniformly **vasodilatory** and **more potent** than PGE_2. **TXA_2** produces vasoconstriction.

3. **PG endoperoxides** (G_2 and H_2) are inherently vasoconstrictor but often produce vasodilatation **(biphasic response)** due to conversion into other PG-PGI_2, etc.

4. **Hypotension** → reflex action → stimulation of heart by PGE_2 and $PGF_{2\alpha}$ → increased CO.

5. **PGE_2 and I_2** maintain **placental** blood flow and are continuously produced locally in **ductus arteriosus** during foetal life to keep it patent and at birth, their synthesis are inhibited → **closure** occurs.

    PG and LT mediate vasodilation and exudation at the site of **inflammation.**

    PGE_1 and **alprostadil** can be used to relax vascular smooth muscle and maintain patent ductus arteriosus. **Alprostadil** injected into penis causes vasodilatation and induces **penile erection**.

6. **TXA_2** produced locally by platelets induces **aggregation** and **release reaction.** Endoperoxides **PGG_2** and **H_2** are proaggregatory. PGI_2 is generated by

vascular endothelium and is **antiaggregatory**. PGD_2 also has antiaggregatory action ($PGI_2 > PGD_2$). PGE_2 has inconsistent effects.

PGG_2, PGH_2, PGI_2 and TXA_2 constitute mutually antagonistic system (antiaggregation in circulation and aggregation on injury).

Aspirin → COX acetylation in platelets → ↓TXA_2 → antiaggregation (lasting >3 days).

Vessel wall synthesizes fresh enzymes within hours but platelets do not synthesize them due to lack of nucleus.

7. $PGF_{2\alpha}$ acts predominantly on **myometrium** while PGE_2 acts mainly on cervix due to its **collagenolytic** property. Both **soften cervix** at low doses. *In vivo*, both enhance **tone** and **amplitude** of uterine contraction and uniformly contract the uterus (more contraction during pregnancy). But *in vitro*, PGE_2 relaxes nonpregnant uterus. **Foetal tissues** produce PG and at term $PGF_{2\alpha}$ is detected in maternal blood. PG mediates initiation and progression of labour (**aspirin** opposes these actions). PG presents in **semen** is absorbed when lodged due to coitus so as to coordinate movement of female genital tract for transportation of **sperm** and facilitation of its **fertilization**.

↑ PG synthesis by endometrium → incoordinated uterine contractions → blood vessel compression → uterine ischaemia → **pain (dysmenorrhoea)**. NSAID is effective in **dysmenorrhoea of most women**. PGE and F Expel Foetus.

8. $PGF_{2\alpha}$, PGD_2, TXA_2 → Bronchoconstrictor **(more potent than histamine)**.
   PGE_2 → Bronchodilator
   PGI_2 → Mild bronchodilator
   PGE_2 and I_2 inhibit histamine release

   Asthmatics are sensitive to constrictor and dilator effects of PG → imbalance between **dilators** (PGE_2 and I_2) and **constrictors** (LT, TXA_2, PGD_2 and $PGF_{2\alpha}$) → asthma.

9. PGE_2 and $PGF_{2\alpha}$ in GIT
   ↓
   Contraction (longitudinal muscle) and contraction/relaxation (circular muscle)
   ↓
   Colic and **watery diarrhoea**

   PGE_2 acts directly on intestinal mucosa → ↑ peristalsis → ↑ **water, electrolyte** and **mucus secretion**. PGI_2 opposes PGE_2 and toxin induced fluid movement. Hence, PG causes **secretory diarrhoea**. PGE_2 reduces acid secretion, juice volume and pepsin content in stomach and inhibits fasting and stimulated secretion (due to feeding, histamine and gastrin). Mucus secretion in stomach and mucosal blood flow are enhanced **(antiulcerogenic)**. PG (specially PGI_2) regulates **gastric mucosal blood flow** and acts as natural ulcer protectives. PGI_2 is mucosal vasodilator.

10. PGE_2 and I_2 enhance H_2O, Na^+ and K^+ excretion (**diuretic effects**), possess a **furosemide like inhibitory effect on Cl^- reabsorption** (↓Cl^- reabsorption), cause renal vasodilation, inhibit tubular reabsorption and **antagonise ADH**

action. TXA$_2$ causes **renal vasoconstriction**. PGD$_2$, E$_2$ and I$_2$ evoke **renin release**. PG regulates intrarenal blood flow and tubular reabsorption. Diuretic action of furosemide is blunted by **indomethacin** (because PG facilitates renal blood flow and inhibits tubular reabsorption). PG facilitates **renin release** due to **sympathetic stimulation. Bartter's syndrome** has decreased sensitivity to **AT II** and enhances production of PG (treatment of the syndrome—**NSAID**).

11. Poor penetration into CNS. **On injection (intracerebroventricularly)**, PGE$_2$ produces sedation, rigidity, behavioral changes and increased body temperature (**PGF$_{2\alpha}$** is not pyrogenic). **NSAID** (PG synthesis inhibitor) is antipyretic. PG is **neuromodulator** in brain by regulating neuronal excitability.

12. PG modulates **sympathetic neurotransmission** by increasing/decreasing NA release from adrenergic nerve endings.

13.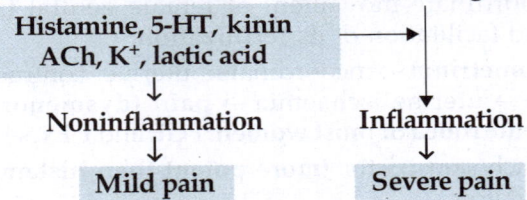

(PGE$_2$ and I$_2$ sensitize afferent nerve ending to cause pain).

14. PGEs are **antilipolytic**, enhance **carbohydrate** metabolism like insulin, **mobilise Ca^{2+}** from bone.

15. PGE$_2$ facilitates release of **anterior pituitary (GH, ACTH, FSH, LH and prolactin)** hormones, **insulin** and **adrenal steroid**. It has **TSH like effect on thyroid**.

LT: **LTB$_4$** is produced by **neutrophils**. **LTC$_4$** and **D$_4$** (cysteinyl LT) are produced by **macrophages**.

Actions

1. **LTC$_4$ and D$_4$** are the **most important allergic mediators** of human allergic asthma, released along with other autacoids during **Ag–Ab reaction** in the lungs, also cause **abdominal colic** during systemic anaphylaxis. LTC$_4$ and D$_4$ contract **most smooth muscles**, are bronchodilators, enhance mucus secretion in airways and induce spastic contraction of GIT.

2. **LTC$_4$ and D$_4$ on injection**—brief **HTN** followed by prolonged **hypotension** (not due to vasodilation) due to coronary constriction induced decrease in CO and decreased circulating volume (because of enhanced capillary permeability).

3. LT is more potent in causing **local edema** than histamine. **LTB$_4$** is **chemotactic** for neutrophils and monocytes and promotes **neutrophils migration** through capillary and their clumping at the site of inflammation. **5-HPETE** and **5-HETE** facilitate histamine release from **mast cells**.

Prostanoid receptor (R): R located at **cell membrane** is specific for **PG, TX, PGI$_2$** and is of **5 types**. Each R has **greatest affinity for a particular PG.** All are G protein coupled R using **IP$_3$/DAG or cAMP** transducer mechanism.
1. **DP: Greatest** affinity for **PGD$_2$** (PGE$_2$ also acts on it).
   Stimulation → ↑ cAMP → **antiaggregation action**.
2. **EP: Greatest** affinity for **PGE$_2$. Enprostil** is a selective agonist.
   Two types of EP
   A. **EP$_1$:** Smooth muscle contraction through **IP$_3$/DAG** pathway.
   B. **EP$_2$:** Smooth muscle relaxation due to → ↑ cAMP → ↑ Cl$^-$ and **water secretion from intestinal mucosa**.
3. **FP: Greatest** affinity for **PGF$_{2\alpha}$. Fluprostenol** is selective agonist.
   Smooth muscle contraction through **IP$_3$/DAG** formation **(most prominent action)**.
4. **IP: Greatest** affinity for **PGI$_2$** (PGE$_2$ also acts on it). **Eicaprost** is selective agonist. Stimulates **adenyl cyclase** in platelets **(antiaggregation)** and in smooth muscle **(relaxation)**.
5. **TP: Greatest** affinity for **TXA$_2$** (PGH$_2$ also acts on it).
   Acts through IP$_3$/DAG.
   Two types: A. TP platelet (platelet aggregation)
   B. TP non-platelet (smooth muscle contraction)
   LT RECEPTORS (act through **IP$_3$/DAG** formation) are: **LTB$_4$ R, LTC$_4$ R** and **LTD$_4$ R**.

ADR of PG
1. Uterine cramps and unduely forceful uterine contraction.
2. Vaginal bleeding, flushing, shivering, fever, malaise.
3. Hypotension, tachycardia, chest pain.
4. Watery diarrhoea, nausea and vomiting.

Uses of PG
1. **Abortion: Procedure of choice for MTP** is **transcervical suction**. Intravaginal **PGE$_2$** pessary inserted 3 hrs before dilatation minimises trauma to cervix by reducing resistance to dilatation. PG converts oxytocin resistant mid-term uterus to **oxytocin responsive one.** PGE$_2$ followed by oxytocin/PGF$_2\alpha$ with hypertonic solution produces **2nd term abortion.**
2. **Induction of labour:** PGE$_2$ and F$_{2\alpha}$ are used in place of oxytocin in toxaemia and renal failure patients because they do not cause **fluid retention.**
3. **Cervical priming:** PGE$_2$ soften the cervix.
4. **PPH: Carboprost** (15-methyl PGF$_{2\alpha}$) controls PPH due to uterine atony in ergotamine/oxytocin resistant cases.

> PGE$_2$ (Dinoprostone)
> PGF$_{2\alpha}$ (Dinoprost)
> 15-methyl PGF$_{2\alpha}$ (Carboprost)

5. **Peptic ulcer:** Stable analogues of PGE$_1$ **(misoprostol, rioprostil)** and PGE$_2$ **(enprostil)** for healing peptic ulcer in smoker/NSAID user.

6. **Patent ductus arteriosus:** It is maintained by PGE_1 (alprostadil).
7. **To avoid platelet damage:** PGI_2 **(epoprostenol)** inhibits aggregation and damage during haemodialysis/cardiopulmonary bypass and improves harvest of platelet for transfusion.
8. a. **PVD:** PGE_2 and I_2
   b. **Bronchial asthma:** PGE_2
   c. **To reduce infarct size:** PGI_2
   d. **Impotence:** PGE_1
9. Menstruation inducing contraceptive.

Platelet activating factor (PAF) is a cell membrane derived **polar lipid** with intense biological activity. **PAF (A**cetyl-**g**lyceryl **e**ther-phosphorylcholine) acts as a signal molecule.

Age

Mech: PAF receptors (G protein coupled) act through $IP_3/DAG \rightarrow Ca^{2+}$ release. Actions are mediated by **PG, TXA, LT** (extracellular messenger).
Proaggregatory actions are due to unmasking of fibrinogen binding sites on platelet surfaces.

Actions
1. **Platelet aggregation** and TXA_2 **release**.
2. **Chemotactic** to neutrophil, eosinophil and monocyte. Stimulates **neutrophil aggregation** to stick to vascular endothelium and migrates across it to **infection site**.
3. Promotes **lysosomal enzymes** and **LT release** and generation of **superoxide radical** by polymorphs.
4. **IV injection** results in intravascular thrombosis.
5. **EDRF release** →**vasodilatation** →**hypotension** and **reduced coronary blood flow** (due to platelet aggregation and TXA_2 release).
6. For enhanced vascular permeability **(most potent agent)**.
7. **Reduces renal blood flow** and Na^+ excretion by direct vasoconstrictor action.
8. Contracts **visceral smooth muscle** by direct action and through release of LTC_4, TXA_2 and **PG**, causes **bronchoconstriction**.
9. **Ulcerogenic** for stomach due to erosion and mucosal bleeding. Gastric smooth muscle contracts.
10. Produces **mucosal edema, secretion** and **bronchial hyper-responsiveness**.
11. Stimulates **intestinal** and **uterine smooth muscle** and promotes **embryo implantation**.

PAF blockers: Ginkgolide B from Chinese plant is PAF blocker. Partial PAF blocker is **alprazolam** and **triazolam**.

Uses of PAF blockers: MI and stroke, shock, GI ulceration, asthma, as contraceptive.

Synthesis and degradation: No preformed store. Ag–Ab reaction stimulates PAF synthesis. Synthesized in **WBC, platelet, kidney cell**, and **vascular endothelium** only (*see* box).

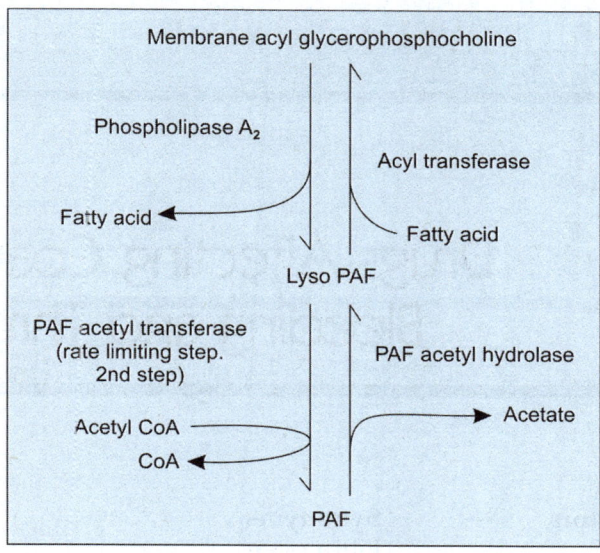

Unit 7
Drugs Affecting Blood

40. Drugs Affecting Coagulation, Bleeding and Thrombosis

Clotting factors	—	Synonyms
I	—	Fibrinogen
II	—	Prothrombin
III	—	Tissue thromboplastin
IV	—	Ca^{2+} C, a, 2, + = 4
V	—	Proaccelerin
VI	—	Unknown
VII	—	Proconvertin
VIII	—	Antihemophilic globulin
IX	—	Christmas factor
X	—	Stuart-Prower factor
XI	—	Plasma thromboplastin antecedent
XII	—	Hageman factor
XIII	—	Fibrin stabilising factor

Hemophilia is **X-linked recessive disorder** due to deficiency of clotting factor **VIII (hemophilia A)** and **IX (hemophilia B)**. Level of clotting factor VIII to be maintained to treat bleeding is **20%** and before surgery **50%. Measure of function of intrinsic system** is PTT (partial thromboplastin time). Normal PTT is **30–40 sec.** Measure of function of **extrinsic system** is **PT** (prothrombin time).

Prolonged PTT
1. **No bleeding:** Deficiency of **HMWK, prekallikrein** and **clotting factor XII**.
2. **Mild bleeding:** Deficiency of clotting factor **XI**.
3. **Severe bleeding:** Deficiency of clotting factor **VIII** and **IX**.

Prolonged PT: Deficiency of clotting factor **VII**, vitamin **K** and **warfarin therapy.**

Prolonged PTT and PT: Deficiency of clotting factor **II, V, X, vitamin K** and **warfarin therapy.**

Prolonged TT (thrombin time)
1. **Mild bleeding:** Afibrinogenemia
2. **Severe bleeding:** Dysfibrinogenemia
3. **Heparin therapy**

Therapeutic products for the treatment of coagulation disorders

Factor	Deficiency state	Concentration (%) relative to normal plasma required for hemostasis	Half-life (days) of infused factor	Therapeutic material
I	Afibrinogenemia, defibrination syndrome	40	4	Plasma fibrinogen, cryoprecipitate
II	Prothrombin deficiency	40	3	Concentrate (factor IX-prothrombin complex)
V	Factor V deficiency	20	1	Fresh-frozen plasma
VII	Factor VII deficiency	Unknown	0.25	Concentrate (some preparations of factor IX)
VIII	Hemophilia A	25–35	0.5	Plasma cryoprecipitate (classic) and other factor VIII concentrate
	von Willebrand's disease	30	Unknown	
IX	Hemophilia B (Christmas disease)	25	1	Plasma, factor IX-prothrombin complex
X	Stuart-Prower defect	25	1.5	Plasma, concentrate (some preparations of factor IX)
XI	PTA deficiency	Unknown	3	Fresh-frozen plasma
XII	Hageman defect	Not required	Unknown	Treatment not needed
XIII	Fibrin-stabilizing factor deficiency	2	6	Fresh-frozen plasma
AT III	Antithrombin III deficiency	80	3	Concentrate (AT III-specific)

Blood clotting factors and drugs that affect them

Component/Factor	Common synonym	Target for the action
I	Fibrinogen	X
II	Prothrombin	Heparin (IIa); warfarin (synthesis)
III	Tissue thromboplastin	X
IV	Calcium	X
V	Proaccelerin	X
VII	Proconvertin	Heparin (VIIa); warfarin (synthesis)
VIII	Antihemophilic globulin (AHG)	X
IX	Christmas factor, PTC	Heparin (IXa); warfarin (synthesis)
X	Stuart-Prower factor	Heparin (IXa); warfarin (synthesis)
XI	PTA	X
XII	Hageman factor	X
XIII	Fibrin-stabilizing factor	X
Protein C and S		Warfarin (synthesis)
Plasminogen		Thrombolytic enzymes, aminocaproic acid

1. **Vitamin K dependent factors** = II, V, VII, IX, X. **Factors** inactivated by heparin are **IIa, IXa, Xa, XIa, XIIa, XIIIa.**

   All numbers having "X" and thrombin (IIa) are inhibited by heparin.

2. **Intrinsic system (slow): All factors** needed for coagulation are present in **plasma.**
3. Factors requiring Ca^{2+} are **IXa, Xa, XIa, XIIa.**
4. Platelet phospholipid (**PL. Ph**) is needed by **IXa** and **Xa.**
5. **Most factors** are protein present in **plasma** in inactive form (**zymogen**). They themselves are activated by **partial proteolysis** to form **active protease** and activate **next factors.**
6. **Antithromboplastin, antithrombin, protein C** and **fibrinolysin** system oppose coagulation and lyse formed clot.

PT (**EXT**rinsic) = Bleeding due to defect in II, V, VII, X
PTT (intrinsic) = Bleeding due to defect in all except VII and XIII

Pure TEXT	→ II + V = VII
	II × V = X
PTT	→ VII, XIII

Protein **S** and Protein **C S**top **C**lotting.
Common disease in bleeding disorders: **HE** (male) gets **HE**mophilia, **HE**mochromatosis, **HE**art attack, **HE**molytic anemia (**HE**inz body), **HE**noch-Schönlein purpura. **SHE** (female) gets **SHE**han's syndrome.

Coagulants: Promote coagulation. Fresh whole blood/plasma provide **all factors** of coagulation and are **best therapy** for deficiency of any clotting factors and act immediately.

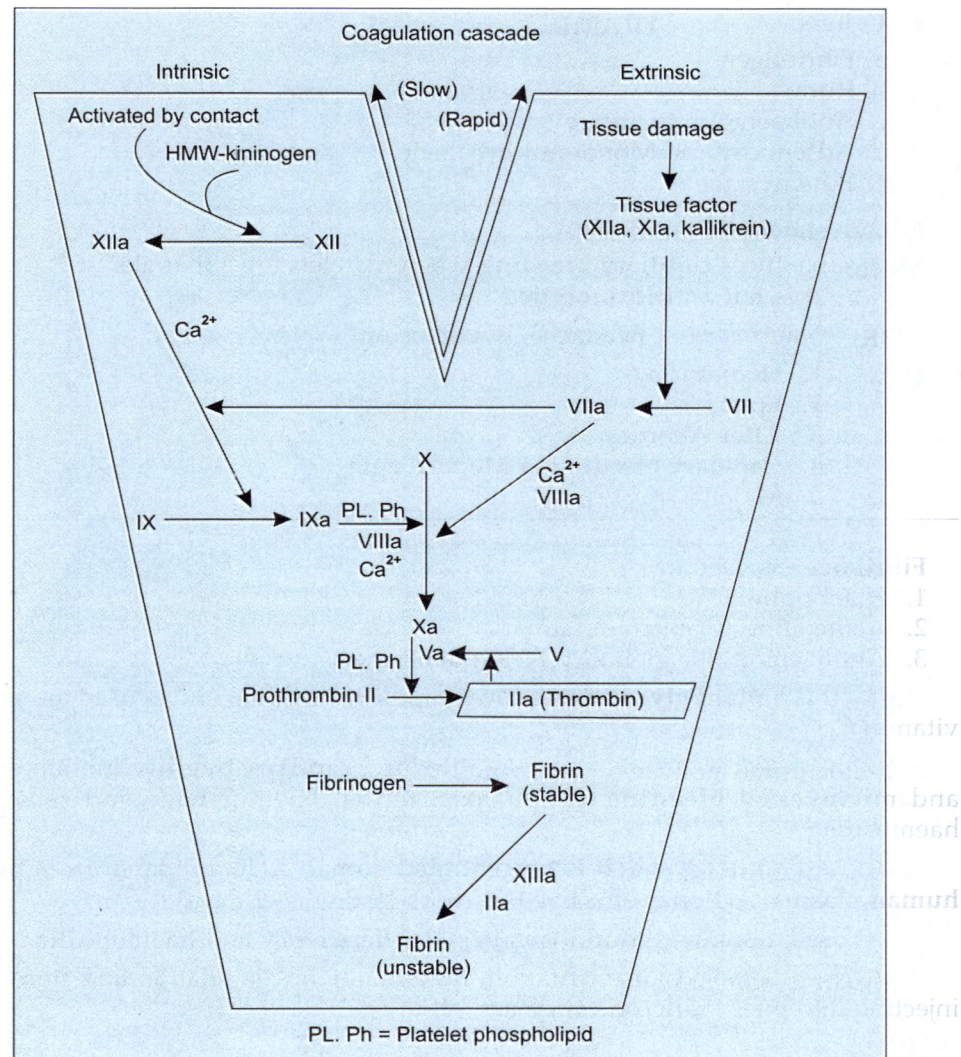

Coagulants are

1. **Fresh whole blood/plasma**
2. **Vitamin K**
   a. **K_1:** Phytonadione or phylloquinone (obtained from plant, fat soluble)
   b. **K_2:** Menaquinone (obtained from bacteria)
   c. **K_3:** (Synthetic, fat and water soluble)
   Fat-soluble — Menadione, acetomenaphthone
   Water-soluble — Menadione sodium bisulfite.
   — Menadione sodium diphosphate.

3. Others **FRAME**
   a. **F**ibrinogen
   b. **R**utin
   c. **A**ntihaemophilic factor
   d. Adreno**c**hrome **M**onosemicarbazone
   e. **E**thamyslate

Ethamyslate: It is a coagulant

Mech: Reduces **capillary bleeding** when platelets are adequate. **It is not antifibrinolytic.**

ADR: Nausea, rash, headache, hypotension.

U:
1. **H**ematuria
2. **E**pistaxis **HEAM**
3. **A**fter Abortion
4. Capillary bleeding in **M**enorrhagia
5. Malena

Fibrinogen is used in:
1. Haemophilia
2. Acute afibrinogenemic state
3. Antihaemophilic globulin (AHG) deficiency.

Rutin: It is a **plant glycoside,** reduces capillary bleeding and is used along with vitamin C.

Adrenochrome monosemicarbazone: Reduces **capillary fragility,** inhibits **oozing** and **microvessel bleeding** in epistaxis, retinal haemorrhage and secondary haemorrhage.

Antihaemophilic factor: It is concentrated human AHG prepared from **pooled human plasma.** Action is effective but short lasting (**1–2 days**).

Uses: Used along with fibrinogen in **AHG deficiency** and **haemophilia.**

Sclerosing agents: Cause irritation, inflammation, coagulation and fibrosis on injection into piles/varicose vein mass.

These are
1. **Phenol (5%)** in almond/peanut oil
2. **Ethanolamine oleate** (5% in 25% glycerine and 2% benzyl alcohol)
3. **Sodium tetradecyl sulfate** (5% in 2% benzyl alcohol)
4. **Quinine** (12.5%) + **urethane** (6.25%)

Local haemostatics (styptics): Substances used to stop bleeding locally particularly from oozing surface that **must never be injected.**

A. **Thrombin:** **Dry powder/solution** applied on bleeding surface. Used in **skin grafting, neurosurgery** and **haemophilia.**
B. **Fibrin:** Used as **sheet/foam** on bleeding surface.
C. **Gelatin foam:** **Sponging gelatin** of various shapes used in **wound packing.**
D. **Astringent:** Used for bleeding gums/piles.
E. **Vasoconstrictors**

Drugs Affecting Coagulation, Bleeding and Thrombosis

F. **Russel viper venom:** Acts as **thromboplastin,** applied locally, used to stop external bleeding in haemophilia.

Anticoagulants (reduce blood coagulation)
Used *in vitro*
1. **Heparin**—1.5 U/ml
2. **Ca^{2+} complexing agents**
   Sodium Edetate – 2 mg/ml → for Investigation
   Sodium Citrate – 5 mg/ml → for Transfusion
   Sodium Oxalate – 10 mg/ml → for Investigation

| C, T | = | Consonants |
| E, I, O | = | Vowels |

Used *in vivo*   DR. END HAD A WEB
1. **Heparin**
2. **LMW heparin**
   — Enoxaprin   (MW 2000–9000)   DR. END
   — Dalteparin ⎱
   — Danaproid ⎰ (MW 2000–9000)
   — Nadoparin
   — Reviparin
3. **Heparinoid:** Heparan sulfate   HAD
   Ancrod
   Dextran sulfate, Lepirudin
4. **Oral anticoagulants**
   A. **Indandione** derivatives : Phenindione
   B. **Coumarin** derivatives : Warfarin sodium
      Ethyl biscoumacetate
             A WEB   Bishydroxycoumarin (dicoumarol)
      Acenocoumarol (nicoumalone)
   C. **Hirulog** and **Hirudin** (newer agents being tested)
5. **Heparin antagonist:** Protamine sulfate
6. **Warfarin antagonist:** Phytonadione (vitamin K)
   Specific antidote of oral anticoagulants: Vitamin K$_1$

Heparin (liquaemin): A medical student (**McLean**) **in 1916** discovered it in **liver.** In 1918, Holt and Howell named it **HEPARIN** (from liver). **In 1937,** it was purified for **clinical use. Heparin** is a **non-uniform mixture** of straight chain **mucopolysaccharide** (MW 10,000–20,000) with polymers of **2 sulfated disaccharide units:**
 A. D-glucosamine-L-iduronic acid
 B. D-glucosamine-D-glucuronic acid

Both disaccharide units vary in length and **proportion.** Some glucosamine residues are **N-acetylated.** It is **the strongest organic acid present in the body,** has strong **electronegative** charges, is found in **all tissues** containing **mast cells** (MW ~ 75000) and is loosely bound to **granular protein.**

Richest sources are: Intestinal mucosa, Lung, Liver.   ILL

Commercially obtained from **pig intestinal mucosa** and **ox lung**. Number of unit of heparin found in **1 mg = 120 units**.

Mech

1. Active both *in vivo* and *in vitro*.
2. **Antiplatelet action** and **lipemia clearing**: It inhibits **platelet aggregation**, prolongs **bleeding time**, clears turbid post-prandial **lipemic plasma**, releases **lipoprotein lipase** from vessel wall and tissues (which hydrolyses TG of chylomicron and VLDL to FFA→ FFA goes into tissue →**plasma looks clear**).
3. Catalyses **AT III activation** (antithrombin III activation) of plasma. AT III is a **serine proteinase inhibitor**. AT III activation →complex binds to clotting factor of intrinsic and common pathways (IIa, IXa, Xa, XIa, XIIa, XIIIa) and inactivates them. AT III is itself a substrate for **protease clotting factor** (but interaction is slow in the absence of heparin). **AT III action is enhanced by heparin by:**
   A. Inducing **conformational** changes in AT III to expose its interactive sites.
   B. Providing **scaffolding** for clotting factor and AT III to get bound and interact with each other. IIa inhibition needs both mechanism (A & B) and Xa inhibition needs only mechanism (A).
4. It prolongs **both PT** (prothrombin time) and **aPTT** (activated partial thrmoboplastin time) at **higher** concentration. It prolongs **only aPTT** at its **lower** concentration (i.e. **lower** concentration of heparin effects only **intrinsic** pathway while **higher** concentration effects **common** pathways).

PT and aPTT test integrity of coagulation cascade

	PT	aPTT
a. Intrinsic pathway interfered	= normal (12–14 sec)	prolonged
b. Extrinsic pathway interfered	= prolonged	normal (26–32 sec)
c. Common pathway interfered	= prolonged	prolonged

Heparin binds to AT III and enhances its proteolytic activity.

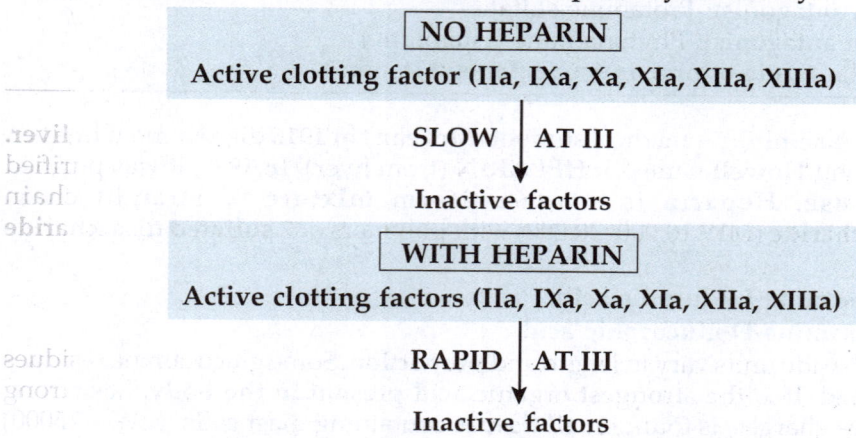

5. It inhibits the action of factor **X** and **thrombin**.

6. It acts by catalysing the reaction between **AT III** and **thrombin** which results in **inactive complex of thrombin.** It also complexes clotting factor **Xa**. Goal of treatment is to enhance **aPTT by 2 times the normal value.**

PK: Not absorbed orally because of large and highly ionised molecule. **Not cross BBB** and **placenta**, hence **anticoagulant of choice in pregnancy. Onset of action** — immediate. **Duration** of action—4 to 6 hrs.

Hepatic metabolism by heparinase and renal excretion: Inactivation due to metabolism follows **zero order kinetics.** Increasing the dose enhances the time to eliminate **50% of the drug. Macrophages degrade** heparin released from **mast cells.**

t½:
    A. **1 hr** when dose is <100 U/kg
    B. **5 hrs** when dose is >100 U/kg
    C. **Longer** in kidney and liver failure
    D. **Shorter** in pulmonary embolism
       (short t½ → hence check aPTT)

Route: IV/SC. Heparin is mostly confined to **vascular system.**

Unitage: 1 unit heparin means prevention of clotting of **1 ml** of citrated sheep plasma for **1 hr** after addition of **0.2 ml of 1% CaCl$_2$ solution.**

1 mg heparin sodium = 120–140 U activity: Heparin alters **shape of RBC** and **WBC**, hence not used in blood count, fragility testing and CFT.

Dose

1. **Conventional dose (IV)**
   a. 5000–10,000 U IV every 6 hourly (**bolus**), (50–100 U/kg children).
   b. 750–1000 U/hr (**continuous**). Dose and frequency controlled by **aPTT measurement** (kept at 50–80 sec) or **by whole blood clotting time** (kept at 2 min).
2. **Conventional dose (SC):** SC if IV is not possible. 10,000–20,000 U every 8–12 hours deep SC. Action starts in 30–60 min. **Haematomas** are common with **IM route** (hence no IM route is considered).
3. **Low dose regimen (5000 U SC every 8–12 hourly):** Start before surgery and continued for 10 days. This inhibits DVT, does not prolong CT/aPTT and is **contraindicated** in neurosurgery or spinal anaesthesia. Patient should not take aspirin or oral anticoagulant.

ADR

1. **Bleeding (most serious complication)** is 1–12%
2. **Hematuria (first sign** of bleeding during heparin therapy)
3. **Thrombocytopenia** due to platelet aggregation
4. **Alopecia** (transient and reversible). Other drugs causing alopecia are oral contraceptive, cytotoxic and ethionamide.
5. **Osteoporosis:** Drugs causing osteoporosis are steroid, GnRH analogue, phenytoin and heparin.
6. **Hypersensitivity reaction** (fever, rigor, urticaria, anaphylaxis) is rare.

CI: Bleeding, thrombocytopenia, HTN (risk of cerebral haemorrhage), threatened abortion, piles, GI ulcer, SABE (embolism), malignancy, TB, ocular and neurosurgery, LP, chronic alcoholism, cirrhosis, renal failure, aspirin/antiplatelet drugs.

IA: Not mix heparin with penicillin, noradrenaline, tetracycline, hydrocortisone.

Uses of heparin (immediate anticoagulant)
1. **Prophylaxis in surgery, MI, CHF, pregnancy** (because it does not cross placenta unlike warfarin), chronic **DIC, warfarin failure**.
2. **Venous thromboembolism** and **pulmonary embolism**.

LMW heparin: MW 3000–7000, **different** anticoagulant profile.
Mech
1. Selectively inhibits factor **Xa** with little effect on **IIa**.
2. Induces **conformational** changes in **AT III** (smaller effect on **aPTT** and **whole blood CT** than unfractionated heparin—UFH).
3. Eno**X**aprin acts on factor **Xa** only (so, monitor **Xa** rather than aPTT).
4. Lesser **antiplatelet** action.
5. Not interact with platelet thus not cause thrombocytopenia.

ADR: Lower incidence of **thrombocytopenia** than heparin.
CI: Renal failure.
PK: Has more predictable **dose-response relationship** than heparin.
Bioavailability **70–90%** compared to **UFH (20–30%)**. Eliminated by **kidney by first order kinetics**. LMWH and UFH are **equally** efficacious.
Better absorbed after **SC injection** than heparin.
Usual dose: 200 U/kg/day (SC). Longer t½.
U: 1. **Prophylaxis of DVT** and **pulmonary embolism**.
2. Treatment of **DVT**.
3. To maintain patency of **cannula** and **shunts** in dialysis.

Heparan sulfate: Heparin like **natural substance** found on cell surface and in intercellular matrix. **Physiological antithrombotic** at the surface of vascular endothelium. **Less potent anticoagulant** than heparin. **Semi-synthetic heparinoids (sulfated mucopolysaccharides)** are potent anticoagulant.

Dextran sulfate: It is **sulfated polymeric sugar 1/7th as potent as heparin** but **duration** of action is **twice**.

Ancrod: It is **enzyme of Malayan pit viper venom**.
Mech: Degrades **fibrinogen** into unstable form of **fibrin** which is taken up by RE cells → depleted fibrinogen (**heparin like effect**).
ADR: Bleeding, hypersensitivity, intravascular obstruction on IV injection.
U: 1. 2 U/kg 6 hourly in **DVT** (developing thrombocytopenia and hypersensitivity reaction to heparin).
2. Use of heparin → to initiate therapy.

Protamine sulfate: It is **strongly basic LMW protein of sperm of fish**.
Mech
1. Causes **rapid reversal of heparinization** (positively charged molecule that acts by binding negatively charged heparin).
2. **Neutralises** heparin weight for weight (1 mg for every 100 U of heparin).
3. Acts as **weak anticoagulant** in the absence of heparin.

4. **Releases histamine** in the body due to its basic nature.

ADR: Hypersensitivity reaction, flushing, dyspnoea.

U:
1. Severe bleeding.
2. Termination of heparin action (after cardiac and vascular surgery).

Coumarin/warfarin: The **most common oral anticoagulant. The most suitable and better tolerated drug. Coumarin derivative, synthetic.**

Mech
1. Inhibits synthesis of **vitamin K dependent clotting factor.**
2. Vitamin K dependent **carboxylase** fixes CO_2 to form **COOH group** on **glutamic acid** and reduced vit K is converted to **KO**. Vitamin K is regenerated from KO by **KO reductase** which is inhibited by **warfarin.**
3. **γ-carboxyglutamyl residues** bind Ca^{2+} and are essential for interaction with cell membrane. Warfarin produces **inactive clotting factor** due to **lack of γ-carboxyglutamyl side chain. KH_2** carries out final step of **γ-carboxylating glutamate residues** of **prothrombin** and **factor VII, IX** and **X. Carboxylation** provides clotting factor to bind Ca^{2+} and to get bound to phospholipid surfaces → **coagulation.**
4. Blockade of reduction of vitamin K to its active form slows **carboxylation** and reduces synthesis of vitamin K dependent clotting factor **(II, VII, IX, X).** Interferes with **normal synthesis** and **γ-carboxylation of vitamin K dependent clotting factor II, VII, IX, X via vitamin K antagonism.**

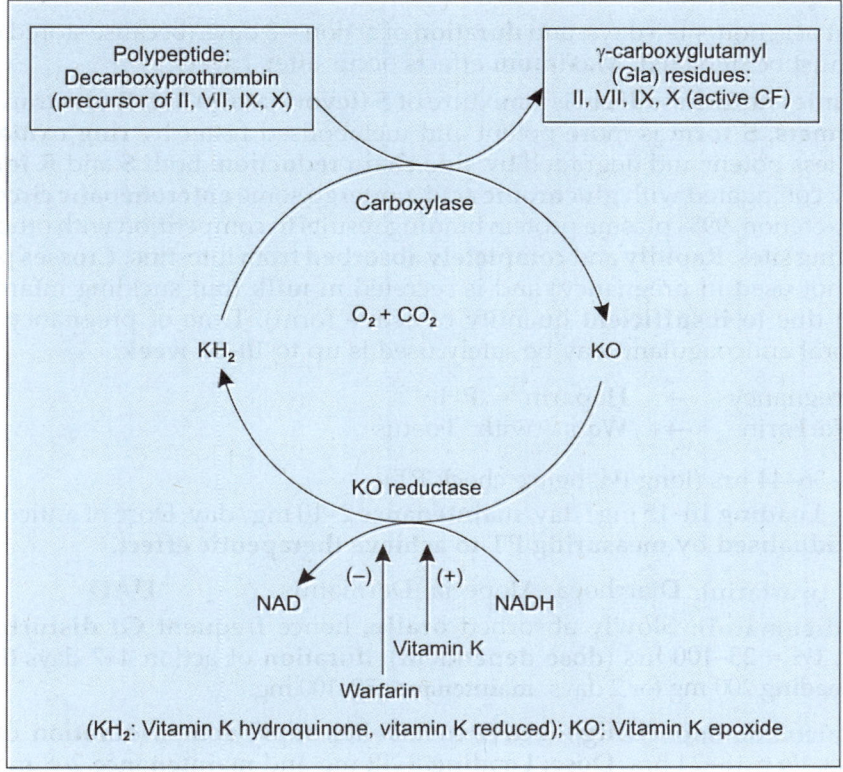

(KH_2: Vitamin K hydroquinone, vitamin K reduced); KO: Vitamin K epoxide

Warfarin is **competitive** Vitamin K blocker and reduces plasma level of **functional clotting factor in dose dependent manner.**

5. Acts only *in vivo* (not *in vitro*) because of indirect interference with **vitamin K synthesis dependent clotting factor in liver.**
6. A. Factor VII—plasma t½ = **6 hrs (shortest)**, its level reduces **first** on warfarin use. Likewise:
   B. Factor VIII   —   plasma t½: 28 hrs   —   2nd
   Factor IX   —   plasma t½: 24 hrs   —   3rd
   Factor X   —   plasma t½: 40 hrs   —   4th
   Prothrombin   —   plasma t½: 60 hrs   —   Last

   So, **order of reduction of level of clotting factor on warfarin use: VII < VIII < IX < X < prothrombin (last).**
7. **Clotting factor synthesis** is reduced in 2–4 hrs but anticoagulant effects develop in **1–3 days** due to gradual decrease of clotting factor already present in plasma. Decrease in clotting factor by **40–50%** causes therapeutic effects.
8. **Protein C** and **S** and **osteocalcin** contain **glutamate residues** that require **vitamin K dependent γ-carboxylation** and are inhibited by **oral anticoagulant.**
9. **Lab. control of PT/prothrombin activity** is essential.

Warfarin affects Extrinsic pathway and prolongs **PT.**   **WEPT**

Therapeutic goal of warfarin is to double PT.

PK (warfarin): Route—**Oral.**

Onset of action = 1–3 days, and **duration** of action = 3 days (because stored clotting factor must be depleted. **Maximum** effects occur after 1 week).

Racemic warfarin sodium is a mixture of **S (levorotatory)** and **R (dextrorotatory) enantiomers. S form** is more potent and metabolised faster by **ring oxidation. R form** is less potent and degraded by **side chain reduction.** Both S and R forms are partially conjugated with **glucuronic acid,** undergo some **enterohepatic circulation. Renal** excretion. **99%** plasma protein binding results in competition with other drugs for binding sites. **Rapidly** and **completely absorbed** from intestine. **Crosses placenta** (hence not used in pregnancy) and is secreted in **milk** (but suckling infant is less affected due to **insufficient** quantity of active form). Time of pregnancy during which oral anticoagulant may be safely used is up to **10–32 week.**

Pregnancy   →   Heparin = PH
WarFarin   →   Wars with Foetus

t½ — 36–44 hrs (long t½, hence check PT).

Dose: Loading 10–15 mg/day, **maintenance** 2–10 mg/day. Dose of anticoagulant is **individualised by measuring PT to achieve therapeutic effect.**

ADR (warfarin): Diarrhoea, Alopecia, Dermatitis.   **DAD**

PK (dicumarol): Slowly absorbed **orally,** hence frequent GI disturbance is present, t½ = 25–100 hrs (**dose dependent**), **duration** of action 4–7 days (**longest**). **Dose: Loading** 200 mg for 2 days, **maintenance** 50–100 mg.

PK (nicoumalone): Drug → active metabolite, rapid action, **duration** of action 2–3 days, t½ = 18–24 hrs. **Dose: Loading** 8–12 mg and **maintenance** 2–8 mg.

ADR (nicoumalone):
1. Dermatitis
2. Urticaria and oral ulceration
3. GI disturbance

DUG

PK (ethyl biscoumacetate): Duration of action 1–3 days, **t½—2 hrs (shortest).**
Dose: Loading 900 mg, **maintenance** 300–600 mg.
ADR (ethyl biscoumacetate): Alopecia and bad taste.
PK (phenindione): Duration of action 1–3 days, **t½—5 hrs.**
Dose: Loading 200 mg, **maintenance** 50–100 mg.
ADR (phenindione):
1. **H**epatitis and **H**ypersensitivity (rash, fever)
2. **A**granulocytosis
3. **L**eukopenia
4. Nephropathy and orange **U**rine

HAUL

ADR of oral anticoagulants
1. **Bleeding (the most important): Hematuria** is a major and the **most frequent sign.** Epistaxis, ecchymosis, bleeding in GIT, internal haemorrhage.
   Treatment: Stop drug, blood transfusion (clotting factor and blood), **fresh frozen plasma** for clotting factor. **Vitamin K** (within 24 hrs, clotting factor is resynthesized). Immediate treatment of choice in severe bleeding due to warfarin toxicity is **fresh blood transfusion.** Increase in Hb level by transfusion of 10 ml/kg = 1 gm% and 15 ml/kg = 2 gm% Hb. Increase platelet count by 1 unit of fresh blood is 10000–15000 dl.
2. **Skin neurosis**
3. **Toxicity** due to phenindione.

Factors increasing effects of oral anticoagulant

a. Malnutrition, malabsorption, prolonged antibiotic therapy	— Due to **decreased vitamin K** **K supply** to liver
b. Liver disease, chronic alcoholism	— Due to **deficient clotting factor** synthesis
c. Hyperthyroidism	— Due to **faster degradation** of clotting factor
d. Newborn	— Due to **low level of vitamin K** and **clotting factor**

Factors decreasing effects of oral anticoagulant
A. **Nephrotic syndrome:** Due to loss of drug in urine bound to plasma protein.
B. **Pregnancy:** Due to higher clotting factor level.
C. **Genetic warfarin resistance:** Due to low affinity of **KO** and **warfarin** to bind to **reductase.**

CI of oral anticoagulants
1. **All contraindications of heparin.**
2. Factors **increasing effects** of oral anticoagulant.
3. **Pregnancy** → increased birth defects specially **skeletal** abnormalities → **foetal warfarin syndrome in early pregnancy (hypoplasia** of nose, eye socket and

bones and **growth retardation**). In **later pregnancy** → CNS defects, haemorrhage and **neonatal hypoprothrombinemia.**

Drugs IA

A. Decreased anticoagulant action
1. **OC** enhances blood clotting factor levels.
2. **All hypnotics except** BZD, rifampicin, griseofulvin enhance metabolism of oral anticoagulant.

B. Increased anticoagulant action
1. **Newer cephalosporin** causes hypoprothrombinemia by additive action like warfarin.
2. **Broad spectrum antibiotics** inhibit gut flora and reduce vitamin K production.
3. **Aspirin** inhibits platelet aggregation → ↑ GIT bleeding.
   Salicylates in high doses cause synergistic hypoprothrombinemic action and displace warfarin from **protein binding site.**
4. **Phenylbutazone** enhances action without change in blood level/t½ of warfarin by reducing protein binding of warfarin and inhibiting metabolism of **more active S enantiomer** while inducing that of R enantiomer.
5. **Probenecid, phenytoin, indomethacin** and long-acting **sulfonamides** displace warfarin from plasma protein binding.
6. **Warfarin, allopurinol, amiodarone, chloramphenicol, erythromycin, cimetidine and metronidazole** inhibit warfarin metabolism.
7. Warfarin inhibits metabolism of phenytoin and tolbutamide and vice versa.
8. **Clofibrate, phenformin, quinidine** and anabolic **steroid** potentiate warfarin action.

		Heparin versus warfarin	
		Heparin	*Warfarin*
1.	**Structure**	Mucopolysaccharide, large anionic polymer, acidic	Coumarin derivative, small lipid soluble molecule
2.	**Route of adm.**	IV/SC	Orally
3.	**Site of action**	Blood	Liver
4.	**Onset of action**	Rapid (sec.)	Slow (1–3 days). Limited by t½ of normal clotting factor
5.	**Duration of action**	Acute (4–6 hrs)	Chronic (3–6 days)
6.	**Source**	Hog lung, pig intestine	Synthetic
7.	**Activity**	*In vitro* and *in vivo*	*In vivo* only
8.	**Mechanism**	Stimulates AT III. Inhibits thrombin and clotting factor X	Inhibits synthesis of vitamin K dependent CF II, VII, IX, X **(vitamin K blocker)**
9.	**Antagonist**	Protamine sulfate	Vitamin K
10.	**Monitoring**	aPTT of intrinsic pathway (desirable)	PT of extrinsic pathway (essential)

9. **Liquid paraffin** reduces vitamin K absorption.
10. **Dipyridamole** inhibits platelet agglutination →bleeding is enhanced.

Uses of anticoagulants: **Heparin therapy** is monitored by estimating **KPTT** of blood (kaolin PTT). **Warfarin therapy** is monitored by estimating **PT**. Normal PT is **12–14 sec. (Quick's method). Warfarin (chronic anticoagulant)** is for **maintenance** therapy and heparin for **initial therapy.** Generally, both are started together, heparin is discontinued after 4–7 days but warfarin is continued. Both heparin and warfarin slow clot production but not dissolve clot. Both inhibit thrombus extension and embolic complication by reducing clot formation (recurrence inhibition). In acute condition, heparin + oral anticoagulants are used.

1. **MI:** It is **arterial** thrombi (platelet aggregation). Heparin/aspirin equally reduces MI occurrence in unstable angina. Currently (aspirin + heparin) are given followed by warfarin.
2. **DVT and pulmonary embolism are venous thrombi (fibrin thrombi):** DOC—anticoagulants for 3 months. LMW heparin (DOC) prophylaxis in elective surgery and prolonged immobilization (due to inhibition of small amount of Xa →inhibition of further amplification of active products such as thrombin).
3. **Cerebrovascular disease:** Anticoagulants inhibit recurrent cerebral emboli but not neurological sequelae.
4. **RHD and AF:** Low dose aspirin/low dose heparin/warfarin inhibits stroke (due to emboli from fibrillating atria). Anticoagulants are given 1 month before and after attempting AF conversion to sinus rhythm.
5. **Thromboembolism** (in vascular surgery, prosthetic heart valve, retinal vessel thrombosis, haemodialysis, extracorporeal circulation): Antiplatelets + anticoagulants are given. For patent long-term intravascular cannulae/catheters—heparin flushes (200 U in 2 ml) every 4–8 hourly.
6. **Defibrination system/DIC** (in malignancy, infection, abruptio placentae): Clotting factor is consumed in the formation of intravascular microclots, hence blood is incoagulable. Heparin preserves clotting factor and checks bleeding.

Summary of uses of anticoagulants
Heparin for DIC/defibrination system,
Embolism (thromboembolism),
Pulmonary embolism and DVT,
AF, and
RHD
Infarction (MI)
Nervous system (cerebrovascular disease)

HEPARIN

Fibrinolytic, Thrombolytic, Antifibrinolytic, Antithrombolytic, Antiplatelet Drugs

Fibrinolytic/thrombolytic agents: Lyse thrombi/clot to recanalyse occluded vessels mainly coronary artery. Venous thrombi are lysed more easily than arterial thrombi.

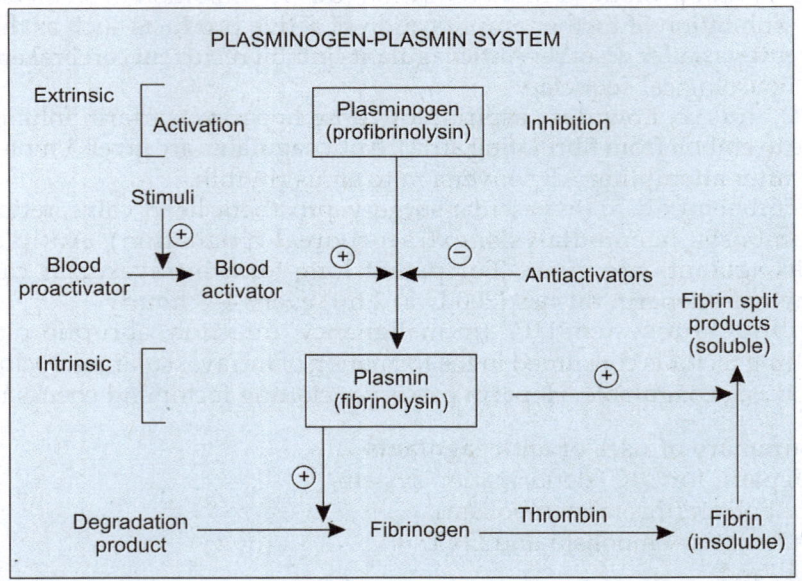

Activator		Source
1. **rt-PA**	:	Recombinant (human protein produced in bacteria)
2. **Pro-urokinase**	:	Melanoma cell culture
3. **Acyl-streptokinase-plasmin**	:	Chemical synthesis
4. **Streptokinase**	:	β-hemolytic streptococci
5. **Urokinase**	:	Human renal tubular cell culture and human urine

Fibrinolytic, Thrombolytic, Antifibrinolytic, Antithrombolytic, Antiplatelet Drugs

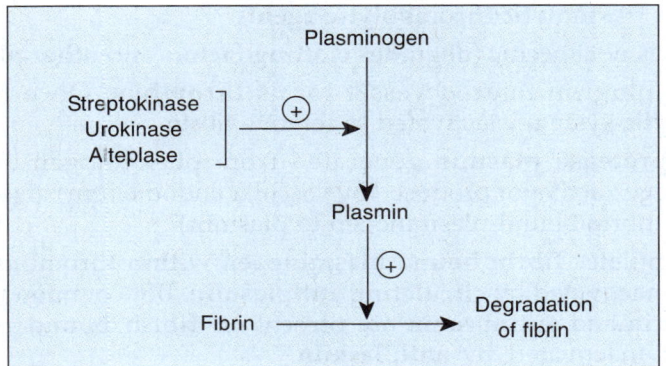

Antigenicity:

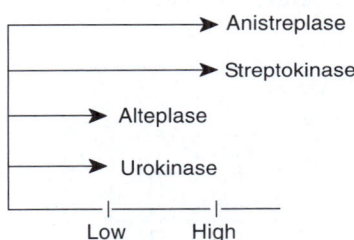

Fibrin specificity:

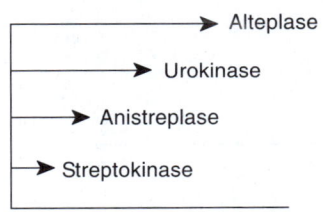

1. **Activators**
   (i) **Extrinsic (available in India)**　　　　　　　　**USA**
      Alteplase (rt-PA), Urokinase, Streptokinase.
   (ii) **Intrinsic:** t-PA, Factor XIIa, kallikrein.

2. **Inhibitors**
   (i) **Extrinsic:** EACA, Aprotinin, Tranexamic acid.　　**TEA**
   (ii) **Intrinsic:** α_2 antiplasmin, α_2 macroglobulin.

3. **Plasmin blocker:** Aminocaproic acid (antidote for fibrinolytics).

Newer fibrinolytics
1. **Anistreplase**
2. **Saruplase:** Recombinant human single chain urokinase type plasminogen activator, fibrin selective, non-pyrogenic, non-antigenic.
3. **Reteplase:** Non-glycosylated mutant of alteplase, 5 times more potent.

Mechanism of fibrinolytic/thrombolytic agents

1. **Plasmin** is not specific (**degrades clotting factors** and **other plasma protein**).
2. Platelet plug on injured vessel forms **thrombus**. Once repair is over, **fibrinolytic system** is activated to remove fibrin.
3. **Serine protease plasmin** generated from plasminogen by **t-PA** (tissue plasminogen activator produced by vascular endothelium) digests **fibrin** (t-PA converts fibrin bound plasminogen to plasmin).
4. **t-PA** stimulates **fibrin bound plasminogen within thrombus**. Plasmin that leaks is inactivated by **circulating antiplasmin**. But common binding site for both **fibrin** and **antiplasmin** are present on **fibrin bound plasmin,** hence it is not inactivated by **antiplasmin**.
5. Stimulation of increase plasminogen → α_2 antiplasmin exhausted → active plasmin persists → **lytic state** → bleeding.

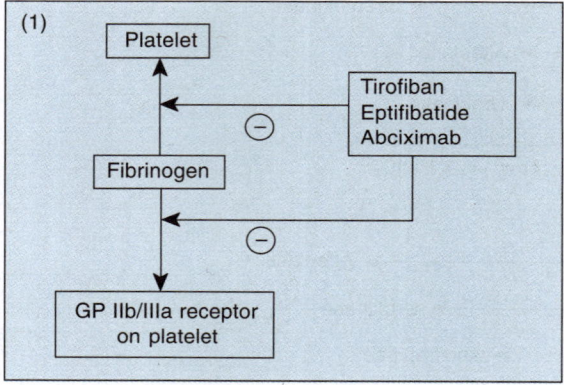

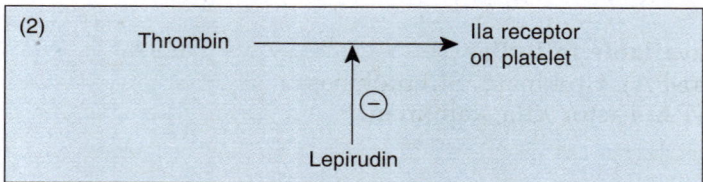

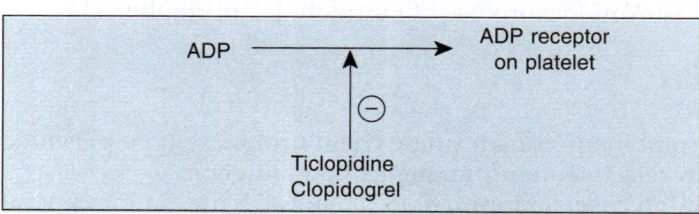

Streptokinase: Source: β-haemolytic streptococci group C. Present in **inactive form**.

Mech

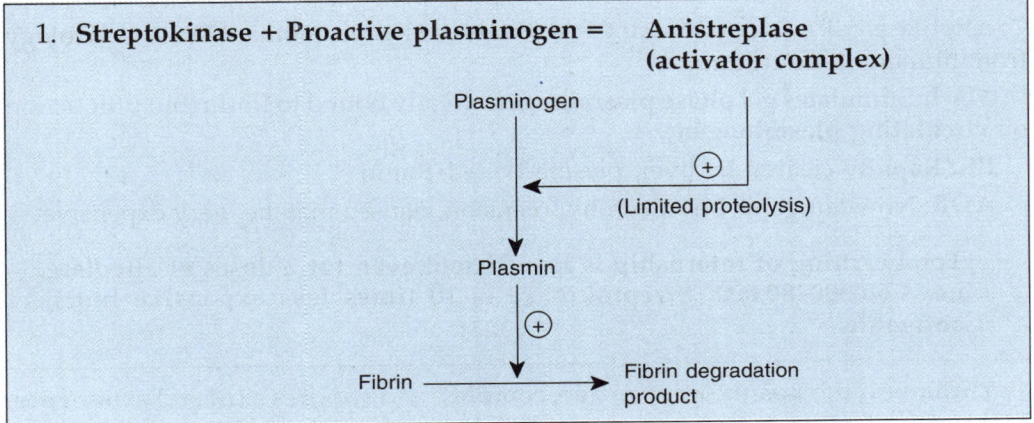

2. **Aminocaproic acid** inhibits plasminogen activation to plasmin.
3. Antistreptococcal Ab inactivates **streptokinase** (hence **less effective**).
4. **APSAC (prodrug)** = Streptokinase + Recombinant human plasminogen.

PK: t½—30–80 min.

ADR of streptokinase

1. **Anaphylaxis** and **hypersensitivity** specially when used **second time** (due to **antigenic** property of streptokinase).
2. Fever
3. Arrhythmia and hypotension.

Advantage of streptokinase: Least expensive of 3 fibrinolytics available in India.

Urokinase: It is **enzyme isolated from human urine** (now produced from cultured human kidney cells).

Mech

1. Stimulates **plasminogen** directly.
2. Streptokinase and urokinase degrade both **fibrin** and **fibrinogen**.

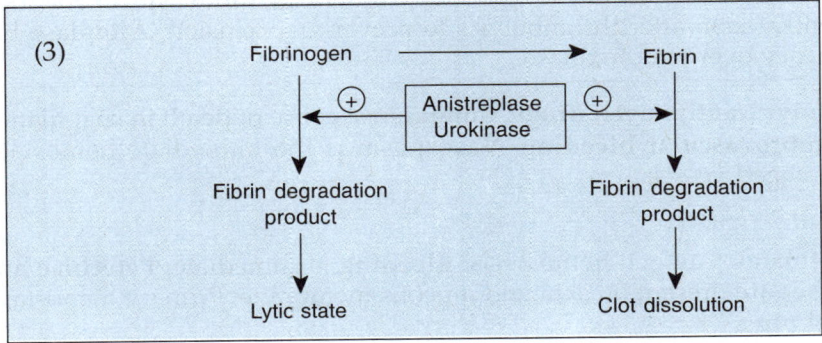

PK of urokinase: Plasma t½ → 10–15 min.

ADR of urokinase: Nonantigenic, hence no allergy and no hypotension. But fever is present during treatment.

Alteplase/rt-PA (recombinant t-PA): Produced by recombinant DNA technology from human tissue culture.

Mech: Stimulates gel **phase plasminogen** already bound to fibrin (but little action on **circulating plasminogen**).

PK: Rapidly cleared by liver, plasma t½ → 4–8 min.

ADR: Now antigenic but fever, hypotension, nausea may be, very expensive.

> Total earning of internship is insufficient even for 2 doses of alteplase, i.e. ₹ 60,000–80,000. Streptokinase is 10 times less expensive but is antigenic.

Thrombolytic therapy is **expensive, complex,** and requires **skill** and **experience.** Main complication is **haemorrhage.** (Alteplase + heparin) is better than (streptokinase + heparin.)

CI of thrombolytic therapy: All causes of bleeding (trauma, surgery, biopsy, stroke, HTN, peptic ulcer, aneurysm, DM, acute pancreatitis, retinal vessel occlusion).

Uses of fibrinolytics

1. **Clot dissolution in brain** by fibrinolytic agent reduces CNS injury after thrombotic stroke but it must be used after haemorrhagic stroke.
2. **Pulmonary embolism**
3. **Peripheral arterial occlusion**
   a. **Recanalyse 40% limb artery occlusion** in patient treated within **72 hrs.**
   b. Indicated if surgical thrombectomy is not possible.
   c. **Thrombolysis** is followed by long-term aspirin therapy and short-term heparin therapy.
4. **DVT** (in leg, pelvis and shoulder). Cure rate—60%.
   Advantage: Venous valve preservation. Reduced pulmonary embolism.
5. **Acute MI: DOC** if fibrinolytic agents instituted within **12 hours** of symptom onset. **Recanalization** occurs in **50–90%** cases. Time factor is very important. Route is **IV** preferably within 3–6 hrs. **Heparin with/without aspirin** is started concurrently/soon after thrombolysis to prevent reocclusion. **Alteplase** has more efficacy over streptokinase.

Antithrombolytic/antiplatelet drugs: Commonest cause of death in coagulation disorder is **cerebrovascular bleeding. Vasospasm** is the immediate hemostatic response of damaged vessels.

Hemostasis is of 2 types

A. **Primary (platelet defect) hemostasis: Bleeding** is immediate. **Petechiae** and **ecchymoses** are present on skin and mucous membrane. Primary hemostasis is **platelet plug.**

B. **Secondary hemostasis (plasma protein): Bleeding** is delayed. **Hematomas** and **hemarthroses** are present on joint and muscle.
Normal platelet count is **2–4 lakh/dl**. Lifespan of platelet in circulation is **10 days**.
   a. Platelet count >100,000 →BT (bleeding time) normal, i.e. **1–6 min (Duke's method)**.
   b. Platelet count 50,000–100,000 →mild ↑ BT.
   c. Platelet count <20,000 → spontaneous bleeding.

Factor responsible for platelet adhesion to vascular endothelium is von Willebrand factor. ADP is powerful inducer of platelet aggregation. Thrombasthenia is defect in platelet aggregation. PG promoting thrombogenesis—TXA_2 from platelet. PG inhibiting thrombogenesis—PGI_2 from vascular endothelium.

BT is a measure of platelet function. Clotting time is measure of clotting factor (normal value 6–10 min by Lee-White method). Platelets stick to damaged vessel wall and to each other (aggregation) → ADP and TXA_2 release → platelet plug. A fibrinous tail is formed in the veins due to sluggish blood flow which traps RBC **(Red tail)**. Platelet mass forms thrombus in artery (hence antiplatelets effective in arterial thrombus and anticoagulant in venous thrombus). PGI_2 (prostacyclin) synthesized in intima of vessels strongly inhibits platelet aggregation. Balance between PGI_2 released from vessel wall and TXA_2 released from platelets controls **intravenous thrombus formation.**

A. **Antithrombolytic/antiplatelet agents**
   1. Ticlopidine and clopidogrel
   2. Dipyridamole and dazoxiben
   3. Sulfinpyrazone
   4. Daxtran-40
   5. Clofibrate
   6. NSAID (aspirin)
   7. Monoclonal antibodies
   8. Peptides (recombinant and synthesized)
   9. Analogues of leech anticoagulant peptide hirudin
   10. **Newer drugs:** Abciximab, tirofiban, eptifibatide
B. **Thrombin inhibitor:** Lepirudin

Dipyridamole: Vasodilator (coronary dilator). Antiplatelet drug.

Mech
   1. Inhibits phosphodiesterase and blocks adenosine uptake to enhance platelet cAMP (cAMP potentiates PGI_2 and inhibits platelet aggregation). TXA_2 and PGI_2 levels are unaltered, antithrombotic drug.
   2. Prevents uptake and degradation of adenosine (a local mediator involved in autoregulation of coronary flow in response to ischaemia). Dilates resistance vessels and abolishes autoregulation.
   3. **Coronary steal phenomenon:** It means direction of blood flow to non-ischaemic area, as occurs with vasodilator. By dilating resistance vessels in non-ischaemic zone, it diverts the already reduced blood flow away from ischaemic zone (pharmacological success but therapeutic failure). Ischaemia itself is the **most** potent vasodilator

	stimulus in skeletal muscle and cerebral beds, vasodilator diverts blood to non-ischaemic area (steal phenomena).
PK:	Extensively protein bound, t½—12 hrs, dose—50 mg/day TDS.
ADR:	Nontoxic, GIT intolerance occasionally, overdose→peripheral vasodilatation and hypotension.
U:	1. Prophylaxis of angina pectoris
	2. Prophylaxis of coronary and cerebral thrombosis in post-MI and post-stroke patients.
	3. Prophylaxis of thrombosis of prosthetic heart valves.
	4. Thromboembolism in prosthetic heart valves (warfarin + dipyridamole).

Dazoxiben: Inhibits TX synthetase→↓TXA_2 formation. But poor antithrombolytic effects are due to longer survival of PGH_2 and G_2 (TXA_2 precursor cyclic endoperoxidase) and platelet stimulation by PGH_2 and G_2.

Ticlopidine

Mech
1. Directly interacts with platelet membrane and inhibits release reaction, aggregation and platelet deposition on fibrin.
2. Alters fibrinogen receptor in such a way that fibrinogen is unable to bind to activated platelets → inhibition of platelet aggregation and clot retraction.
3. Inhibits platelet aggregation by irreversibly inhibiting ADP pathway involved in fibrinogen binding.
4. Prolongs bleeding time and enhances platelet survival.

ADR:
1. Diarrhoea, abdominal pain, vomiting
2. Headache and tinnitus
3. Rash
4. Bleeding
5. Rarely, neutropenia and jaundice

U:
1. Reserved for those who cannot tolerate aspirin
2. Stroke (thrombotic stroke/recurrence)
3. TIA
4. Intermittent claudication
5. Unstable angina
6. Coronary artery bypass grafts
7. Secondary prophylaxis of MI

Heparinoids: Danaparoid (heparan sulphate mainly), lepirudin.

Danaparoid (LMW heparinoid contains mainly heparan sulfate of pig gut mucosa for heparin induced thrombocytopenia).

Uses of antiplatelets

1. **Cononary artery disease**
   a. **MI:** Aspirin (reduces mortality, inhibits reinfarction and reocclusion). Heparin + aspirin in PTCA (percutaneous transmural coronary angioplasty).

b. **Unstable angina:** Aspirin (100–150/day) + heparin followed by warfarin for maximum benefit.
c. **Primary and secondary prevention of MI.**
2. **Cerebrovascular disease:** TIA, stroke
3. **Coronary bypass implants:** Patency of implanted bypass vessel improved by aspirin/ticlopidine. Best choice is aspirin started just after operation.
4. **PVD:** Intermittent claudication and thromboembolism.
5. **Venous thromboembolism**
6. **Prosthetic heart valve and arteriovenous shunts:** Antiplatelets + warfarin reduce microthrombi formation on the artificial heart valve and risk of embolism. Antiplatelets prolong patency of chronic arteriovenous shunts (implanted for haemodialysis) and of vascular grafts.

Abciximab: It is a **monoclonal Ab** composed of **Fab** fragment of **murine monoclonal Ab** directed against **glycoprotein GP IIb/IIIa complex** joined to constant regions of **human Ig**.

GP IIb/IIIa receptor antagonists (block platelet aggregation induced by all platelet agonists) block receptor for platelet aggregation. GP IIb/IIIa is receptors (integrin) for fibrinogen and vWF through which agonists (ADP, TXA_2, thrombin, collagen, etc.) induce platelet aggregation.

Fibrinogen and vWF + platelet surface →anchor platelets to one another by agonist action. These drugs are antithrombotic monoclonal Ab or platelet aggregation inhibitor (by binding GP IIb/IIIa receptors).

Mech: By binding to **GP IIb/IIIa, Ab** blocks **fibrinogen binding** and **vWF** and consequently, **aggregation** does not occur.

$$\text{Abciximab, eptifibatide, tirofiban inhibit} \xrightarrow{\text{Fibrinogen} \downarrow} \text{GP IIb/IIIa receptor on platelet}$$

PK : Antiplatelet effect = **1–2 days**
ADR : Bleeding
U : Cardiac ischaemic complication (IV).

Tirofiban and eptifibatide: These are drugs having **antiplatelet action**.
Mech
    1. Block **GP IIb/IIIa receptor** (action **similar** to abciximab).
    2. Both mimic **arginine-glycine-aspartic acid sequence of fibrinogen**.
    3. Both reduce **thrombotic complications**.
PK: Rapidly cleared from **plasma**.
    Duration of effects—**4 hrs**.
    Eptifibatide and its metabolites excreted by **kidney**. Tirofiban excreted **unchanged by kidney**.
ADR: Bleeding.

Clopidogrel: It is analog of **ticlopidine**.
Mech: **Selectively** and **irreversibly** blocks ADP binding to platelet. It thus prevents **ADP-mediated activation of glycoprotein complex GP IIb/IIIa**, thereby inhibiting platelet aggregation. Also inhibits **cytochrome**.

PK: Extensively metabolised by **liver. Renal** and **faecal** elimination.
ADR: Bleeding. **CLOPI**dogrel = **CLO**t (Platelet)/Oral Platelet Inhibitor.
IA: Interferes with metabolism of phenytoin, tolbutamide, warfarin, fluvastatin and tamoxifen if taken **concomitantly.**

Lepirudin: It is a **polypeptide** that is highly specific **thrombin blocker.** Produced by **recombinant DNA technology in yeast cells.** It is recombinant form of hirudin (polypeptide of salivary gland of leech) and inhibits thrombin used in heparin-induced thrombocytopenia.

Mech: **One molecule** of lepirudin binds to **one molecule of thrombin,** resulting in blockade of **thrombogenic** activity of thrombin.

Thrombin → IIa receptor
  ↑(−)
  Lepirudin

PK: t½—1 hr, Undergoes **hydrolysis, renal** elimination.
ADR: Bleeding
U: HIT (IV)

HIT (heparin-induced thrombocytopenia) Types I and II and HAT (heparin-associated thrombocytopenia) are due to heparin use

HIT
 — Type I (nonimmunogenic)
 — Type II (immunogenic, platelet count drops by <50%, life-threatening)

Antifibrinolytics inhibit plasminogen activation and clot dissolution.

EACA (epsilon aminocaproic acid): It is analogue of amino acid **lysine** and is specific **antidote** of fibrinolytic agents.

Mech: Combines with **lysine binding site of plasminogen** and **plasmin→** unable to bind to fibrin → lysis → **bleeding.**

ADR
1. Hypotension, bradycardia, arrhythmia
2. Myopathy (rarely)

U: Dose 5 gm oral/IV stat + 1 gm hourly **(maximum 30 gm/day)**
1. **Overdose** of fibrinolytic (urokinase/alteplase/streptokinase)
2. **Trauma** and surgical bleeding (prostatectomy in haemophilics)
3. **Menorrhagia,** PPH, abruptio placentae
4. **Recurrent** subarachnoid and GI bleeding
5. **Haematuria** (but causes ureteric obstruction by clots)

Tranexamic acid: **7 times** more potent than EACA.

Mech: Binds to **lysine** binding site on plasminogen→inhibits its combination with fibrin.

ADR:
1. **Thrombophlebitis** of injected vein
2. Nausea, vomiting, giddiness
3. **Diarrhoea**

U: Inhibits excessive bleeding in
— Overdose of fibrinolytics
— Surgery in haemophilias
— Menorrhagia specially due to IUCD
— Epistaxis
— Peptic ulcer
— Trauma

Aprotinin is a **polypeptide** isolated from **bovine** tissues with **polyvalent protease inhibitory activity.**
Mech: Inhibits **trypsin, chymotrypsin, plasmin and kallikrein.**
Pk: Route — Only IV
t½ — 2 hrs
U: 1. In the beginning of cardiopulmonary bypass **surgery** (reduces blood loss).
2. Traumatic, hemorrhagic and endoscopic shock **(adjunct value).**
3. **Acute pancreatitis** (trypsin released may be fatal).
4. Carcinoid, prostatic surgery and fibrinolytic states.

> **Risk factors for coronary disease**
> 1. Smoking, HTN, DM
> 2. Men >45 yrs, women >55 yrs not receiving HRT
> 3. HDL <35 mg%
> 4. Family history of MI/sudden cardiac death before 55 years of age in **first** degree relative

1. Platelet (Pla**TE**let) inhibitors are **T**irofiban, **E**ptifibatide, and **A**bciximab.
2. **E**rythromycin, **N**icotinic acid, **G**emfibrozil, and **C**lofibrate are contraindicated with statins **ENG**lish Contraindicated
3. **N**oonan's syndrome, **E**llis–van Creveld syndrome, **D**own's syndrome, **T**AR, **P**KU, **H**alt-Oram syndrome **NE** for **DTPH** cause ASD.

42. Drugs for Hyperlipidemia

Antihyperlipidemic drugs reduce lipid and lipoprotein from blood.

6 classes of lipoprotein (on the basis of particle size and density)					
Major apolipoprotein	Class	Diameter (nm)	Electrophoretic mobility in Agarose gel	Functions	Core lipid
A-I and II (HDL formation)	HDL	5–10 (smallest)	α (highest)	CH removal from tissue	CHE
B-100 (secretion)	LDL	20–25	β	CH transport to liver and tissue	CHE
B-100, E (mediates remnant uptake by liver)	IDL	20–25	β	TG and CHE transport to liver. LDL source	CHE > TG
A-I and II, C protein, B-48 (secretion)	Chylomicron	100–500 (largest)	Remains at origin (least)	Dietary TG transport	TG >> CHE
B-100, C protein, E	VLDL	40–80	pre-beta	Endogenous TG transport	TG >> CHE
	Chylomicron remnant	30–50	pre-beta	Dietary CH transport	CHE >> TG

Marker in serum which predicts atherosclerosis at an early age is **apoprotein B-100**.

Chylomicron has **largest** diameter and **least** mobility while **HDL** has **smallest** diameter and **highest** mobility on electrophoresis.

> By same amount of force, smaller body moves faster, hence HDL, according to Newton's laws of motion.

Drugs for Hyperlipidemia

Lipid transport: Lipid is carried in **plasma** after getting associated with **apoproteins**. Plasma Lipid Level depends on Lipoprotein Levels.

Structure of lipoprotein globules
– **Core** = TG + CHE (cholesteryl ester).
– **Outer polar layer** = phospholipid + free CH + apoprotein.

Dietary lipid absorption in intestine with the help of **bile** acid → **chylomicron** formation → **lacteals** → **thoracic duct** → **bloodstream**.

During its passage through capillaries, **endothelial bound lipoprotein lipase** hydrolyses TG into FA which passes into **muscle cell** to be used as **energy** source and into fat cell to be again convered into **TG (and stored)**. **Hepatocyte** has receptor for surface apoprotein of chylomicron remnant (remaining part), hence engulfs **chylomicron remnant containing CHE (mainly)** and **TG (little)** and digests it. **Free CH** liberated is either **stored in hepatocytes** after esterification/**incorporated** into different lipoprotein and released into blood/**excreted** in bile as **CH (cholesterol)/bile acids.**

Liver secretes **VLDL** having TG + CHE into blood.

VLDL $\xrightarrow{\text{Endothelial lipoprotein lipase}}$ FA → adipose tissue and muscle.

Its remnant is **IDL** (intermediate DL) and has **CHE > TG**. **50% IDL** is taken back to hepatocyte by attachment to LDL receptor and rest **50%** loses remaining TG gradually and becomes LDL containing only **CHE. Rate of LDL uptake** is regulated by rate of **LDL receptor synthesis** in particular tissue. **CHE of LDL** is de-esterified and used mainly for **cell membrane formation.** CH released into blood from membrane degradation is incorporated into **HDL**, esterified with the help of enzyme **LCAT** (lecithin cholesterol acyl transferase) and transported back to **VLDL** and **IDL** completing cycle. Excess lipoprotein is phagocytosed by **microphage** for disposal but due to overload, CH is deposited in **xanthomas (in skin** and **tendon)** and **atheromas** (in arterial wall). Increased level of VLDL, IDL, LDL, chylomicron and chylomicron remnant are **atherogenic** while **HDL** is **protective** (because it facilitates CH removal from tissues).

> HDL is Healthy: Tissue to Hepatocyte.
> LDL is Lousy: Liver to tissue
> HDL and LDL carry **most CH** (LDL carries from Liver to Tissue and HDL from Tissue to Hepatocyte).

Hyperlipoproteinemia is **Primary** and **Secondary**.

Primary hyperlipoproteinemia is due to **single gene defect/monogenic/genetic/familial, or multiple gene defect/polygenic/multifactorial.**

Secondary hyperlipoproteinemia is associated with **DM, myoedema, nephrotic syndrome, chronic alcoholism** and **drugs** (OC, steroid, beta blocker). **LDL** is primary carrier of plasma **CHE** and **VLDL** is primary carrier of plasma **TG**.

> LDL + CHE = 6 letters
> VLDL + TG = 6 letters

Type of primary hyperlipoproteinemia						
Type	Disorder	Cause	Increased plasma lipoprotein	Plasma lipid		
				CH	TG	DOC
I	Familial lipoprotein lipase deficiency	Genetic	Chylomicron	↑↑	↑↑↑	Dietary management
II A	Familial hyper-cholesterolemia (LDL receptor deficiency)	Genetic	LDL	↑↑	X	Lovastatin ± resins
II B	Polygenic hyper-cholesterolemias (**commonest**)	Multifactorial	LDL	↑	X	Lovastatin ± resins
III	Familial dysbetalipopr-oteinemia. Abnormal apoprotein in IDL + chylomicron remnant	Genetic	IDL + chylo-micron rem-nant (slow clearance)	↑	↑	Gemfibrozil, bezafibrate
IV	Hypertriglyceridemia	Genetic < multifactorial	VLDL	X	↑↑	Gemfibrozil, nicotinic acid
V	Familial combined hyperlipidemia	Genetic	VLDL, LDL	↑	↑	Gemfibrozil, nicotinic acid

Types of hyperlipidemia in which
  a. Hypertriglyceridemia is present — **Types I, III, IV, V**
  b. Hypercholesterolemia is present — **Type II**

Increase LDL–CH is **atherogenic** and increase HDL–CH level is either **protective** or indicates a **low atherogenic state.**

All subjects are given drug therapy
  a. At LDL–CH level **≥190 mg%**
  b. At **≥130 mg% with CAD**
  c. At serum **TG >200 mg%** (if CAD, total blood CH ≥240 mg%, HDL >35 mg%, types III and IV hyperlipidemia, multiple risk factor and acute pancreatitis are present).

Hypercholesterolemia is said to exist when serum CH level exceeds **200 mg%**.

Classification of total, LDL and HDL–CH value (mg%)			
Serum TG	Total plasma CH	LDL–CH	HDL–CH
<200 = **Desirable**	<200	<130	<35
200–400= **Borderline**	200–239	130–159	35–60
400–1000= **Undesirable**	≥240	≥160	≥61
>1000= **Very high**	>239	>159	>60

Classification of hypolipidemic drugs

1. **HMG–CoA reductase inhibitors (statin)**
   Fluvastatin
   Lovastatin   "FLAPS cut body fat"
   Atorvastatin
   Pravastatin
   Simvastatin
2. **VLDL production and lipolysis inhibitors**
   Nicotinic acid (niacin/vitamin B$_3$).
3. **Antioxidant:** Probucol
4. **Fibric acid (isobutyric acid) derivatives**
   Bezafibrate
   Clofibrate   **BCG Failure**
   Gemfibrozil
   Fenofibrate
5. **Resins**
   Colestipol
   Cholestyramine
6. **Others**
   Neomycin
   Gugulipid

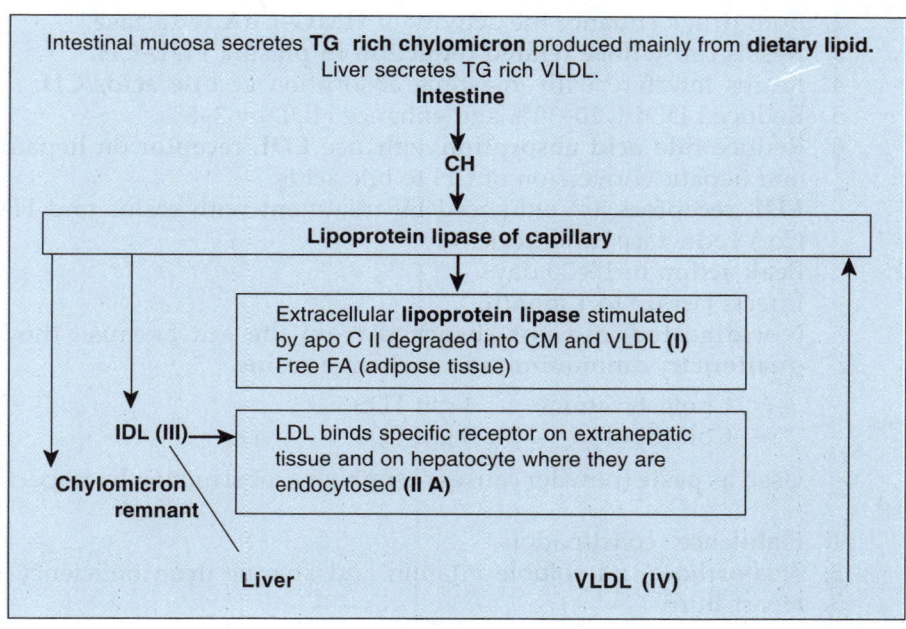

Lipid lowering drugs	Effects on LDL (bad CH)	Effects on HDL (good CH)	Effects on TG	ADR
Bile acid resins	↓↓	No effect	↑ (slight)	Bad taste, GIT discomfort
HMG–CoA reductase inhibitors	↓↓↓	↑	↓	Myopathy, reversible increase in LFT
Niacin ↓↓	↑↑	↓		Red flushed face (treatment—**aspirin**)
Probucol	↓	↓	No effect	↓ HDL
Lipoprotein lipase stimulator (gemfibrozil)	↓	↑	↓↓↓	Muscle damage, ↑ LFT

Cholestyramine and colestipol: These are **bile acid sequestrants (resins)/basic ion exchange resins** supplied in the **chloride** form.

Mech
1. Bind **bile acid** in the intestine interrupting their **enterohepatic circulation. Faecal excretion** of bile salts and CH is enhanced due to their absorption with the help of bile salts. This leads to enhanced **hepatic metabolism** of CH to bile acid, more **LDL receptor** expression on hepatocyte, increased **clearance** of plasma IDL, LDL and VLDL. Though hepatic **HMG–CoA reductase** synthesizes more CH, **overall body pool of CH is reduced.**
2. Both drugs enhance the activity of **HMG–CoA reductase.**
3. Resins cause **dose related reduction in plasma LDL–CH.**
4. Resins interfere with intestinal absorption of **bile acids/CH.**
5. Reduce LDL by **10–30%** and enhance HDL by **3–5%.**
6. Reduce **bile acid absorption,** enhance **LDL receptor** on hepatocyte and hepatic conversion of CH to bile acids.
LDL receptors are enhanced by treatment with resins and HMG–CoA reductase inhibitors.

PK: Peak action in 15–20 days.
Effects last up to **1 month.**
Not digested and not absorbed from the gut because they are **quarternary ammonium ion exchange resins.**

Dose: Cholestyramine — 4 gm TDS
Colestipol — 8 gm TDS

Used as **paste** (powder causes oesophageal obstruction by impaction).

ADR
1. Flatulence, constipation
2. Steatorrhoea, fat soluble vitamin and anionic drug deficiency.
3. Heart burn

Drugs for Hyperlipidemia

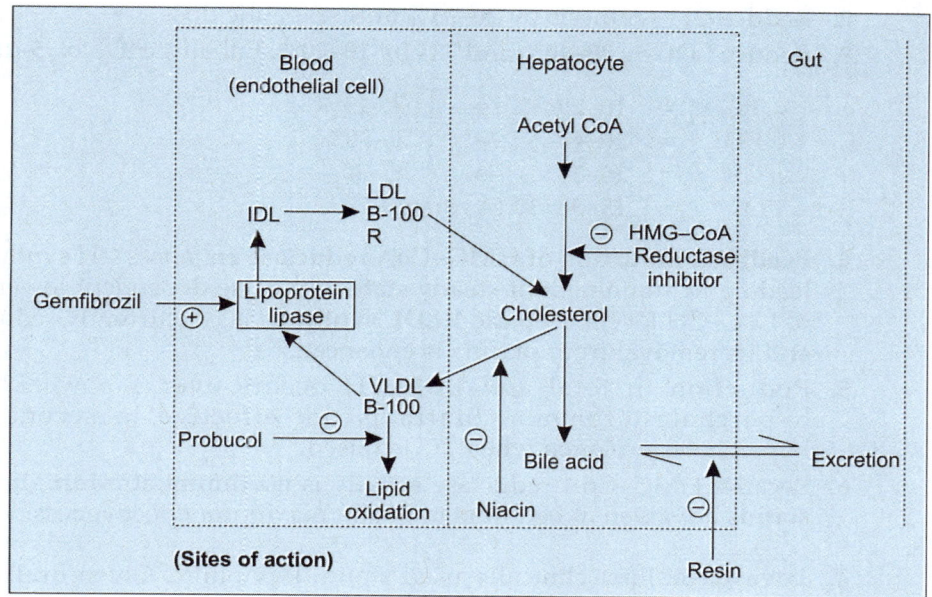

(Sites of action)

4. Worsening of piles
5. Nausea, ↑ TG and VLDL

IA

1. Bind and reduce absorption of **orally** administered drugs (digoxin, thiazide, barbiturate, phenylbutazone, warfarin, HMG–CoA reductase inhibitors).
2. **Resin + (nicotinic acid/HMG–CoA reductase inhibitors)** cause **synergistic** lowering of plasma CH.

U

1. In increased **LDL–CH** level (type IIa, IIb, and V).
2. **Prophylaxis** of angina and MI: Cholestyramine reduces raised LDL–CH level.
3. **Itching** of obstructive jaundice.
4. Bile salt mediated **diarrhoea.**

Statin

Statin is the most efficacious and **the best tolerated hypolipidemic drugs.**

Mech

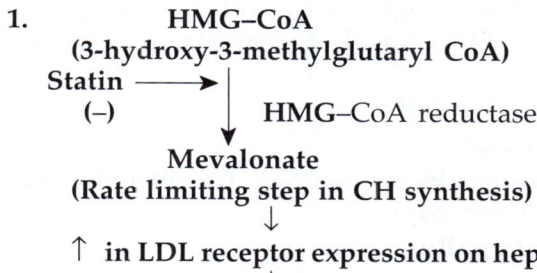

↑ in LDL receptor expression on hepatocyte
↓
↑ uptake and catabolism of IDL and LDL

2. Reduce CH synthesis by **20–35%** at therapeutic dose.
3. Reduce LDL by **20–40% and TG by 10–20%**. Enhance HDL by **5–15%**.

↓ TG	=	10–20 →	T–15%
↓ LDL	=	20–40 →	L–30%
↓ CH	=	20–35 →	C–30
TLC	=	15, 30, 30 (Average)	

4. **Feedback induction of HMG–CoA reductase** enhances CH synthesis leading to attainment of **steady state** with dose dependent lowering of LDL–CH levels. **Hepatic VLDL synthesis** is concurrently reduced and its removal from plasma is enhanced.
5. Reduction in total and LDL–CH occurs over 4–6 weeks in hypercholesterolemia. **Statin** is not effective in secondary hypercholesterolemia when TG is raised.
6. Because HMG–CoA reductase activity is **maximum at midnight, all statins** are given at bed time to obtain **maximum** effectiveness.

PK

1. **Lovastatin:** First clinically used statin. Lipophilic. Given **orally** in precursor lactone form.
   Decrease in LDL–CH by **25%** at **20 mg/day.**
   Decrease in LDL–CH by **32%** at **40 mg/day.**
   Decrease in LDL–CH by **40%** at **80 mg/day.**

25	—	20
32½ = (25 + 7½)	—	40
40 = (25 + 7½ + 7½)	—	80

   Concurrent decrease in plasma **TG** level by **10–20%** due to decrease in VLDL level also occurs, along with **5–15%** increase in HDL–CH level.
   (Bile salt + sequestrant + lovastatin) cause decrease in LDL by **60%** and (nicotinic acid + lovastatin) by 70%.
   Incomplete absorption. Extensive first pass metabolism. Metabolite excreted mainly in **bile.**
   Dose: 10–40 mg/day.
2. **Simvastatin**
   Twice as potent as **lovastatin. Lipophilic** and given in **lactone precursor form.** Better **oral** absorption, Extensive **first pass metabolism.**
   Dose: 40 mg/day (**maximum**).
3. **Provastatin: Hydrophilic**
   Equipotent to **lovastatin** at low doses. CH lowering effect is less at **highest doses (40 mg/day).**
4. **Fluvastatin: Hydrophilic**
   Nearly **half as** potent as **lovastatin. Maximum** dose (40 mg/day) achieves less LDL reduction than lovastatin.

ADR

ADR of statin (HMG–CoA reductase inhibitor):

Hepatic damage, **MyopathoGENIC** (aggravated by Gemfibrozil, Erythromycin, Niacin, Itraconazole, Cyclosporine)
Gestational problem (not to be used)
Coumarin like Action (bleeding tendency)

1. **Lovastatin: Hepatotoxicity, myopathy** (myositis, skeletal muscle inflammation).
2. **Headache, rashes, nausea, bowel upset.**
3. **Sleep disturbance** more with lipophilic drugs.
4. Increase **serum transaminase** (but rare liver damage).
5. Muscle tenderness and increase in **CPK level**. Myopathy **more common** in combination with erythromycin/cyclosporine/gemfibrozil/nicotinic acid.

U:

1. **DOC** in **primary** hyperlipidemias with increase LDL and total CH level (types IIa, IIb, and V) and **secondary** hypercholesterolemia (DM, nephrotic syndrome) on the basis of the **most significant study.**
2. **4S study** (Scandinavian Simvastatin Survival Study).

Fibric acid derivatives

Mech

1. Stimulate **lipoprotein lipase**—a key enzyme in the degradation of VLDL resulting in decreased circulating TG.
2. Reduce **FFA** in the periphery and release of FA from adipose tissue.
3. Reduce LDL by **10–15%** and TG by **20–50%** and enhance HDL by **10–15%** (due to transfer of surface lipid components from catabolised **VLDL to HDL**).

Gemfibrozil: Newer fibric acid derivative, more effective, better tolerated than clofibrate.

Mech

1. Reduces **VLDL** secretion by liver and enhances production of **HDL** apoprotein.
2. Shifts small dense **LDL** particles (more atherogenic) to larger less dense particle (like bezafibrate).
3. Reduces the level of **clothing factor VII—phospholipid complex.**

PK

Completely absorbed **orally**
Renal excretion
Elimination t½—8 hrs
Dose: 600 BD

ADR

1. **Epigastric distress** and loose motion
2. Bodyache and headache
3. Skin rash

    4. Eosinophilia
    5. **Impotence**
    6. **Blurred vision**
    7. Myopathy (uncommon)

U

1. Type III hyperlipoproteinemia **(most effective)**.
2. MI without known CAD →**34% reduction.**
3. **DOC** in raised TG level types IV and V disease.
4. **Adjuvant** during type IIa patient.

Clofibrate

Mech
1. Reduces **VLDL, IDL, LDL, TG and CH.**
2. Enhances **ADH secretion** and reduces urine volume in **nephrogenic DI** →water retention occurs.

PK: Completely absorbed **orally.**
Clofibrate → active metabolite → **renal excretion (partly after glucuronidation and partly unchanged).** t½ →12–18 hrs.

ADR
1. **Diarrhoea** and abdominal pain
2. Enhanced appetite →**weight gain**
3. Skin **rashes,** myalgia, and **flu-like syndrome due** to allergy
4. **Gallstone** due to enhanced uric acid level
5. **Cardiac arrhythmia**
6. **Loss of libido**

IA:
1. Potentiates **oral anticoagulants**
2. **Displaces** sulfonylurea, phenytoin, furosemide and phenothiazine.

CI:
1. **Liver** and **kidney** disease
2. **Pregnant/lactating** women

U: Not used now

Fenofibrate

Fenofibrate has greater action on **LDL** than other fibrates.

Bezafibrate has greater action on **LDL–CH** than gemfibrozil.

Mech:
1. Reduces circulating **fibrinogen** and **glucose.**
2. Slows **atherosclerotic process.**

ADR:
1. GI upset
2. Myalgia
3. Rashes

U
1. Alternative for gemfibrozil in **mixed hyperlipidemias** (types III, IV, and V).
2. **Hypercholesterolemia** (type II) but inferior to statin and resin.

Probucol

Probucol is **hypocholesterolemic drug** with **antioxidant** property and is **lipophilic** compound.

Mech
1. Causes **antiatherogenic** effect by inhibiting **LDL oxidation** rather than decreasing CH level.
2. Oxidised LDL is taken up by **macrophages** and deposited in **atheromas** and **xanthomas**.
3. Causes **modest lowering** of total plasma CH (more due to reduced HDL–CH). CH lowering is due to suppression of formation of major **apoprotein** of HDL.

PK:
1. **Lipophilic**
2. **1/10th** of oral dose is absorbed.
3. **Accumulates** in the body fat and persists for months after discontinuation.
4. t½—**47 days**.
5. Slowly excreted in **bile**

ADR:
1. Bowel upset and abdominal pain **common**
2. Hypersensitivity (rare)
3. Foetal effects due to **lipophilicity**
4. Prolonged **QT interval** (cautious use in arrhythmia)

U: Hyperlipoproteinemia (type IIa and IIb): **Second line drug.** Given with another drugs. It regresses **xanthomas** and reduces plasma CH in **familial homozygous hypercholesterolemia**.

Gugulipid

Gugulipid is a **mixture of sterones** obtained from **"gum guggul"** (used in **Ayurveda**).

Mech: **Modest** lowering of plasma CH and TG.
ADR: Loose stools

Guidelines for selection of hypolipidemic drugs

1. ↑ **LDL and normal TG**

   Monotherapy
   A. Statin
   B. Bile acid sequestrant
   C. HRT
   D. Nicotinic acid

   Combination therapy
   A. Statin + Bile acid sequestrant
   B. Nicotinic acid + Bile acid sequestrant
   C. Statin + Nicotinic acid

   NSB →SB, NB, SN

2. ↑ **LDL and TG (200–400 mg%)**

   Monotherapy
   A. **Statin**
   B. Gemfibrozil
   C. Nicotinic acid

   Combination therapy
   A. Statin + Gemfibrozil
   B. Statin + Nicotinic acid
   C. Nicotinic acid + Gemfibrozil
   D. Nicotinic acid + bile acid sequestrant

   NSG →SG, NG, NS

3. TG (>400 mg%): Gemfibrozil, nicotinic acid.

Summary of lipid lowering drugs

Class	Drugs	Mechanism of action	Main lipoprotein decreased	Adverse effects
Nicotinic acid	Nicotinic acid	↓ VLDL synthesis	VLDL	Gallstones, myopathy
Fibric acid derivatives	Clofibrate, Gemfibrozil	↓ VLDL synthesis, ↑ lipoprotein lipase activity	VLDL, LDL	GI-upset, flushing, hyperglycemia, hepatic dysfunction
Probucol	Probucol	Not known	LDL	Diarrhoea, low HDL
Estrogens	Premarin,	Not known estradiol	LDL	High VLDL, endometrial carcinoma
HMG-CoA reductase inhibitors	Lovastatin, simvastatin, pravastatin	Block cholesterol synthesis	LDL	GI-upset, myopathy
Bile acid binding resins	Cholestyramine, colestipol	Promote sterol excretion	LDL	GI-upset, High VLDL

43 Plasma Expanders

High molecular weight substance exerting **colloidal (oncotic) pressure** and retaining **fluid** in vascular compartment on **IV infusion**.

Human plasma may transmit **AIDS, hepatitis** and reconstituted human albumin is **expensive**. Hence, **synthetic** colloid is used **commonly**.

The best plasma expander is **human plasma and reconstituted human albumin**. Desirable property of plasma expander: It should be **stable, cheap, easily** sterilizable, pharmacodynamically **inert, not antigenic, not pyrogenic,** not interfering with **grouping** and **cross-matching** of blood and **not leaking out** (remains in circulation).

Plasma expanders are
a. Dextran
b. Human albumin
c. PVP (polyvinyl pyrrolidone)
d. HES (hetastarch/hydroxyethyl starch)
e. Polygeline (degraded gelatin polymer)

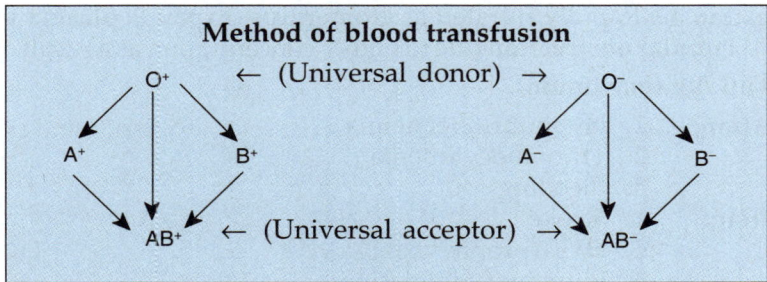

Human albumin: It is obtained from **pooled human plasma**.
Osmotic equivalence: 100 ml of 20% human **albumin** solution
= 400 ml of fresh frozen **plasma**
= 800 ml of **whole** blood

Properties
a. Not interfere with **coagulation**, hence used without regarding patient's blood group.
b. Not transmit serum **hepatitis** due to **heat treated** preparation.

c. **20% solution** holds additional **fluid** from tissues. Hence, **crystalloid solution** is concurrently used in **dehydrated** patient.

ADR: Feverile reaction

Disadvantage: Expensive

U:
1. **Dialysis**
2. **Burn, shock, hypovolemia**
3. **Acute hypoproteinemia**
4. **Acute liver failure**
5. Dilution of blood using albumin and crystalloid solution are used before **cardiopulmonary bypass.**

Dextran: Commonest used plasma expander, cheap, stored for **10 years,** and a **polysaccharide** obtained from **sugar beet.**

Two forms: — **Dextran 70** (MW–70000), common.
— **Dextran 40** (MW–40000).

Dextran has nearly **all poperties of ideal plasma expander except**
a. Its **interference** with blood grouping and cross-matching.
b. Increase **BT** by interfering with coagulation and platelet function.
c. Due to **structural similarity to antigenic polysaccharide,** it reacts with **polysaccharide reacting Ab** (though not antigenic) →**anaphylaxis** (itching, hypotension, urticaria, bronchospasm).

Mechanism (dextran 70): Expands plasma volume for nearly **24 hours.**

PK (dextran 70): Slowly excreted by **glomerular filtration** and **oxidised** in the body over weeks, some deposited in **RE cells.**

Mechanism of dextran 40

1. Acts more **rapidly than** dextran 70.
2. Reduces blood **viscosity** and inhibits **RBC sludging** that occurs in shock by coating them and maintaining their **electronegative change.**

PK of dextran 40: Rapidly filtrated at **glomerulus.** Expands **plasma volume** for short period. **Tubular obstruction** due to higher concentration as a result of **oliguria.**

Dose: 20 ml /kg (maximum).

CI of dextran:
1. Hypofibrinogenemia
2. Thrombocytopenia
3. Bleeding

U of dextran:
1. Stroke
2. DVT (prophylaxis)
3. Pulmonary infarction

Polygeline/degraded gelatin polymer: It is a **polypeptide** with **MW–30,000** exerting **oncotic pressure similar to albumin, not antigenic.**

No interference with blood grouping or cross-matching, **stable** for 3 years.

PK: Not metabolised in the body, excreted **slowly** by kidney.
Plasma volume expansion lasts for **12 hrs.**

ADR: Hypersensitivity reaction (flushing, rigor, urticaria, wheezing, hypotension).

Disadvantage: More expensive than dextran.
U: Priming of heart-lung and **dialysis machine.**

HES: It is a **complex mixture of ethoxylated amylopectin** of average **MW–4.5 Lac** (range 10,000 to one million). It has **colloidal property.** In colloidal property, 6% HES = Human albumin. It has slight plasma volume expansion in excess of volume infused. **Hemodynamic status** is improved for **24 hrs.**
PK: MW <50,000, excreted rapidly by **kidney, 40%** infused dose appears in **urine/day,** larger molecules →smaller molecules (**t½—17 days**).
- **ADR:** 1. **Anaphylactoid reaction** (urticaria, bronchospasm, periorbital edema).
  2. **Salivary gland swelling**
  3. **Flu-like symptoms,** chills, itch, fever, vomiting.
- **U:** 1. **Volume expansion**
  2. To improve harvesting of granulocytes because it accelerates **erythrocyte sedimentation.**

PVP: Synthetic polymer (MW–40000). Used as **3.5% solution.**
Mech: 1. Releases **histamine**
2. **Interferes** with blood grouping and cross-matching.
PK: Slowly excreted by **kidney** and small amount by liver into **bile.** A fraction is stored in **RE cells** for prolonged periods.
IA: Binds with **penicillin** and **insulin** in circulation so that the same is not available for action.
U: Less commonly used as plasma expander.

U of plasma expander
1. As **plasma expander** in burns, hypovolemia, trauma and endotoxic shock.
2. **Temporary measure** in case of whole blood loss (O_2 carrying capacity is absent).

CI of plasma expander
1. Severe **anemia**
2. **Cardiac** failure
3. Pulmonary **edema**
4. **Renal insufficien**cy

Magic of **3** and **4** in blood cells:
1. Iron/gram Hb = **3.4 mg**
2. Bilirubin formed/gram Hb = **34 mg**
3. Oxygen carried/gram Hb = **1.34** cm^3
4. Average lobe/neutrophil = **3.4**
5. HbS (the first and the most common), haemoglobinopathy
   Homozygous = 0.3%   Heterozygous = 13%
6. Maximum oxygen carried/Hb = **4**
7. Hb chain/Hb = **4** (2 α and 2 β)
8. Energy bonds of 2 ATP/glucose = **4**
9. Pyrrole/Hb chain = **4**

10. MW of Hb = 64000
11. MW of erythropoietin = 34000
12. Total Fe in the body = 4 gm
13. % of total Fe in Hb = 64
14. % of total Fe in myoglobin = 4
15. Distance of Fe from heme plane in deoxy Hb = 0.4 Å
16. Difference of residues of (β–α) = >4 (146–141)
17. RBC/ml blood = >4 billion (5 billion)
18. Period of Hb A1c as blood glucose indicator = 4 months (maximum)
19. Power of vessel radius in PVR = 4th
20. Mean pressure in vena cava = 4 mm Hg
21. Hb molecule per RBC = 70 × 4 million
22. TLC = >4000 per mm^3
23. Platelet count = 4 lakh (maximum)/dl
24. Types of lymphocytes = 4

Unit 8
GIT Related Drugs

44. Drugs for Peptic Ulcer

Peptic ulcer (= gastric ulcer + duodenal ulcer) is due to exposure of stomach and duodenum to **pepsin** and **gastric acid**. **Imbalance** occurs between **aggressive** (acid, pepsin, and *Helicobacter pylori*) and **defensive** (gastric mucus, HCO_3^-, PG and innate resistant of mucosal cells) factors.

Regulation of HCl secretion

H^+, K^+-**ATPase (proton pump)** secretes H^+ in apical canaliculi of parietal cell and is stimulated by **ACh, histamine** and **gastrin** via their own **receptors** located on **basolateral membrane of** the cells. Paracrine enterochromaffin like cell called **histaminocyte** is located in **oxyntic gland**.

H_2 **receptor** generates **cAMP** then acts on proton pump involving Ca^{2+}. But **M** and **G receptors** act on **phospholipase C**.

$M_{2/3}$ and G R → phospholipase C → IP3 – DAG → mobilise intracellular Ca^{2+}.

(**MR subtype** on histaminocyte is undefined)

H_2 blockers suppress **histamine, ACh, pentagastrin** and **any gastric acid secretory stimulus. PGE_2** is cytoprotective in gastric mucosa by increasing **mucus** and HCO_3^- secretion and by inhibiting **acid secretion** (by opposing cAMP generation in parietal cell and gastric release from antral cells).

> ### Goals of antiulcer therapy
> Pain relief, ulcer healing, inhibition of release and complication, etc. Duodenal ulcer is chronic remitting and relapsing disease lasting several years. **Mainly 2 goals** (pain relief and ulcer healing) are achieved **most effectively** by H_2 blocker/proton pump inhibitor. **Benign gastric ulcer** should be reduced by **50% after 4 weeks** of treatment, otherwise malignancy should be ruled out by endoscopy, cytology and biopsy. **70% malignant gastric ulcer** also heals by medical treatment. **Most duodenal ulcer** heals within **4–6 weeks** of treatment.

Classification

A. Drugs for reduction of gastric acid secretion
  1. **PG analogues:** Rioprostil, Enprostil, Misoprostol. **REM**
  2. **Proton pump inhibitors:** Pantoprazole, Rabeprazole, Omeprazole, Lansoprazole, Esomeprazole. **ROLE**
  3. **H$_2$ antihistaminics/H$_2$ blockers/H$_2$ antagonists (reversible blockers)**

     RANItidine ⎫
     ROXAtidine ⎬ **RANI RUKJA NAJA**
     NIZAtidine ⎬ Competitively
     Cimetidine ⎭
     Famotidine   (Competitively and non-competitively).
     Loxatidine   (Non-competitively).

     (Except loxatidine and nizatidine, all are available in india).
  4. **Anticholinergic:** Pirenzepine, Oxyphenonium, Trimipramine, Doxepin, Propantheline. **TOP**

B. Ulcer protective: Sucralfate, CBS (colloidal bismuth subcitrate).

C. Ulcer healing drugs: Cabenoxolone sodium, Deglycyrrhizinised liquorice.

D. Antacid (neutralization of gastric acid)
  a. **Systemic:** NaHCO$_3$, sodium citrate.
  b. **Nonsystemic**
     Mg(OH)$_2$
     MgCO$_3$
     Al(OH)$_3$ gel
     CaCO$_3$
     Mg trisilicate
     Magaldrate

E. Anti-*H. pylori* drugs: Clarithromycin, amoxicillin, tetracycline, tinidazole, metronidazole.

Cimetidine (the prototype): H$_2$ blocker is **the most popular** drug for peptic ulcer, and inhibits **all phases** of gastric acid secretion. **First H$_2$ blocker** introduced clinically is **cimetidine. Sir James Black** developed the **first H$_2$ blocker (Burimamide) in 1972.**

  Mech: 1. H$_2$ blockers block **histamine-induced gastric secretion, cardiac stimulation, uterine relaxation** and **bronchial relaxation.**
  2. Attenuates hypotension due to histamine.
  3. H$_2$ blockers reduce **acid secretion** in response to ACh and gastrin.
  4. **All phases** (basal, psychic, neurogenic and gastric) of secretion have dose-dependent suppression. Secretory response to histamine, ACh, insulin, gastrin, alcohol and food is attenuated. The **most prominent** action is on acid output **(antiulcerogenic effects).**
  5. Ulcer healing dose produces **60–70%** inhibition of acid output/day.

PK: Cimetidine is absorbed **orally.** Bioavailability—**60%** due to first pass hepatic metabolism. **Crosses placenta** and reaches milk. Poor penetration in **brain** due to its **hydrophilic** nature. **2/3 excreted** unchanged in urine and bile and the rest as oxidised metabolites. Elimination t½ → **2–3 hours.**

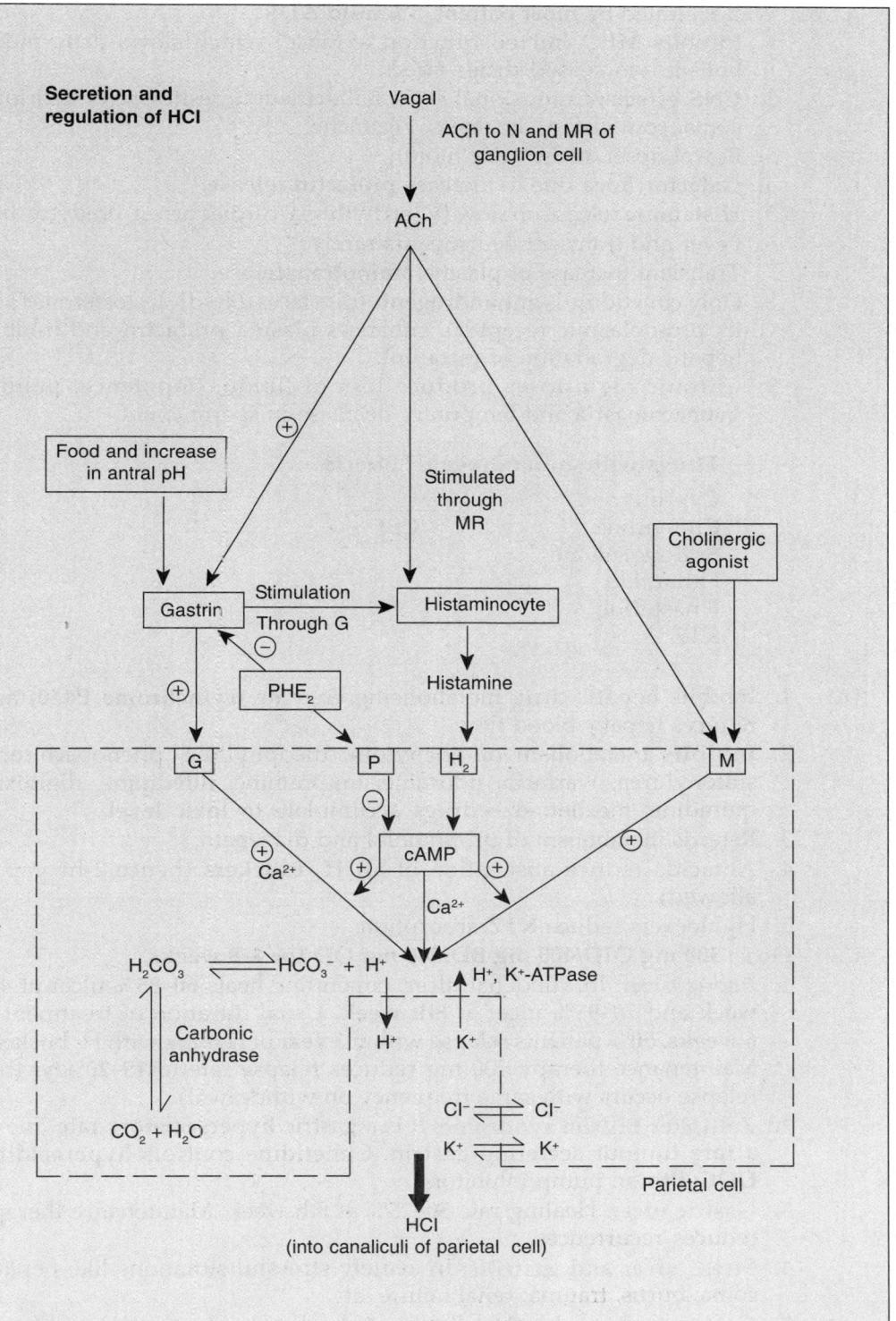

ADR: Well tolerated by **most patient, 5% mild ADR.**
1. Inhibits **MFO** (mixed function oxidase) which slows drug metabolism →increased drugs effect.
2. **CNS effects:** Confusional state, hallucination, restlessness, delirium, coma, convulsion, dizziness, headache.
3. Bowel upset, rashes, dry mouth.
4. **Galactorrhoea** due to increase **prolactin release.**
5. **Histamine** release on slow IV (arrhythmia, cardiac arrest, bradycardia).
6. Fever and transient neutropenia rarely.
7. Transient increase of plasma **aminotransferase.**
8. Only cimetidine is **antiandrogenic** (displaces dihydrotestosterone from its protoplasmic receptor), enhances plasma **prolactin** and inhibits hepatic degradation of **estradiol.**
9. Chronic high doses produce loss of libido, impotence, painful **gynaecomastia** and temporary decrease in sperm count.

> **Drugs with antiandrogenic effects**
> Cyproterone
> Cimetidine   CSF
> Spironolactone
> Flutamide
> Finasteride
> KTZ

IA:
1. Inhibits hepatic drug metabolising enzyme **(cytochrome P450)** and reduces hepatic blood flow.
2. **Inhibits** metabolism of phenytoin, theophylline, phenobarbitone, sulfonylurea, warfarin, lidocaine, imipramine, nifedipine, digitoxin, quinidine, mexiletine → drugs accumulate to **toxic level.**
3. Retards metabolism of propranolol and diazepam.
4. Antacids reduce absorption of **all H$_2$ blockers** (hence 2-hr gap is allowed).
5. H$_2$ blockers reduce **KTZ** absorption.

U: Dose: **300 mg QID/400 mg BD/800 mg OD for 4–8 weeks.**
1. **Peptic ulcer:** In duodenal ulcer, cimetidine heals **60–85%** ulcer at 4th week and **70–95%** ulcer at **8th week.** Usual duration of treatment is **6 weeks. 50%** patients relapse within **1 year** of healing with H$_2$ bockers. Maintenance therapy 400 mg reduces relapse rate to **15–20%/yr** (but relapse occurs with same frequency on withdrawal).
2. **Zollinger-Ellison syndrome:** It is a gastric **hypersecretory rate** due to a rare tumour secreting gastrin. Cimetidine controls **hyperacidity. DOC:** Proton pump inhibitors.
3. **Gastric ulcer:** Healing rate **50–75%** at 8th week. Maintenance therapy reduces recurrences.
4. **Stress ulcer and gastritis:** In acutely stressful situations like hepatic coma, burns, trauma, renal failure, etc.
5. **Gastroesophageal reflux:** Facilitates healing by decreasing acidity.

Drugs for Peptic Ulcer 517

6. **Prophylaxis of aspiration pneumonia:** H_2 blocker reduces aspiration of acidic gastric content during surgery and anaesthesia.

Gastritis Type A	4A
Autoimmune disorder characterised by Autoantibodies to parietal cells, pernicious Anemia and Achlorhydria.	
Gastritis Type B: It is due to *H. pylori*.	

Ranitidine: It was introduced after cimetidine as **second H_2 blockers/nonimidazole H_2 blocker having furan ring. It is 5 times** more potent than cimetidine without having antiandrogenic effect, and without increasing prolactin secretion with lesser permeability into brain and lower incidence of ADR.

Dose: 300 mg OD/150 mg BD, maintenance therapy—150 mg.

Famotidine: The most potent H_2 blocker. 8 times more potent than ranitidine. No antiandrogenic action. Healing **same** as with cimetidine. It is a thiazole ring having H_2 blockade which binds to H_2 R.

Mech: Binds to H_2 receptor.

Thiazole ring with H_2 blockade.

PK: Longer duration of action. Elimination t½—**3 hours**, oral bioavailability → 40–50%, renal excretion (**70% in unchanged form**).

Dose: 20 mg BD for healing and 20 mg OD for maintenance. **Maximum 480 mg/day** in Zollinger-Ellison syndrome.

ADR: Headache, dizziness, bowel upset.

U: ZE syndrome and Aspiration Pneumonia } Due to higher potency and longer duration. **ZAP**

Roxatidine: PK, pharmacodynamic, ADR are **similar** to ranitidine but **twice** as potent and longer acting as ranitidine.

Nizatidine: Same to ranitidine in potency and **properties.** It is a **thiazole** ring having H_2 blocking property.

PK: Bioavailability—**90%**, plasma t½ = 1–1.5 hr.

Loxatidine: Powerful **non-competitive H_2 blocker.** Completely inhibits gastric secretion.

Omeprazole

Omeprazole is a **prototype** of new class of **substituted benzimidazole.** H^+, K^+-ATPase is present in **apical membrane** and **tubulovesicular apparatus of parietal cells.**

Mech: 1. **Irreversibly** inhibits H^+, K^+-ATPase in stomach cells.
2. Inhibits final common step in **gastric acid secretion** (dose dependent suppression of gastric secretion) → **totally abolishes HCl secretion.**
3. Inactive at **neutral pH** but rearranges to **two forms (sulphenic acid** and **sulphenamide configuration) at pH <5** (as it is inactive at neutral pH) that react covalently with **"SH group"** of H^+, K^+ ATPase enzyme and inactivate it irreversibly (specially when **two molecules** of omeprazole react with **one molecule of enzyme).**

4. It is concentrated at **acidic pH** in canaliculi after diffusing into **parietal cells** from blood (because charged forms generated at acidic pH are unable to diffuse back).
   Drugs → blood → parietal cell → canaliculi (charged form).

Acid secretion is resumed after new **H$^+$, K$^+$-ATPase molecule synthesis.**
PK: Oral absorption **50%** (but at higher gastric pH, more absorption occurs).
Hepatic metabolism, **renal** excretion, **plasma t½—1 hour.**
Binds tightly to its target enzyme, hence detected in gastric mucosa long after its disappearance from plasma.

ADR:
1. Compensatory **hypergastrinemia** due to marked and long lasting acid secretion.
2. Headache and dizziness
3. Bowel upset and nausea

IA: Inhibits **oxidation** of morphine, diazepam, phenytoin, and **enhances their levels.**

U:
1. **Peptic ulcer:** 20 mg OD for 4–8 weeks heals ulcer, useful in H$_2$ inhibitor resistant case, integral component of anti-*H. pylori* therapy.
   Best drug for treatment of peptic ulcer—**omeprazole.**
2. **Reflux oesophagitis (DOC)**
3. **Gastritis**
4. **ZE syndrome: Omeprazole (DOC):** More effective than H$_2$ blocker in controlling hyperacidity in ZE syndrome. **Dose:** 60–120 mg BD.

Lansoprazole: More potent than omeprazole (**similar in properties**).
Mech: Less persistent inhibition of acid secretion because H$^+$, K$^+$-ATPase is **partly reversible.**
ADR: Same as omeprazole
IA: Less significant
Pantoprazole: **Similar** in potency, properties and clinical efficacy to **omeprazole.**
Mech: Newer H$^+$, K$^+$-ATPase inhibitor. Lower affinity for **cytochrome P450** than omeprazole/lansoprazole.
Rabeprazole causes fastest acid suppression and helps in gastric mucin synthesis. Potency and efficacy similar to omeprazole.
Esomeprazole: S-enantiomer of omeprazole. Better control of intragastric pH and better GERD symptom relief plus more healing of erosive esophagitis than omeprazole. ADR and IA similar to parent drugs.

> **Anticholinergic (atropine):** Reduces **gastric juice volume** without raising its pH (unless there is food in stomach to dilute secreted acid).
> **Antacids:** Given concurrently act for longer period due to **delayed gastric emptying** caused by atropine.
> **Pirenzepine (selective M$_1$ anticholinergic):** It is **hydrophilic** (not produce CNS effects), reduces **gastric secretion**, inhibits **acid secretion** only by **40–50%** (less than H$_2$ blockers) with narrow therapeutic range (ADR with slight excess) and is used in **ulcer + flatulent dyspepsia.**
> **Trimipramine** and **doxepin:** These are TCA with **anticholinergic** properties and **weak proton pump inhibitory** action (reduce gastric acid secretion).

PG analogues: **PGE₂** and **I₂** are effective in **ulcer** treatment.
Mech:
1. **Exogenous PG** enhances mucosal resistant by:
   a. Stimulating gastric **mucus** secretion.
   b. Increasing mucosal **blood** flow and mucosal **cell restitution.**
   c. Increasing gastric and duodenal HCO_3^- secretion.
2. PGE₂ and I₂ produced in gastric mucosa inhibit **acid secretion + gastrin** production and promote **mucus plus HCO_3^-** secretion. Reinforce **mucus layer** covering gastric and duodenal mucosa buffered by HCO_3^- secreted into this layer by underlying epithelial cells (**the most important function**).
3. **Weaker** than H₂ blocker.
4. Enhance **mucus** resistance to tissue injury.
5. **Misoprostol** (PGI analogue) inhibits ulcer due to NSAID.

ADR:
1. Abdominal cramp and diarrhoea.
2. Uterine bleeding and abortion.

CI: **Women** of child-bearing potential.

U:
1. **Gastric ulcer**
2. **Reflux esophagitis**
3. **Ulcer** healing in arthritis using NSAID.
4. Treatment and inhibition of NSAID associated GI injury and blood loss.

Antacids: Basic substances neutralising gastric acid and **raising pH** of gastric contents (**at pH >4,** peptic activity is reduced because pepsin secreted as complex dissociates **below pH 5** → optimum peptic activity occurs between **2 and 4**).

Ideal antacids: They are potent in neutralising acid, inexpensive, not absorbed from GIT, palatable, and contain negligible Na.

ANC (acid neutralising capacity): Number of mEq of 1 N HCl brought to pH **3.5 in 15 min** by unit dose of antacid preparation (using determination of weight/equivalent weight of agent and rate of dissolution). Unit–mEq/gm.

Mech
1. Not reduce acid production.
2. Agents raising antral pH to 4 evoke **gastrin release** → increase acid secreted specially in hyperacidity and duodenal ulcer→**acid rebound** →gastric motility.

PK: Single dose acts for ½–1 hr, with meal, it acts for **2–3 hrs (maximum).** Food reduces the rate of HCl neutralisation.

NaHCO₃: It is **systemic** antacids, **water soluble,** acts **instantaneously** and is a **potent neutraliser** (1 gm neutralises 12 mEq HCl).

ADR
1. **Metabolic alkalosis** at high doses (compensated by alkaline urine secretion).
2. **Enhanced blood pH** in renal insufficiency.
3. **Acid rebound** (usually short lasting due to increase pH).
4. **Hypernatremia** →**CHF** and **edema.**
5. NaHCO₃ + HCl (gastric) →(CO₂ + H₂O + NaCl) → **CO₂ production in stomach** → discomfort, bloating and eructation, distension, risk of ulcer perforation, LES relaxation.

CI: HTN and cardiac disease
U:
1. Heart burn (for symptomatic treatment)
2. To alkalinise urine
3. To treat acidosis

Sodium citrate: Same as $NaHCO_3$ (1 gm neutralise 10 mEq HCl). But CO_2 production is **absent**.

Non-systemic antacid: It is **insoluble** and poorly absorbed **basic** compound. Reacts in stomach to form corresponding **chloride salt** → chloride salt reacts with intestinal HCO_3^- → no absorption → **no acid–base disturbance.** Small absorbed amount has **same** alkalinising effects as $NaHCO_3$.

Aluminium hydroxide/$Al(OH)_3$: Bland weak slowly reacting antacid. **Polymerizes** into less reactive form → ANC of preparation gradually **declines** on storage. ANC usually is 1–2.5 mEq/gm.

Mech
1. Al^{+++} **relaxes** smooth muscle.
2. Delays **gastric emptying** (unlike other antacids).
3. Causes **constipation** due to its smooth muscle relaxant and mucosal astringent action. Large doses cause intestinal **obstruction.**
4. $Al(OH)_3$ absorbs pepsin at **pH >3** but releases it at lower pH → **inactive pepsin.**
5. Coats and protects ulcer (acts as **demulcent**).
6. Binds PO_4^{3-} in intestine and inhibits its absorption → **hypophosphatemia** on regular use → osteomalacia, anorexia, malaise, weakness.

ADR
1. **Hypokalaemia**
2. **Hypophosphatemia**
3. **Constipation** Al → Constipation = AC
                         alu**MINIUM** amount of faeces
4. Al^{3+} **toxicity** in renal impairment (because small amount of Al^{3+} absorbed is excreted by kidney)
5. **Osteomalacia, anorexia, malaise, weakness.**

U:
1. Hyperphosphatemia.
2. PO_4^{3-} stones

Other **alum salts** (PO_4^{3-}, aminoacetate, glycinate) have **similar** antacid properties.

$Mg(OH)_2$: Low water solubility. Its aqueous suspension (milk of magnesia) has low OH^- concentration and thus low alkalinity. 1 gm neutralise 30 mEq HCl. Mild acid rebound.

ADR:
1. Hypokalaemia
2. Diarrhea   Mg = Must go to bathroom

$MgCO_3$: Crystalline, water soluble, slow reaction with HCl, CO_2 evolved.

Mg trisilicate: Low solubility and reactivity. 1 gm neutralise 10 mEq HCl (but clinically only 1 mEq is neutralised before it is passed into duodenum. pH is usually < 3). **Silica** produced by reaction with HCl is **gelatinous** (absorbs and inactivates pepsin and protects ulcer base).

Mech: All Mg salt have **laxative** action (by generating osmotically active $MgCl_2$ in stomach and through Mg^{++} induced **cholecystokinin** release). **5%** of administered Mg is absorbed **systemically.**

U: 1. As **laxative**
2. As osmotic **purgative** (soluble Mg salt).

Magaldrate: It is **hydrated** complex of **hydroxy magnesium aluminate.** ANC = 28 mEq/gm.

Mech: Reacts rapidly with **acid** and releases **Al(OH)$_3$** which is slow reacting but **freshly released alum hydroxide** is unpolymerised (more reactive form).

CaCO$_3$: It is potent and rapidly acting acid neutraliser. ANC = 20 mEq HCl/gm. But ANC of **commercial** preparation = 13 mEq HCl/gm.

Mech: Liberates **CO$_2$** in stomach at slower rate than NaHCO$_3$.

ADR
1. **Distension and discomfort**
2. **On chronic use:** Renal stone, hypercalcemia, hypercalciuria and alkalosis.
3. **Hypokalemia**
4. **Milk alkali syndrome (hypercalciuria):** It is due to **CaCO$_3$/NaHCO$_3$** for peptic ulcer characterised by headache, anorexia, weakness and renal stone.
5. **Acid rebound** is marked. Total antacid requirement and gastric motility are enhanced.
6. **Constipation in most individuals.**
7. **Hyperacidity (greatest drawback):** Ca^{2+} diffuses into gastric mucosa →increase HCl production by parietal cell and by releasing gastrin **(greatest drawback).**

ANC of antacids	
CaCO$_3$	— 20 mEq HCl /gm
	— 13 mEq HCl/gm (commercial)
Magaldrate	— 28 mEq HCl /gm
Mg trisilicate	— 10 mEq HCl /gm
Al(OH)$_3$	— 1 to 2.5 mEq/gm
Mg(OH)$_2$	— 30 mEq HCl /gm
Na citrate	— 10 mEq HCl /gm
NaHCO$_3$	— 12 mEq HCl /gm

Antacid combination (↓dose reduces toxicity)
a. Fast Mg(OH)$_2$ + slow Al(OH)$_3$.
   Al(OH)$_3$ (constipation) + Mg(OH)$_2$ (loose stool).
   Most widely used antacid mixture. Prompt and sustained effect.
   Combination neutralises each other's side effects.
b. Mg salt (laxative) + aluminium salt (constipation). Bowel movement **least** affected.
c. Gastric emptying **least** affected: Aluminium salt (slow emptying) + Mg/Ca salt (fast emptying).

IA of antacids
1. IA is due to **enhanced pH** and **nonabsorbable antacid.**
2. Antacids **reduce absorption** of tetracycline, iron salt, fluoroquinolone, H$_2$ blocker, KTZ, diazepam, phenytoin, phenothiazine, INH, indomethacin, ethambutol and nitrofurantoin.
3. Efficacy of nitrofurantoin is reduced by **alkalinization of urine.**

U of antacids

1. **Z-E syndrome and giant duodenal ulcer.** Antacid is **adjuvant** in them.
2. **Gastroesophageal reflux:** As adjuvant, antacids promptly relieve **heart burn** due to reflux of acid gastric contents into esophagus. Increase pH improves LES tone (lower esophageal sphincter tone).
3. **Prophylaxis** of aspiration pneumonia, during endoscopy, surgery, comatose patient.
4. **Duodenal ulcer:** 30 ml antacid mixture **1** and **3 hrs** after meals and at **bedtime**. Healing rate = **80%**.

Sucralfate

Sucralfate is **basic Al salt of sulfated sucrose (sucrose sulfate).** Efficacy is **similar** to antacid and H_2 blockers.

- **Mech:**
    1. **Al sucrose sulfate** polymerizes in **acid** environment of stomach, selectivity binds **neurotic peptic ulcer tissue** and acts as **barrier** to acid, pepsin and bile but does not work in the presence of H_2 blockers/antacids.
    2. Has **viscous consistency** in acidic medium. Polymerises by **cross-linking** of molecules at **pH <4** and adheres to **ulcer base for >6 hrs.**
    3. Acts as **physical barrier** by preventing acid, pepsin and bile from coming in contact with ulcer base due to precipitation of **surface protein** at this ulcer base.
    4. **Dietary proteins** form another layer by deposition.
    5. Delays gastric emptying but has **no acid neutralizing action.** Promotes healing of gastric and duodenal ulcer (efficacy is **similar** to cimetidine at **4 weeks** for **duodenal** ulcer). SucralFATE Sacrifices phosFATE.
- **ADR:**
    1. **Constipation** (2% patient)
    2. **Hypophosphatemia** by binding PO_4^{3-} ion in intestine.
    3. Dry mouth and nausea rarely.
- **IA:**
    1. **Antacids** reduce sucralfate efficacy.
    2. Sucralfate **interferes** with absorption of tetracycline, digoxin, fluoroquinolone, phenytoin and cimetidine.
- **PK:** Minimum oral absorption.
- **U:**
    1. **Peptic ulcer:** 1 gm 1 hr before 3 major meals and at bed-time for 4–8 weeks.
    2. **Recurrent ulcer:** 1 gm BD for 6 months.
    3. **Gastritis** and **bile reflux:** 4 daily doses are needed.

CBS /Tripotassium dicitratobismuthate (colloidal bismuth subcitrate): It is **water soluble colloidal bismuth compound** and precipitates at **pH <5**. Heals 60% ulcer at **4 weeks** and 90% at 8 weeks. Cimetidine resistant ulcer heals by subsequent 4 weeks CBS treatment.

- **Mech**
    1. Inhibits **pepsin** activity, binds to gastric **mucus gel layer**, and eradicates *H. pylori* hence gastritis.
    2. Stimulates **mucosal PGE_2** production → increased secretion of **mucus** and HCO_3.

3. **CBS** and **mucus** form **glycoprotein-Bi complex** which coats ulcer and acts as **diffusion barrier to HCl**.
4. Detaches *H. pylori* from mucosal surface and kills it.
5. Absorbs **pepsin** and reduces its output.
6. Colloidal Bi forms **Bi protein coagulant**.

PK: Mostly **faecal** excretion. **Small renal** excretion.
Dose: CBS 120 mg taken as Bi_2O_3 30 min before 3 meals for 4–8 weeks.
ADR
1. **Osteodystrophy** and **encephalopathy** due to bismuth toxicity.
2. Headache and dizziness
3. **Diarrhoea**
4. Patient acceptance of CBS is compromised by **blackening of tongue, dentures** and **stools**.

U:
1. **Gastritis and nonulcer dyspepsia:** Due to *H. pylori*. Ulcer recurrence is due to *H. pylori*. Outstanding feature of CBS is—**lower relapse rate of ulcer**.
2. *H. pylori*: **Triple therapy combination** = CBS + metronidazole + amoxycillin/tetracycline (up to **90% eradication** in 1 month).

Carbenoxolone sodium: It is **steroid like triterpenoid derivative of glycyrrhetinic acid of liquorice root** for gastric ulcer healing.

Mech:
1. Augmentation of **mucus** production (**most important action**).
2. Enhances **glycoprotein** synthesis by gastric mucosa.
3. Interferes with activation of **pepsinogen**.
4. Increases lifespan of gastric **epithelial cells**.
5. Inhibits bile reflux by enhancing **pyloric tone** → enhanced back diffusion of H^+ in gastric mucosa.
6. Slows **PG degradation** in gastric mucosa.

PK: Complete **oral** absorption. **Biliary excretion**. Highly **plasma protein** bound.

ADR:
1. **Mineralocorticoid like** action → Na^+ and water retention and K^+ loss.
2. **Edema** and **HTN**.

Drugs causing hypokalemia
AMB, carbenicillin, gentamicin, carbenoxolone, steroid, diuretic.

CI:
1. Hepatic and renal disease
2. HTN and CHF

U: Gastric ulcer

Deglycyrrhizinized liquorice: Mechanism **same** as carbenoxolone (but **less** effective). But **Na** and **water** retention is **absent**.

Anti-*H. pylori* drugs: These are for **all ulcer** patients. *H. pylori* (**Gram-negative**) is **lifelong host** and attached to surface epithelium beneath mucus having **urease activity** → produces NH_3 to maintain microenvironment around bacteria and to promote back diffusion of H^+. *H. pylori* bacillus acts as **commensal in 20–70% normal individuals** and causes chronic gastritis, gastric CA, gastric lymphoma, peptic ulcer, dyspepsia. **90% gastric** and **duodenal ulcer** has *H. pylori* infection. H_2 blocker/proton pump inhibitor eradicates *H. pylori*, heals peptic **ulcer,** and lowers **relapse** rate.

Drugs for *H. pylori* — TACT

- Tetracycline
- Amoxycillin
- Clarithromycin
- Tinidazole/metronidazole

Single drug is ineffective and resistance develops rapidly.

1 week regimens

a. Amoxycillin + Clarithromycin + Omeprazole.   CO, CMO
b. Amoxycillin/Clarithromycin + Omeprazole + Metronidazole/tinidazole.

2-week regimens   CO, TBM, ARM

a. Amoxycillin/Clarithromycin + Omeprazole.
b. Amoxycillin/Tetracycline + Bismuth + Metronidazole/Tinidazole.
c. Amoxycillin + Ranitidine + Metronidazole.

Meckel's diverticulum
(**commonest** congenital anomaly of GIT)
The **"FIVE 2s"** about it are:
1. 2 inches long
2. 2 feet from **ileocecal valve**
3. 2% **population**
4. Commonly in first **2 yrs of life**
5. May have **2 types** of epithelia

45. Emetics, Antiemetics, Digestants, Carminatives and Gallstone Dissolving Drugs

Emesis/vomiting is due to stimulation of **vomiting centre or emetic centre** found in **medulla oblongata**. **CTZ** (chemoreceptor trigger zone) found in **NTS** (nucleus tractus Solitarius) and **area postrema** are the **most important relay areas for afferent** impulses arising in GIT, throat and other viscera. CTZ is **unprotected** by BBB. Cytotoxic drugs, radiation, and irritants release **5-HT** from **enterochromaffin** cells which acts on **5-HT₃ receptors** found on **vagal afferent** and sends impulse to **NTS** and **CTZ**.

Receptor on CTZ and NTS are

| 1, 2, 3, M, μ | H₁ (histamine)
D₂ (DA)
5-HT₃ (serotonin)
M (cholinergic)
μ (opioid) |

Receptors relay emetic **signals** and **antiemetic drugs** act on them. **Vestibular apparatus** generates impulse on disturbance which reaches the emetic centre, mainly relayed from cerebellum and acts on H₁ and M R.

Unpleasant sensory stimuli (bad odour, severe pain, fear, ghastly sight, recall of obnoxious events, anticipation of emetic stimulus) cause nausea and vomiting through higher centre.

Decreased gastric tone, and peristalsis accompany **nausea**. In the emetic response, fundus and body of stomach, esophageal sphincter and esophagus **relax** while duodenum and pyloric stomach **contract** in a retrograde manner. Rhythmic contractions of **diaphragm** and **abdominal muscle** then compress the stomach and evacuate its contents via the mouth. Conditions inhibiting gastric emptying predispose to **vomiting**.

Emetics

A. **Acting on CTZ:** Apomorphine.
B. **Acting on CTZ and reflexly:** Ipecacuanha.
C. **In emergency such as poisoning:** Powdered mustard suspension.

Apomorphine: It is a **semisynthetic** derivative of morphine.
Mech: It acts as **dopaminergic agonist** on CTZ.
PK: 6 mg IM/SC within 5 min induces **vomiting. No oral use** (because dose is larger, slow to act, and inconsistent in action).

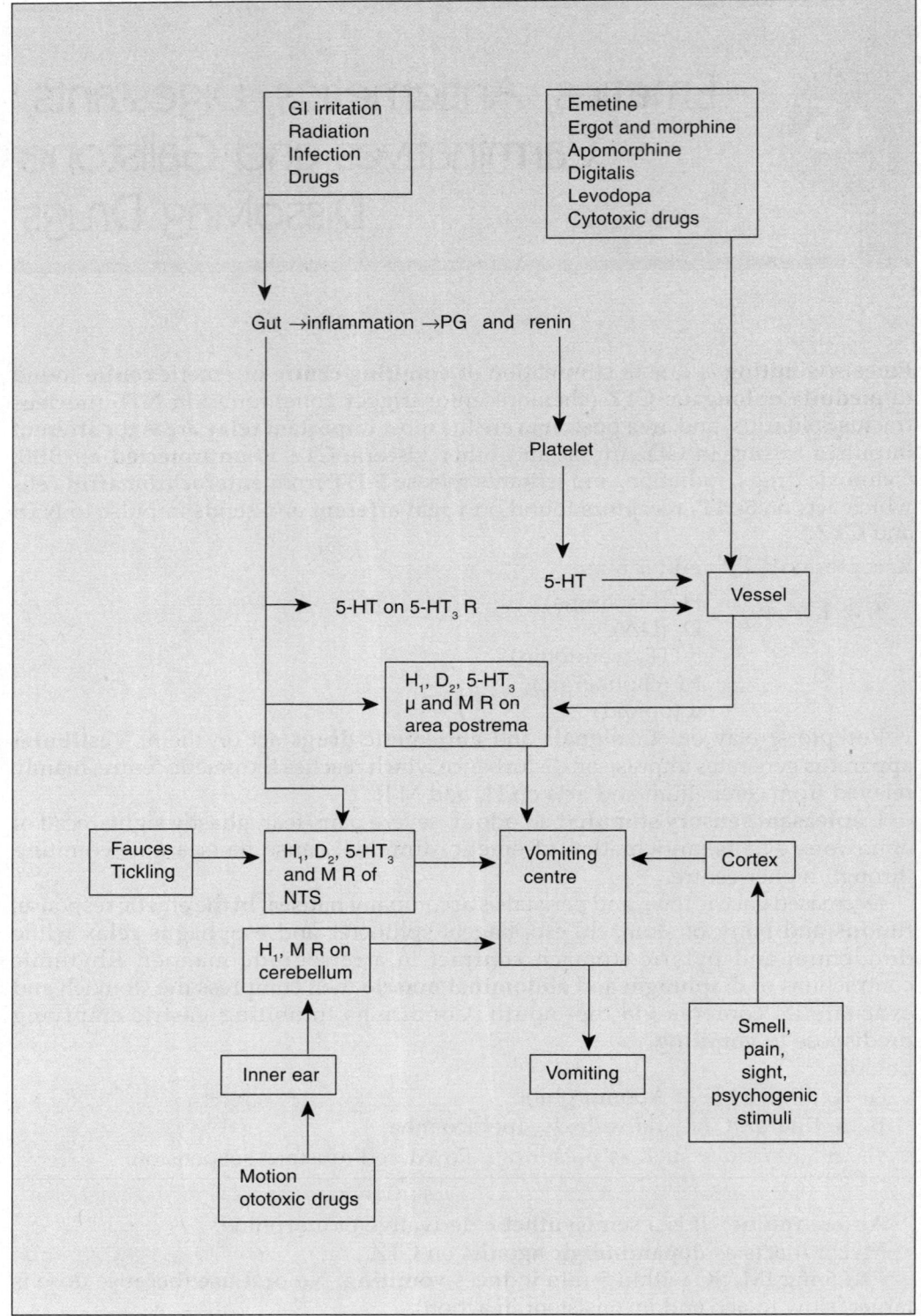

Emetics, Antiemetics, Digestants, Carminatives and Gallstone Dissolving Drugs

ADR: Respiratory and CNS depression
U: To induce vomiting
Ipecacuanha: Dried root of Cephaelis ipecacuanha has **emetine.**
Mech: Acts by irritating **gastric mucosa** and through **CTZ.**
PK: Safer, less dependable, takes 15 minutes for the effects.
U: Used as **syrup Ipecacuanha.**
Dose: — 20 ml adult.
 — 10 ml children.
 — 5 ml infant.

CI of all emetics

1. **CNS stimulant drug poisoning** (precipitates convulsion).
2. **Kerosine (petroleum) poisoning** due to high chemical pneumonia and liquid aspiration (because of low viscosity).
3. **Unconscious patient.**
4. **Morphine** and **phenothiazine poisoning** (due to emetic ineffectivity).
5. **Corrosive (acid, alkali) poisoning** (due to injury and perforation to esophageal mucosa).

Antiemetics

1. **Anticholinergics:** Hyoscine, dicyclomine.
2. **H₁ blocker:** Promethazine
3. **Neuroleptic:** CPZ, prochlorperazine, haloperidol, thiethylperazine.
4. **Prokinetic:** Metoclopramide
    Domperidone
    Cisapride, mosapride   MD Cardiology
5. **5-HT₃ blocker:** Granisetron
    Ondansetron   GOT
    Trapisetron
6. **Adjuvant antiemetics:**   BZD   BDC
    Dexamethasone
    Cannabinoids

Neuroleptics: These are potent **broad spectrum antiemetics.** Antiemetic **dose** is much lower than antipsychotic dose. They inhibit **D₂ R in CTZ** and antagonise apomorphine induced vomiting.

Uses

1. **Nausea** and **vomiting**
    (Drug induced and postanaesthetics)
2. **Vomiting:** Malignancy, cancer chemotherapy and radiation induced. Disease induced such as gastroenteritis, uremia, migraine and liver disease.
3. **Morning sickness of hyperemesis gravidarum**
    Ineffective in other motion sickness due to absence of involvement of dopaminergic link in vestibular pathway.

Prochlorperazine: It is **labyrinthine suppressant,** has **selective antivertigo** and **antiemetic action** (better antiemetics than antipsychotic action).

> Extrapyramidal ADR such as muscle dystonia is the **most important limiting features**.
> **Cannabinoids** are **antiemetics** against moderately emetogenic chemotherapy. **Nabilone (synthetic cannabinoid)** is less hallucinogenic and more antiemetic than cannabinoid.

Metoclopramide: Prokinetic drugs promote gastroduodenal **peristalsis** and speed up **gastric emptying**. Metoclopramide is **only chemically (not pharmacologically)** related to **procainamide**. Introduced in **1970** as gastric emptying agent.

Actions

1. Enhances **gastric peristalsis** and relaxes **pylorus** plus **first part of duodenum** →speeds up gastric emptying. **LES tone** is increased and **gastroesophageal reflux** is inhibited. Also enhances **intestinal peristalsis**.
2. Acts on **CTZ** and inhibits apomorphine induced vomiting.

Mech

1. Enhances **ACh release** from myenteric neurones → ACh acts on M_3 R of smooth muscle → **peristalsis** is increased (gastric prokinetic and LES tonic action).
2. Inhibits $5-HT_3$ R of vagal afferent in GIT and NTS/CTZ.
3. D_2 blockade in CTZ causes central antiemetic action.
4. DA through D_2 R delays gastric emptying if **food** is found in the stomach and mediates gastric dilatation/LES relaxation. Drug enhances gastric emptying and LES tone (**blockade of DA action**). Metoclopramide + domperidone inhibit DA on D_2 R (which normally inhibit ACh release).

PK: Rapidly absorbed **orally**, enters **brain**, crosses **placenta** →secreted in milk, partly **conjugated in liver** and **excreted in urine** within **24 hrs, t½** → 3–6 hrs.

ADR:
1. Sedation and dizziness
2. **Diarrhoea**
3. Muscle dystonia
4. **On chronic use:** Galactorrhoea, gynaecomastia, parkinsonism.

IA:
1. Enhances absorption of diazepam and aspirin by facilitating **gastric emptying**.
2. Reduces **digoxin** absorption by allowing less time for it.
3. Reduces **cimetidine** bioavailability.
4. Based on anticholinergic, sedative and antihistaminic effects, H_1 **blockers** inhibit extrapyramidal ADR of metoclopramide and supplement its antiemetic action due to central anticholinergic action.
5. **BZD** has weak antiemetic property due to sedative action and suppress **ADR** of metoclopramide.

U:
1. **Antiemetic:** Postoperative, migraine, radiation sickness, morning sickness (**unsafe in pregnancy**) and cancer therapy induced vomiting. **Pyridoxine** is also used in morning sickness and hyperemesis gravidarum. **BZD** is used as **adjuvant** to metoclopramide/ondansetron in vomiting. Dexamethasone alleviates nausea and vomiting due to moderately emetogenic chemotherapy and reduces ADR of primary antiemetic.

2. **Gastrokinetic (to accelerate gastric emptying):** When food is taken <4 hrs before emergency GA. In facilitating duodenal intubation and in relieving postvagotomy/DM associated gastric statis.
3. **Dyspepsia**
4. **Gastroesophageal reflux** (heart burn and acid erructation)

LES tone is governed by
A. Inherent tone of **sphincteric smooth muscle.**
B. **Smoking** (relaxes LES)
C. **Diet** (protein rich food enhances LES tone while fat, alcohol, coffee and chocolates reduce the tone).
D. **Drugs** (opiates, anticholinergic, and CCB reduce LES tone).
E. **Neurogenic** (vagus is motor to sphincter and promotes esophageal clearing).
F. **Hormonal** (gastrin enhances and progesterone reduces the tone).

Delayed gastric emptying: Enhances chance of reflux. Acidity of gastric contents is **the most important** aggressive factor in causing ulcers and esophagitis. **Metoclopramide** enhances LES tone, facilitates gastric emptying and improves esophageal closure. **Cisapride** is **equally** effective and **domperidone** is less effective. **Prokinetic drugs** are adjuvant to H_2 blockers/proton pump inhibitors in reflux disease. H_2 **blockers** reduce activity of gastric content, inhibit nocturnal acidic exposure and produce esophageal healing in 50–70% patient. **Omeprazole/ lansoprazole** is DOC for severe reflux disease (rapid relief and higher healing due to more complete acid suppression) but there is **"recurrence after stoppage."** Proton pump inhibitor and H_2 blocker inhibit **acid secretion** but antacid **neutralizes** it. **Sodium alginate** forms **thick frothy** layer which **floats on gastric content** and inhibits **contact** of acid with esophageal mucosa. Antacids neutralise acid, improve tone and help in healing.

Cisapride: Effects on **gastric motility,** are **similar** to metoclopramide (but it is not D_2 **agonist** and has no action on CTZ). **No hyperprolactinemia.**

Mech: 1. Restores and facilitates **motility** throughout GIT.
2. Acts on **5-HT$_4$ R** to enhance ACh release from myenteric plexus.

PK: Oral bioavailability—**33%,** inactivated by **hepatic** metabolism, t½ = 10 hrs.

ADR: 1. Diarrhoea
2. Abdominal cramps (**commonest**)
3. **QT prolongation** leading to torsade de pointes.

CISAPRIDE is PRIDE of CISA: Cardiotoxicity due to K⁺ channel blockade if taken with **I**nhibitors of CYP4503A4 (azoles, macrolides and protease inhibitors) and **S**timulates 5-HT$_4$ R raising **A**denyl cyclase level.

Precaution
1. In **liver disease,** dose is to be reduced.
2. Combined use of cisapride and macrolides/imidazole.

IA: Atropine blocks its prokinetic action due to **ACh release** from myenteric plexus through **5-HT$_4$ R agonism.**

U: 1. Gastroesophageal reflux
2. Constipation

Advantage: Prokinetic action without antidopaminergic ADR.

Mosapride: Congener of cisapride
Same gastrokinetic and LES tonic action due to 5-HT$_4$ agonistic and 5-HT$_3$ antagonistic action in myenteric plexus. ADR due to absent D$_2$ blockade and uses similar to cisapride.

Domperidone: Chemically related to **haloperidol** but pharmacologically related to **metoclopramide**.
  Mech: 1. D$_2$ blocker
  2. Acts on CTZ
  3. Lower antiemetic and prokinetic actions are present.
PK: Crosses **BBB poorly,** absorbed **orally,** bioavailability—15% due to first pass metabolism, completely **biotransformed, renal** excretion, plasma t½—7.5 hrs.
  ADR: 1. Hyperprolactinemia and galactorrhoea
  2. Dry mouth   3. Diarrhoea
  4. Cardiac arrhythmia   5. Rashes and headache
  IA: Interacts with **levodopa/bromocriptine.**
  U: 1. **Similar** to metoclopramide **except** with high emetogenic chemotherapy. It has lower antiemetic efficacy.
  2. **Parkinsonism: Antiemetic of choice** with levodopa.

Ondansetron: Effective in **60–80% cases.**
Mech
  1. **5-HT$_3$ blocker**
  2. Inhibits depolarising action of 5-HT$_3$ R on **vagal afferents** in GIT and CTZ plus NTS. Centrally acting antiemetic.
  3. Inhibits emetogenic impulses both **peripherally** and **centrally.**
PK: Oral bioavailability → 60–70%, **hydroxylated by (CYP1A2, 2D6, 3A),** metabolites excreted in **urine** and **faeces,** duration of action → 4–12 hrs, t½—3–5 hrs.
  Dose: 8 mg oral/IV
  ADR: Well tolerated
  1. Headache
  2. Constipation
  3. Diarrhoea
  4. Abdominal discomfort

> You will not vomit so you can go **ON-DANC**ing

U
  1. **DOC** preoperatively
  2. Postoperative nausea and vomiting **(adjuvant drugs** used for optimum benefit are dexamethasone, promethazine or diazepam).
  3. **Cancer chemotherapy/radiotherapy induced vomiting.**
  Mech: Cellular damage by drugs/radiation
                        ↓
        5-HT release from intestinal mucosa
                        ↓
          Stimulation of vagal afferent of GIT
                        ↓
      NTS and CTZ activation by emetogenic impulses
Granisetron is **10 times** more potent than ondansetron, but has **same ADR** profile.

Carminative: Promotes **expulsion of gases** from GIT leading to warmth and comfort in epigastrium.

Classification

1. $NaHCO_3$—**1 gm** (range 0.6–1.5 gm).
2. Tincture ginger
3. Tincture cardamom CO. } 1 ml
4. Oil of dil
5. Oil of peppermint } 0.1 ml → 0.1 = Oil

Condiments and spices: Contain volatile oil.

Mech: Relax LES and enhance GIT motility due to irritation action and flavour → feeling of warmth and comfort in abdomen.

U:
1. **Flatulent dyspepsia**
2. **Milk regurgitation** in infant is inhibited.

Bitters: Promote **gastric secretion** causing **increase appetite.** Used in dyspepsia before meal.

Classification

A. **Simple bitters:**
1. Chirata
2. Ethyl alcohol
3. Picrorhiza
4. Tincture gentian

B. **Aromatic bitter:** Orange peal (as tincture aurantil 2–4 ml).

Digestant: Promotes **food digestion,** and is used in **pancreatic insufficiency.**

Classification

1. HCl (used in **achlorhydria**) 10 ml of 10% HCl in 200 ml H_2O.
2. Pepsin used in **gastric achylia.**
3. Papain used in **row papaya.**
4. Pancreatin
5. **Diastase** and **takadiastase** (amylolytic enzyme of *Aspergillus oryzae*).

Pancreatin

Pancreatin is pancreatic enzyme of hog and **pig pancreas** and contains **amylase, lipase** and **trypsin.**

U:
1. **Chronic pancreatitis:** Reduces pancreatic duct pressure and pain.
2. **Diarrhoea and steatorrhoea:** Reduces fat and nitrogen of stools.

It is **enetric coated** as pepsin of stomach digests it.

Methyl polysiloxane (dimethyl polysiloxane or dimethicone/simethicone): It is **silicon polymer—a viscous amphiphilic liquid.**

Mech: Reduces **surface tension** and collapses **froth antifoaming agents.** Collapse froth, water repellant.

PK: Pharmacologically **inert,** not absorbed from GIT.

U:
1. Flatulence (antifoaming property).
2. Ulcer surface protection (coats ulcer to protect from HCl).
3. Gastroesophageal reflux.
4. Antacid dispersion in gastric content.

Gallstone dissolving drugs (ursodiol and chenodiol): Bile salts (salts of **cholic** acid and **chenodeoxycholic** acid conjugated with **glycine** and **taurine**) dissolve **CH** (cholesterol) because of its amphiphilic action. Increase CH/bile salt ratio crytallises CH in bile →crystal acts as **"nidi"** for stone formation. **Chenodiol** (chenodeoxycholic acid) and **ursodiol** (ursodeoxycholic acid) reduce CH level of bile due to CH solubilization from stone surface. Ursodiol is **hydroxy epimer** of chenodiol.

Mech
A. **Ursodiol**
  1. Reduces **CH secretion** and **CH saturation index** of bile.
  2. Inhibits intestinal **CH absorption.**
  3. Promotes **solubilization** by liquid crystal formation.

B. **Chenodiol**
  1. **HMG–CoA reductase inhibitor** (inhibits CH synthesis in liver).
  2. Reduces **LDL R** in liver (plasma LDL-CH level is enhanced).
  3. Reduces **CH secretion** in bile.
  4. Promotes micellar **solubilization** of CH.
  5. Generates **litholytic bile acid pool.**

> **Stone**
> Types: Cholesterol stone, mixed stone and pigmented stone.
> **Risk factors for stone**   **5 Fs**
>   Female, Fat, Forty, Fertile, Flatulent.

ADR
A. **Ursodiol:** Not significant
B. **Chenodiol:** Diarrhoea and ulceration (of both gastric and esophageal mucosa).
U: Dose = Ursodiol 7–10 mg/kg/day
           = Chenodiol 10–15 mg/kg/day

Efficacy is enhanced by single daily bedtime dose and low CH diet

A. **Ursodiol**
  1. Complete dissolution of CH stone in **50% patients.**
  2. **Bile salt** and **acid** are also used as **replacement therapy** in cholestasis, biliary fistula and liver disease.
B. **Chenodiol:** Partial/complete dissolution of **cholesterol gallstone in 40%** over ½—2 yrs

CI: Pregnancy

Limitations
1. Stone >15 mm in diameter is not dissoluted by the drugs.
2. Functional gallbladder with stone dissolves the stone as bile entry is needed for dissolution.

> **Motilin** acts on **motilin R** of myenteric plexus neurones of gastric **antrum** and **duodenum** to enhance **ACh release. Erythromycin** is **motilin R agonist.**

For quick dissolution: Direct instillation of **liquid ether, methyl terbutylether** into gallbladder through percutaneous pigtail catheter. **Recurrence** after drug discontinuation due to supersaturation is common.

46. Drugs for Constipation and Diarrhoea

With vomiting both pH and food come up.
With diarrhoea both pH and food go down.

Number of peristaltic waves produced in
  A. Stomach   —   3 waves/min
  B. Duodenum   —   10 waves/min

Gastric acid secretion is **maximum** with:
  Protein diet.   **PG**
  Parietal cell produces HCl and Intrinsic factor of castle. **HIP**
  Chief cells produces **pepsinogen**. H^+, K^+-ATPase leads to H^+ **ion secretion**.
  Brunner's gland is related to Alkaline Duodenal Exocrine secretion.

BEAD

Gastrin is **the most potent stimulant for gastric acid secretion**.
Chronic duodenal ulcer causes normal/hyposecretion of acid.
Stress ulcers are 1. Curling's ulcer (Burns)
                     2. Cushing's ulcer (head injury)

Commonest cause of upper GI bleeding is peptic ulcer. **Commonest cause of death** in peptic ulcer is bleeding. **Mucoprotective PG** is PGE_2 and I_2. PG I and E Inhibit Erosin.

Laxatives (Purgatives/Cathartics/Aperients): Promote **evacuation** of bowels. **Laxative/Aperient:** Milder action (elimination of soft but formed stool). **Purgatives/cathartic: Stronger** action (means increase fluid evacuation).
  Drugs in: = Low dose act as Laxative.
              = High dose act as Purgative

Classification
  1. **Stool softener**   — DOSS (docusates)
  2. **Lubricant**   — Liquid paraffin
  3. **Osmotic purgative** — $MgSO_4$
                             $Mg(OH)_2$
                             Na_2SO_4
                             Na_3PO_4

                                   Sod pot tartrate
                                   Lactulose
4. **Bulk forming**   — Dietary fibre (bran)
                                   Ispaghula
                                   Methyl cellulose
                                   Psyllium/Plantago
5. **Stimulant (contact) purgatives**
   A. **Castor oil**
   B. **Diphenyl methane:** Bisacodyl, Phenolphthalein.
   C. **Anthraquinones/Emodins:** Senna, Caseara.

Mech. of all purgatives: All **purgatives** enhance **water** content of faeces by:
   A. Acting on intestinal mucosa to decrease net absorption of water and electrolyte.
   B. Increasing **propulsive** action **(primary action)** allowing **less time** for salt and water absorption **(secondary effects)**.
   C. **Hydrophilic/osmotic action** retaining water and electrolytes in intestinal lumen.

Mech. of laxatives: Laxatives accumulate fluids in gut lumen by:
   A. Inhibiting **Na^+, K^+-ATPase** of villous cells (impairing water and electrolyte absorption).
   B. Increasing **PG synthesis** in mucosa →increase secretion.
   C. Stimulating **adenylyl cyclase** in crypt cells → increasing water and electrolyte secretion.
   D. **Structural injury** to absorbing intestinal mucosal cell.

Bran

Bran is **byproduct of flour industry** (40% dietary fibre). Dietary fibres consist of **unabsorbable cell wall and polysaccharides** (pectin, cellulose and glycoprotein).

Mech: 1. Absorbs **water** in intestines.
       2. Supports **bacterial** growth in colon.
       3. Some dietary fibres (gums, lignin, pectins) bind **bile acids** and promote their excretion in faeces (CH degradation in liver is enhanced). Hence plasma **LDL-CH** is reduced.
       4. Reduces **rectosigmoid intraluminal pressure** (relieves irritable bowel disease and colonic diverticulosis).

CI: Gut ulceration   **GAS**
       Adhesion
       Stenosis

U: Functional constipation (increased intake of dietary fibre is **the most approriate method** for prevention and treatment)—**DOC for most patient.**

Dose: 20–40 gm/day for 4 days.

Ispaghula and plantago/psyllium
- **Mech:** Contain **natural colloidal mucilage** → forms gelatinous mass by absorbing water.
- **U:** **3–12 gm husk** mixed with water/milk per day for **1–3 days**.
- **Precaution:** No dry use due to esophageal impaction.

Methyl cellulose and carboxy methyl cellulose: These are **semisynthetic, colloidal** and **hydrophilic** derivatives of **cellulose**.
- **Dose:** 5 gm/day in most individual.
- **DOSS:** It is **anionic detergent**.
- **Mech:** Softens stools by net water accumulation in intestinal lumen by action on intestinal **mucosa. Emulsifies** colonic contents. Disrupts **mucosal barrier** and enhances drug **absorption**.
- **ADR:**
  1. Cramps and abdominal pain.
  2. Bitter
  3. Hepatotoxicity

Liquid paraffin
Liquid paraffin is **viscous liquid** (mixture of **petroleum hydrocarbon**) and pharmacologically **inert**.
- **Mech:** Softens stools.
- **Disadvantages**
  1. Unpleasant to swallow.
  2. Lipid pneumonia.
  3. Carries away **fat soluble vitamin**.
  4. Passes into intestinal mucosa → lymph → **foreign body granulomas** in intestinal submucosa, spleen, liver and mesenteric lymph node.

Stimulant purgatives
- **Mech:**
  1. They produce **griping and irritate intestinal mucosa** but stimulate motor activity. They enhance **motility** by acting on **myenteric plexuses. Accumulate water and electrolyte in lumen.**
  2. Inhibit **Na$^+$, K$^+$-ATPase** at basolateral membrane of villous cells → transport of Na$^+$ and water into interstitium is reduced. **Secretion** is enhanced by **cAMP** stimulation in crypt cells and by **PG** synthesis.
- **ADR:**
  1. Colonic atony
  2. Hypokalemia
- **CI:**
  1. Pregnancy
  2. Subacute/chronic intestinal obstruction

Phenolphthalein
Phenolphthalein is **indicator and purgative** and turns **alkaline urine to pink**.
- **PK:** Partly absorbed and re-excreted in bile (**enterohepatic circulation**).
- **ADR:**
  1. **Leaky mucosa.**
  2. **Fluid evacuation** and cramps.
  3. **Irritable bowel syndrome** on prolonged use.
  4. **Allergic** reaction (rashes, eruption, S-J syndrome).

Bisacodyl
- **Mech:** Irritates oral and rectal mucosa → reflux enhances motility → evacuation occurs in 30 min.
- **PK:** Activation by **deacetylation** in the intestine (colon).
- **ADR:** Inflammation and mucosal damage.

Anthraquinones: Senna **(the most popularly used)** is leaves and pod of Cassia and Cascara is powdered bark of buck-thorn tree. They contain **emodins** (Anthraquinone glycoside).
- **Mech:**
  1. **Unabsorbed** in small intestine, they are passed to colon where **bacteria** liberate **active anthrol form.**
  2. Act locally or may be absorbed in circulation (purgative action and uses are **similar to diphenylmethane**).
  3. Anthrol enhances **peristalsis** and reduces **segmentation.**
  4. Inhibit salt and water absorption in colon.
- **PK:** Excreted in **bile.** After getting secreted into milk, they cause **purgation** in suckling infant.
- **ADR:**
  1. Cramps
  2. Colonic Atony   **CREAM**
  3. Melanosis
  4. Rashes
  5. Eruption

Castor oil is **the oldest** purgative, is bland vegetable oil of **Ricinus communis** seeds and contains **triglyceride of ricinoleic acid** (a polar long chain FA).
- **Mech:**
  1. Hydrolysed in ileum by **lipase** to ricinoleic acid and glycerol. **Nerve ending irritation** enhances peristaltic contraction. **Ricinoleic acid** irritates mucosa and stimulates intestinal **contraction.**
  2. Reduces intestinal **absorption** of water and electrolyte and enhances **secretion** by detergent like action on mucosa.
- **ADR:**
  1. **Irritable bowel syndrome** on prolonged use.
  2. Enhanced **peristalsis.**
  3. **Structural damage** to villous tips.

Osmotic purgatives: Mg^{2+} releases **CCK.** All organic **salts** used as purgative have **similar** action. Salts are:
  1. $MgSO_4$ (epsom salt)
  2. $Mg(OH)_2$ called milk of magnesia (used as antacid)
  3. Na_2SO_4 (Glauber's salt)
  4. Na_3PO_4
  5. Sod pot tartrate
- **CI:**
  1. Renal insufficiency (**Mg salt**)
  2. CHF patient (**sodium salt**)
- **U:**
  1. Preparation of bowel before surgery and colonoscopy.
  2. Food/drug **poisoning**
  3. **As afterpurge** in treatment of tapeworm infestation.

Lactulose
Lactulose is **semisynthetic disaccharide (fructose + lactose).**

Mech: Retains **water**. Broken down by bacteria in colon to more active product.
ADR: 1. Flatulence and cramps.
2. Colonic bacteria convert **NH_3** into **NH_4^+ salt** (non-absorbable) → blood NH_3 level and pH of stool are reduced.
U: Hepatic coma. Other drugs used to reduce blood NH_3 in hepatic coma are **sod. benzoate and sod. phenylacetate**.
Na benzoate + NH_3 → hippuric acid → **urine**.
Na phenylacetate + NH_3 → phenylacetic glutamine → **urine**.

CI of all laxatives

1. Undiagnosed abdominal pain, colic/vomiting.
2. **Organic constipation** due to stricture or obstruction in bowel, hypothyroidism, hypercalcaemia, malignancy, drugs (opiates, sedatives, CCB, clonidine, Fe, TCA, antihistaminic, anticholinergic and antiparkinsonism).

Danger of purgative abuse

1. Rupture of inflamed appendix
2. Hypokalemia
3. Steatorrhoea
4. Malabsorption syndrome
5. Spastic colitis
6. Protein losing enteropathy

Uses of purgatives

1. **Functional constipation:** Inadequate fibre, lack of exercise, sedentary life and irregular bowel habit cause a **symptom** called constipation. They are **2 types:**
   A. **Spactic constipation** (irritable bowel).
      Bulk forming agent – **DOC**.
      Osmotic agent – **contraindicated**.
   B. **Atonic constipation:** (Sluggish bowel) due to **old age**, etc. Treated by exercise, etc.
2. **Bedridden patient** (MI, stroke, fracture, postoperative).
3. **To avoid straining at stools** (hernia, CVS disease, eye surgery, piles and fissure).
4. **Bowel preparation:** For surgery, colonoscopy and abdominal X-rays.
5. **After anthelmintics**
6. **Food/drug poisoning**

Treatment of diarrhoea: >5 million (>1 million in India) per year children **under age of 5 years** die of diarrhoea. Antidiarrhoeal drugs reduce loss of fluid and electrolytes that occur with diarrhoea. These drugs should not be used to treat diarrhoea that is caused by **poison/infection/chronic/ulcerative colitis. Water and electrolyte** are passively absorbed secondary to nutrient (glucose, amino acid) absorption. **Active Na^+, K^+-ATPase** mediated salt absorption occurs in ileum and colon, mainly in villous cells, water follows iso-osmotically. **Glucose facilitated Na^+ absorption** occurs in ileum. **One Na^+ ion** is transported along with **each molecule of glucose absorbed** (this mechanism is intact even in severe diarrhoea).

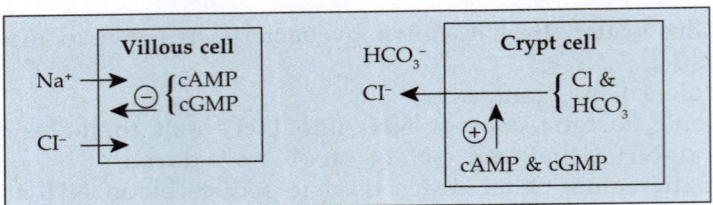

HCO_3^- and Cl^- absorption is passive **(paracellular)** and by exchange of HCO_3^- for Cl^- **(transcellular)**, HCO_3^- is absorbed by H^+ **secretion (similar** to that in PT of kidney) and Na^+ accompanies it. K^+ is excreted in faecal water, by exchange with Na^+ and by secretion into mucus and in **desquamated cells.** Na^+, K^+-ATPase **inhibition and structural damage to mucosal cell by Rotavirus** cause diarrhoea by reducing absorption. Stimuli enhances **cAMP and cGMP** causing net loss of salt water. Cholera toxin, ETEC exotoxin, *S. aureus* and *Salmonella* stimulate Adenyl Cyclase **ACCESS** →Enhances secretion (peak in 24 hrs) and persists until stimulated cells shed in normal turnover, i.e. 36 hrs after single exposure. **PG and intracellular Ca^{2+}** stimulate secretory process. **All acute enteric infections** produce secretory diarrhoea. **Heat stable toxin (ST) of ETEC,** *C. difficile* and *E. histolytica* cause **cGMP** accumulation which stimulates anion secretion and inhibits Na^+ absorption. Diarrhoea associated with **carcinoid** (secreting 5-HT) and **medullary CA of thyroid** (secreting calcitonin) is mediated by **cAMP. Bile acids** cause diarrhoea by stimulating **adenyl cyclase.**

Therapeutic treatment of diarrhoea: Most diarrhoeas are **self-limiting.**

Therapeutic measures are

   A. Treatment of **fluid depletion, shock** and **acidosis.**
   B. **Nutrition** maintenance.
   C. **Drug** therapy.

Rehydration (orally/IV) is needed in **most diarrhoeas. IVF (infusion over 2–4 hrs)** is indicated in:
   A. >10% body weight loss.
   B. >10 ml /kg/hour loss.

Composition of IVF (Dhaka fluid)

NaCl	— 5 gm	= 85 mM		
KCl	— 1 gm	= 13 mM	in 1 L of H_2O/5% glucose solution.	
$NaHCO_3$	— 4 gm	= 48 mM		
This gives	— Na^+	= 133 mM	+	→13
	— K^+	= 13 mM	–	→8
	— Cl^-	= 98 mM		
	— HCO_3^-	= 48 mM		

Alternatively (IVF)

Ringer lactase recommended by WHO–1991 gives

   Na^+ = 130 mM
   K^+ = 4 mM
   Cl^- = 109 mM
   Lactate = 28 mM

Drugs for Constipation and Diarrhoea

ORT (oral rehydration therapy)
- Mild = 5–7.5% fluid loss of body weight.
- Moderate = 7.5–10% fluid loss of body weight.
- Severe = >10% fluid loss of body weight.

Excess glucose facilitates Na$^+$ absorption.

Principles of ORS (oral rehydration salt/solution)
1. Should be **isotonic.**
2. **Molar ratio of glucose/Na$^+$ should be higher.**
3. **K$^+$ and HCO$_3^-$ provided,** make up the losses.

Universal formula of WHO (ORS)

NaCl	=	3.5 gm
Citrate	=	2.9 gm
KCl	=	1.5 gm
Glucose	=	20 gm

in 1 L of water.

This gives:
- Na$^+$ = 90 mM
- K$^+$ = 20 mM
- Cl$^-$ = 80 mM
- Citrate = 30 mM
- Glucose = 110 mM

ORS recommended by WHO causes **periorbital edema** due to **excess Na$^+$ absorption.**

Electrolyte composition of diarrhoea

Diarrhoeas	Na$^+$	Cl$^-$	K$^+$	HCO$_3^-$
Cholera (adult)	140	104	13	44
Cholera (infant, children)	88	86	30	32
ETEC	53	24	37	18
Rotavirus	37	22	38	06

Maximum water absorption occurs in **slight hypotonic** solution and in **glucose** concentration between **80 and 140 mM. Stool volume** is enhanced if its concentration is higher. **K$^+$ loss** is substantial in **most diarrhoea.** The base(HCO$_3^-$, citrate, lactate) corrects **acidosis** due to alkaline loss in stools. **ORS** is given at ½–1 hourly. ORS restores and maintains **hydration, electrolyte** and **pH balance. It is the best approach to IV hydration.** >300 million litre of ORS prevents >0.5 million death annually.

U:
1. **Diarrhoea**
2. **Non-diarrhoeal uses of ORT**
   A. Heat stroke
   B. Postsurgical, postburn, post-trauma.

Super ORS
Function
A. Rehydration
B. Decrease in purging rates
C. Improvement in diarrhoea by enhanced absorption.

Boiled rice powder 40–50 gm/L: It is substitute for **glucose. Rice starch** is slowly hydrolysed at brush border or in lumen into glucose which is absorbed. Rice has **7% protein** → amino acid stimulates salt and water absorption. It reduces stool volume compared to **WHO-ORS** in cholera patient. Rice is **cheap and widely available. Rice, maize, potato, wheat based ORS** appears desirable for developing countries.

Maintenance of nutrition: Diarrhoea patient should not be starved because **fasting** reduces **brush border disaccharidase enzymes, salt, water and nutrients. Feeding** during diarrhoea enhances intestinal digestive enzymes and cell proliferation in mucosa. **Breast milk, ½ strength buffalo milk, boiled potato, rice, chicken soup and banana sago** should be given as soon as possible.

Two categories of diarrhoea patient

A. If diarrhoea is **waterly without mucus and blood having dehydration and vomiting but no fever; causes may be:** Adhesive but noninvasive entrotoxigenic organisms such as cholera, ETEC, Rota and *Salmonella* → stimulate massive secretion by stimulating **cAMP**. Maintenance therapy is **ORS.**

B. If diarrhoea is **slightly loose,** smaller volume with **mucus/blood, dehydration, fever and abdominal pain but no vomiting; causes may be:** Enteroinvasive organisms like *Shigella*, EPEC, *C. jejuni, Salmonella, Yersinia, E. histolytica, C. difficile*. Antimicrobial is needed but no need in noninfective causes (thyrotoxicosis, coeliac disease, irritable bowel syndrome, pancreatic enzyme deficiency, tropical sprue). Diarrhoea caused by **viruses** (Rotavirus, etc.) needs **no chemotherapy.** *Salmonella* **food poisoning** is **self-limiting** but treated patients pass organism in stool for longer period than untreated patient.

1. *Y. entrocolitica*—cotrimoxazole (**the most suitable drug**). Alternative—Tetracycline.
2. Cholera—**tetracycline** (DOC-reduces stool volume to half). Alternative—Cotrimoxazole.
   MDR cholera—ciprofloxacin/norfloxacin.
3. Fluoroquinolones eradicate *C. jejuni* and *C. difficile* and produce pseudomembranous enterocolitis (**DOC—metronidazole).** Alternative—vancomycin.
4. Amoebiasis and giardiasis—metronidazole, furazolidone, diloxanide furoate.

Nonspecific antidiarrhoeal agents

A. **Absorbants:** Ispaghula, psyllium and methylcellulose.
B. **Antisecretory:** Bismuth subsalicylate
   Atropine
   BAMS=O Mesalazine
   Sulfasalazine
   Octreotide
C. **Antimotility:** Diphenoxylate—atropine   **DLC**
   Loperamide
   Codeine.

Sulfasalazine/salicylazosulfapyridine: It is **5-ASA-Azo bond—sulfapyridine.**

> **Sulfasalazine**
> ↓   Colonic bacteria (split azo bond)
> **Sulfapyridine** and **5-ASA (5-Aminosalicylic acid).**

Mech: 1. 5-ASA exerts **local anti-inflammatory** effect by inhibiting PG, LT and PAF synthesis and reduces **mucosal secretion, number of stools, fever** and **abdominal cramps (corticosteroid** is better than sulfasalazine in acute exacerbation).
2. **Sulfapyridine** carries **5-ASA** to colon without being absorbed proximally.

ADR: It is due to **sulfapyridine** absorbed in colon:
1. Haemolysis, blood dyscrasias and **anemia.**
2. Nausea, vomiting, headache, fever
3. **Rashes** (4) Joint pain (5) **Male infertility.**

U: Ulcerative colitis **(DOC).**

Mesalazine/Mesalamine: It is the **official name of 5-ASA.** It is absorbed in small intestine and does not reach large bowel. It is **coated by acrylic polymer,** so that 5-ASA should be delivered to distal small bowel and colon. **1 gm** sulfasalazine gives **400 mg** mesalazine.

ADR: 1. Abdominal pain and diarrhoea.
2. Headache and nausea.

CI: **Renal** and **hepatic** inpairment.

IA: Enhances gastric toxicity of **glucocorticoid** and hypoglycaemic action of **sulfonylurea.**

Olsalazine

Olsalazine consists of **2 molecules of 5-ASA** coupled together by **azo bond** and is **the most reliable** preparation for delivery of 5-ASA to colon.

Balsalazine is **5-ASA** linked to **4-aminobenzoyl beta alanine** as the carrier.

Octreotide

Octreotide is **somatostatin** analogue (synthetic peptide).

Mech: **Antisecretory** and **antimotility** action on gut.
PK: Plasma t½—90 min. Route — S.C. injection.
U: 1. **Diarrhoea** in carcinoid and VIP secreting tumour.
2. **Refractory diarrhoea** in AIDS.
3. **A**cromegaly, **B**leeding peptic ulcer, **C**arcinoid metastasis, **D**iabetic ketoacidosis, **E**sophageal varices, **F**istulae (pancreatic, biliary, intestinal).   **ABCDEF**

Uses of antisecretory drugs: Ulcerative colitis, traveller's diarrhoea, diarrhoea in AIDS, diarrhoea in carciniod and VIP secreting tumour, drug induced diarrhoea.

> **Opioids:** These have **antimotility** and **antisecretory** action. Enhance small bowel **tone, absorption** and **segmenting activity.** Reduce **propulsive**

movements and intestinal **secretion**. Act on **μ-receptor** of enteric neuronal network (also act on **δ-opioid R**). Enhance resistance to luminal transit and allow **more time** for absorptive processes.

Diphenoxylate—atropine: It is opioid related to **pethidine** and is **constipating** agent.
- **Mech:** Same as codeine. **The most prominent action—anti-diarrhoeal.**
- **PK:** Absorbed **systemically. Crosses BBB.**
- **ADR:** 1. Atropine discourages abuse. **Diphenoxylate (2.5 mg)—atropine (0.025 mg).**
    2. Respiratory depression.
    3. Paralytic ileus.
- **CI:** <6 yrs due to **toxic megacolon.**
- **U:** Diarrhoea.

Loperamide

Loperamide is opiate analogue.
- **Mech:** 1. **Weak anticholinergic** property. Inhibits secretion.
    2. Interacts with **calmodulin** (antidiarrhoeal action).
    3. Improves **faecal continence** by increasing anal sphincter tone.
    4. **The most suitable antimotility drug.**
- **ADR:** 1. Abdominal cramps and rashes (**the most common).**
    2. **Paralytic ileus** and **toxic megacolon** with abdominal distension (serious complication in young children).
- **CI:** 1. **Chidren <4 yrs.**
    2. **CI of antimotility drugs**
        A. Acute **infective** diarrhoea (because they delay clearance of pathogen from intestine).
        B. Diverticulosis, ulcerative colitis and irritable bowel syndrome enhance intraluminal pressure.
- **Dose:** 10 mg (**max**)/day.

Uses of antimotility drugs

1. Traveller's diarrhoea.
2. Idiopathic diarrhoea in AIDS.
3. Non-infective diarrhoea.
4. After anal surgery, colostomy, etc. to induce short-term constipation.

Unit 9
Respiratory System

47. Drugs for Respiratory System

Cough is a **symptom** and **protective reflex for expulsion** of secretion/foreign body from air passages and occurs due to **stimulation of mechanoreceptors and chemoreceptors in throat, respiratory passages/stretch receptors in lungs.**

Cough is A. **Useful (productive)** → drains the airway. Should not be suppressed.

B. **Useless (nonproductive)** → should be suppressed. Drains no airway.

Classification
1. **Mucokinetic (expectorant)**
    - A. **Directly acting:** Na/K citrate/acetate, KI, guaiacol, guaiphenesin (glyceryl guaiacolate), balsum of tolu, vasaka, terpin hydrate.
    - B. **Reflexly acting:** KI, NH_4Cl, $(NH_4)_2CO_3$, Ipecac (ipecacuanha).
    - C. **Mucolytics:** **A**cetyl cysteine, **A**mbroxol, **B**romhexine and **C**arbocisteine. **ABC**

2. **Antitussives (cough centre suppressant)**
    - A. **Opioid:** Codeine, pholcodine, morphine and ethyl-morphine.
    - B. **Nonopioid:** **P**ipazethate
        Oxeladin   **POND**
        Noscapine
        Dextromethorphan, carbetapentane, chlophedianol.
    - C. **Antihistaminics:** Chlorpheniramine, diphenhydramine, promethazine.

3. **Pharyngeal demulcents:** Lozenges, linctuses, liquorice, glycerine.
4. **Antibiotics.**

Pharyngeal demulcents
Pharyngeal demulcents sooth the throat directly and by promoting salivation and **reduce afferent impulses** from irritated/inflamed pharyngeal mucosa.

Mucokinetics

Mucokinetics enhance bronchial **secretion** and reduce its **viscosity** facilitating its removal (**cough is lost**).

- **Na and K citrate/acetate:** It enhances bronchial secretion by salt action.
- **KI:** It is secreted by **bronchial gland,** enhances volume of secretion and is gastric irritant.
- **ADR:** Goitre and hypothyroidism on chronic use.

Guaiacol
- **Mech:** Enhances **bronchial secretion** and **mucosal ciliary action.** After absorption from gut, it is secreted by **tracheobronchial gland.**
- **ADR:** Gastric upset.

Tolu balsum, vasaka, terpin hydrate act in the same way.
Ammonium salt and **syrup ipecac:** Gastric irritant.
- **ADR:** Reflexly enhance sweating and bronchial secretion.

Bromhexine

Bromhexine is derivative of **alkaloid varicine** of Adhatoda vasica (vasaka) and is **mucokinetic + mucolytic.**
- **Mech:** **Depolymerises** mucopolysaccharides directly and by lysosomal enzyme.
- **ADR:** 1. Lacrimation, and
  2. Rhinorrhoea
- **U:** **Removal of** mucus plug.

Ambroxol: Metabolite of bromhexine with actions, uses and ADR similar to it.

Acetyl cysteine

Acetyl cysteine is a **mucolytic** agent breaking the network of fibres in tenacious sputum.
- **Mech:** Opens **disulfide bonds** in mucoproteins of sputum.
- **U:** As cough elixir.

Carbocisteine

- **Mech:** **Same** as acetyl cysteine.
- **ADR:** 1. Rashes
  2. GI irritation
- **U:** Combined with **amoxicillin/cephalexin**
  1. Bronchitis
  2. Bronchiectasis
  3. Sinusitis

Antitussives

Antitussives act in CNS to **raise threshold of cough centre**. Also act peripherally in respiratory tract to reduce **tussal impulses.**
- **Codeine:** **Less potent** than morphine.
- **Mech:** 1. Suppresses cough for 6 hrs.
  2. **Naloxone** blocks its antitussive action, i.e. it acts through **opioid receptor** in brain.

ADR: 1. Constipation
2. Respiratory depression
3. Drowsiness
CI: 1. Asthma
2. Diminished respiratory reserve.

Ethylmorphine and **pholcodine** are **similar** to codeine in efficacy.

Narcotine

Narcotine (noscapine) is **opium alkaloid of benzoisoquinoline series. Equipotent** antitussive as codeine
Mech: Releases histamine leading to **bronchoconstriction in asthma.**
ADR: Nausea and headache
U: As cough elixir

Dextromethorphan

Dextromethorphan is **synthetic** compound. Its 2 forms are **l-isomer** for analgesic action and **d-isomer** for antitussive action (enhances threshold of cough centre).
ADR: Dizziness and nausea.

Carbetapentane is **non-opioid synthetic antitussive with local anaesthetic** and **anticholinergic actions.**

Oxeladin is **synthetic centrally** acting antitussive.

Chlophedianol is **similar** to oxeladin.
ADR: 1. Vertigo
2. Irritability
3. Dryness of mouth.

H_1 **antihistaminics** afford relief in cough due to their **sedative** and **anticholinergic** actions.

DRUGS FOR ASTHMA

1. **Bronchodilators**
   A. **Anticholinergic**
   B. **Sympathomimetics:** Adrenaline, ephedrine, isoprenaline, orciprenaline, terbutaline, salbutamol and salmeterol, bambuterol, formoterol.
   C. **Methylxanthine:** Theophylline, aminophylline, theophylline ethanolate, choline theophylline and hydroxyethyl theophylline.
2. **Corticosteroids**
   A. **Systemic**—prednisolone.
   B. **Inhalational:** Beclomethasone dipropionate, budesonide, flunisolide, fluticasone propionate, triamcinolone acetomide.
3. **Mast cell stabilisers:** Ketotifen, nedocromil, Sod. cromoglycate.
4. **Anti-LT (anti-LUKotrienes):** Zileuton (Inhibits LOX **hence** no LT formation).
   Zafir**LUK**ast (Inhibits LT R).
   Monte**LUK**ast and cina**LUK**ast.

Bambuterol: Biscarbamate ester prodrug of terbutaline.
Mech: Hydrolysed in plasma and lungs by pseudo-ChE to release active drug in 24 hours.
U: Chronic bronchial asthma 20 mg OD.

Formoterol: Bronchodilator.
Mech: Selective β_2 agonists.
PK: Long-acting (12 hours) but faster onset of action (10 minutes). Inhaled 20 µg BD.
U: For rapid bronchodilation.

Methylxanthenes

Methylxanthenes are **methylated xanthene alkaloids,** consumed as **beverages.**

Drugs are:
1. Theophylline
2. Theobromine
3. Caffeine

All 3 alkaloids have qualitatively **similar** action.

Action:
1. **Stimulant** at **low** dose and **toxic** at **high** dose in CNS. **Caffeine** produces a sense of **well-being, alertness** and **beats boredom, allays fatigue, clears thinking, improves performance** and **enhances motor activity.**
   Order of action: Caffeine > Theophylline > Theobromine.
   They stimulate **respiratory, vasomotor** and **medullary vagal centres. At high doses,** they cause nervousness, restlessness, pain, insomnia, excitement, tremor, convulsion, etc.
   Vomiting is due to CTZ stimulation and gastric irritation. Only caffeine is used as **CNS stimulant** and is more effective on it (but **theophylline** and **theobromine** act on **peripheral sites).**
2. Stimulant effect on **heart rate:** Increase **force** of contraction. Increase **heart rate** by **direct** action. Decrease **heart rate** by **vagal** stimulation.
3. **Vasodilatation. Caffiene** is used in migraine because it **constricts** cranial vessel. **Variable BP (increase systolic** and **decrease diastolic BP). HTN** is due to **vasomotor** centre and **direct** heart stimulation. **Hypotension** is due to **vagal** stimulation and **direct** vasodilatation.
4. **All smooth muscles** are relaxed **(most prominent effects** are exerted on bronchi specially in asthma due to release of **adrenergic transmitter** and direct action).
5. **Mild diuresis** by inhibiting tubular reabsorption of Na^+ and water and by increasing GFR and renal blood flow.
6. Enhance **contractile power of smooth muscle.** Increased Ca^+ **release** from sarcoplasmic reticulum by direct action. Increased **ACh release** relieves fatigue and enhances muscular work.
7. Enhance **acid** and **pepsin secretion** in stomach.
8. Inhibit **mediator release** from mast cells.
9. Enhance **BMR** → Increased plasma FFA.

> **Functions of methylxanthenes**
> 1. CNS and myocardial stimulation
> 2. Bronchodilation
> 3. Diuresis
> 4. Cerebral vessel constriction (reduce headache)

Mech:
1. **Ca²⁺ release** from sarcoplasmic reticulum in skeletal and cardiac muscle.
2. Inhibit **adenosine receptor**. Adenosine **contracts smooth muscle,** dilates cerebral vessels and **inhibits** gastric secretion.

    ATP/GTP
    ↓ Adenyl cyclase/Guanyl cyclase
    Increase cAMP/cGMP (intracellularly).
    ↓ Phosphodiesterase ←(-)
    5-AMP/5-GMP   Theophylline

    Theophylline enhances **adrenaline** induced cAMP accumulation. Increased cAMP causes **vasodilatation, bronchodilation,** and **cardiac stimulation.**
3. Theophylline **dilates** systemic blood vessel.
4. Increase **diaphragmatic contractility** with theophylline at therapeutic concentration contributes the beneficial effects in dyspnoea.

PK:
A. **Caffeine:** <50% bound to plasma protein. **Distributed** all over the body.
Volume of distribution **0.5 L/kg.** Complete hepatic metabolism by demethylation and oxidation. **Renal** excretion. Plasma t½ → 3–6 hrs.

B. **Theophylline:** Well absorbed **orally.** Distributed in **all tissues.** Crosses **placenta** (secreted in **milk**). Volume of distribution— 0.5 L/kg. 50% protein bound. Extensively metabolised in **liver** by oxidation and demethylation. **Smoker** metabolises it faster than nonsmoker. **10%** excreted unchanged in urine. **t½ 7–12 hrs (adults)** at therapeutic concentration and 3–5 hrs **(children).**

AT high doses, **t½ is enhanced to 60 hrs** because kinetics change from **first to zero order** (i.e. theophylline metabolizing enzymes are **saturable** as kinetics change from first order to zero order). Therapeutic rang is **5–20 µg/ml.** Its concentration in blood should be monitored due to its **low therapeutic index.**

Factors which need dose reduction are
1. CHF (× 0.6)
2. Pneumonia (× 0.4)
3. Liver failure (× 0.3)
4. Age >60 yrs (0.6)

ADR: Drugs causing **hyperventilation syndrome** are:
Methylxanthene, salicylate, beta agonist, progesterone.

A. Caffeine
1. Nervousness, insomnia, agitation, delirium, convulsion, tremor.
2. Muscular twitching, rigidity
3. Increased body temperature
4. Tachycardia, palpitation
5. Diuresis
6. **Contraindication**—peptic ulcer

B. **Theophylline**
1. **Orally** → Gastric pain
   IM → Rectal pain
2. Precordial pain
3. Syncope
4. **Sudden death** due to ventricular arrhythmia. Hypotension/asystole.

Toxicity of theophylline: ADR of theophylline occurs in GIT, CVS and CNS (mainly in children).
1. Convulsion, delirium
2. Shock
3. Arrhythmia (CVS worsens), extrasystole and hypotension.
4. Flashes of light seen
5. Flushing, tachyapnoea and agitation
6. Increased muscle tone

IA of theophylline

1. Allopurinol, cimetidine, OC, ciprofloxacin and erythromycin **inhibit** theophylline metabolism and **enhance** its plasma level (dose of theophylline should be reduced by **2/3**).
2. Theophylline **enhances** the effects of furosemide, digitalis, oral anticoagulants, hypoglycaemics and sympathomimetics but **reduces** the effects of Li and phenytoin.
3. Aminophylline should **not be mixed** with ascorbic acid, CPZ, morphine, promethazine, pethidine, phenytoin, penicillin G, insulin, tetracycline, phenobarbitone, erythromycin, but can be given with furosemide only.
4. Agents inducing theophylline metabolism reduce its plasma level and its dose is to be increased by the **factor** (i.e. factors in which theophylline dose is to be increased are): Smoking (1.6), Phenytoin (1.5), rifampin (1.5), phenobarbitone (1.2).

U:
1. In analgesic mixture.
2. **Migraine** (due to cranial vessel constriction): Caffeine.

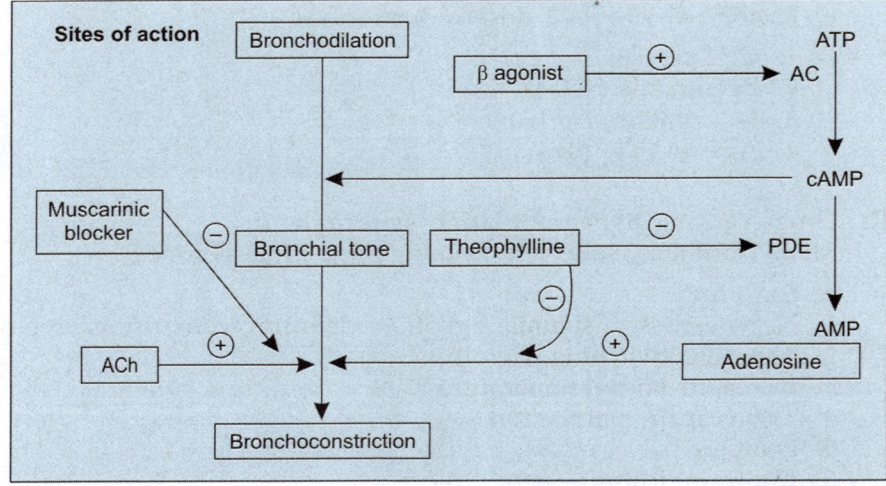

3. To counteract **hypnotic** overdose.
4. **Apnoea** in premature infants.
5. **Bronchial asthma and COPD:** Theophylline causes bronchodilatation, reduces mediator release, improves mucociliary clearance, stimulates respiratory drive and enhances diaphragmatic contractility.
6. Status asthmaticus: Aminophylline (IV).
7. The **second commonest** drug used in asthma—theophylline.

Anti-LT drugs (zafirlukast, montelukast, cinalukast and zileuton): LT is product of 5-lipoxygenase pathway. **5-lipoxygenase is found in cells of myeloid origin** (mast cells, basophil, neutrophil). LT B_4 is chemoattractant to neutrophil and eosinophil.

Mech: **Zileuton** inhibits 5-lipoxygenase selectively. zafirlukast and montelukast selectively and reversibly inhibit **cysteinyl LT-1 receptor.**

PK: All are orally active. >90% plasma protein bound. Extensively metabolised.
Renal excretion—zileuton. **Biliary** excertion—zafirlukast and montelukast.

Oral dose: Zafirlukast   — 40 mg twice daily
Montelukast — 10 mg daily
Zileuton   — 600 mg 4 times daily

ADR:
1. Elevation of serum hepatic enzyme.
2. **Churg-Strauss syndrome** (eosinophilic vasculitis).
3. **Dyspepsia**
4. Zafirlukast and zileuton inhibit **CYP450.** Both enhance serum level of **warfarin.**

U:
1. Prophylaxis of asthma.
2. Reduction of beta agonist and steroid dose.

Sodium cromoglycate

Sodium cromoglycate/cromolyn sodium is **mast cell stabilizer** and **synthetic chromone derivative.**

Mech:
1. Inhibits mast cell **degranulation** → release of mediators of asthma (histamine, LT, IL, PAF).
2. Inhibits **chemotaxis** of inflammatory cells.
3. Reduces Ca^{2+} **influx** during mast cell degranulation.

PK: Excreted unchanged in **urine** and **bile.** Not absorbed **orally** (so given as aerosol through metered dose inhaler delivering **1 mg per dose**→2 puffs 4 times a day).

ADR: Bronchospasm, throat irritation and cough.

U:
1. **Allergic rhinitis** and **allergic conjunctivitis.**
2. **Bronchial asthma:** Specially in atopic (extrinsic) and exercise induced asthma.
3. **Prophylaxis of asthma** (not effective in active attack).

Nidocromil sodium: Similar in action and use to cromoglycate.

Ketotifen

Ketotifen is **orally** active **nonchromone** prophylactic drug and is H_1 **blocker.** It is neither bronchodilator nor anti-inflammatory.

- **Mech:**
  1. H_1 blocker.
  2. Stimulation of **immunogenic** and **inflammatory cells** and **mediator** release are inhibited.
  3. Inhibits **phosphodiesterase.**
  4. Restricts Ca^{2+} entry and blocks LTC_4/LTD_4.
- **PK:** Absorbed **orally.** Bioavailability—**50%** due to first pass metabolism. t½—22 hrs. Dose →1–2 mg BD.
- **ADR:**
  1. Sedation and dizziness.
  2. Dry mouth
  3. Nausea
  4. Weight gain
- **U:**
  1. Bronchial asthma: Reduces respiratory symptoms in **50–70% asthma** after 6–12 weeks.
  2. Produces **symptomatic relief** in atopic dermatitis, rhinitis, conjunctivitis, urticaria and food allergy.

Corticosteroids: Inhibit LT synthesis, reduce bronchial **hyper-irritability, mucosal edema** and **Ag: Ab reaction,** restore responsiveness to resistant **sympathomimetic. Inhalational steroid** (high topical and low systemic activity) reduces bronchial hyperactivity and enhances **PEFR.**

ADR of beclomethasone: Commonest in 30% (dysphonia, sore throat, oropharyngeal candidiasis, hoarseness of voice→treated by nystatin, gargling and Spacer). Beclomethasone is used in severe chronic asthma. **Systemic steroid** is used in severe chronic asthma, status asthmaticus or acute asthma exacerbation in resistant intensive bronchodilator therapy. **ADR of systemic steroid** is ulcer, osteoporosis and adrenal suppression.

Budesonide has high topical: System activity ratio and is better than beclomethasone (indicated in **rhinitis** and **nasal polyposis** but **contraindicated** in infection and nasal ulcer). **Aerosols** are used in solution by metered dose inhaler and nebuliser but used as dry powder by spinhaler and rotahaler.

Bronchial asthma (inflammation with hyper-reactivity): It is **hyper-responsiveness** of tracheobronchial smooth muscle to various stimuli, resulting in narrowing of air tubes, increased secretion, mucosal edema and mucosal plugging. Allergy is only in 10% adult.

- **Two types:**
  - **A. Extrinsic asthma:** Mostly episodic. Less prone to status asthmaticus.
  - **B. Intrinsic asthma:** Perennial. Status asthmaticus is common.

Mast cells of lungs and inflammatory cells produce mediators:
  A. Histamine, TNF-α and protease enzyme from granules (immediate).
  B. Phospholipid release from membrane followed by mediator synthesis within minutes (LT, PG, PAF).
  C. Gene activation followed by protein synthesis within hours (IL, TNF-α).

Drugs for Respiratory System

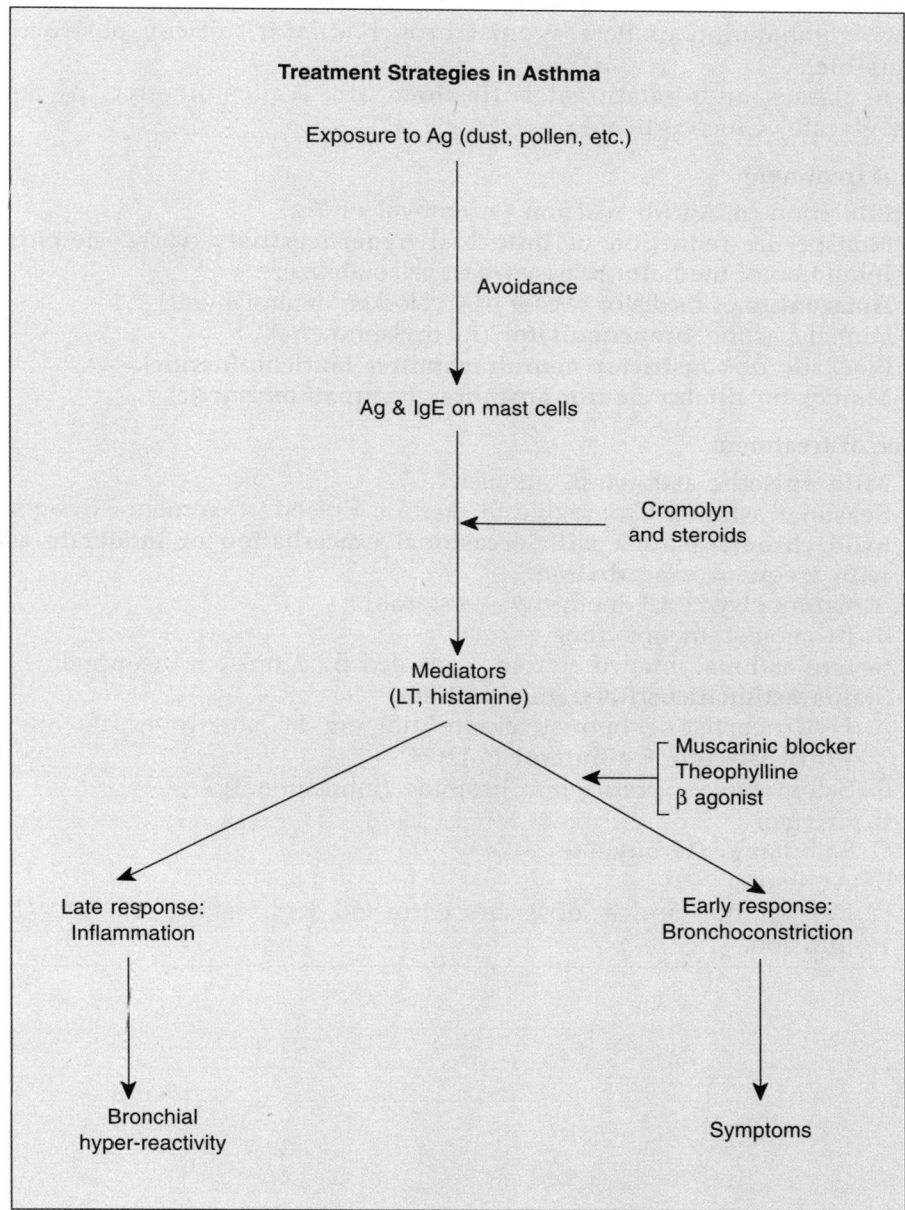

These **mediators** constrict bronchial smooth muscle→mucosal edema, hyperemia and viscid secretion → reversible airway obstruction. **Hyperactivity** is enhanced by bronchial epithelial damage. **Vagal** discharge to bronchial muscle is enhanced **reflexly**.

COPD (a disorder of expiratory air flow limitation) is due to emphysema, chronic bronchitis and peripheral airway disease, and is common in smoker and after 40 yr. Patients derive less than 15% improvement in FEV in 1 Sec (FEV1) following inhalation of beta agonist bronchodilator (airway obstruction is **irreversible**).

Four classes of inhalational antiasthma are: Anticholinergic, β_2 agonist, Cromoglycate, Glucocorticoid.   ABCG

Aim of treatment
1. Inhibition of **Ag:Ab** reaction → removal of Ag.
2. Nonspecific **reduction of bronchial hyper-reactivity** (corticosteroid).
3. Inhibition of **mediator** release (mast cell stabilizer).
4. **Antagonism** of mediator release (PAF blocker, antihistaminic).
5. Directly acting **bronchodilator** (methylxanthene).
6. Blockade of **constrictor neurotransmitter (anticholinergic).**
7. Mimicking **dilator neurotransmitter (sympathomimetic).**

Choice of treatment
1. **Mild episodic asthma:** β_2 agonist.
2. **Seasonal asthma:** Cromoglycate/steroid. Episode treatment—β_2 agonist
3. **Mild chronic asthma with occasional exacerbation or moderate asthma with frequent exacerbation.**
   A. Cromoglycate, if ineffective → steroid.
   B. β_2 agonist/theophylline.
4. **Severe asthma:** Inhaled steroid + inhaled β_2 agonist + theophylline.
5. **Status asthmaticus/Refractory asthma**
   A. Hydrocortisone hemisuccinate 100 mg IV stat then 100 mg TDS. **Corticosteroid + albuterol is DOC.**
   B. Salbutamol + ipratropium bromide (inhalational).
   C. Oxygen
   D. Salbutamol/terbutaline
   E. Antibiotic
   F. Dehydration and acidosis are corrected with saline, $NaHCO_3$/lactate infusion.

Unit 10
Antimicrobial Agents

48
Principles of Chemotherapy

Antimicrobial drugs or agents (AMA) refer to **all natural, synthetic and semisynthetic** substances able to kill/inhibit microorganisms, are the **greatest** contribution of the present century to therapeutics.

Antibiotics are substances produced by microorganisms able to suppress/kill microorganisms at **low** doses/concentrations.

Chemotherapy: It means treatment of systemic infection and malignant cell (the term coined by **Paul Ehrlich**).

Classification
  I. **Based on mechanism of action**
   1. **Cell wall synthesis inhibitors**
      Ristocetin   **RBC, PVC**
      Bacteriocin
      Cephalosporin
      Penicillin
      Vancomycin
      Cyclosporin
   2. **Causing cell membrane leakage**
      A. **Polypeptide** — Polymyxin   **PCB**
                           Cilastatin
                           Bacitracin
      B. **Polyenes** — AMB, nystatin, hamycin
      C. **Imidazole** — Not antibiotic
   3. **Protein synthesis inhibitors**
      30s inhibitors
      Aminoglycoside (bactericidal).
      Tetracycline (bacteriostatic).
      50s inhibitors —
      Chloramphenicol (bacteriostatic)
      Erythromycin (bacteriostatic)   **Buy AT 30 and**
      Lincomycin (bacteriostatic)   **CELLS at 50**
      cLindamycin (bacteriostatic)
      Streptogramins

4. **Interfering with DNA synthesis**
   Zidovudine
   Idoxuridine   ZIA
   Acyclovir
5. **Interfering with DNA function**
   Metronidazole
   Norfloxacin   MNR
   Rifampicin (inhibits DNA dependent RNA polymerase).
6. **DNA gyrase inhibitors:** Quinolone.
7. **Misreading of mRNA code:** Aminoglycoside.
8. **Interfering intermediate metabolism**   PEST
   P = PAS and pyrimethamine
   E = Ethambutol
   S = Sulfone and sulfonamide
   T = Trimethoprim

II. **Based on chemical structures**
   1. **Aminoglycoside:** Streptomycin
   2. **Macrolide:** Erythromycin
   3. **Nitrobenzene:** Chloramphenicol
   4. **Nitrofurans:** Nitrofurantoin

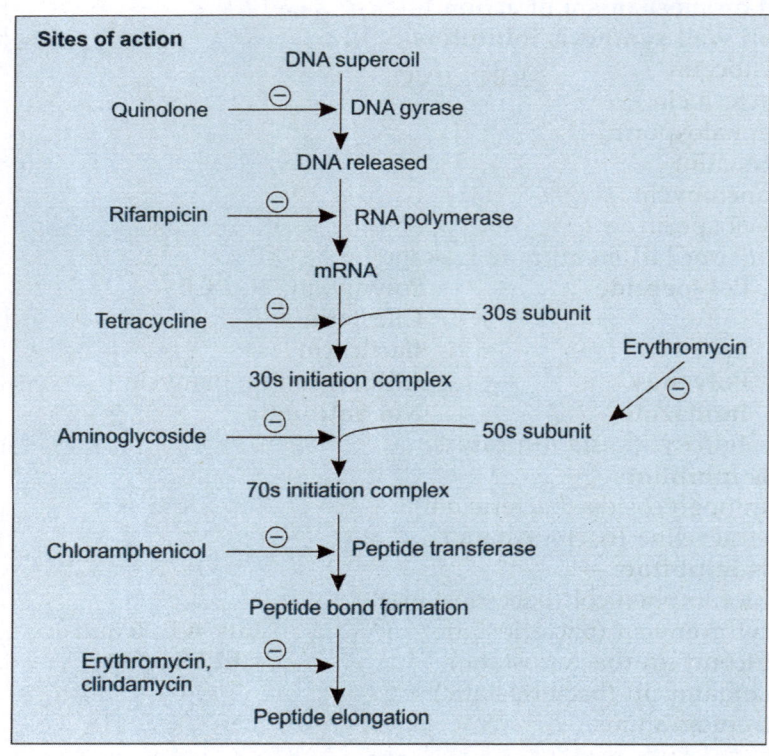

5. **Nitroimidazole:** Metronidazole
6. **Imidazole derivative:** KTZ
7. **Nicotinic acid derivative:** INH, Pyrazinamide
8. **Diaminopyrimidine:** Trimethoprim
9. **Quinolones:** Ciprofloxacin, gatifloxacin
10. **Polypeptides:** Polymyxin B
11. **Tetracycline:** Oxytetracycline
12. **β-lactam antibiotics:** Penicillin
13. **Sulfonamide:** Dapsone, sulfadiazine
14. **Polyene:** AMB
15. **Other:** Rifampicin, clindamycin, vancomycin, ethambutol and griseofulvin.

Antimicrobial therapy

Mechanism of action	Drugs
1. Block cell wall synthesis by inhibition of peptidoglycan cross-linking	Penicillin, cephalosporins, imipenem, aztreonam
2. Block peptidoglycan synthesis	Bacitracin, vancomycin
3. Block protein synthesis at 50s ribosomal subunit	Chloramphenicol, erythromycin/macrolides, lincomycin, clindamycin
4. Block protein synthesis at 30s ribosomal subunit	Aminogylcosides, tetracylines.
5. Block nucleotide synthesis	Sulfonamides, trimethoprim
6. Block DNA topoisomerase	Quinolones
7. Block mRNA synthesis	Rifampin
8. Block bacteria/fungal cell membrane	Polymyxins
9. Disrupt fungal cell membrane	Amphotericin B, nystatin, fluconazole/azoles
10. Unknown	Isoniazid, metronidazole, pentamidine

III. **Based on type of action**
   Bacterostatic   **CL TENSE**
   Chloramphenicol
   Lincomycin
   Tetracycline
   Erythromycin (at low dose)
   Nitrofurans (at low dose)
   Sulfonamide (at low dose)
   Ethambutol

Bactericidal: Penicillin, cephalosporin, ciprofloxacin, vancomycin, polypeptide, aminoglycoside, cotrimoxazole, INH, rifampicin, nalidixic acid.

IV. Spectrum of activity

Broad spectrum:	Tetracycline
	Chloramphenicol
Narrow spectrum:	Penicillin G
	Erythromycin
	Streptomycin
	Cephalosporin

V. Based on source

A. Fungi: Penicillin
  Cephalosporin
  Griseofulvin

B. Actinomycetes   `PACT`
  Polyene
  Aminogylcoside and macrolide.
  Chloramphenicol
  Tetracycline

C. Bacterial   `BACTerial`
  Bacitracin and polymyxin B
  Aztreonam
  Colistin
  Tyrothricin

D. DNA recombinant technology
  Chloramphenicol

ADR due to AMA use   `SHIRT`
  Superinfection
  Hypersensitivity
  Masking of **I**nfection
  Resistance of drug
  Toxicity.

A. Toxicity: All AMAs are irritant and cause systemic toxicity.

1. **Drugs of high therapeutic index** means **more dose without host cell damage**, e.g. penicillin, cephalosporin, erythromycin.
2. **Drugs of low therapeutic index**   `ACT`
   Aminoglycosides—8th CN damage and kidney toxicity.
   Chloramphenicol—bone marrow depression or BMD (granulocytosis **commonest**).
   Tetracycline—liver and kidney damage, antianabolic effect.
3. **Drugs of very low therapeutic index**
   AMB: Neurotoxic, nephrotoxic and bone marrow toxicity.
   Polymyxin B: Neurotoxic, nephrotoxic.
   Vancomycin: Alopecia and kidney damage.

B. **Hypersensitivity:** All AMAs cause hypersensitivity reaction ranging from rashes to anaphylactic shock.

C. **Drug resistance:** Means unresponsiveness of microorganism to AMA
   2 types: (a) Natural. **(b)** Acquired.
   Natural resistance: Negative bacilli to penicillin G. *M. tuberculosis* to tetracycline.

   Acquired resistance is due to **rapeated** use of drugs. Drug resistant develops by mutation/gene transfer.

   Mutation (heritable genetic change occurring randomly and spontaneously) may be in:
   I. **Single step** (means **single gene** mutation), e.g. *E. coli* and Staphylococcus to refampicin. Enterococci to streptomycin.
   II. **Multiple step:** A **number of gene mutation** leads to resistant in stepwise manner, e.g. resistant to tetracycline, erythromycin, etc.
   Gene transfer occurs by —

   Conjugation
   Transduction
   Transformation

(1) **Conjugation** means **sexual** contact through sex pilus, involves **R factor, RTF,** extrachromosomal DNA **(Plasmid)/chromosomal DNA,** occurs in **colon** among **negative** bacilli of **same/another species** e.g.,
   a. **Acetyl transferase** producing bacteria (*S.typhi, E.coli, H. influenzae*) destroy chloramphenicol. Chloramphenicol to typhoid bacilli. Penicillin to gonococci and streptomycin to *E.coli*.
   b. **β-lactamase** producing bacteria (Gram +ve) destroy β-lactam antibiotic (penicillin, cephalosporin) under control of plasmid.
(2) **Transduction** means transfer of **resistance causing gene (R factor)** through **bacteriophage** to another bacteria, e.g. penicillin, erythromycin and chloramphenicol resistance.
(3) **Transformation:** Release of **resistance causing gene into medium** which is **imbibed** by another organism becoming resistant to drugs, e.g. pneumococcal resistant to penicillin G.

   Cross-resistance is **acquisition** of resistance to one drug conferring resistance to another drug to which organism has not exposed, is seen in **chemically** and **mechanically similar** drugs, e.g. resistant to one tetracycline means resistant to **all others.**

   Resistance may be **prevented** by:
   a. Preventing inadequate, indiscriminate and unduly prolonged use.
   b. Using rapidly acting, cidal, and **selective** drug.
   c. Using **combination** of drugs of different mode of actions (synergistic/additive activity).

D. **Superinfection:** Which means **new** infection development due to AMA therapy, is due to reduced host **defence** (AIDS, SLE, malignancies, anticancer therapy, DM, steroid therapy). It is the **most common** with **broad spectrum** antibiotics, long-term therapy, and severe illness.

Pharmacology Review

Organism causing super infection	Clinical feature	Treatment
Proteus	Enteritis	Cephalosporin
Pseudomonas	UTI	Carbenicillin
C. difficile	Colitis	Vancomycin
C. albicans	Enteritis	Nystatin
Resistant Staphylococcus	Enteritis	Cloxacillin

Normal flora also secretes **bacteriocin** (which inhibits pathogenic oganism to help host defence) and synthesizes vitamins B and K.

E. **Masking of infection:** Occurs due to the use of AMA to treat sufficiently to one infection and suppressing others, e.g. penicillin masks syphilis and treats gonorrhoea.

Choice of AMA

1. **Age:** Antibiotics **contraindicated** in children are: **CATS**
   A. Chloramphenicol causes **gray baby syndrome** when dose exceeds 100 mg/kg per day.
   B. Aminogylcosides: cause **deafness** (8th CN toxicity).
   C. Tetracycline: causes discolouration of permanent **teeth** hence contraindicated in pregnancy and children below 8 yrs.
   D. Sulphonamides displace **bilirubin** from protein binding site and cause **Kernicterus** due to more permeable **blood–brain barrier (BBB)**.

2. **Pregnancy:** All AMAs are contraindicated in pregnancy due to risk to foetus. However some **safe AMAs are:**

   Miconazole   **MEN = Not Contraindicated in Pregnancy.**
   Erythromycin
   Nitrofurantoin
   Nystatin
   Cephalosporin
   Penicillin

3. **Hepatic and renal function**
   A. Drugs used without dose reduction in renal failure are
      Doxycycline
      Rifampicin   **DR**
   B. Antimicrobials needing dose reduction in renal failure.

Even in mild failure	Only in severe failure
Cephalexin **CAVE Failure**	Carbenicillin **Multi-National Company**
Aminoglycosides	Cotrimoxazole
Vancomycin	Norfloxacin
Ethambutol	Cefotaxime
Flucytosine	Metronidazole
Amphotericin B	Ciprofloxacin
Acyclovir	

C. **Drugs avoided in renal failure are:** Cephalothin, cephaloridine, nitrofurantoin, nalidixic acid, Tetracycline **except** doxycycline.
D. **Drugs avoided in Hepatic failure are:** Pyrizinamide and Pefloxacin, Erythromycin, Nalidixic acid, Tetracycline and Talampicillin.

PENT House

4. **Genetic factors**   CSF
   Chloramphenicol
   Sulfonamide
   Fluoroquinolone
   Primaquine and nitrofurantoin cause haemolysis in G6PD deficient patients.
5. **Organism sensitivity**

MIC (minimum inhibitory concentration) is the **lowest** concentration which prevents visible growth of bacteria determined in micro well culture plates using serial dilution of antibiotics.

MBC (minimum bactericidal conc) is the concentration of antibiotic which kills **99.9% of bacteria**. A **small** difference between **MIC** and **MBC** indicates that antibiotic is primarily **bactericidal** while a large difference indicates **bacteriostatic** action. **Break point concentration** of antibiotics is the concentration that demarcates between **sensitive** and **resistant bacteria**.

Postantibiotic effect: Depending on antibiotics and organism, the organism starts multiplying in free medium after a brief exposure and a lag period. This lag period is called **postantibiotic effects**.

6. AMA should be **narrow** spectrum for **definitive** therapy and **broad** spectrum for empirical therapy.

Most antibiotics are given at **2 to 4 half-life intervals** to attain therapeutic concentration **intermittently** for **optimum** action.

Concentration dependent inhibition means inhibitory effects depend on **ratio of peak concentration to the MIC**. The **same daily dose** produces **better** action when given as **single** dose than as **divided** dose, e.g. aminoglycosides.

Time dependent inhibition means inhibition depends on the **length of time** the concentration remains **above MIC**. The **division** of daily dose has better effect but doses should be so spaced that the surviving organism again starts **multiplying** and a **cidal** action is exerted, e.g. β-lactams.

Penetration: Drugs should be present in **sufficient concentration** for adequate **length of time** at the **site of action**.

Fluoroquinolones penetrate soft tissues, joints, lungs, prostates. **Ciprofloxacin** and **rifampicin** have **intracellular** penetration. Ampicillin, Cephalosporin, Erythromycin have **biliary** penetration.   ACE

Cefuroxime
Ceftriaxone
Chloramphenicol   have **CSF penetration**   5Cs
Ciprofloxacin

Advantages of combination of AMAs

A. **Synergism** (supradditive effect) means **decrease in MIC** of one AMA in the presence of another or MIC of both may be lowered. In **synergism, MIC** of each AMA is reduced to $\leq 25\%$. In **additive** effect, MIC of each AMA is reduced to **25–50%**. In **antagonism**, MIC of each AMA is reduced to >50%.

Two **static agents** are often additive and exert **cidal** action, e.g. sulfonamide + trimethoprim in typhoid. **Two cidal agents** are often **additive,** e.g. rifampicin + INH in TB. **Cidal** and **static** drugs may be **synergistic** and **antagonistic** depending on organism. If the organism is highly **sensitive** to cidal drug, **antagonism** is seen bacause **cidal** drugs act primarily on **rapidly** multiplying organsim and **static** retards multiplication, e.g. penicillin + chloramphenicol in pneumococci. If organism is **low sensitive to cidal** drug, **synergism** is seen, e.g. rifampicin + dapsone in leprosy.
B. It reduces **resistance** in chronic infection, broadens spectrum and reduces ADR.

		Mechanism of action and resistance		
Sl. No.	Drugs	Target	Mechanism of action	Mechanism of resistance
1.	Bacitracin	Cell wall	Inhibits recycling of membrane lipid carrier, preventing addition of cell wall subunit	Not known
2.	Vancomycin	Cell wall	Inhibits addition of new cell wall subunits (muramyl pentapeptides)	Change in target substitution of terminal amino acid of peptidoglycan subunit
3.	β-lactams (penicillins, cephalosporins)	Cell wall	Inhibit cell wall cross-linking	Drug inactivation by β-lactamase, insensitive site Decreased permeability
4.	Polymyxins	Cell membrane	Interferes with membrane permeability by charge alteration	Not known
5.	Gramicidin	Cell membrane	Forms pores	Not known
6.	Sulfonamides and trimetrioprim	Cell metabolism	Inhibit enzymes involved in folic acid synthesis competitively	Formation of insensitive target that bypass metabolic block
7.	Quinolones	DNA synthesis	Inhibit DNA gyrase (β subunit)	• Insensitive target

Mechanism of action and resistance (Contd.)

Sl. No.	Drugs	Target	Mechanism of action	Mechanism of resistance
				• Decreased intracellular accumulation (active efflux)
8.	Novobiocin	DNA synthesis	Inhibit DNA gyrase (β subunit)	Not known
9.	Metronidazole	DNA synthesis	Shortlived intermediates are generated by election transfer system intracellularly	Not known
10.	Rifampicin	DNA synthesis	Inhibits DNA dependent RNA polymerase	Mutation of polymerase gene causing insensitive target
11.	Macrolides	Protein synthesis	Bind to 50s ribosomal subunit	Change in target (ribosomal methylation)
12.	Clindamycin	Protein synthesis	Binds to 50s ribosomal subunit	Change in target (ribosomal methylation)
13.	Chloramphenicol	Protein synthesis	Binds to 50s ribosomal subunit	Drug inactivation (chloramphenicol acetyl transferase)
14.	Tetracyclines	Protein synthesis	Bind to 30s ribosomal subunit	• Decreased intracellular drug accumulation (active efflux) • Insensitive target
15.	Aminoglycosides	Protein synthesis	Bind to 30s ribosomal subunit	Drug inactivation
16.	Mupirocin	Protein synthesis	Inhibits isoleucine t-RNA synthetase	Insensitive target (mutation of target gene)

Pharmacology Review

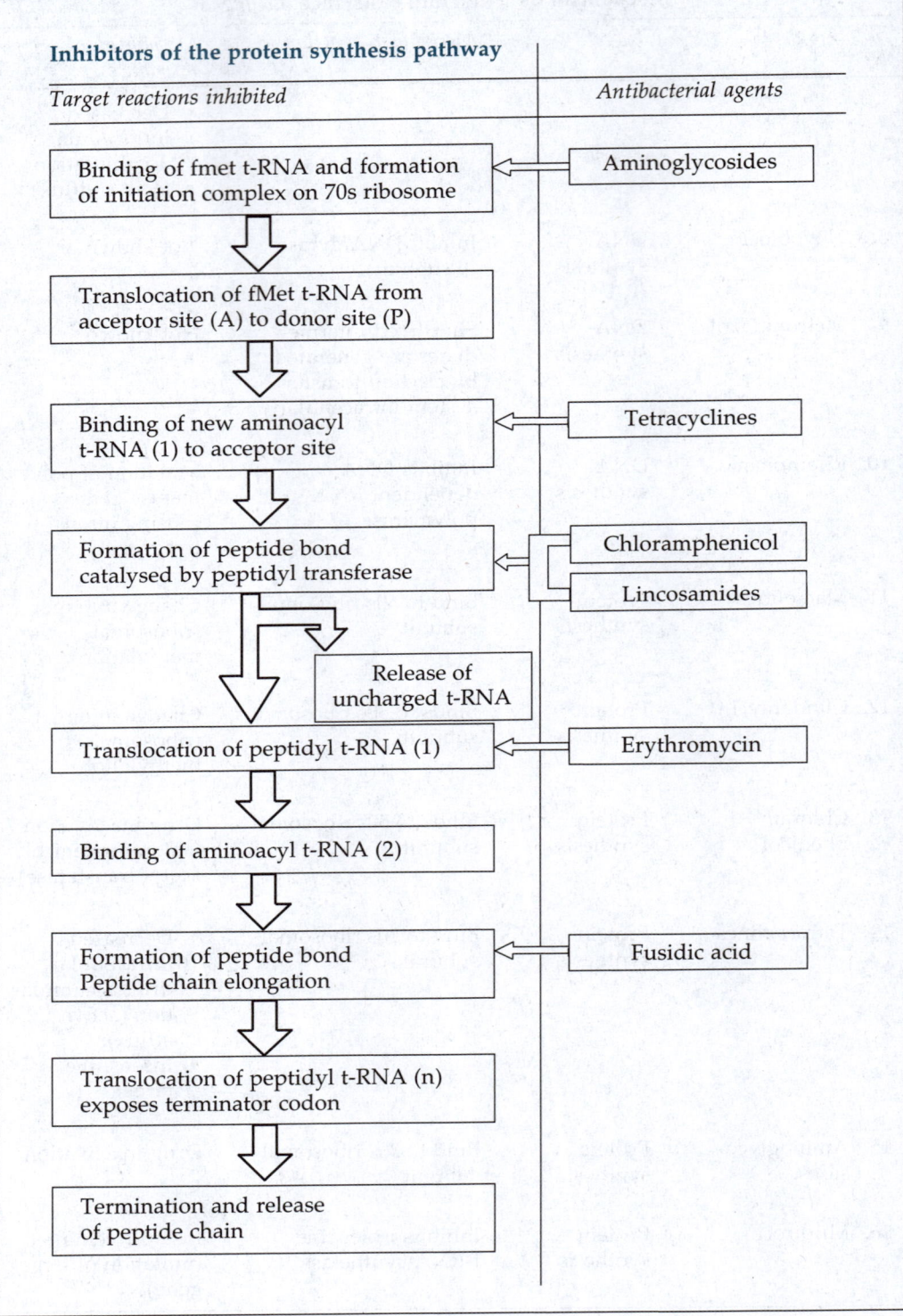

1. **Stopping codons**
   UGA = U Go Away
   UAA = U Are Away
   UAG = U Are Gone
2. **Initiation codon**
   AUG = inAUGurates protein synthsis.
3. Gram-Negative secretes endotoxin: | N-dotoxin |
4. These bugs do not **Gram stain** well:
   Treponema (**too thin** to be visualised).
   Rickettesia (intracellular parasite).
   Mycobacteria (high lipid content wall).
   Legionella (intracellular → silver stain).
   Chlamydia (intracellular parasite).
   | These Rascals May Microscopically Lack Colour |
5. A. **Gram +ve microorganisms**
     a. Gram +ve **Cocci**–*Staph., Strept.*
     b. Gram +ve **Bacilli**–*Bacillius, Clostridium, C. diph.*
     c. **Actinomycetes** | ABC |
   B. **Gram –ve micoorgansim:**
     a. Gram –ve **Cocci**—*Neisseria*
     b. Gram –ve **Bacilli**—*E. coli, Salmonella, Shigella, Klebsiella, Proteus, Pseudomonas, Vibrio, Haemophilus, Yersinia, Francisella, Rickettsiaceae.*
     c. **Brucella, Bordetella** (coccobacillus)
     d. **Chlamydiae**
     e. **Spirochetes**

β-Lactam Antibiotics

β-lactam antibiotics are as follows:
1. **Penicillin**
2. **Cephalosporin**
   Both the above antibiotics are destroyed by **β-lactamase (penicillinase and cephalosporinase)** of bacteria.
3. **Carbapenems** and **monobactam** (parenterally).

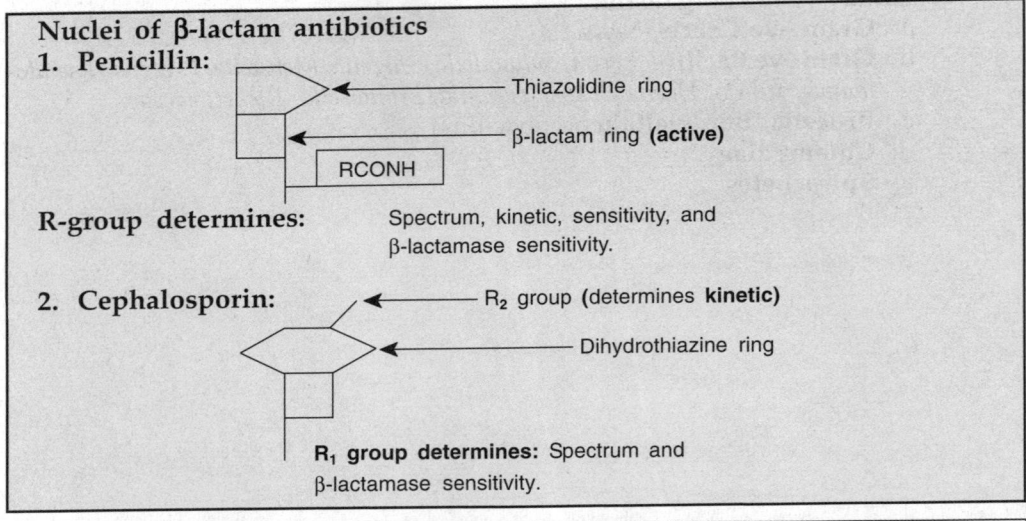

Nuclei of β-lactam antibiotics
1. Penicillin: — Thiazolidine ring; β-lactam ring (active); RCONH
   R-group determines: Spectrum, kinetic, sensitivity, and β-lactamase sensitivity.
2. Cephalosporin: — R_2 group (determines **kinetic**); Dihydrothiazine ring
   R_1 group determines: Spectrum and β-lactamase sensitivity.

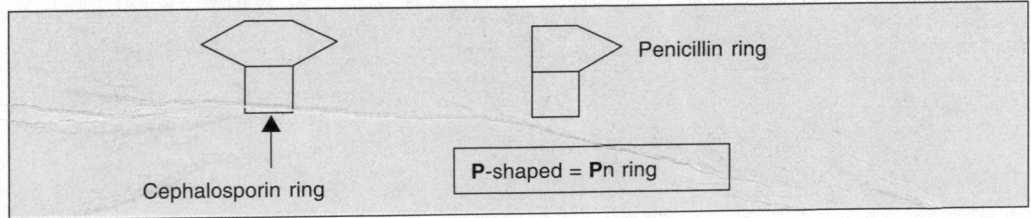

Cephalosporin ring | Penicillin ring | P-shaped = Pn ring

Penicillin

Penicillin was discovered by **A. Fleming (1929)** from **Penicillium notatum**, purified by Chain and Florey and commercially extracted from *P. chrysogenum*.

Basic nucleus of all penicillins is 6-aminopenicillanic acid.

β-lactamase inhibitors: clavulanic acid and sulbactam.
Best combination: (1) Amoxicillin + clavulanic acid. (2) Ampicillin + sulbactam. (3) Taz**OBAC**tum + **PIPE**racillin **TOBAC**co **PIPE**
Unitage of penicillin: 1U of crystalline sod. benzyl penicillin is **equal to 0.6 mg** of standard preparation.
Route: Penicillin G → IV form and penicillin V → oral form.

> PnG not go to GIT
> PnV not go to IV.

Natural penicillin (Narrow spectrum):
(1) Benzyl penicillin, (2) phenoxymethyl penicillin, (3) phenethicillin.

Mech. of action of penicillin

1. **Cidal,** acts on **cell wall.** Bacteria form **UPD-N-Acetyl glucosamine. Peptidogylcan** is linked together to form long strands splitting off **UDP. Final step** is cleavage of terminal **D-alanine** of peptide chain by **transpeptidase** for cross-linking. This transpeptidase is inhibited by **β-lactam** antibiotics by binding on **PBP** (penicillin binding protein) found on the enzyme. **PBP varies** in organism hence affinity for β-lactam varies in organism. This is effective against multiplying organism because resting organism is not making new cell wall.
2. **CWD** (cell wall deficient) forms of bacteria are produced due to **hyperosmotic** effect and **bacterial autolysin, cells burst causing bacteriolysis.**
3. It also inhibits **carboxypeptidase.**
4. **Peptidogylcan cell wall** is **absent in man** and **mycoplasma,** hence β-lactam is **nontoxic to man** and mycoplasma. The cell wall is **entirely** of peptidogylcan in Gram +ve but in **Gram –ve** bacteria, alternating layers of **peptidoglycan** and **lipoprotein** are present. That is why positive bacteria is **more** sensitive to β-lactam than negative bacteria. Positive = Penicillin = Peptidoglycan.

> **Summary of mechanism**
> 1. Binds **penicillin binding protein**
> 2. Inhibits **transpeptidase** cross-linking of cell wall.
> 3. Activates **autolytic enzyme.**

Benzyl penicillin/penicillin G (PnG): Narrow spectrum (Gram-positive bacteria: Gram-positive **cocci except** group D streptococci or enterococci and Gram-positive **bacilli**).

Resistance due to penicillinase

Bacteria — Gram +ve → enzyme in surrounding
— Gram –ve → enzyme in between lipoprotein and peptidoglycan mainly.

Gram –ve bacteria has **porin channel** and **ampicillin** crosses better than PnG. **Permeability** of **beta-lactam** antibiotics varies, hence **sensitivity** also. Therefore sensitivity of ampicillin is better than PnG.

PK: Acid labile (destroyed by gastric acid). $<1/3$ **of oral dose is** absorbed in active form. More absorbed by **elderly** and **infants** due to lower gastric acidity. Absorption through **IM** route is rapid and complete. Distributed **extracellularly** (reaches **most**

body fluids). 60% plasma protein bound. A little metabolised due to rapid excretion by **kidney (10% by glomerular filtration** and **the rest by tubular secretion)**. Plasma t½—**30 min** (t½ longer in neonates due to imperfect tubular secretion). At 3 months, t½ of neonates becomes **30 min.**

IA: **Probenecid** block tubular secretion of PnG and enhances its plasma concentration.

ADR: **Most nontoxic antibiotic.**
Pn ⇒ Hypersensitivity reaction = Hapten (Pn) + Serum protein.
1. Skin rashes **(commonest).**
2. Local irritancy and spinal cord degeneration.
3. **Microembolism (insoluble).**
4. **Most common allergic drugs (highest** with procaine PnG).
5. Contact dermatitis on topical use (hence not used **except** in gonococcal ophthalmia).
6. **Anaphylaxis:** It occurs within 20 min in **0.1% patient** (mediated by IgE), **most serious** reaction due to **penicilloic acid** (treated by adrenaline). Skin test to check for hypersensitivity is **PnG or penicilloyl–polylysine.**
7. **Jerisch–Herxheimer reaction:** Penicillin injection in secondary **syphilis** causes fever, shivering, lesions, cardiovascular collapse due to **spirochetal lytic product release** lasting about **12–72 hrs** in first dose. Treated by **aspirin** and **sedation.**

ADR of PENICILLINS

Penicilloyl moiety (hapten) for allergy and penicilloate for anaphylaxis, Exfoliative dermatitis, Negative Coombs' reaction rare (+ve common), IgE for anaphylaxis, Commonest (allergy 1–4%), IgM for allergy, Lips, tongue, face and periorbital swelling (angioedema), Low BP (shock), Increased body temperature, Nephritis, SJ syndrome, skin rashes of all types, serum sickness.

Uses: (A) DOC is in
1. **Gram +ve cocci**
   a. **Pneumococci (commonest** cause of ASOM)
   b. **Streptococci** (*S. viridans*—**commonest** cause of SABE)
   c. **Staphylococcus** (penicillinase resistance penicillin is used). *S. aureus* is the commonest cause of acute bacterial endocarditis.
   d. **Peptococci, Peptostreptococci, Clostridia.**
2. **Gram –ve cocci (aerobic)**
   a. Meningococci (meningitis with acute adrenal insufficiency cause **Waterhouse–Friderichsen syndrome**).
   b. Gonorrhoea.

Rheumatic fever   SPEC
Subcutaneous nodules
Polyarthritis
Erythema marginatum
Carditis and Chorea

3. **Gram –ve bacilli** (Fusobacterium)
4. **Gram +ve rods/Bacilli:** B. anthracis, C. diphtheriae
5. **Spirochetal:** Treponema, Leptospira
6. **Actinomycosis** (commonest site is faciocervical)

> U of Pn **CABS**
> Cocci
> Actinomycosis
> Bacilli
> Spirochetes

B. **Prophylaxis** **GRASSED**
   1. Gonorrhoea
   2. Rheumatic fever
   3. Agranulocytosis
   4. Surgical infection
   5. Syphilis
   6. Endocarditis due to bacteria
   7. Diphtheria due to C. diphtheriae

> C. Diphtheriae produces exotoxin encoded by β-prophage and inhibits protein synthesis via ADP ribosylation of **EF-2**. **Symptoms:** Greyish white membrane with lymphadenopathy.
> **Lab diagnosis:** Gram +ve rods with metachromatic Granules.
> ADP ribosylation, Beta prophage, Corynebacterium Diphtheriae, Elongation Factor-2, Granules and Greyish white membrane
> **ABCDEFG**

Semisynthetic penicillin: Amidase acts on natural Pn to form 6-Aminopenicillanic acid + benzyl side chain.

In place of benzyl side chain, other side chain can be attached to it resulting in various semisynthetic penicillin production.

Procaine Pn and **benzathine Pn** are salts of Pn (not semisynthetic Pn).

Classification
A. **Acid resistant**   **A CAP For DON**
   Cloxacillin
   Ampicillin
   Penicillin V (phenoxy methyl Pn)
   Flucloxacillin
   Dicloxacillin
   Oxacillin
   Nafcillin
   Amoxycillin
B. **Penicillinase resistant**   **MCQ For DON**
   Methicillin
   Cloxacillin
   Quinacillin

Flucloxacillin
Dicloxacillin
Oxacillin
Nafcillin

C. **β-lactamase inhibitors:** Sulbactam and clavulanic acid.
D. **Antistaphylococcal Pn/β-lactamase resistant:** Cloxacillin, flucloxacillin and methicillin.
E. **Extended spectrum Pn**
   1. **Aminopenicillin:** Ampicillin, amoxycillin and bacampicillin.
   2. **Antipseudomonal**
      a. **Carboxy Pn**
         Carbenicillin
         Carbenicillin indanyl
         Carbenicillin phenyl (Carfecillin)
         Ticarcillin
      b. **Ureido Pn:** Mezlocillin, azlocillin and piperacillin.
   3. **For Gram –ve except *P. aeruginosa*:** Mecillinam (Amdinocillin).

Special features

1. **PnV** dissolves in **duodenum** and is used **(as K⁺ salt) only orally.**
2. **Penicillinase resistance Pn** has side chain to protect β-lactam ring from **staphylococcal penicillinase** hence used against penicillinase producing staphylococci. This is not resistance to Gram –ve **β-lactamase.**
3. **Methicillin** is **acid labile,** hence only injected. It is **inducer of penicillinase production.**
   MRSA (methicillin resistant *Staphylococcus aureus*) is **resistant to all β-lactam,** erythromycin, aminogylcoside and tetracycline. MRSA is treated by **vancomycin/ciprofloxacin.** It causes albuminuria and haematuria. **Commonest** cause of drug induced allergic nephritis is methicillin.
4. **Cloxacillin** is more active against **penicillinase** producing Staphylococcus. It is **acid and penicillinase resistant.** Oxacillin, floxacillin (flucloxacillin) and dicloxacillin are isoxazolyl penicillin **similar** to cloxacillin.
5. **Piperacillin is 8 times** more potent than carbenicillin. Active against Klebsiella and neutropenic/immunocompromised patient.
6. Amdinocillin inhibits **cell wall synthesis** by a different mechanism than other penicillin. Used in typhoid, UTI, dysentery.
7. **Carbenicillin is** active against *A. aeruginosa* **and indole +ve proteus** insensitive to PnG.

Used as **sodium salt** in proteus and Pseudomonas infection (burn, UTI, septicemia). **Sodium loading from Pn** is **commonest** with carbenicillin and ticarcillin which are disodium salt.

Ampicillin: It is active against **all organisms sensitive to Pn** in addition to many **Gram –ve bacteria.** More active against *Strep. viridans* and **enterococci than PnG,** equally active against pneumococci, gonococci and meningococci. Less active **against other** Gram +ve cocci.

β-Lactam Antibiotics

PK: Not degraded by **gastric acid. Incomplete oral absorption. Food** interferes with absorption. Excreted partly in **bile** and reabsorbed leading to **enterohepatic circulation.** Sulbactam + AMPicillin   SAMPle

Renal excretion (mainly). Plasma t½ —**1 hr.**

Dose: 10–30 mg/kg/day orally/IV/IM 6 hourly.

ADR:
1. **Nonallergic** rashes in patient with infectious mononucleosis.
2. **Diarrhoea**

U:
1. Cholecystitis   C GETS DRUM
2. Gonorrhoea
3. Endocarditis (SABE)
4. Typhoid
5. Septicemia
6. Dysentery
7. RTI
8. UTI
9. Meningitis, polyarthrosis, acute glottis due to *H. influenzae.*

IA:
1. **Hydrocortisone mixed in IV solution of ampicillin inactivates it.**
2. **Probenecid** retards its renal excretion.

Coverage: Ampicillin/Amoxycillin:
Haemophilus influenzae **(commonest)**   HELPS
E. coli
Listeria
Proteus mirabilis
Salmonella and *Shigella*

Amoxycillin: Similar to ampicillin except:
1. Its **oral** absorption is better
2. **Diarrhoea** is less
3. Less **active** against *H. influenzae* and Shigella.

Clavulanic acid: Inhibits **class II to V** of β-lactamase by forming **covalent bond** with the enzyme, called **"suicidal inhibition"** (after binding to the enzyme, it gets **inactivated**). It is a **progressive inhibitor** (inhibition changes from **reversibility** to **covalent** bond formation). It is obtained from *Streptomyces clavuligerus.*

Mech: Inhibits **class II to V** of **β-lactamase** produced by Gram **+ve** and **gram −ve** bacteria.

PK: Elimination t½—**1 hr**, rapid **oral** absorption, bioavailability—**60%**, tissue distribution matches **amoxycillin.**

Best combination: Amoxycillin + clavulanic acid = co-amoxyclav.

After **hydrolysis** and **decarboxylation,** clavulanic acid is excreted by **glomerular filtration.** Amoxycillin is excreted **unchanged** by **tubular** secretion. Clavulanic acid + amOXycillin   COX

ADR:
1. GI intolerance
2. Hepatitis
3. Rashes
4. Candida stomatitis/vaginitis.

U: Clavulanic acid re-establishes **amoxycillin activity** against β-lactamase producing organisms:

1. *B. Fragilis*
2. *H. Influenzae*
3. *N. Gonorrhoea.*
4. *Salmonella and Shigella*
5. *Proteus*
6. *E. coli*
7. *S. Aureus (not MRSA that has altered PBP)*
8. *Klebsiella*

U of co-amoxyclav
1. Skin and soft tissue infection
2. Intra-abdominal and gynaecological sepsis, gonorrhoea.
3. RTI and UTI
4. Biliary infection.

Sulbactam

Sulbactam is **semisynthetic. Uses** and **actions** are **similar** to clavulanic acid. Active against **Class I to V β-lactamase.**

Best combination: Ampicillin + sulbactam salt = **sultamicillin tosylate.**

2–3 times less potent than clavulanic acid on **weight basis** (but **same** level of inhibition is at higher concentration). Inconsistent **oral** absorption.

ADR: Diarrhoea, rashes and thrombophlebitis.

Cephalosporin

Cephalosporin is **more toxic** than Pn. It is **semisynthetic** antibiotic derived from **cephalosporin C** obtained from **fungus cephalosporium.**

Common nucleus: 7-aminocephalosporanic acid. **Bactericidal:** Cell wall synthesis inhibition (**same** mechanism as Pn but binds to different proteins than those bound by Pn).

Spectrum: Active against Gram **+ve** and Gram **−ve** bacteria except MRSA and enterococci.

Basis of resistance to cephalosporin
1. **Altered PBP** reducing affinity for antibiotic.
2. **Impermeability** to antibiotic.
3. **Cephalosporinase (β-lactamase)** production by bacteria against cephalosporin.

Route: Oral and parenteral (IV).

Classification
First generation
A. **Parenteral**
   Cephalothin
   Cephaloridine
   Cefazolin
   Cephapirin

Common structure and mech. (inhibition of synthesis of bacterial peptidoglycan cell wall) are shared by beta-lactam.

FIGures SPEAK

B. Oral
Cephalexin
Cephradine
Cefadroxil

Second generation
A. Parenteral
Cefotetan
Cefuroxime
Cefoxitin
Cefamandole
Cefonicid
Ceforanide and cefmetazole

4 Cefo
2 Cefu
2 Cefa

B. Oral
Cefuroxime axetil
Cefaclor
Cefprozil
Loracarbef

Third generation
A. Parenteral
Ceftazimide
Ceftizoxime
Ceftriaxone
Cefotaxime
Cefoperazone

Cefta
2 Cefti
Ceftri
2 Cefo
Cefi

B. Oral
Cafixime
Cefpodoxime and **Cefti**buten

Fourth generation
Parenteral
Cefepime
Cefpirome

Mech. of cephalosporin: Inhibition of **transpeptidase leading to** inhibition of wall synthesis → Bactericidal.

First generation: Cephaloridin is **the most nephrotoxic** cephalosporin. Cefazolin is used in **most surgery.** First generation cephalosporin is the **most effective** cephalosporin for Gram +ve bacterial infection.

Coverage: Gram +ve cocci *(Staphylococcus, Streptococcus, Pneumococcus).*
Cephalothin is effective in the **most PnG sensitive organism,** but resistant to staphylococcal β-lactamase. **Cephalexin** is **the commonest** used cephalosporin. IV cephalosporin is used in surgical prophylaxis.

Second generation: Active against **Gram +ve** and **−ve** bacteria **except** enterococci and *P. aeruginosa.* Cefaclor, cefuroxime and cefamandole are highly active.
Only 2nd generation cephalosporins cross **BBB** and **most important** use is against **meningitis** caused by *H. influenzae, Pneumococcus,* and *Meningococcus.* **Most active** against **bacteroides.**

Coverage of cephalosporin
A. **First generation**   PEcK
   Proteus mirabilis
   E. coli
   Klebsiella pneumoniae
B. **Second generation**   HEN PEcKS
   Haemophilus
   Enterobactor
   Neisseria
   Proteus
   E. coli
   K. pneumoniae
   Serratia

Cefotetan is active against *B. disiens* (**most common** in pelvic infection), *B. fragilis*, and *B. bivius*.

Third generation cephalosporin: **Broad** spectrum. Cefotaxime, ceftizomixe and ceftriazone possess **highest** activity against Gram +ve organism. **Most active** against *E.coli, Klebsiella, Proteus* and *P. aeruginosa*.

Relative action: **Cefotaxime, ceftizoxime, ceftrixone > cefoperazone > ceftazidime.** Ceftizoxime is most active against **anaerobes.** Cefotaxime, ceftizoxime and ceftriaxone penetrate **CNS** hence used in **meningitis.** Cefotaxime and ceftizoxime are used in meningitis, multiresistant hospital acquired infection, septicemia, urethritis and infection of immunocompromised patient.

Ceftriaxone has **longest t½—8 hrs** and **equally** eliminated in **urine** and **bile**. It is used in **meningitis,** multiresistant typhoid, UTI, abdominal sepsis, septicemia, gonorrhoea. **Ceftazidime** is the **most active** cephalosporin against **Pseudomonas (best antipseudomonal cephalosporin).** It is used in febrile neutropenia with haematological malignancies, burn, etc. **Gentamicin + ceftazidime** is the **most effective combination** against Pseudomonas meningitis. **Cefoperazone** has **hypoprothrombinemic action** and **disulfiram like** action. Eliminated in bile (**70%**): hence useful in **renal failure. Used in** UTI, RTI, meningitis, biliary infection, septicaemia and soft tissue infection. **Cefixime** is used in RTI, UTI and biliary infection.

Fourth generation: Cefpirome enters **porin channel** due to **zwitterion character** and is used in RTI, multiresistant hospital acquired infection, septicemia. **Most cephalosporin** are eliminated by **active tubular secretion by kidney.**

As a group, third generation cephalosporin have
1. **Broadest** spectrum
2. **Highest** activity against Gram-Negative bacteria
3. **Lowest** activity against Gram +ve bacteria
4. **Highest** resistant to β-lactamase
5. **Highest** lipid Solubility
6. **Best** penetration into CSF.

Highest → SNB = Short Note Book

ADR of cephalosporin (more toxic than Pn)
1. **1st generation**—seizures
2. **Cefamandole**—rare **disulfiram**-like reaction after alcohol.
3. **Cefotetan**—anaphylaxis
4. **Cefmetazole**—**disulfiram**-like reaction after alcohol.
5. **Ceftriazone**—hypoprothrombinemia, pseudocholelithiasis and bleeding.
6. **Cefoperaxone**—disulfiram-like reaction after alcohol.
7. **Ceftazidime**—**blood urea** and **plasma transaminase** are enhanced. Neutropenia and thrombocytopenia are produced.
8. Patient with history of **IgE-mediated allergic reaction to Pn** (anaphylaxis, urticaria, angioneurotic edema) have **near to same** effect to cephalosporin.
9. **Cefaclor**—serum sickness-like reaction, arthralgia, rash, erythema multiforme.
10. **Cefpodoxime**—rarely nephritis, hepatitis, eosinophilia and bloody diarrhoea.
11. **Cefixime**—stool change and diarrhoea (**most prominent**).
12. Hypoprothrombinemia ⎫ Cefoperazone
    Disulfiram-like reaction ⎬ Cefamandole
    Bleeding ⎭ Moxalactam
13. **Bleeding** with **cephalosporin** having **methylthiotetrazole at position 3** (ceftriaxone and cefoperazone). Bleeding is due to **hypoprothrombinemia** caused by same mechanism as **warfarin** commonly in patient with cancer, renal failure and intra-abdominal infection.
14. **Pain** after IM injection.
15. **Hypersensitivity reaction : Rash—most frequent,** anaphylaxis, angioedema, asthma, urticaria, positive Coombs' test with rare haemolysis.
16. **Nephrotoxicity highest with cephaloridine.**

ADR of CEPHALOSPORIN
Commonest (hypersensitivity reaction), Exfoliative dermatitis, Positive Coombs' reaction, Haemolysis, Alcohol intolerance (disulfiram like reaction). Low prothrombin, Old age causes Serious bleeding, Platelet loss, Oral-anal loss in diarrhoea, Rash, Immediate reaction (anaphylaxis, bronchospasm, urticaria), Nephrotoxicity.

U of cephalosporin
1. **Alternate to PnG in allergic** patient.
2. Gram –ve bacteria: RTI, UTI, **soft tissue** infection.
3. **Penicillinase** producing Staphylococcus.
4. **Mixed aerobic-anaerobic** infection.
5. Typhoid
6. Gonorrhoea
7. Meningitis
8. **Most surgical prophylaxis: Cefazolin.**
9. Septicemia
10. **Neutropenic patient:** Prophylaxis and treatment.

> Cephalosporin have differences from Pn because **Spectrum** is broader, resistance to β-lactamase is **more** and only a few are effective when taken **orally.**

Aztreonam (monobactam because other ring is missing): Bactericidal.
Active against **enteric** bacilli (Gram –ve), *H. influenzae* and Pseudomonas.

Mech: 1. **Binds to PBP3** → inhibition of cell wall synthesis.
2. **Synergistic** with aminoglycoside.
3. **Resistant to most** β-lactamase.
4. **Most promising feature**—lack of cross-sensitivity.

PK: Same as Pn. No cross-allergenicity with Pn.

ADR: GI upset, vertigo and headache.

U: **(Only parenterally used)**
1. **Gram –ve rod:** Klebsiella, Pseudomonas, Serratia **KPS**
2. Hospital acquired infection, UTI, biliary infection, GIT infection, female genital tract infection.

Carbapenems (imipenem–cilastin): Extremely potent and **broadest spectrum** β-lactam antibiotic among any antibiotics.

Mech
1.

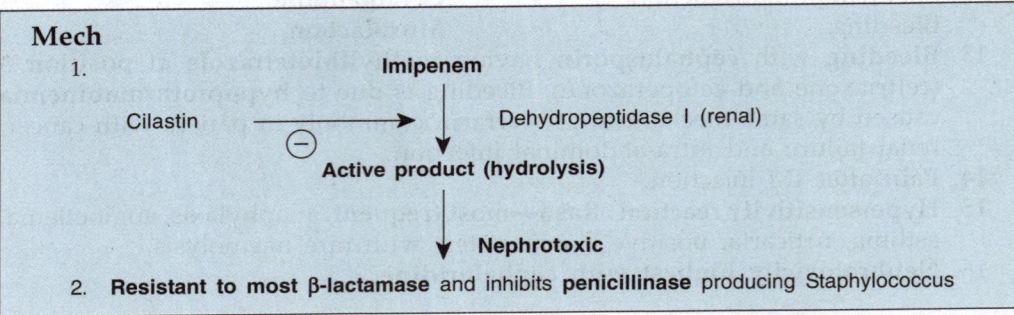

2. **Resistant to most β-lactamase** and inhibits **penicillinase** producing Staphylococcus

PK: Distributed to most tissues. t½—1 hr. Route: Only parenterally.

ADR: 1. Seizures
2. Rash
3. GI intolerance

U: (Imipenem + cilastin):
1. Hospital acquired infection.
2. Infection in immunocompromised

ENDOTOXIN (features): Endothelial cell/Edema
Negative (Gram), DIC, O-Ag, TNF, Outer membrane, eXtremely heat stable, IL-I, NO/Neutrophil chemotaxis.

P. AERUGINOSA (features)
Aerobic, Exotoxin A, Resistance/rod, UTI, Green-blue dressing, Iron containing lesion, Negative (Gram) Odor of grapes, Slime capsule, Adherin pilli.

Antipseudomonal drugs   ABC
Aminoglycosides
Beta-lactam (third gen. cephalosporin, aztreonam, imipenem, morepenem), Ciprofloxacin, colistin, polymixin B.

50. Tetracycline

Tetracycline means **nucleus of 4 cyclic rings**. **All** are obtained from **soil actinomycetes**. All are **semisynthetic except** chlortetracycline + demeclocycline (from *S. aureofaciens*) and **oxytetracycline** (from *S. rimosus*).

First tetracycline is **chlortetracycline**. **Minocycline** is the **most potent** tetracycline.

Classification

Group I (Low potency)	Group II (Intermediate potency)	Group III (Highest potency)
1. **C**hlortetracycline	1. Demeclocycline	1. Doxycycline
2. **O**xytetracycline	2. Methacycline	2. Minocycline
3. **T**etracycline	3. Lymecycline	

COT

Spectrum: Except fungi and viruses, it inhibits **all types** of pathogenic microorganism:
- All Gram +ve bacilli
- All Gram –ve bacilli
- All Gram +ve cocci
- All Gram –ve cocci
- Spirochetes
- Rickettsiae
- Mycoplasma
- Actinomyces
- *E. histolytica*
- Plasmodium
- Chlamydia

> Spirochetes are:
> **B**orrelia (Big size)
> **L**eptospira
> **T**reponema
>
> **BLT-B is Big**

Exceptions:
1. Fungi
2. Viruses
3. Few Gram –ve bacilli such as

Bact. fragilis
P. aeruginosa
Klebsiella
Proteus
Salmonella typhi

> **Big Precipitate–KPS**

Mech:
1. **Static.**
2. Inhibit **30s** → peptide chain fails to grow.
3. Bacteria concentrate drugs **intracellularly** by active transport. Gram-negative bacteria has **porin channel** for drug diffusion.
4. **Lipid soluble** drugs **(Group III)** enter by **passive** diffusion into bacteria.
5. **Carrier** involved in active transport of tetracycline is **absent** in host cell. Hence, host cells are **insensitive** to drugs.

Resistance
1. **Pumping out** mechanism of bacteria.
2. **Plasmid** mediated synthesis of **protection protein** is the **commonest** cause of resistance which protects **ribosomal binding site from drug.**

PK: All tetracyclines are used **orally (commonest).** Doxycycline and minocycline are **completely absorbed** even from full stomach. Tetracycline has **chelating** property. Therefore, absorption is impaired due to Ca^{++}, Mg^{2+}, Al^{3+} and Fe^{3+} present in **milk** and **antacids.** They concentrate in **liver** and **spleen** and bind to **mitochondria** of bone and teeth. **Minocycline** concentrates into the **fat** of the body. **CSF** concentration of most tetracycline is **¼th of that of plasma.** Most are **excreted** in urine **except** doxycycline (which is excreted in **faeces**) and **minocycline** (which is excreted in **bile** and **urine**).

$t½$		
	– Group I	→ 6–10 hrs
	– Group II	→ 16–18 hrs
	– Group III	→ 18–24 hrs

IA: Phenobarbitone and phenytoin **enhance metabolism of tetracycline** (hence action of doxycycline is reduced).

ADR:
1. **Kidney damage:** All tetracyclines enhance renal failure (except doxycycline) causing **PCT damage** by **outdated** drugs which are degraded into **epitetracycline, anhydrotetracycline** and **epianhydrotetracycline.** PCT damage causes **Fanconi syndrome.**
2. Antianabolic effect:
   Reduced protein synthesis
   Increased negative **nitrogen** and **urea** balance
3. Phototoxicity: Nail distortion
   Highest with demeclocycline
4. Intracranial pressure
5. Liver damage
6. a. Diarrhoea:
   Group I drug — High
   Group II drug — Intermediate
   Group III drug — Low
   b. **Diabetes insipidus:** Demeclocycline antagonises **ADH**
7. Enhanced sensitivity **(hypersensitivity)**
8. Vestibular toxicity: Ataxia, vertigo and nystagmus common with minocycline.
9. Superinfection:
   Commonest AMA — Tetracycline
   Commonest site — Intestine
   Most serious problem — Pseudomembranous enteritis.

10. **Bone And Teeth damage:** Due to **chelating** property (Ca^{2+}—tetracycline chelate gets deposited in developing teeth and bone).

>   **KAPIL DEV'S BAT**

CI: 1. Pregnancy
2. Children <8 years
3. Hepatic and renal failure
4. With penicillin (inactivation)
5. Not take with **milk/antacid** because **divalent cations** inhibit absorption of tetracycline in gut.

U: Tetracycline is used in **mixed** infection although combination with β-lactam and **aminoglycoside**/FQ are also used.

A. **DOC in**
1. Relapsing fever and Rickettsial infection
2. Brucellosis
3. Chlamydial infection: Trachoma, **inclusion** conjunctivitis, ophthalmia neonatorum, psitticosis.
4. Plague and atypical Pneumonia
5. Cholera
6. Venereal disease: Lymphogranuloma venereum, urethritis, endocervicitis.
   Most effective in granuloma inguinale.

>   **RBC—PCV (Packed Cell Volume)**

B. **Second choice in**
1. Chancroid
2. Urethritis
3. Tularemia
4. Syphilis
5. Actinomycosis
6. Tetanus
7. Gonorrhoea
8. Listeria

>   **CUTS AT Growing Listeria**

C. **Other uses**
UTI
Amoebiasis
Traveller's diarrhoea (doxycycline as prophylaxis in this and in renal failure).
COPD
Acne
Meningitis
P. falciparum

>   **U AT cAMP**

Uses of tetracycline
Borrelia
Chlamydia
Ureaplasma
Mycoplasma

>   **Become rats = B CUM RATC**

Rickettsiae
Acne
Tularemia
Cholera

Clostridia with exotoxin (Gram +ve, spore forming, anaerobic bacilli)
1. *C. tetani*: **T**etanus is **T**etanic paralysis (inhibits glycine).
2. **B**otulinum is from **B**ad bottles of food (cause flaccid paralysis).
3. **P**erfringenes **P**erforate gangrenous leg.
4. **D**ifficile cause **D**iarrhoea.

A. **Food poisoning is due to:** Vomit Big Smelling Chunks
   Vibrio in contaminated seafood.
   Bacillus in reheated rice.
   S. aureus in custard and meats.
   Clostridium perfringens in reheated meat.
B. Enterobacteriaceae (*E. coli*, Salmonella, Klebsiella, Proteus, Serratia, Enterobacter) have somatic **(O)** Ag, Capsular Ag (K for virulence), Flagellar Ag. All **F**erment glucose and are oxidase negative
   COFFEE
C. e**P**idemic typhus (*R. Prowazekii* = Tetracycline DOC) is transmitted by **P**ediculosis corporis (contrast to endemic typhus).

Antibiotics inhibiting biochemical steps

Penicillin	— Transpeptidase
Gentamicin	— Proper reading of mRNA codons
Doxycycline	— Aminoacyl tRNA binding
Chloramphenicol	— Peptidyltransferase
Erythromycin	— Amino acid translocation
Clindamycin	— Peptide bond formation
Linezolid	— 70s formation
Ciprofloxacin	— DNA gyrase
Bactrim	— Dihydrofolate reductase
Rifampin	— RNA polymerase
INH	— Mycolic acid synthesis

51 Chloramphenicol

It is **obtained from**
A. **Streptomyces** venezuelae.
B. **DNA recombinant technology** from *E. coli* (commercially all are **synthetic**).
It is **yellow white crystalline solid** and needs protection from **light**. It is **the first completely synthetic** antibiotic.

Spectrum: **Broad** spectrum **(same range as tetracycline plus active** against Salmonella and **inactive against** Entamoeba, Plasmodium, fungi, Mycobacterium, Pseudomonas, Proteus, and virus).

Mech:
1. Bacteriostatic.
2. **Inhibit 50s ribosome** → inhibition of aminoacyl tRNA to acceptor site for amino acid incorporation **and inhibition of peptide bond formation.**
3. Inhibits **mitochondrial protein synthesis** especially in bone marrow.
4. Inhibit **50s peptidyl transferase.**

Resistance
1. Decreased **permeability** to bacteria and **low affinity for drug.**
2. Transfer of **R factor by conjugation** → acquisition of **R plasmid encoded for acetyl transferase** (which inactivates the drug by **acetylation**) e.g. Gram −ve bcteria such as *S. typhi*. → **acetyl-chloramphenicol** is unable to bind to the **bacterial ribosome.**

PK: Orally active **(commonest** route**).** 55% plasma protein bound. Penetrates serous cavity, **BBB** and crosses **placenta**. Goes into **milk** and **bile**. Plasma t½—4 hrs. Metabolised by **glucuronide transferase** through **glucuronide conjugation** in the liver. Excreted mainly in **urine** and a little excreted unchanged in urine. **Neonates** and **cirrhotics** need low dose due to low conjugating ability.

ADR:
1. **Gray baby syndrome: 100 mg/kg/day** in neonates leads to
   A. Hypotonia, hypothermia
   B. Ashen gray cyanosis
   C. Blockade of **electron transport** in liver and muscle
   D. Irregular respiration and cardiovascular collapse. This **syndrome** is due to **inability** of newborn to metabolise the drug which is due to **lack of liver UPD-glucuronyl transferase**. The dose in neonate should be **limited to 25 mg/kg/day.**

2. Hypersensitivity reaction
3. Superinfection
4. Irritation
5. Bone marrow depression **(BMD):** Chloramphenicol is the **most important** and **most common** cause of aplastic anemia **(commonest manifestation),** agranulocytosis, thrombocytopenia or pancytopenia.

ADR of CHLORAMPHENICOL

Colour (gray baby syndrome), **H**ypothermia, **L**ess blood cells, **O**ccurrence of encephalopathy and cardiomyopathy, **R**efusal to suck, **A**shen gray colour, **M**ost common (BMD), **P**aresthesia of digits, pleasant taste absent, **H**ypersensitivity (rash, JH reaction), **E**ye (blurred vision), **N**ausea, **I**nhibitor of protein synthesis of inner mitochondrial membrane, **C**yanosis, **O**ptic neuritis, **L**oss of ganglion cell of retina.

IA: It prolongs t½ of: Warfarin
Tolbutamide
Chlorpropamide
World Trade Centre   Cyclophosphamide and phenytoin.

U: 1. **Typhoid (enteric) fever:** It causes **relapses and no cure of carrier** due to **bacterostatic** property of the drug. In MDR, **4-FQ** and **ceftriaxone** are **DOC** in adult. Other drugs are cotrimoxazole, ampicillin/amoxycillin and ceftriaxone **(fastest cidal** drug for typhoid for **all isolates).**

Dose of ceftriaxone
A. 4 gm/day IV for 2 days, followed by 2 gm/day IV for 3 days.
B. 75 mg/kg/day in children.
   These doses prevent **carriers** and **relapses.** For relapse in AIDS→4-FQ.
   1. **Meningitis** due to *H. influenzae*, Neisseria, streptococci.
   2. **Anaerobic** infection (wound, pelvic and brain abscess).
   3. **Intraocular** infection, conjunctivitis, ear infection (ENT infection).
   4. **Plague**
   5. **UTI**
   6. **Second choice**
      Rickettsia
      Brucellosis
      Cholera
      Shigellosis
      Chlamydiae
      B. pertussis (whooping cough)
      Pneumococcal meningitis

RBCs
CBP = Complete blood picture

Obligate intracellular: Rickettsia and Chlamydiae.
They cannot make their **own ATP.**

Stay inside cells when it is Really Cold.

Chlamydiae
A. **E**lementary body **E**nters cell via **E**ndocytosis.
B. **R**eticulate body **R**eplicates in cell by fission.
C. *Chlamydia trachomatis* **ABC**
   = Chronic infection causes Blindness in Africa

ABC = Africa/Blindness/Chronic infection

52 Aminoglycosides

Aminogylcosides are obtained from **actinomycetes**. **Streptomycin** is the **first** aminogylcosides discovered by **Waksman in 1944** and it is the **least nephrotoxic aminogylcosides**. **Gentamicin** is the **cheapest** and the **first line** aminoglycosides. Neomycin and framycetin are **topically** used due to **systemic** toxicity. **All are water soluble, used as sulfate salt, not absorbed orally,** distributed **extracellularly,** not penetrate **brain,** excreted unchanged in **urine, bactericidal, 20 times more active in alkaline than acidic medium** interfering with bacterial **protein synthesis,** active primarily against **aerobic** negative bacilli having **narrow** safety margin between therapeutic and **toxic concentration** (**narrow therapeutic** index). **All are nephrotoxic** (PCT damage), and **ototoxic** (destroy sensory hair cells of vestibule and cochlea of inner ear **permanently** leading to loss of **hearing** and **equilibrium**). **All reduce ACh release** (neuromuscular block) and prolong action of curare like muscle relaxant. Tobramycin causes **least blockade.** This blockade is partially antagonised by IV **Ca^{2+}** (used in UTI). (Aminoglycosides + β-lactam antibiotic) combination is **broad** antibiotic treatment and is used in **septicemia.**

Classification:

FATS

Framycetin and kanamycin
Amikacin, neomycin and netilmicin
Tobramycin, gentamicin
Sisomycin

Mech: 1. Through **porin channels,** they enter cell and bind **irreversibly to ribosome (cidal action).** Cidal action is due to **secondary change** in integrity of cell membrane because other antibiotics inhibiting protein synthesis are **satic** (erythromycin, tetracycline, chloramphenicol).
2. They **leak out proteins** leading to cell death due to **defective protein incorporation** into the membrane.
3. They bind **ribosomes** (streptomycin inhibits **30s** ribosome and others inhibit **50s** and **30–50s** interface), **freeze initiation** and inhibit **polysome formation.** Misreading of codon is due to **30–50s** interface binding.

Summary of Mech: Inhibit **initiation** complex formation, cause **misreading** of mRNA, need **O$_2$** for uptake (hence ineffective against anaerobes).

Aminoglycosides

Resistance: It is by **R-factors** transmitted by **conjugation (commonest** cause), by inactivating antibiotic and by reducing its uptake.

Streptomycin
Streptomycin is obtained from *S. griseus*.

PK: 2/3 excreted by **glomerular filtration. t½ → 2–4 hrs.** Distributed **extracellularly** (volume of distribution 0.3/kg). Highly **ionised**.

Uses:
1. Tularemia
2. TB
3. SABE
4. Plague

STP

A. **ADR of aminoglycosides:** amiNOgylcosides = Nephrotoxic, Ototoxic.
B. **Precaution of aminogylcosides**
   1. Pregnancy
   2. Ototoxicity
   3. Nephrotoxicity
   4. Not mixed with any other Drug.

POND

(aminogylcoside is nephrotoxic with cephalosporin and ototoxic with loop diuretic).

Gentamicin: It is obtained from *M. purpurea*.

PK: Broader spectrum, t½ → 2–4 hrs. More potent (MIC for **most** organism is **4–8** times lower). Ineffective against TB, *Strep. pyogenes* and *Strep. pneumoniae*.

Dose:

Creatinine clearance	Dose interval
1. <10 ml/min	48 hours
2. 10–30 ml/min	24 hours
3. 30–70 ml/min	12 hours
4. >70 ml/min	8 hours

Dose of gentamicin is dependent on **body weight** and **renal function** such as average adult dose **with** normal renal function (creatinine **clearance** >70 ml/min) is **1–1.5 mg/kg/IM/IV 8 hourly**. Septopal (gentamicin—PMMA) is a new drug delivery system of **gentamicin sulfate** in osteomyelitis.

U: Gentamicin is the **cheapest** and the **first line** aminogylcoside.

SPERMS BLUES

1. SABE
2. Peritonitis
3. ENT infection
4. RTI in all patient of impaired host defence
5. Meningitis
6. Septicaemia
7. Burns
8. Lung abscess
9. UTI
10. Conjunctivitis in the Eye
11. Pneumonia
12. OsteoMyelitis

Amikacin

Amikacin is **semisynthetic, widest** spectrum among aminoglycosides. **More hearing loss than vestibular disturbance. Dose:** 7.5 mg/kg/day.

Resistance: It is **resistant to bacterial aminoglycosides inactivating enzyme** and induces lower microbial resistance than other aminoglycoside.

U: Same as gentamicin.

Tobramycin

Tobramycin acts against *P. aeruginosa*, etc. It was obtained in **1970 from** *S. tenebrarius*. Antibacterial, pharmacokinetic properties and dosage are **identical** to gentamicin. It produces **equal** cochlear and vestibular damage (but ototoxicity and nephrotoxicity are lower than gentamicin). It is **2–4 times more** active against Pseudomonas and Proteus than gentamicin.

Dose: 1–15 mg/kg IM/IV TDS.

Neomycin

Neomycin is obtained from *S. fradiae*. Active against **most Gram IM/IV bacilli** and **some Gram +ve cocci.**

- **Mech:** 1. Inhibit **30s** ribosome.
  2. Reduces **plasma LDL-CH** by complexing bile acid in intestine and inhibiting its absorption.
- **ADR:** 1. Intestinal mucosal damage.
  2. Diarrhoea.
  3. Malabsorption syndrome.
  4. Steatorrhoea.
  5. Apnoea (muscle paralysis when applied to peritoneum).
- **U:** 1. Alternative to bile acid binding **resins.**
  2. **Topically** in skin, ear and eye infection in combination with polymyxin and bacitracin.
  3. **Hepatic coma:** NH_3 produced by colonic bacteria is converted to **urea** by liver. Neomycin suppresses intestinal flora →↓ NH_3 **production** →↓ NH_3 level in blood.
  If no detoxification of NH_3 in hepatic failure →↑ blood NH_3 → encephalopathy.

Framycetin: Similar to neomycin. Systemically highly toxic. Hence, used only **topically** in skin, ear and eye infection.

Spectinomycin: Inhibit **30s** ribosome, is **static** and acts alternatively in gonorrhoea.

---

1. **Lactose fermenting enteric bacteria:** Lactose is **KEE**
   Klebsiella   E. coli   Enterobacter
2. **PSEU**domonas **AER**uginosa (**AER**obic) causes:

   PSEU
   - Pneumonia in cystic fibrosis.
   - Sepsis (black lesion on skin).
   - Extended otitis (swimmer's ear).
   - UTI.
3. A. ty**PHU**s has centri**PHU**gal spread of rash (outward).

B. sPotted fever is centriPetal (inward).
C. Q fever is Queer (no rash and vector).
4. FTA–ABS (= Find The Ab–ABSolutely) versus VDRL:
   Most specific
   Earliest +ve
   Remains +ve the longest
   VDRL is less specific

TPHA = Test Positive Hamesha Aayega

ADR of aminoglycoside is GENTAMICIN

General (hypersensitivity reaction, neuropathy), **E**ye (optic nerve dysfunction), **N**ephropathy. **T**oxicity (vestibular and cochlear), **A**uditory dysfunction, **M**uscular paralysis, **I**on imbalance of endolymph, **C**oncentration of drug in otic fluid 6 times > plasma, **I**ncreased blind spot (scotoma), **N**MJ blockade.

Nephrotoxic drugs

Aminoglycosides, **V**ancomycin, **O**pioid, **I**NH, **D**igoxin, **A**ZT, **β** **b**locker, **C**hloroquine, **C**lofibrate, **C**ephalosporin, lithium, sulfonylurea.

AVOID ABC

53. Macrolide and Other Antibiotics

Macrolide: It has **macrocyclic lactone ring** with attached **sugar**.

Classification **CARES**

- Clarithromycin
- Azithromycin
- Roxithromycin
- Erythromycin and Spiramycin

Erythromycin was obtained from *S. erythreus* in **1952,** though it was in use from the **1950s**.

It is **slightly water soluble, bacteriostatic, narrow** spectrum (**broad** spectrum against **Gram +ve**).

Mech:
1. **Static** at low and **cidal** at high concentration. Cidal action also depends on **organism** and its **multiplication**.
2. Gram +ve bacteria accumulates it **intracellularly** by active **transport**. It is slightly **water soluble** (non-ionised or penetrable) and active in alkaline medium.
3. Binds to **23s rRNA of 50s ribosomal subunit** and inhibits translocation of peptide chain from **A to P-site on mRNA** (inhibition of protein synthesis).

Resistance: Plasmid-mediated resistance to all cocci due to less permeability and to enterobacteriaceae due to esterase and methylase. Change in **50s ribosome** is also due to chromosomal **mutation**.

PK: Acid labile hence **enteric coated tablet** is used leading to incomplete absorption. Crosses placenta and **serous membrane only.** 70–80% protein bound. Excreted in **bile** in active (unaltered) form. t½—**1.5 hr. Dose**—8 gm/day **(maximum).**

ADR:
1. **GIT disturbance** (burning, nausea, vomiting) is the **commonest** ADR. **Drug binds to motilin R of GIT** →increase gut motility.
2. Hearing loss
3. Hypersensitivity
4. Hepatitis
5. Cholestatic jaundice.

ADR of MACROLIDES

Most striking ADR (cholestatic hepatitis), increased QT interval, Cardiac arrhythmia, Raised aminotransferase and transaminase, Oral (epigastric distress), Leukocytosis, IV (abdominal cramp, diarrhoea, emesis), Deafness, Eosinophilia, Skin eruption.

IA: 1. Causes rise in **plasma** level of Warfarin, Theophylline, Carbamazepine

WTC = World Trade Centre

2. **Reduction of MFO** (mixed function oxidase) activity enhances drug effect because the drug is **metabolised by MFOs** (e.g. theophylline).

U: 1. As **alternative** to Pn in allergic patients.
2. **DOC** in Pertussis
Chlamydia   **PCM**
Mycoplasma
  A. **Whooping** cough →**most effective** in 2 weeks.
  B. **Pneumonia** —atypical due to **mycoplasma** and **legionnaires**—(DOC).
3. **Second choice in**
  A. Chanchroid.
  B. Campylobacter enteritis.
  C. Pn resistant Staphylococcus.
  D. **Chlamydia trachomatis** in urogenital tract when tetracycline is **contraindicated**.

Azithromycin: Acid stable. **Expanded spectrum:** Accumulates in **fibroblast** and macrophages and inhibits **penicillinase** producing *S. aureus* but not MRSA.

PK: **Acid stable,** rapid oral absorption, t½ >50 hrs due to **slow** release from intracellular sites. **Excretion <10% in** urine and **rest** in bile.

ADR: 1. GI upset
2. Headache and dizziness.

U: **Primary indications**
1. Pharyngitis, tonsilitis, sinusitis, bronchitis, pneumonia and otitis media.
2. Staphylococcus and Streptococcus infection.
3. MAC infection in AIDS.

Roxithromycin: Has **no affinity** to cytochrome P450 and clinically **no interaction** with Warfarin, Theophylline and Carbamazepine. **WTC** t½ is **12 hrs.** Used as **alternative to erythromycin** in RTI, GTI, ENT and skin infection.

Clarithromycin: Spectrum, ADR and IA similar to erythromycin.

PK: Rapidly absorbed **orally.** Oral bioavailability—**50%** due to first pass metabolism (food delays absorption). **Greater** tissue distribution than erythromycin.

Metabolised by **saturation kinetics** (t½ 3–6 hrs at **low** dose and **6–9 hrs** at **high** doses). **1/3 of oral dose** is **excreted unchanged in urine.**

U: 1. Skin, ear, RTI, and MAC (AIDS).
2. **Second choice** in atypical mycobacteria and leprosy.

Spiramycin

Spiramycin is **macrolide**.

Actions and properties resemble erythromycin.

ADR: Rash, diarrhoea, gastric irritation.
U: *T. gondii* (other uses similar to erythromycin). Dose = 3 MU 3 times for 3 weeks (repeated after 2 weeks).

Other antibiotics:
A. Clindamycin and lincomycin
B. Glycopeptide: Vancomycin and teicoplanin
C. Spectinomycin
D. Fusidic acid and linezolid
E. Polypeptide antibiotics
F. Urinary antiseptic and streptogramins

Clindamycin

Clindamycin is a **Lincosamide** antibiotic **similar** in mechanism and spectrum to **erythromycin**. It inhibits **cocci except MRSA** by inhibiting **50s**.

Mech: 1. Inhibit **50s** ribosome →inhibition of protein synthesis.
2. Penetrates **skeletal** and **soft tissues**. Accumulates in **neutrophils** and **macrophages**.

PK: **Orally** absorbed. Excreted in **urine** and **bile**. t½—3hrs.

ADR: 1. Rashes, urticaria.
2. Abdominal pain, diarrhoea and pseudomembranous enterocolitis.

U: 1. **Anaerobic and mixed infecion:** Clindamycin + aminoglycoside/cephalosporin.
Alternative to clindamycin in anaerobic infection is **metronidazole** and **chloramphenicol**.
2. **Bone and joint infection.**
3. **AIDS: Toxoplasmosis** (clindamycin + pyremethamine) and *P. carinii* (clindamycin + primaquine).

Vancomycin

Vancomycin is a **Pn substitute glycopeptide antibiotic** and was discovered in 1956 as **Pn substitute**. Bactericidal

Coverage
Clostridia
Diphtheroids
C. difficile
Enterococcus
Neisseria
MRSA
Strept. viridans

Mech: 1. Inhibits **cell wall synthesis** by binding terminal **dipeptide** sequence of peptidoglycan units and preventing their release from the **carrier** and their **cross-linking**.
2. Has **bactericidal** action.

PK: Not absorbed **orally**. On **IV administration**, it is widely distributed (**crosses** meninges and **serous** cavities). t½—**6 hrs**. Excreted by glomerular filtration.

ADR
1. Redman syndrome (anaphylaxis, intense flushing, fever, chill).
2. Allergy
3. Hypotension due to **histamine release.** Erythema (Redneck syndrome) is also due to **histamine release.**
4. Thrombophlebitis
5. Nephrotoxicity   **NOT HEAR**
6. Ototoxicity

U: Systemically toxic but used in:
1. MRSA **(most effective).**
2. Pn allergic patient. Pn resistant pneumococci and diphtheroid.
3. Cancer therapy.

Spectinomycin: Bacteriostatic. Coverage—Gram –ve bacteria.
Mech: Inhibit **30s** ribosome →no protein synthesis.
ADR: Urticaria, fever and CNS effects.
U: **Gonorrhoea** (Pn allergic patient) in pregnancy when FQ is **contraindicated.**

Fusidic Acid

Fusidic acid is **narrow** spectrum **steroidal antibiotic** for **staphylococci** and is used **topically.**

Polypeptide Antibiotics

Polypeptide antibiotic is **LMW cationic** polypeptide and **bactericidal** antibiotic.

Polypeptide antibiotics are
1. Polymyxin B and polymyxin E
2. Colistin
3. Bacitracin
4. Tyrothricin

Coverage: Colistin and **polymyxin B** and **E** are active against **gram-negative cocci** and **rods** except:
Proteus
Neisseria   **PNS = Peripheral Nervous System**
Serratia

Colistin is more potent against Shigella, Salmonella and Pseudomonas. **Resistant** to polypeptide antibiotic is **absent.**

Mech:
1. Polymyxins are **cationic** and **basic** proteins that act like **detergents.**
2. Polypeptide antibiotics have **detergent like action** on membrane by forming **pseudopore** →ions leak out. The membrane is distorted and the **endotoxin** is inactivated. These occur due to **high affinity for phospholipid.**

ADR:
1. Acute renal **tubular necrosis.**
2. **Neuromuscular** blockade.
3. **Neurological** disturbances (nausea, vomiting, diarrhoea).
4. **Histamine release.**

U:
1. **Topical:** Skin, ear and eye infection.
2. **Oral:** Enteritis.

Bacitracin
Bacitracin is obtained from *Bacillus subtilis*. **Bactericidal**
- Coverage: Active against Gram +ve cocci and bacilli.
- Mech: Inhibits **cell wall synthesis** at a **step earlier than that inhibited by Pn.**
- PK: **Not absorbed orally. Systemically** toxic (parenterally not given).
- U: **Topically** in skin and eye infection.

Tyrothricin: It is obtained from *Bacillus bravis* and is water soluble, **thermostable,** active against Gram +ve and few Gram –ve bacteria.
- Mech: 1. **Leakage of cell membrane.**
  2. **Uncoupling** of oxidative phosphorylation in bacteria.
- PK: Not absorbed orally.
- ADR: 1. **Systemically toxic** (used only parenterally).
  2. **Haemolysis.**
- U: **Topically** in skin infection.

Urinary antiseptics: Nalidixic acid, nitrofurantoin, phenazopyridine and methenamine.

Nitrofurantoin
Nitrofurantoin is **bacteriostatic** but **bactericidal** at higher concentration. More active in **acidic** media. Acts against **Gram –ve bacteria.**
- Resistant: Develops **slowly** but **cross-resistance is absent.**
- Mech: Susceptible bacteria enzymatically reduces nitrofurantoin to generate **reactive intermediates** which damage **DNA of bacteria.**
- PK: Absorbed orally. Hepatic metabolism. >50% excreted unchanged in urine. Plasma t½ → 30–60 min.
- IA: 1. Antagonises the action of **nalidixic** acid.
  2. **Probencid** prevents its tubular secretion → reduces concentration attained in urine → urinary antiseptic action is interfered.
- CI: 1. Renal excretion is reduced in **azotemic** patient→toxicity is enhanced. Hence, **contraindicated** in renal failure
  2. **Pregnancy and neonates**
- ADR: 1. **GI intolerance** (commonest)
  2. **Acute reaction** (chill, fever, leucopenia)
  3. **Peripheral neuritis**
  4. **Haemolytic anemia except** in G6PD deficiency.
  5. **Liver damage** and pulmonary reaction **with fibrosis** on chronic use.
  6. **Dark brown urine** on exposure to air.
- U: UTI 50–100 mg TDS/QID.

Hexamine
Methenamine (hexamine) is a **hexamethylenetetramine.**
- Mech: 1. Inactive but decomposes slowly in **acidic urine (pH <5.5)** to release **formaldehyde** which inhibits **all bacteria.**

2. Antimicrobial activity is **absent** in blood, tissues and kidney parenchyma.
3. Urine pH <5.5 is maintained by administering **mandelic acid/ascorbic acid.**
4. **Formaldehyde** is **bactericidal** against Gram –ve bacteria.
5. Used **orally** in the form of **enteric coated tablet** so that it must be protected from **gastric juice.**
6. **Mandelic** acid itself is urinary antiseptic and acts by lowering pH of urine.

ADR:
1. Gastritis due to **formaldehyde.**
2. Cystitis, haematuria and CNS symptoms.

CI:
1. **Renal failure:** Mandelic acid of methenamine mandelate accumulates in the blood causing acidosis.
2. **Liver disease:** Released NH_3 is not detoxified.

IA: Sulfonamide antagonises methenamine.
U: Chronic resistant UTI not involving kidney substance.

Phenazopyridine: Has **analgesic** action. Antimicrobial action is absent.
U: Symptomatic relief in cystitis (but causes epigastric pain).

Oxazolidinone (linezolid): Static. Approved by FDA (2000). First member.

Mech: Bind to 50s subunit of bacterial ribosomes (prevents union of 50s and 30s subunits into 70s pre-initiation complex) to inhibit protein synthesis.
Spectrum: Gram +ve (MRSA, VRSA, VRE) bacteria.
ADR: Anemia, thrombocytopenia and gut upset (commonest).
PK: Absorbed orally, metabolised nonenzymatically, renal excretion. Plasma t½ = 5 hrs.
U: All Gram +ve organisms (VRE and MRSA).
IA: Inhibits MAO (interacts adrenergic/serotonergic drugs and tyramine).

Lincomycin: The forerunner of clindamycin (same mechanism and ADR, less potent, but more colitis and diarrhoea).
PK: Absorbed orally, excreted in bile, plasma half-life = 5 hrs.

Teicoplanin: It is a glycopeptide (a mixture of 6 similar compounds). For Gram +ve bacteria.
Mech: Mechanism and spectrum similar to vancomycin.
ADR: Rash, fever, ↓ WBC, histamine release.
U:
1. Enterococci (more active than vancomycin).
2. MRSA
3. Penicillin resistant streptococci. Dose is reduced in renal insufficiency due to its renal excretion. Single dose due to long t½ (4 days) = 400 mg IV/IM

Streptogramins (Dalfopristin/Quinapristin): Static. Combination of 2 semisynthetic pristinamycin (synergism).
Mech: Bind to 50s subunit of bacterial ribosomes, inhibiting protein synthesis.
Resistance: Gram-negative and *E. faecalis* intrinsically resistant.

ADR: Thrombophlebitis.
U: Most Gram-positive cocci (MRSA, VRE and VRSA), Neisseria, Legionella, Chlamydia. Combination is cidal for Staph. and Strept.

Nonsurgical antimicrobial prophylaxis
1. Meningococcal infection—rifampicin (**DOC**)
2. Gonorrhoea—ceftriaxone.
3. Syphilis—benzathine PnG
4. Recurrent UTI—trimethoprim-sulfamethoxazole (TMP-SMX)
5. PCP—**DOC (TMP-SMX)**, Pentamidine.

UTI: It is due to **Gram-negative** bacteria specially coliforms. Acute infection is due to single organism (**commonest**—*E. coli*). Chronic and recurrent infection is **mixed**.
For lower UTI—3 day regimen.
For upper UTI—longer treatment.

Treatment of chronic and recurrent infection
Sulfonamide
Cotrimoxazole
Trimethoprim
Nitrofurantoin
Ampicillin
Cephalexin
Norfloxacin
FQ (for complicated cases)
Gentamicin (effective against **most** urinary pathogen)

UTI Bugs: **SEEK PP**
Serratia and **S**taphylococcus
E. coli
E. cloacae
Klebsiella
Proteus
Pseudomonas

WHooping cough = **H**undred day fever
Amio**D**arone = Hun**D**red **D**ay Drug (half-life = 100 day)
Tetanus = Eigh**T** day disease
Herpes = Six day disease HERPES = 6 Letters
Exanthum of parvovirus = 5th disease. E = 5th letter
HBV → **D**ouble shelled **D**NA virus = **D**ane particle.

54. Sulfonamides and Cotrimoxazole (Bactrim)

Sulfonamide is derivative of **sulfanilamide** (P-aminobenzene sulfonamide). Sulfonamide was the **first** AMA for pyogenic infection. It is not antibiotic.

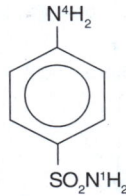

N^1 **(sulfonamido-N)** governs **solubility, potency** and **PK** and the individual member **differs** in the nature of N^1 substitution.

N^4 governs **antibacterial** action. Prontosil red (sulfonamidochrysoidine) was **first synthesized** by **Klarer** and **Mietzsch**. Efficacy **first demonstrated** by **Domagk**. Prontosil red is converted to sulfanilamide.

Spectrum: Bacteriostatic for Gram-positive and -negative bacteria. **Bactericidal** concentration in urine in selective absence of thymine. Sensitivity changes from time to time and place to place. Spectrum is **broad**.

Resistance to sulfonamide is **R-factor** mediated. **Causes** of resistance:
A. Increased **PABA** production.
B. Low affinity of **folate synthetase** to drugs.
C. Adoption of **alternative pathway** in folate metabolism.
But **cross-resistance** is absent.

Classification
A. Highly absorbed
1. Short-acting (4–8 hrs):   Sulfadiazine
   Sulfamethizole
   Sulfasomidine
   Sulfasoxazole
2. Intermediate-acting (8–16 hrs): Sulfaphenazole
   Sulfamethoxazole
3. Long-acting (1–7 days): Sulfamethoxypyridazine
   Sulfadimethoxine

4. Ultralong-acting (>1 week): Sulfadoxine
   Sulfamethopyrazine
B. **Poorly absorbed:** Succinyl sulfathiazole
   Phthalyl sulfathiazole
C. **Special purpose:** Mafenide (burn)
   Sulfasalazine (RA and ulcerative colitis)
   Silver sulfadiazine (topical)
   Sulfacetamide sodium (eye drop)

Mech of sulfonamide

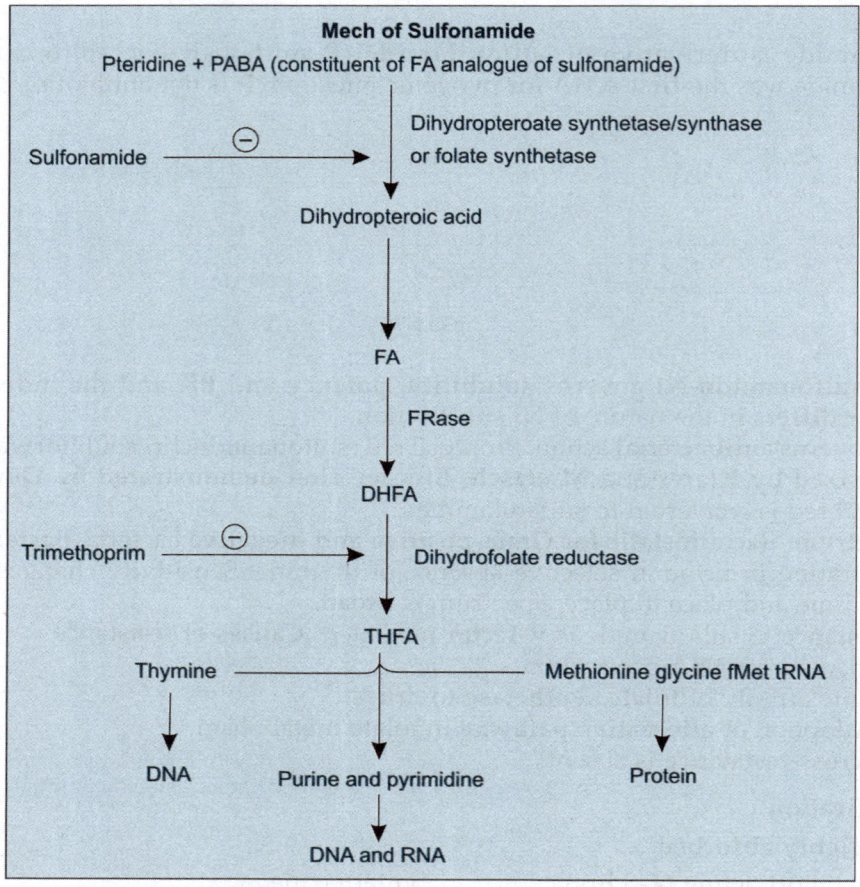

Bacteria have **no active transport** for folate and must synthesize it. Humans have active transport for folate and obtain it from diet. Hence, inhibition of folate synthesis has no effect on host cells.

PK: Completely absorbed orally. Distributed to **all body fluids.** Metabolism is by **acetylation** at N^4 by non-microsomal enzyme primarily in liver.

Sulfonamides and Cotrimoxazole (Bactrim)

Slow and **fast acetylator** is present but it is clinically insignificant. Acetylated derivative is inactive, less soluble in acidic urine and causes **crystalluria**. Plasma protein binding varies **10–95%**.

Excreted in **kidney** through glomerular filtration.

ADR — HCG
1. Hypersensitivity with long-acting drugs: photosensitization. **Stevens-Johnson syndrome** is the **most severe** form of erythema multiforme. Sulfonamide is the **commonest** drug for SJ syndrome and exfoliative dermatitis.
2. Crystalluria: Sulfadiazine, sulfapyrine, sulfathiazole.
3. GIT intolerance
4. Hepatitis
5. Haemolysis in **G6PD deficient**.
 Kernicterus in newborn due to removal of bilirubin from plasma albumin binding site.

IA:
1. Inhibit phenytoin and warfarin.
2. Drugs having **sulfonamide group or causing cross-allergenicity** are:
    Furosemide
    Acetazolamide
    Chlorothiazide   FACTS
    Tolbutamide
    Sulthiame (antiepileptic)

U:
1. UTI (acute and uncomplicated)
2. Conjunctivitis
3. Recurrent otitis media
4. Pharyngitis and gum infection
5. **Malaria:** Fansidar (long-acting sulfonamide + pyrimethamine) is for treatment and prophylaxis in chloroquine resistance malaria.
6. Burns
7. Nocardiosis
8. Toxoplasmosis (sulfadiazine + pyrimethamine)

> **Sulfasalazine:** It is a compound of **sulfapyridine** and **5-ASA** (5-aminosalicylic acid), has **anti-inflammatory** activity. Sulfapyridine splits off in the **colon by bacterial** action and is absorbed systemically (active moiety). Efficacy is **similar** to hydrochloroquine and better tolerated than gold/penicillamine in RA/ulcerative colitis.

Cotrimoxazole (bactrim)

Cotrimoxazole = Trimethoprim + sulfamethoxazole
Cotrimazine = Trimethoprim + sulfadiazine

Use of cotrimazine is **same** as cotrimoxazole.

Trimethoprim is a **diaminopyrimidine** related to pyrimethamine. Individually **static,** combination becomes **cidal** and is due to **same t½—10 hrs.**

> 11/9 hr = half-life of TMP/SMX = WTC and **Pentagone on 11/9.**

Optimal synergy is at the concentration ratio of **TMP : SMX (1 : 20)**. This ratio in plasma is obtained when the drug is given in the form **TMP : SMX (1 : 5)** because trimethoprim (TMP) has larger volume of distribution.

PK: TMP is **more rapidly** absorbed than sulfamethoxazole (SMX). Plasma protein bound = TMP **40%** and SMX **65%**.
Half-life of TMP = 11 hrs and **SMX = >9 hrs**.
TMP is partly metabolised in liver and excreted in urine.

ADR: (**Same** as sulfonamides):
1. **Anemia:** Combination induces folate deficiency in host leading to anemia (treatment—**folinic acid**).
2. **Bone marrow depression,** megaloblastic anemia, thrombocytopenia.
3. **Teratogenic** risk
4. 50% incidence of fever, rash and **bone marrow hypoplasia** among AIDS patient with *P. carinii* infection.
5. Selective toxicity occurs because **bacterial reductase** is **20,000** times as sensitive as human reductase.

U:
1. UTI (acute and uncomplicated)
2. RTI
3. Diarrhoea and dysentery
4. Chancroid
5. Typhoid
6. *P. carinii*
7. Prostatitis

Trimethoprim (TMP): It is **diaminopyrimidine** derivative and causes selective toxicity because bacterial reductase is **20,000 times** as sensitive as human reductase.

Mech: Competitive inhibitor of dihydrofolate reductase. It is alone as effective as combination.

PK: 40% plasma protein bound. Hepatic metabolism. Renal excretion.

ADR: It is due to **sulfonamide:**   **LAG**
1. Leukopenia
2. Anemia (megaloblastic)
3. Granulocytosis   **TMP = Treats Marrow Poorly**
4. BMD

ADR of SULFONAMIDE

SJ syndrome and skin rash, pruritis, Urine (crystalluria), Low bilirubin due to displacement from plasma albumin, Fever, Oral hypoglycemics/oral anticoagulants/hydantoin commonly inhibited, Necrosis of liver, Anemia and BMD, Malaise, Increased bilirubin in CNS (kernicterus), Dermatitis and Erythema.

ADR of Cotrimoxazole is TRIMETHOPRIM

Thrombocytopenia, Rash, Increased gut upset, Megaloblastosis, Exfoliative dermatitis, Toxic epidermal necrolysis, Hepatitis, Occurrence of SJ and Sweet's syndrome, Purpura (HS), Renal dysfunction, Infiltration of lung, Myelosuppression.

U: 1. UTI (acute, chronic and recurrent cases).
2. **DOC** in AIDS for prophylaxis and treatment against *P. carinii* (TMP/SMX).
3. **DOC** for prophylaxis against **secondary** infection due to *T. gondii* in AIDS is SMX/TMP and due to *C. neoformans* and *C. albican* is fluconazole.

Drugs for typhoid or enteric fever (4Cs)
1. Ciprofloxacin: DOC in adults
2. Cephalosporins: DOC in children
3. Chloramphenicol ⎤ Resistance
4. Cotrimoxazole ⎦ has developed

Antidote drugs are cotrimoxazole, proguanil, pyrimethamine, methotrexate, etc.

55. Quinolones and Fluoroquinolones

Quinolones: These are **synthetic** antibiotics.
  Coverage—Gram-positive and Gram-negative bacteria.
  First member—Nalidixic acid active against Gram-Negative bacteria.
  Mech: Inhibits bacterial **DNA gyrase** and is **bactericidal** (inhibition of replication).
  PK: Absorbed orally. Hepatic metabolism producing active metabolite. Plasma t½—8 hrs. Renal excretion. For systemic infection, concentration of free drug in plasma and most tissues is **non-therapeutic,** i.e. MIC value for susceptible bacteria is nearer to "break point concentration". But urine concentration of drug is **20–50 times** that in plasma, hence lethal to urinary pathogen.
  ADR:
  1. **GI intolerance (commonest).**
  2. **Neurological disturbance** (headache, vertigo, visual loss): **Most important**
  3. Parkinsonism like symptoms, leukopenia, biliary statis.
  4. Haemolysis in G6PD deficient patient.
  CI: Infants
  IA: Nitrofurantoin antagonises its effect.
  U: UTI and diarrhoea (Gram –ve bacteria).
Rosoxacin: It is **quinolone derivative** acting against gonococcal infection.

Fluoroquinolones: These are **bactericidal** and are quinolones having **fluorine** substitution. **First generation** has **one** and **second** generation **> one** fluorine substitutes.

Mech: Inhibit **DNA gyrase** by binding its **A subunit** and inhibiting its cutting and resealing function. Cidal action is through digestion of DNA by **exonuclease** (its production is signalled by damaged DNA). Mammals have **Topoisomerase II** in place of DNA gyrase with low affinity for FQ.

Resistance: Chromosomal mutation producing gyrase with low affinity for FQ. **Less permeability** to drug uptake. FQ has low mutational resistance (slow mutational development). Less active at **acidic pH.**

  Coverage:
  1. Active against Gram +ve and Gram –ve bacteria.
  2. Active against β-lactam and aminoglycoside resistant bacteria.

Dose: Generally 400 mg BD orally; ciprofloxacin, pefloxacin and ofloxacin IV also.

Classification

A. **First generation**
   Pefloxacin
   Ofloxacin   `PONC~PONS`
   Norfloxacin
   Ciprofloxacin

B. **Second generation**
   Fleroxacin
   Amifloxacin   `FALSe`
   Lomefloxacin
   Sparfloxacin

C. **Newer FQs:**   Moxifloxacin   `Must Get TLC`
   Gatifloxacin
   Trovafloxacin
   Levofloxacin
   Clinafloxacin
   Grepafloxacin

Ciprofloxacin: **Most** active against Pseudomonas among FQ.

Has **widest** spectrum. It is the **prototype** and the **most potent** first generation FQ. **Most susceptible** bacteria are aerobic Gram-negative bacilli.

Resistant bacteria of ciprofloxacin are:

   Anaerobic cocci
   B. *fragilis*   `ABC`
   Clostridia

PK (of all FQs)

A. Absorbed orally. **Most important** feature is high tissue penetratibility. Excreted in urine (both by glomerular filtration and tubular secretion).

B. **Ciprofloxacin:** 30% palsma protein bound. **Most potent** and **widest FQ**. 20% metabolised. Rapidly absorbed orally **(70%)**. Vol. of distribution **4 L/kg**. Synergism with **aminoglycoside** and **anti-Pseudomonas β-lactam**. Elimination t½—4 hrs. `4 L/kg + 4 hrs`

C. **Pefloxacin:** Methyl derivative of norfloxacin, completely absorbed orally. **Highest** penetration of CSF among FQ. t½ →8–16 hrs. **85%** metabolised and excreted in urine. Oral bioavailability is **95%**.

D. **Ofloxacin: Intermediate** between ciprofloxacin and norfloxacin in activity against Gram –ve becteria. **More potent** than ciprofloxacin for Gram +ve bacteria, excreted unchanged in urine, oral bioavailability **90%**, plasma protein binding is **25%**, elimination t½—7 hrs.

ADR of ciprofloxacin

1. GI intolerance and CNS manifestation (headache, dizziness): **Commonest** but mild.
2. Hypersensitivity: Sparfloxacin also causes photosensitivity and prolongation of QT interval.
3. **Tendonitis** and **tendon rupture**.

ADR of QUINOLONES

QT interval prolonged by grepafloxacin and sparfloxacin, **U**pset of gut (commonest), **I**ncreased serum transaminase, **N**eurosis of liver by trovafloxacin, **O**ccurrence of rash, **L**eukopenia, **O**ther rare ADR (diarrhoea, colitis), **N**ausea, **E**osinophilia, **S**eizures.

CI: (FQ):
1. In childern due to cartilage damage in weight bearing joints of BONES.
2. Pregnancy

FluoroquinolONES
BONES

IA of FQ:
1. Enhance plasma level of
   Theophylline
   Caffeine
   Warfarin

WTC = World Trade Centre

2. Enhance CNS toxicity by NSAIDs.
3. Absorption of FQ is reduced by antacid and iron salts.

U of ciprofloxacin   CUT The GERMS
1. Chancroid (alternative to cotrimoxazole)
2. UTI
3. TB
4. Typhoid (**DOC** even in chloramphenicol resistant case)
5. Gonorrhoea
6. Enteritis and eye infection
7. RTI
8. Meningitis (though CSF penetration is not good)
9. Septicemia and skin infection (Bone infection also). In septicemia, ciprofloxacin is combined with aminoglycoside/cephalosporin of 3rd generation.
10. Norfloxacin is used in UTI, diarrhoea, etc.

Gatifloxacin: It is a **newer fluoroquinolone** effective against **Gram +ve, Gram –ve** and **anaerobic** bacteria, **mycoplasma** and **intracellular organisms**. It is **synthetic, broad spectrum methoxy FQ** having a unique **8-methoxy structure** that appears to enhance **bactericidal** action and reduces the rate of development of resistance of Gram +ve, Gram –ve and anaerobic bacteria. Newer quinolones (moxifloxacin and gatifloxacin) are safe and effective treatment for CAP. Newer FQs have enhanced activity against Gram +ve and anaerobes. Gatifloxacin and sparfloxacin have enhanced activity against **MRSA**.

Mech: Inhibits bacterial **topoisomerase II (DNA gyrase)** and **topoisomerase IV** which are essential for **duplication, transcription** and **repair** of bacterial DNA.

PK: Well absorbed **orally** (not effected by food).
Peak plasma concentration → **1–2 hrs** after dosing.

Absolute bioavailability—**96%**.
Distributed widely to **most target tissues**.
(concentration higher in tissues than serum).
Protein binding **20%** (independent of conc). **80% excreted** unchanged in urine through glomerular filtration and tubular secretion.
Elimination t½ → **7–14 hrs** (independent of dose and route). Renal clearance is independent on dose and is reduced in renal insufficiency.
Route: Oral and IV dose—interchangeable **(bioequivalent)**.
Drug metabolism in liver is **<1%**.
Longer t½ than ciprofloxacin, hence longer duration of action than ciprofloxacin.
Same PK and antimicrobial properties through **oral/IV** route. Now banned due to toxicity.

IA: Free from clinically important drug interactions.

> **Gatifloxacin highlights**
>
> Extremely broad spectrum of antibacterial activity.
> Longer half-life than most other quinolones and hence longer action.
> Single daily dosing ensures better patient compliance.
> Oral and interavenous dosages are bioequivalent.
> Quick onset of action—peak plasma concentrations occur 1–2 hours after oral administration.
> A higher C max (3.79) resulting in faster action.
> Low protein binding (only about 20%).
> Higher MICs than most other quinolones.
> Minimal hepatic metabolism (less than 1% is metabolized in the liver) and hence the action is not affected by liver dysfunction.
> It has an extremely good bioavailability (96%) and hence is reliable in its action. Longer postantibiotic effect.
> Effective against all respiratory pathogens.
> Low incidence of side effects and good patient safety profile.
> Hinders resistance mechanism to quinolones.

MIC of gatifloxacin

<0.25 mg against most micro-organism. It has **lowest MIC** against respiratory pathogens and **least MIC** against anaerobes as compared to ciprofloxacin.

U: Dose: 400 mg OD for 7–10 days.
1. Acute sinusitis
   Acute pyelonephritis
   Acute exacerbation of chronic bronchitis
   Community Acquired pneumonia (CAP)

   Commonest cause of CAP: Legionella, S. pneumoniae, H. influenzae, Mycoplasma

   Longitudinal **SHM**

   Gatifloxacin is active against **all RT** infection. Success in CAP—**96%**.

2. UTI
3. Gonorrhoea   **AUG**

Trovafloxacin: Newer FQ. Active against most anaerobes.

PK: T½ is **10 hrs**, hence OD is given up to 14 days only. **23%** is conjugated with **glucuronide** and excreted in urine. **63%** is excreted in faeces as mixture of metabolites and unchanged drug.

ADR of newer FQ

1. **Trovafloxacin: Similar** ADR profile as FQ
   A. GI intolerance and hepatotoxicity
   B. Dizziness
   C. Insomnia
2. **Grepafloxacin**
   A. Taste perversion
   B. Prolongation of QTc interval
3. **Levofloxacin**
   A. Diarrhoea
   B. Nausea

Disease/causative organism	First choice (DOC)	
1. **Gonorrhoea** Nonpenicillinase producing	Amoxycillin 3 g oral or Ampicillin 3.5 g oral, or Proc. Pen G 4.8 MU IM	+ Probenecid 1 g oral
Penicillinase producing	Ceftriaxone 250 mg IM or Cefuroxime 250 mg IM	+ Probenecid 1 g oral
2. **Syphilis** Early (primary, secondary and latent <1 yr) Late (>1 yr)	Benzathine Pen. 2.4 MU IM, 1–3 weekly inj. or Proc. Pen. G 1.2 MU IM × 10 days Benzathine Pen. 2.4 MU IM weekly × 4 weeks, or Proc. Pen. G 1.2 MU IM × 20 days	
3. *Chlamydia trachomatis* Nonspecific urethritis Lymphogranuloma venereum	Tetracycline 500 mg QID × 7 days oral, or Doxycycline 100 mg BD × 7 days oral -do- for 2 weeks (aspirate fluctuent lymph node)	
4. **Granuloma inguinale/ Donovanosis** (*Calymmatobacterium granulomatis*)	Tetracycline 500 mg QID × 10 days oral, or Doxycycline 100 mg BD × 3 days oral	
5. **Chancroid** (*H. ducreyi*)	Cotrimoxazole 960 mg BD × 7 days oral, or Erythromycin 500 mg QID × 7 days oral	
6. **Genital Herpes simplex** Early cases Late cases Recurrent cases	Acyclovir 5% oint. locally 6 times a day × 10 days (does not prevent recurrence) Acyclovir 200 mg 5 times a day × 10 days oral Acyclovir 200 mg 3–5 times a day for 6 months	
7. *Trichomonas vaginalis*	Metronidazole 2 g single dose or 400 mg TDS × 7 days, or Tinidazole 2 g single dose or 600 mg OD × 7 days (treat the male partner also if recurrent)	

Causes	DOC
1. *H. ducreyi*	Bactrim/erythromycin
2. *C. trachomatis*	Tetracycline/doxycycline
3. Syphilis	Penicillin
4. Gonorrhoea	Penicillin/ceftriaxone + probenecid 1 gm OD
5. *C. granulomatis*	Tetracycline/doxycycline
6. Genital HSV	Acyclovir
7. *Trichomonas vaginitis*	Metronidazole (tinidazole)

56. Antitubercular and Antileprotic Drugs

> 6 million Indians suffer from TB; 6 million children never see the school. 6 million women have only one saree and they die for political fool.

33% world's population is infected with *M. tuberculosis*. **Commonest** health problem in India is pulmonary TB.

Classification

A. **First line drugs** (high efficacy with low toxicity):
   Pyrazinamide (Z)
   Ethambutol (E)   **PERIS**
   Rifampin (R)
   Isoniazid (INH)/iso-nicotinic acid hydrazide (H).
   Streptomycin (S)

B. **Second line drugs:** (low efficacy and high toxicity):
   Amikacin, azithromycin   **A ROCK**
   Rifabutin
   Ofloxacin
   Ciprofloxacin, capreomycin, clarithromycin
   Kanamycin

Tuberculostatic

PAS (para-aminobenzoic acid)   **PET**
Ethambutol
Thiacetazone
Ethionamide
Cycloserine

Isoniazid/INH (iso-nicotinic acid hydrazide)/(H)

The **most** widely used antitubercular drug. **Safe** in pregnancy. **Cidal** for rapid growing and **static** for slow growing acting extracellularly/intracellularly (macrophage) and **equally** in both acidic and basic medium.

Cheapest drug for TB, and ineffective for **most atypical** bacteria.

Resistance: Developed rapidly due to **mutation.**

Mech: Inhibits **nucleic acid, glycolysis, lipid membrane** and **mycolic acid** of cell wall.

PK: Completely absorbed and distributed to **all tissues** and **all sites** of infection. **Acetylation** in the liver is the **most** important pathway of INH metabolism.
35% Indians are fast acetylators →t½—1 hr (causes hepatitis).
65% Indians are slow acetylators →t½—3 hrs (causes peripheral neuritis due to competition of INH with **pyridoxine for apotryptophanase** enzyme). Excreted in **urine.**

IA:
1. Al(OH)$_3$ inhibits absorption.
2. INH inhibits phenytoin, diazepam, warfarin and carbamazepine.
3. Only INH Increases phenytoin level (most drugs reduce phenytoin level).

ADR:
1. Peripheral neuritis due to loss of pyridoxine (**commonest**). Pyridoxine (vitamin B$_6$) 10 mg/day prophylactically inhibits neurotoxicity and 100 mg/day is the treatment.
2. Hepatitis: Toxicity is due to toxic metabolites (**acetyl isoniazide**). Alcohol and barbiturate induce CYP450 causing hepatitis.

> **INH** = **I**njures **N**erves and **H**epatocytes.

3. Reduced Ab response.
4. Thrombocytopenia.

ADR of ISONICOTINIC ACID HYDRAZIDE

Inhibition of parahydroxylation of phenytoin, **S**tupor, **O**totoxic (tinnitus), **N**ecrosis of liver due to acetyl hydrazine (metabolite), **I**mpaired memory, **C**ommonest (peripheral neuritis especially paresthesia), **O**ptic neuritis and atrophy, **T**emperature raised (1–2%), **I**ncreased glucose in overdose, **N**europathy (slow acetylator), **I**dea and reality separation, **C**ontrol on one-self lost, **A**nemia, **C**oncentration of plasma aspartate and alanine transaminase activities Increas**D**, **H**epatitis, **Y**ellow (Jaundice), **D**istress (epigastric), **R**ash 2%, **A**rthralgia and shoulder hand syndrome, diz**ZI**ness, **D**ecreased platelet, **E**ruption and eosinophilia.

U:
1. TB.
2. Only agent used as solo-prophylaxis against TB. In renal failure, INH is given 3 times weekly in the dose of 300 mg.

Rifampicin/rifampin: It is **semisynthetic** derivative of refamycin B obtained from *S. mediterranei*. Bactericidal.

Efficacy **same** as INH and better than other drugs. Effects both organism residing intracellularly/extracellularly.

It is the only antitubercular drug for **dormant bacilli** in caseous lesion.

Ceftriaxone and rifampin are **least** nephotoxic drugs.

Mech:
1. **Bactericidal** action
2. Inhibits β-subunit of DNA dependent **RNA polymerase** enzyme → RNA synthesis is reduced.

PK: Absorbed orally, widely distributed goes through **enterohepatic** circulation, t½ → 2–5 hrs, excreted mainly in **bile.**

IA:
1. Enhances elimination of HIV protease inhibitors, anticoagulants and methadone.

Pharmacology Review

2. Microsomal enzyme inducer (enhances its own metabolism and warfarin, steroid, digoxin, sulfonylurea and OC metabolism).
3. **Most** drugs reduce phenytoin level except INH (increases phenytoin level).

ADR:
1. **Orange** colour of tears, sweat and urine. Secretion is **orange-red**. ADR is **same** as INH.
2. Hepatotoxic, Influenza like illness, Nephrotoxic   **INH**
3. Syndromes
   Cutaneous
   Abdominal   **SCARF**
   Respiratory
   Flu-like
4. Haemolysis
5. Shock
6. Renal failure but **least** nephrotoxic

Rifampin's	4Rs

RNA polymerase inhibitor
Revs up microsomal P450
Red/orange body fluid
Rapid resistance if used alone

ADR of RIFAMPICIN: **R**ash (most common), **I**njury to liver, **F**ever, **A**nemia and acute tubular necrosis, **M**icrosomal enzyme induction, **P**latelet loss, **I**nterstitial nephritis, **C**NS (fatigue, ataxia, numbness, loss of conc), **I**g light chain proteinuria, **N**eonate (crosses placenta), **S**kin sensitive and gut upset.

U: In patient, TB bacilli exists in **3 pools**
   A. Metabolically extracellular pool
   B. Metabolically intracellular pool
   C. Necrotic caseous pool

Rifampin is **the only cidal drug** active against **all the 3 pools.**

INH and streptomycin are **cidal** against metabolically extracellular active organism. INH and pyrazinamide are cidal for intracellular organism. Rifampin is the drug active against **dormant** bacilli in caseous lesion.

Uses are
1. TB (taken before breakfast due to solubility in organic solvent and water at acidic pH).
2. Leprosy: It delays resistance to DDS.
3. Prophylaxis of meningitis and *H. influenzae*.
4. MRSA and diphtheroids: Second choice.
5. Brucellosis (**DOC**)
6. Systemic fungal infection.

Ethambutol: It is **static** for rapid growing bacteria.
Mech: Inhibits **mycolic acid** and **RNA synthesis**.
PK: 3/4 absorbed orally. Widely distributed but poorly crosses BBB.

Temporarily accumulated in **RBC**.
<50% metabolised. Plasma t½—4 hrs.
Renal excretion by glomerular filtration and tubular secretion.

ADR:
1. Optic neuritis (**commonest**): Dose and duration dependent. Impairs red green vision and causes field defects (reversible).
2. Hyperuricemia, rash and neuropathy.

ADR of ETHAMBUTOL
Exfoliative dermatitis, rash, pruritis, **T**emperature raised, **H**allucination, **A**naphylaxis (rare), **M**ost important (optic neuritis), **B**lood (leukopenia), **U**rate in blood raised, **T**ingling **o**f **L**imb/fingers.

CI: Child <12 yrs.

Thiacetazone (Tzn/amithiozone): Cheap, bacteriostatic, inhibits emergence of resistance.

PK: Orally active. Excreted unchanged in urine. t½—12 hrs. **Dose:** 2.5 mg/kg OD.

ADR:
1. Hepatitis
2. Exfoliative dermatitis
3. Stevens-Johnson syndrome
4. Bone marrow depression

PAS (para-aminosalicylic acid): Chemistry and mechanism same as sulfonamide. Least active antitubercular drug. **Tuberculostatic**

PK: Distributed **all over the body except** CSF.
50% **acetylated,** t½—1 hr, excreted in urine.

ADR:
1. Goitre
2. Liver dysfunction
3. Blood dyscrasias

Ethionamide (Etm): Tuberculostatic of moderate efficacy. Acts both on **extracellular** organism and **intracellular** organism. Sensitive to **atypical** mycobacteria.

PK: Absorbed orally, distributed to **all tissues,** t½—2–3 hrs, dose—1 mg/day.

ADR:
1. Abdominal intolerance
2. Hepatitis
3. Mental disturbance
4. Impotence

Cycloserine: Obtained from *S. orchidaceus*. **Tuberculostatic.**

Mech: It is analogue of D-alanine (inhibits cell wall synthesis by inhibiting enzyme recemizing L-alanine).

PK: Absorbed orally, distributed to **all tissues, 2/3** excreted unchanged in urine. CSF concentration is **equal** to plasma concentration 33% metabolised.

ADR: CNS toxicity (treated by **pyridoxine** 100 mg/day).

Pyrazinamide (Z): **Most** effective against slow growing intracellular bacilli. **Weakly cidal,** active in **acid,** cross-resistance is **absent, resistance develops rapidly when used alone.**

PK: Absorbed orally, CSF penetration is **maximum,** t½ →6–10 hrs.

> Pyrazinamide **P**enetrates **C**SF

ADR:
1. Hepatotoxicity (**commonest**)
2. Loss of DM control
3. Hyperuricemia (gout)

Drugs causing hyperuricemia
A. Aspirin
B. Diuretics (thiazide, furosemide, ethacrynic acid, chlorthalidone)
C. Pyrazinamide
D. Cytotoxic drugs

CI:
1. Liver disease
2. Corticosteroid is used in TB and AIDS + TB but is contraindicated in intestinal TB due to causing **silent perforation.**

Treatment of TB: At least **two drugs** are used to prevent resistance:

INH 300 mg OD
+ Rifampin 600 mg OD } for 9–12 months

This combination is **most effective** with the synergistic effect and **99%** cure rate. **Most experts** advice addition of third drug (ethambutol or pyrazinamide) in initial treatment.

INH 300 mg OD + thiacetazone 150 mg OD for 12–18 months is the **cheapest regimen** with **80–90%** cure rate.

INH 300 mg OD + ethambutol 15 mg/kg OD for 12–18 months is **the least toxic regimen** and **safest** in pregnancy. HRZ and E are safe to foetus and 2 HRZ + 4 HR are given for 6 months in TB of pregnancy. **Strongest** risk factor for latent TB is AIDS. **Regimen for AIDS with TB:** Initial 2 HRZE + continuous 7 HR/4 HRE. For MAC in HIV, ethambutol + clarithromycin are the **most effective** regimen. In HIV positive, **rifabutin** is the lifelong prophylaxis. **Commonest** cause of drug resistance is patient's default. Relapse rate after successful antitubercular treatment (ATT) is <1%. Symptomatic relief occurs in **2–3 weeks** of ATT in **most patient.** X-ray findings disappear after about 4 months of ATT. Streptomycin + ethambutol is the regimen for **hepatitis.**

Chemoprophylaxis of TB: INH 5 mg/kg for 12 months is given in:
A. Nonvaccinated T. test positive child of <3 yrs.
B. Unvaccinated T. test positive.
C. Tuberculin sensitive
D. Immunosuppressed patient. INH for 6 months is given to infants of highly infectious patient.

Categorywise alternative treatment regimen for tuberculosis

TB category	Initial place (daily/3 × per week)	Continuation phase	Total duration
I	2 HRZE (S)	4 HR/4(HR)₃ or 6 HE	6 / 8
II	2 HRZES + 1 HRZE	5 HRE or 5 (HRE)₃	8 / 8
III	2 HRZ	4 HR/4(HR)₃ or 6 HE	6 / 8
IV	**Chronic case**		

A. 2 HRZE initially then 7 HR/4 HRE (**AIDS**)
B. **Most** effective regimen for MAC: E + clarithromycin/azithromycin
C. 12 RZE in **H** resistance
   ZE + S/E + Cipro/Ofl. in **HR** resistance   ZESECO
D. 2 HRZ + 4 HR (TB in **pregnancy**)
   BCG + INH prophylaxis for infant
E. S + E in hepatitis due to hepatotoxicity (**commonest** ADR and more frequent with HRZ regimen)

Resistance
```
    20  10   1% (primary)
    H   S   R
    50  25  25% (secondary)
```

2 (HRZE) 3 where 2 means **months**, and 3 means **thrice weekly**

Treatment category and sputum exam. in DOTS chemotherapy

Category I:	New smear +ve, seriously ill smear −ve or extrapulmonary	2 (HR ZE)₃ 4 (HR)₃	
Category II:	Smear +ve, relapse, failure, default 5 (HR E)₃	2 (HR ZES)₃ 1 (HR ZE)₃	ZE ZES, ZEE Z
Category III:	Smear +ve, not seriously ill, extrapulmonary	2 (HR Z)₃ 4 (HR)₃	

Standard drug regimen

2 HRZE — 2 PERI
4 HR — 4 RI   } 06 months

2 HRE — 2 ERI
7 HR — 7 RIs } 09 months

Twice weekly PIS
Daily   IT   } 12 months

P = Z
H = I
Tzn = T

IT IS Pyridoxine
Daily Twice weekly

12 months regimen is **inexpensive** and reasonably effective.

Twice weekly **P**yridoxine (100 mg OD), **I**NS and **S**treptomycin (**PIS**) is **100% effective** if primary resistance is absent and if INH + streptomycin is used in first 2–3 months.

INH + Thiacetazone is **80–95% effective** when taken daily for 12 months.

Dose: PERIS (=ZERHS) → P E S R I **(mg/kg/day OD)**
                              25 20 15 10 5

Antileprotic drugs

M. leprae (effects skin, mucous membrane and nerves) was discovered by **Hansen (1873)**, hence the disease is called Hansen's disease. **1/3 Leprosy** of the world is in India.

Nerves effected in leprosy are

A. All nerves of upper limb (ulnar, median, radial)
B. Post-tibial nerve
C. Lateral popliteal nerve
D. Facial nerve

Radial nerve (great extensor nerve) supplies to   **BEST**
    Brachioradialis
    Extensor of wrist and finger
    Supinator
    Triceps

Classification

A. Sulfones: Dapsone (DDS)
              Acedapsone (DA-DDS)
              Solapsone
              Sulfadoxine
B. Phenazine derivatives: Clofazimine
C. Antitubercular drugs: Rifampin
                               Ethionamide
                               Thiacetazone
D. Antibiotics: Clarithromycin
                               Ofloxacin
                             Minocycline

DDS: Though **most potent** drug for *M. leprae* is rifampin, **DDS is DOC.**

Cochrane **first** time used DDS in India. It was discovered by **Cockate (1941).** It is **cheapest, simplest, commonest** and **oldest antileprotic and is a 4,4-diamino diphenyl sulfone.** It is **most** effective (patients become non-infectious in 3 months). It is **cidal** at high doses and **static** at low doses like sulfonamide. Rifampin is the **fastest** acting cidal against *M. leprae* (patients become non-infectious in 3 months).

Mech: Same as sulfonamide (inhibition of PABA incorporation into folic acid). Sulfone (DDS) is PABA analogue that reduces **folic acid** synthesis.

PK: Completely absorbed orally. Widely distributed in the body.

70% plasma protein bound. Concentrated in lepromatous skin, muscle, liver, kidney.

                      LEpromatous = LEthal

Acetylated, glucuronide and **sulfate** conjugated in liver, excreted in bile and ultimately in urine.
t½—>24 hrs. Dose—1–2 mg/day.

ADR: 1. Tolerated up to 100 mg/day but causes **anaemia** (haemolytic) in G6PD deficient which is **commonest** and **the most important.**
2. Methaemoglobinemia
3. Hepatitis
4. Gastric intolerance
5. Cutaneous reaction

CI: 1. **Anaemia (Hb <7 gm%)**
2. Sensitive person.

U: DMRD—AIIMS
1. Dermatitis herpetiformis
2. Madura foot, malaria of chloroquine resistance.
3. Rhinosporidiosis
4. Dermatitis artifecta
5. Actinomycosis and Hansen's disease
(In malaria DDS + pyrimethamine is given).

Clofazimine (CLO): Leprostatic. Lipophilic: Anti-inflammatory.
Mech: Inhibits template function of DNA.
PK: 40–70% absorbed orally.
Deposited in skin, fat, monocyte, macrophage and gut in crystalline form, t½—70 days, dose—50–200 mg/day.

ADR: 1. Skin: Clo disColourises
Reddish black discolouration of skin, urine and sweat.
Phototoxicity: Eruption.
Conjunctival pigmentation, discolouration of hair and body secretion.
2. GIT: Enteritis.
Late syndrome (deposition of crystal in intestinal submucosa).

CI: Kidney and ⎫
    Liver   ⎬ Damage   KLPD
    Pregnancy ⎭

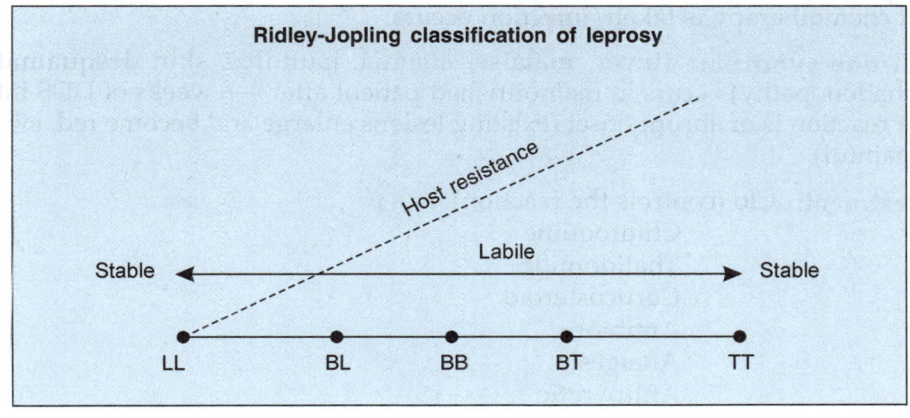

Ridley-Jopling classification of leprosy

Based on immunity of host

Tuberculoid leprosy (TT): Causes early, severe but localised deformity.
Lepromatous leprosy (LL): Causes late, mild and widely spread deformity.
Most severely deformed patient is borderline patient (BT, BB, BL) with **Lepra/Type I reaction.**

Paucibacillary leprosy (PBL)

A. TT: Lepromatous test positive. **CMI normal,** polar type.
   Anaesthetic patch. Causes early, severe but localised deformity.
B. BT
C. I (intermediate)

Multibacillary leprosy (MBL)

A. LL: Diffuse skin and mucous membrane infiltration. Nodules, polar type **CMI absent.** Lepromatous test negative. Causes late, mild and wide deformity.
B. BL

For **all forms,** only DDS is used.
MDT (multidrug therapy) is the **regimen of choice for all** cases of leprosy due to:
  a. Effectiveness in primary DDS resistance.
  b. Prevention of emergence of DDS resistance.
  c. Rapid symptomatic relief.

For MBL (2 yrs):   DDS 100 mg/day   **DR CM**
                       Rifampin 600 mg/month
                       Clo 50 mg/day

For PBL (6 months): DDS 100 mg/day   **DR**
                       Rifampin 600 mg/month

Alternative regimens: Clo (50 mg/day) + Ofl 400 mg/minocycline 100 mg/clarithromycin 500 mg daily (any two) for 6 months followed by Clo (50 mg/day) + any one of Ofl 400 mg/minocycline 100 mg daily for 18 months. Resistance to Clo is **absent.**

All *M. leprae* isolated from relapse cases are fully sensitive to rifampin.

Lepra reaction II: In LL, Jarisch-Herxheimer (arthus) type of reaction takes place due to release of **Ag from killed bacilli** and causes **erythema nodosum leprosum** when chemotherapy is taken/infection occurs.

Sulfone syndrome (fever, malaise, anemia, jaundice, skin desquamation, lymphadenopathy) occurs in malnourished patient after 4–6 weeks of DDS intake. Lepra reaction is of abrupt onset (existing lesions enlarge and become red, swollen and painful).

Treatment: Clo (controls the reaction)
              Chloroquine
              Thalidomide
              Corticosteroid
              Antibiotic
              Analgesic
              Antipyretic

Reversal reaction/leprae reaction I: In TT, delayed hypersensitivity to *M. leprae* Ag causes neuropathy and cutaneous ulceration.
Treatment: Corticosteroid and clofazimine.

Type 1
Seen in 1 condition = Borderline
Due to 1 mechanism = Hypersensitivity (CMI)
Responds to 1 drug = Corticosteroid
Type 2 (DOC = Thalidomide):
Seen in 2 conditions = Borderline and lepromatous
Due to 2 mechanism = Arthus phenomena and immune complex
Responds to 2 C = Corticosteroid and Clofazimine.

Adverse effect of first line anti-tubercular drugs
1. **INH: I**nsanity, i.e. psychosis, **N**euritis, **H**epatitis.
2. **RIF**ampicin: **R**ed discolouration of urine, **I**nduction of liver enzymes and its toxicity, **F**lu-like symptoms.
3. **P**yrazinamide: **P**ain in the joints which may also be gout due to hyperuricemia (**P**lus hepatotoxicity).
4. **E**thambutol: **E**ye toxicity—field defects, loss of visual acuity and colour vision.
5. **S**treptomycin: **S**imilar to all aminoglycosides, i.e. nephro-neuro-ototoxicity.

Most important side-effect of antileprotic drugs (C, D, E)
1. **C**lofazimine: **C**utaneous discolouration, e.g. on **C**heeks is **C**osmetically unacceptable, is a **D**ye with **D**ual action (bacteriostatic and anti-inflammatory) and causes **D**ryness of skin and **D**iscolouration of body cover.
2. **D**apsone: **D**egradation of RBCs (due to methemoglobinemia).
3. **E**thionamide: **E**mesis.

57
Antimalarial Drugs

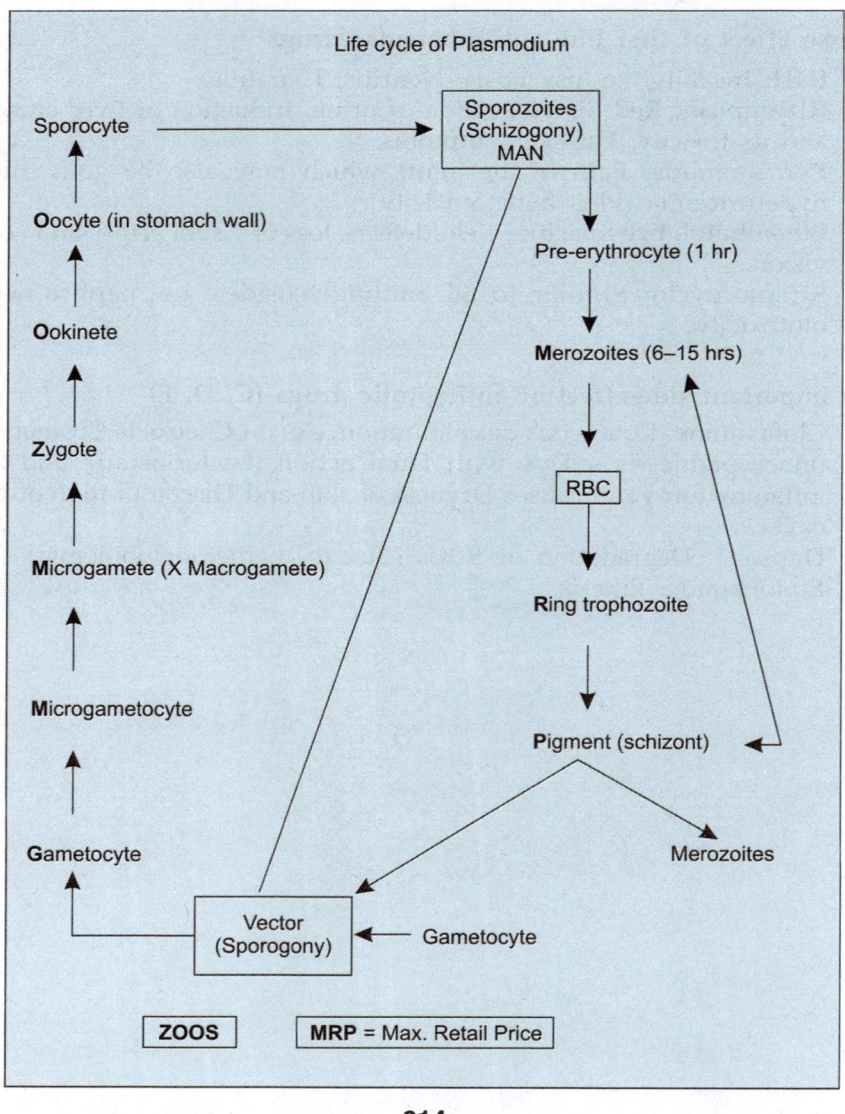

Antimalarial Drugs

Classification

1. **4-A**minoquinoline: Chloroquine, amodiaquine
2. **8-A**minoquinoline: Primaquine, bulaquine
3. **A**cridine: Mepacrine (quinacrine, atabrine)
4. **B**iguanides: Chloroguanide (proguanil)
5. **C**inchona alkaloid: Quinine
6. **Q**uinoline–methanol: Mefloquine
7. **D**iaminopyrimidines: Pyrimethamine
   Trimethoprim
8. **S**ulfonamide and Sulfone: DDS
   Sulfadoxine
   Sulfamethopyrazine
9. **T**etracycline: Tetracycline, doxycycline
10. **N**ewer drugs: Halofantrine, pyronaridine, Artemisinin (artesunate, artemether and artether), atovaquone

ABC Quinine TDS

Objectives of drugs: Are to prevent/treat/eradicate/reduce infection.

Uses:
1. **Causal prophylaxis** (pre-erythrocytic phase in liver): **Primaquine** is causal prophylaxis for **all species** of malaria, and kills **sporozoites** within infected liver cells. **Dose:** 0.5 mg/kg. but it is toxic.
   Other drugs are **pyrimethamine** and **proguanil.**
2. **Suppressive prophylaxis** (erythrocytic schizogony is blood schizonticides):
   Mefloquine (250 mg/week) is for chloroquine resistant *P. falciparum*. Other drugs are quinine, pyrimethamine, proguanil, amodiaquine. In **pregnancy,** prophylaxis is given after Ist trimester.
3. **Gametocidal: Primaquine** (0.75 mg/kg) for **all plasmodia.**
   Chloroquine acts against *P. vivax* and *P. ovale*. Quinine and mepacrine acts against *P. vivax*. Pyrimethamine and proguanil acts against **all stages** of Plasmodium.
4. **Radical cure** (exoerythrocytic phase/hypnozoites): In **relapsing** malaria *(P. vivax/P. ovale)*, primaquine **15** mg OD for 2 weeks/**15** days (DOC) is given. **Relapse of vivax/ovale** is treated like primary attack.
5. **Suppressive cure:** Pyrimethamine 25 mg/chloroquine 300 mg is given weekly for 10 weeks, after leaving endemic area.
6. **Clinical cure** (erythrocytic schizonticide): **One of the following regimen is used.**
   Fast acting high efficacy drugs (for *P. falciparum/P. falciparum* resistant):
   A. Quinine 8 mg/kg TDS for 7 days
   B. Chloroquine 600 mg stat + 300 mg after 8 hrs + 300 mg OD for next 7 days.
   C. Mefloquine
   D. Mepacrine 15 mg/kg single dose
   E. Halofantrine

F. Artemisinin 4 mg/kg on first day followed by 2 mg/kg for 5 days (OD).
Artesunate (IV/IM) 2 mg/kg on first day followed by 1 mg/kg for 4 days.
Artemether (IM) 2 mg/kg for 5 days.

Slow acting low efficacy drugs
A. Chloroquine 600 mg stat followed by 300 mg after 8 hrs and 300 mg OD for next two days (DOC).
B. Pyrimethamine 25 mg + sulfonamide 500 mg single dose for chloroquine resistant cases.

Chloroquine: Chloroquine resistant to *P. vivax* was **first** reported in 1989 in Papua New Guinea. Amodiaquine is **similar** to chloroquine.

Mech: 1. Rapidly acting erythrocytic schizonticide (**ring stage**) against **all species** of plasmodia but does not inhibit **relapses** in *P. ovale* and *P. vivax*.
Active against **gametocytes** of *P. vivax, P. ovale* and *P. malariae*.
2. *P. falciparum* resistant is due to reduced ability of the parasite to accumulate chloroquine. **Verapamil** restores both concentrating ability and sensitivity to this drug.
3. Acts on **all Plasmodium infected RBC except** chloroquine resistant *P. falciparum*.
4. **Commonest** schizonticide and 4-aminoquinoline. Inhibits DNA and RNA synthesis.
5. 50% remission in RA (inhibits B lymphocyte due to decrease in monocyte IL-I).

PK: 50% plasma protein bound. Has high affinity for **melanin nuclear chromatin.** Good oral absorption. Concentrated in liver, spleen, kidney, retina, lungs, leucocytes and skin. **Route**—oral/IM/IV. Partly hepatic metabolism, slowly excreted in urine, $t_{½}$ →3–10 days.

ADR: 1. **On chronic use:** corneal opacity, retinal damage and myopathy due to drug accumulation in retina and tissues (**most disturbing**).
2. Ototoxicity, bitter taste and hypotension due **to CVS depression (common). Parenteral route causes CNS toxicity** and **cardiac depression.**
3. **Acute ADR:** CNS toxicity, uncontrollable itching, GI intolerance, headache.
4. Graying of hair, rashes.

ADR of **CHLOROQUINE** (concentrates in lysosome of phagocytic cells):
Anemia, **C**orneal deposits, **H**ypotension (arrhythmia and cardiac depression), **L**ichenoid skin eruption, **O**totoxicity, **R**etinopathy (bulls eye), **O**ver the top (gray hair), **Q**RS wide, **U**rticaria, **I**ncreased seizures, **N**ail discoloured, **E**rythematous rash.

Caution: 1. Liver damage
2. GIT disease
3. Neuropathy
4. Haematological disease

CI:	1. Psoriasis
	2. Porphyria
	3. Parenteral route in chlidern → convulsion and death.
U:	**(Safe in pregnancy)** My DEAR

1. Suppressive prophylaxis and clinical cure of **all types of malaria except** caused by resistant *P. falciparum* **(DOC).**
2. **Falciparum** and **cerebral malaria with coma:** CVS ADR is due to **parenteral** route, but prevented by slow IV infusion → 10 mg/kg in 5% **dextrose** infused over 8 hrs followed by 15 mg/kg infused over 24 hrs. Then **oral** route is adopted.
   (3 mg/kg 6 hourly IM is also adopted).
3. **D**LE and SLE
4. **E**xtraintestinal amoebiasis, giardiasis, taeniasis.
5. Rheumatoid **A**rthritis (50% remission)
6. **R**eaction (lepra and photogenic)
7. Infectious **M**ononucleosis

Mefloquine: It is for suppressive prophylaxis/multiresistant *P. falciparum*.
Most effective drug for chloroquine resistant *P. falciparum*.
Mech: Rapidly acting **erythrocytic schizonticide but slower** than chloroquine and quinine.

PK:	Oral absorption. Accumulated in liver, lung and intestine. Hepatic metabolism. t½ → 2–3 weeks due to enterohepatic circulation and its tissue binding. Secreted in bile. **Only antimalarial excreted in faeces.** No parenteral preparation of mefloquine.
IA:	1. Halofantrine/Quinidine/Quinine+Mefloquine cause **QTc lengthening.**
	2. CCB/β blocker/digitalis/antidepressant + mefloquine cause bradycardia/arrhythmia.
ADR:	1. **Encephalitis** and **neuropsychiatric** reaction (disturbed sense of balance, ataxia, anxiety, strange dream, hallucination) are **serious ADR.**
	2. Bitter taste, diarrhoea, vomiting nausea, abdominal pain.
	3. Sinus bradycardia
	4. Hepatic and cutaneous toxicity

ADR of Mefloquine
Motor function altered
Eye dysfunction, emesis
Frequently (diarrhoea, dysphoria, dizziness)
Loss of consciousness
Ototoxicity (mild)
Quinine + mefloquine contraindicated
Unusual psychotic problem
Increased seizures
Nausea
Encephalopathy

CI: Safe in pregnancy but is avoided in first trimester.
U: 1. Multiresistant *P. falciparum*. 15 mg/kg (max 1 gm) single dose.
2. Prophylaxis of malaria among travellers to areas with MDR (5 mg/kg).

Mepacrine: More toxic and less effective than chloroquine.
Mech: Erythrocytic schizonticide.
ADR: 1. Cramps
2. Vertigo and psychosis
3. **Skin** and **eye discolouration** on chronic use.
CI: 1. Pregnancy
2. Psoriasis
3. Along with primaquine
U: 1. Malaria: 600 mg/week for prophylaxis. 3 gm over 6 days for clinical cure.
2. Giardia
3. Tapeworm

Quinine: It is the **levorotatory alkaloid** of cinchona bark. Its **d**-isomer quini**d**ine is antiarrhythmic and antianginal.
Mech: 1. **Erythrocytic schizonticide for all species of plasmodia** (less effective and more toxic than chloroquine)
2. Though mechanism is not known, it accumulates in **acidic vacuole** and causes pigment changes, possibly by inhibiting **heme polymerase**.
3. It acts as **"General protoplasmic poison"** acting on **all living cells** causing pain + necrosis + fibrosis of muscle, thrombosis of vein and paralysis of nerves due to local irritant and anaesthetic action.
4. Reduces skeletal muscle power, enhances gastric secretion, depresses CNS and CVS, releases insulin causing **hypoglycaemia** and stimulates myometrium causing abortion (hence **contraindicated**).
PK: Complete oral absorption. 70% plasma protein bound. Low CSF penetration, hepatic metabolism, renal excretion, t½ →10–12 hrs, noncumulative.

ADR (CINCHONISM)
Common (hypoglycaemia, cinchonism, bitter taste), **I**schaemic retinal vessel, **N**eurotoxic (8th CN), **C**olour perception disturbed, **O**totoxic, **N**ight blindness. diarrhoea, **I**nsulin level raised, **S**kin hot and flushed (**M**ost common). Hypotension and arrhythmia. Haemolysis and thrombocytopenia.

Cinchonism: It is due to large single doses (ringing of ears, nausea, vomiting due to gastric irritation and CTZ stimulation, confusion, vertigo, headache, loss of hearing and vision due to neurotoxicity and retinal plus auditory vasoconstriction, diarrhoea, flushing and perspiration) and subsides on stopping the drug. Poisoning at higher doses additionally causes delirium, fever, respiratory depression, cyanosis and arrhythmia + hypotension leading to **death**. Haemolysis and hence haemoglobinuria (**black water fever**) plus kidney damage specially during pregnancy and falciparum malaria occur.

Hypersensitive person develops rashes, **itching**, purpura, angioedema and bronchospasm.

CI: Pregnancy (due to abortion)
U: 1. Nucturnal muscle cramp
2. Myasthenia gravis diagnosis (single dose causes weakness in myasthenia gravis)
3. Septicidal
4. Varicose vein (thrombosis and fibrosis)
5. **Cerebral malaria** (*P. falciparum* with impaired consciousness): **Quinine (DOC) 600 mg (10 mg/kg) diluted in 5% glucose (200–500 ml)** solution and infused over 2–3 hrs and repeated every 8 hrs till consciousness then the patient is switched over to oral therapy to complete 7 days course.
Hypoglycaemia (most important ADR due to hyperinsulinemia) is prevented by **5% dextrose** infusion. Cooling of fever, IV diazepam for convulsion, correction of fluid, electrolyte balance and acidosis are instituted.
6. Resistant falciparum malaria: Acts more rapidly than pyrimethamine + sulfadoxine. After schizonticidal action of quinine, parasitemia clearance is achieved by slower acting drugs.

Regimens are

A. Quinine (3 days) + sulfadoxine 1500 mg single dose + pyrimethamine 75 mg.
B. Quinine (3 days) + tetracycline 250 mg QID × 7 days/doxycycline 100 mg OD × 7 days (for complicated malaria).

Treatment of malaria

A. **Signet ring *P. vivax***
Radical: Primaquine 15 mg × 5 days + chloroquine 600 mg single dose.
High doses: Primaquine 15 mg × 5 days + chloroquine 600 mg first day, then 600 mg 2nd day and 300 mg 3rd day

B. ***P. falciparum***
Presumptive: Chloroquine 600 mg single dose (adult).
Radical: First day chloroquine 600 mg + primaquine 45 mg.
Second day chloroquine 600 mg. Third day chloroquine 300 mg.
Resistant case: Pyrimethamine 50 mg + sulphalene 1 gm + primaquine 45 mg.
If again resistance: 1. Quinine 1800 mg × 7 days, or
2. Quinine 1800 mg × 3 days + tetracycline 1–2 gm × 7 days, or
3. Mefloquine 750 mg + pyrimethamine 750 mg + sulfadoxine 1500 mg + primaquine 45 mg.

Chloroguanide/proguanil: Erythrocytic schizonticide.
Mech: 1. Schizonticide.
2. **Cyclysed** in body to cycloguanil →inhibits plasmodial **DHFRase**.
PK: Absorbed from gut, partly metabolised.
Renal excretion, t½ → 16–20 hrs.
ADR: 1. **Megaloblastic anemia (in renal failure).**

    2. Mouth ulcer
    3. Renal loss
    4. Stomatitis
    5. Hematuria
    6. Rashes
    7. Transient hair loss
U: Causal prophylaxis

Pyrimethamine: Action **similar** to chloroguanide but it is more potent.
Mech:
1. Slowly acting erythrocytic schizonticide.
2. Inhibits **DHFRase** and has **2000 times** greater affinity for plasmodial enzyme but poor action on bacterial DHFRase.
3. Acts on **mature form (blood stage)**
4. Inhibits *T. gondii*

Resistance: It is by **mutation** in DHFRase.

PK: Absorbed from gut. Accumulated in lung, liver, kdiney, and spleen. Metabolised and excreted in urine with t½ of 4 days.
Duration of prophylactic concentration in blood is 2 weeks.

ADR:
1. Megaloblastic anemia
2. Granulocytopenia
3. Rashes

CI: Pregnancy and lactation

U:
1. Pyrimethamine + sulfonamide/DDS in attacks of malaria (**supradditive synergism** due to sequential block) and in *P. falciparum*.
2. Pyrimethamine +sulfadiazine: **DOC** in *T. gondii* of CMI reduced patient.
3. Chronic resistant *P. falciparum*:
   A. Fansidar = Pyrimethamine (t½—100 hrs) + sulfadoxine (t½—170 hrs).
   B. Maloprim = DDS + pyrimethamine.

Primaquine: Differs from **all other antimicrobial agents** due to effect on primary and secondary tissue phase of malaria parasite.

Mech:
1. Acts against pre-erythrocytic stage of *P. falciparum* than that of *P. vivax*.
2. Highly active against gametocyte and hypnozoites. **Gametocidal for all plasmodia.** Radical cure for *P. ovale* and *P. vivax* to eradicate exoerythrocytic stage. It is **the only drug** which eliminates tissue forms of parasite and is active on exoerythrocytic forms and gametes of *P. vivax* and *P. ovale*.

PK: Orally absorbed, hepatic oxidation, plasma t½ → 3–6 hrs. Renal excretion in 24 hrs.

ADR:
1. GI upset
2. Dose-related haemolysis, cyanosis and methemoglobinemia due to **oxidant property** of drug. But dose <60 mg produces no haemolysis. Haemolytic anemia occurs in G6PD deficient even with the dose of 15–30 mg/day. **Dark urine** indicates haemolysis. Risk of haemolysis is enhanced in RA, SLE and acutely ill.

ADR of PRIMAquine
Primarily in G6PD and NADH met Hb reductase deficiency
Raised BP
Increased HR
Methemoglobulinemia
Anemia.

CI:
1. Pregnancy because foetus is G6PD deficient.
2. Connective tissue disorder.

U:
1. Radical cure of relapsing malaria.
2. *P. falciparum*: 45 mg primaquine + chloroquine 300 mg kill gametes (give once a week for 10 weeks).

Artemisinin derivatives: Active against *P. falciparum* resistant to **all other** antimalarial drugs. They are sesquiterpine lactone of *A. annua*.

Mech:
1. **Artemisinin + heme** cause iron mediated cleavage of peroxide bridge and generation of organic **free radical** that binds to membrane protein resulting in damage to parasite.
2. Not kill hypnozoites but it is **schizonticide**.

PK: Prodrugs { Artesunate (t½ = <1 hr)
Artemether (t½ = 3–12 hrs) }
↓
Dihydroartemisinin

Dose: Artesunate (oral)—4 mg/kg 1st day + 2 mg/kg/day × 5 days.
Parenteral—2 mg/kg 1st day + 1 mg/kg × 4 days (IM).

ADR:
1. Itch and drug fever.
2. Abnormal bleeding and dark urine.
3. S-T segment changes and first degree AV block.
4. Neurotoxicity, QT prolongation.

U: Acute attack of multi-resistant *P. falciparum* (reserved drug).

Halofantrine: It is phenanthrene methanol blood schizonticide.

Active against *P. falciparum* resistant to chloroquine and sulfa-pyrimethamine and against *P. vivax*. Cure rate 84–97% with doses 8 mg/kg TDS.

Mech: **Same** as quinine.

PK: **Water insoluble.** Erratic orally (low oral absorption).

Plasma t½—24 hrs (drug).
Plasma t½—3 days (active metabolite).

ADR:
1. GI upset, diarrhoea.
2. Itching, rashes.
3. Serum transaminase elevation.
4. Prolongation of QTc interval, ventricular arrhythmia.

U: Multiresistant *P. falciparum*.

1. Antimalarial drugs acting on all stages of development of Plasmodium are **pyrimethamine** and **proguanil**.
2. Antimalarial drugs safely used in **pregnancy** are

   | CAP | Chloroquine
Amodiaquine
Proguanil |

3. Drugs causing **retinopathy** are chloroquine and phenothiazine (thioridazine).
4. Drugs causing **corneal opacities** are chloroquine, mepacrine, vitamin D and indomethacin.
5. Drugs causing **hypoglycaemia** are quinine, aspirin, pentamidine, propranolol, oral hypoglycaemic, insulin, etc.

Neuromuscular blocking antibiotics: Low ATP Clearance Lincomycin, Aminoglycoside, Tetracycline, Polypeptide antibiotic, Clindamycin.

Bulaquine: Developed in India like arteether.
Congener of primaquine. Antirelapse action in vivax (hence given with chloroquine for 5 days). Partly metabolised to primaquine.
CI and precaution: Same as primaquine.
Atovaquone: It is naphthoquinone.
Spectrum: Plasmodium (erythrocytic schizonticide), *T. gondii* and *P. carinii*.
Mech: Interferes with ATP production and collapses plasmodial mitochondrial membrane. Proguanil potentiates its action and inhibits resistance.
ADR: Diarrhoea, vomiting, rash, fever.
U: 1. *P. falciparum* and *P. vivax* (proguanil + atovaquone for 3 days orally).
2. *T. gondii* and *P. carinii* in AIDS.

Chloroquine resistance: It is due to CG_2 (altered chloroquine—transporter protein of parasite). Mostly low grade resistance (RI) is present in India. 8–16% is RII and RIII (1978–2002). Highest RII and RIII in N-E region of India (hence sulfa-pyrimethamine is preferred in NAMP). RI 16% and RII 6.7% in vivax has been reported from Bihar in 2000.

58

Antiprotozoal Agents

Classification
1. **Tissue amoebicides**
   A. For both intestinal and extraintestinal amoebiasis:
      a. Nitroimidazole : Tinidazole
         Nimorazole
         TN MOSS Metronidazole, Ornidazole
         Secnidazole, Satranidazole
      b. Alkaloid : Emetine
         Dehydroemetine
   B. For extraintestinal amoebiasis: Chloroquine
2. **Luminal amoebiasis**
   A. Amide: Diloxanide furoate.
   B. 8-hydroxyquinolines:
      Quiniodochlor (clioquinol, iodochlorohydroxyquin).
      Diiodohydroxyquin (iodoquinol)
   C. Antibiotic: Tetracycline

Metronidazole: Introduced in 1959.

Coverage: Protozoa (**cidal** activity)
Anaerobic bacteria
B. fragilis
C. perfringens
Fusobacterium
H. pylori
Streptococci.

Mech: 1. Diffuses into microorganism
↓
Reduction of nitro group
↓
Intermediate compound formation
↓
Damage of DNA
(cytotoxic action)

2. Interferes with **electron transport** from reduced substrate **(NADPH)**.
3. Inhibits **CMI** to induce **mutagenesis** and to cause **radiosensitization**.

PK: Completely absorbed from small intenstine. Widely distributed in the body attaining **therapeutic** concentration in CSF, saline, semen, and vaginal **secretion**. **Hepatic metabolism by oxidation** and **glucuronide conjugation**.

Renal excretion. Plasma t½—8 hrs.

ADR: Most common (anorexia, nausea, abdominal cramp, metallic taste, headache, dry mouth), Thrombophlebitis. Emesis, Rash, Occurrence of numbness/paraesthesia, Neuropathy, Increased PT, Disulfiram like rxn and diarrhoea, Abdominal stress, **Z(S)**ence of pelvic pressure, **O**nly temporary neutropenia, **L**ithium toxicity, **E**stablished ADR in first trimester.

METRONIDAZ(S)OLE

CI:
1. Chronic alcoholism
2. Blood dyscrasias
3. Neuropathy
4. Pregnancy (due to mutagenic potential, teratogenic effect **absent**).

IA:
1. Disulfiram like intolerance to alcohol.
2. Cimetidine reduces the metabolism of metronidazole.
3. Metronidazole reduces renal elimination of lithium.
4. Enzyme inducers (rifampin, phenobarbitone) reduce its therapeutic effect.

Uses:
1. Anaerobic infection. Colorectal/pelvic surgery. Appendicectomy, brain abscess and endocarditis.
2. *H. pylori*: Gastritis/peptic ulcer.
3. Infestation: Guinea worm
4. Nonspecific bacterial vaginosis
5. Amoebiasis: **DOC** for all amoebic infection.
   Dose: (invasive dysentery and liver abscess):
   800 mg TDS × 8 days.
   40 mg/kg/day children.
6. Giardiasis **(DOC)**
   Dose: 200 mg TDS × 7 days is equally effective to 2000 mg/day × 3 days.
7. Trichomonas vaginitis **(DOC with 100% cure)**
   Dose: 400mg TDS × 7 days.
8. Pseudomonas Enterocolitis: **CHINA GATE**

Tinidazole: Similar to metronidazole except t½—12 hrs (hence more suited for single dose) and better tolerated.

U:
1. Amoebiasis
2. Anaerobic infection
3. *H. pylori*
4. Giardiasis
5. Trichomoniasis

Antiprotozoal Agents

Emetine: It is alkaloid from **Cephaelis ipecacuanha**. It is **amoebicide** (kills trophozoites but not cysts). **Reserved drug** for amoebiasis (intestinal and extraintestinal).

Mech:
1. Inhibits intraribosomal translocation of tRNA - amino acid complex → inhibition of protein synthesis.
2. Not curative, as the patient passes the cyst in the stool.

PK: Not given orally because it is **vomited. Route:** 60 mg OD SC/IM. Concentrated in liver, lung, kidney and spleen. Excreted in urine in 1–2 months.

ADR:
1. **Most serious complication:** Hypotension, tachycardia, change in ECG and myocarditis.
2. Abdominal cramp, nausea, vomiting (due to CTZ stimulation on IM/SC and gastric irritation).
3. Irritation (pain, stiffness, eczema)

CI:
1. Pregnancy
2. Renal failure
3. Cardiac failure

Diloxanide furoate: Directly kills trophozoites.

PK: **Furoate ester (by hydrolysis in intestine)** → **diloxanide (weak amoebicide).** Diloxanide is largely absorbed. Hepatic metabolism by **glucuronidation** and excreted in urine.

ADR:
1. Flatulence
2. Itching, urticaria, nausea

U:
1. **DOC** in amoebiasis (mild)
2. Diloxanide furoate + metronidazole/tinidazole for severe cases.

8-hydroxyquinolines: Kill cysts forming **trophozoites** in the intestines but are ineffective in extraintestinal amoebiasis.

Coverage: Entamoeba
Giardia
Trichomonas
Fungi (dermatophytes, Candida)
Bacteria

PK: **Least** absorbed from intestine (10–30%). **Hepatic conjugation with sulfate** and **glucuronic** acid. Renal excretion. Unabsorbed part reaches lower bowel and acts on luminal cycle of amoebiae.

ADR:
1. Green stools
2. Pruritis
3. Goitre
4. **Iodism** (furunculosis, mucous membrane inflammation) due to chronic iodine overload.
5. **Acute reaction** (angioedema, fever, chills and cutaneous haemorrhage).
6. **SMON** (subacute myelo-optic neuropathy).

U: Used as an alternative to diloxanide furoate.
1. Entamoeba
2. Giardia

3. Trichomonas
4. Candida and dermatophytes
5. Bacterial skin infection
6. Traveller's diarrhoea

Secnidazole: Same spectrum of activity and potency as metronidazole but oral absorption is rapid and plasma t½ is **24 hrs.**
U: 1. Single dose 30 mg/day in intestinal amoebiasis, giardiasis, trichomonas vaginitis and bacterial vaginosis.
2. 1.5. gm/day × 5 days in hepatic amoebiasis.

Protozoa	DOC
1. Balantidium coli	— Tetracycline
2. Babesia	— Clindamycin + quinine
3. *Dientamoeba fragilis*	— Idoquinol
4. *Giardia lamblia*	— Quinacrine
5. *Isospora belli*	— Cotrimoxazole
6. *Leishmania braziliensis* *L. donovani* *L. tropica*	Sodium stibogluconate
7. *Pneumocystitis carinii*	— Cotrimoxazole
8. *Toxoplasma gondii*	— Pyrimethamine + trisulfapyrimidines
9. *Trypanosoma cruzi*	— Nifurtimox
T. gambiense *T. rhodesiense* (African trypanosomiasis hemolymphatic stage)	Suramin
10. Late disease with CNS involvement	Melarsoprol

Ornidazole: Half-life = 14 hrs.
ADR, dose and duration similar to tinidazole.
U: Amoebiasis, giardiasis, trichomoniasis, bacterial vaginosis and anaerobic infection.
Satranidazole: Half-life = 14 hrs.
Advantage: Emesis, nausea, metallic taste, CNS symptoms and disulfiram like reactions absent. Acetamide metabolite (carcinogen) is not produced.
Furazolidone: It is nitrofuran compound.
PK: Partly absorbed orally and excreted in urine (orange colour).
ADR: Nausea, headache and dizziness.
U: Gram-negative bacilli, Giardia and Trichomonas.

Treatment of amoebiasis
1. **Invasive intestinal amoebiasis (amoebic dysentery)**
   A. Metronidazole/tinidazole—**DOC**
   B. Secnidazole 2 gm single dose—alternative.
   C. Dehydroemetine—rarely used in **most severe case** for faster relief. Also used in metronidazole **contraindication** (rashes/neuropathy).

2. **Chronic intestinal amoebiasis (asymptomatic cyst passer)**
   A. Diloxanide furoate—**DOC**
   B. Metronidazole/tinidazole—alternative
3. **Hepatic amoebiasis**
   A. Metronidazole/tinidazole **(DOC)**
   B. Dehydroemetine
   C. Chloroquine given after metronidazole or dehydroemetine to finish intestinal reservoir of infection.

Treatment of giardiasis

1. **DOC:** Metronidazole 10 mg/kg/day × 7 days.
   OR   Tinidazole 10 mg/kg/day × 7 days.
   OR   Secnidazole 2 gm single dose.
2. **Mepacrine:**   5 mg/kg/day × 5 days.
3. **Quiniodochlor:** Alternative.
4. **Furazolidone:** 5 mg/kg/day × 5 days.

Treatment of trichomoniasis (Vulvovaginitis)

1. **DOC** with 100% cure (given orally):
   Metronidazole 10 mg/kg/day × 7 days.
   OR   Tinidazole 10 mg/day × 7 days.
   OR   Secnidazole 2 gm single dose.
2. **Nimorazole** 2 gm single dose given orally.
3. **Intravaginally**
   — Diiodohydroquin
   — Quiniodochlor
   — Clotrimazole
   — Hamycin
   — Natamycin
   — Povidone iodine

Drugs for leishmaniasis: Macocutaneous leishmaniasis (*L. braziliensis*), dermal leishmaniasis (*L. tropica*) and visceral leishmaniasis (kala-azar by *L. donovani*) → carrier is **female sandfly phlebotomus** (**promastigote** = flagellate extracellular form) →transmitted to MAN (intracellularly within macrophage in nonflagellate form=**Amastigote**).

   Classification: a. Diamidine—pentamidine
   b. Antimonial—sodium stibogluconate
      Meglumine antimonate
      Urea stibamine
   c. Other—amphoterecin B (AMB), ketoconazole (KTZ), allopurinol and miltefosine

---

Sodium stibogluconate: Water soluble pentavalent antimonial containing 1/3 antimony by weight.
   Mech: Blocks **G**lycolytic and fatty acid (**L**ipid) pathways.
         stibo**GL**uconate
   PK: Cumulative. Absorbed from IM route. Excreted unchanged in urine within 6–12 hrs. **Dose:** 20 mg/kg (max. 850 mg) daily by IM (in

buttock)/IV × 25 days (according to **WHO**). Patient is cured if no parasite is detected in splenic/bone marrow aspirates. IV sodium stibogluconate is incorporated in **lyposome** also, from where drug is taken by **macrophages**.

ADR:
1. Metallic taste
2. Abdominal pain, nausea, vomiting
3. Stiffness of injected muscle
4. Sterile abscess
5. CNS symptom
6. Liver and kidney damage
7. ECG changes

U:
1. **DOC** in kala-azar
2. Dermal leishmaniasis (oriental sore) (KTZ/mepacrine is also given).

Pentamidine

Mech:
1. Interferes with **kinetoplast** DNA and inhibits **topoisomerase II**.
2. Interferes aerobic **glycolysis**.
3. Interferes with uptake and use of **polyamines**.

PK: Absorbed from injection site. Stored in liver and kidney for months. Excreted unchanged in urine.

Dose: 4 mg/kg on alternate day IM/IV over 1 hr for 5–25 weeks till parasites are cleared. **98% cure** rate achieved after **40 injections.** Dry powder in vials is dissolved to yield 10% solution before injection.

ADR: **Histamine** is released due to its basic nature causing acute reactions (**IV route > IM route**).
1. Cardiovascular collapse, hypotension
2. Dyspnoea and fainting
3. Rigor, rashes, fever
4. Mental confusion
5. Liver, kidney damage
6. **Cytolysis of β-cells**
   ↓
   Insulin release
   ↓
   Hypoglycaemia
   ↓
   IDDM.
7. Necrosis through IM route

U:
1. *L. donovani*: Sod. stibogluconate resistant kala-azar.
2. Trypanosomiasis
3. **P. carinii** in **AIDS**
   Pentamidine + cotrimoxazole
4. Blastomyces
5. Bacteria

Antifungal Agents

Drugs are for **superficial** and **deep (systemic)** fungal infection.
AMB for systemic mycosis and griseofulvin for dermatophytes were introduced in **1960**.

Human mycoses are
1. Deep
2. Superficial (keratin digestion)
3. Opportunistic: **A**spergillosis
   Aculomycosis
   Mucormycosis   O AMPere
   Penicillosis
   Otomycosis.

Superficial infection
A. Surface infection: On dead layers, e.g. tinea.
B. Cutaneous infection: On living skin, e.g. dermatophytes, Candida.

Deep infection
A. Subcutaneous/intermediate
B. Systemic/deep seated/internal organ:
   Blastomycosis
   Histoplasmosis   BHC
   Cryptococcosis, **C**occidioidomycosis and paracoccidioidomycosis.

Classification
1. **Antimetabolite** : Flucytosine
2. **Allylamine** : Terbinafine
3. **Antibiotic**
   A. **Polyenes**: AMB, nystatin, hamycin, natamycin (pimaricin).
   B. **Heterocyclic benzofuran**: Griseofulvin.
4. **Azoles:** A. **Imidazoles**
   a. **Topical**   KTZ   K COMES
                            Clotrimazole
                            Oxiconazole
                            Meconazole

Econazole
Sulconazole
   b. **Systemic**—KTZ (ketoconazole)
 B. **Triazole:**
   a. **Topical**—terconazole
   b. **Systemic**—fluconazole and itraconazole
5. **Other topical agents**
Naftifine
Tolnaftate
Undecylenic acid
Ciclopirox olamine
Haloprogin
Benzoic acid.

Weak antifungal: Quiniodochlor, sod thiosulfate

Never ToUCH B

Amphotericin B (AMB): Obtained from *S. nodosus.* **Polyene** has macrocyclic ring with one side (**lipophilic**) and other side (**hydrophilic**). Insoluble in water and unstable in aqueous medium.

Mech:
1. Binds with **sterol** of cytoplasmic membrane to enhance permeability.
2. High affinity for **ergosterol** present in cell membrane, forming **micropore**. **Hydrophilic** side forms **interior** of the pore through which substances of the cell move out. The pore is stabilised by membrane sterols filling up the **spaces** between AMB molecules on lipophilic side forming **outer** surface of the pore and increasing cell permeability.
3. Pores disrupt **homeostatis**.
4. **Cholesterol** of host cell resembles **ergosterol** and has higher affinity for it (hence one of the **most toxic** systemically used antibiotic and **least** toxic polyene).
5. Bacteria is **insensitive** to polyene due to absence of sterols.
6. Enhances **immunity**, hence useful in immunocompromised patient. Binds to ergosterol and forms micropores in cell membrane through which ions are lost.

Spectrum: Yeast, fungi, leishmania.
Fungicidal at high and **fungistatic** at low doses.

PK: Not cross BBB. Not absorbed **orally** but given orally for intestinal candidiasis and intestinal moniliasis, elimination t½—15 days, **60%** hepatic metabolism, excreted in **urine** and **bile**. Widely distributed in the body on IV as **suspension with deoxycholate**.

Raute and dose:
A. **Oral** 50–100 mg QID.
B. **Parenteral** 0.7 mg/kg (max. 3–4 gm × 2–3 months) suspension made with bile salt (deoxycholate) for systemic mycosis (IV **commonest**).
C. **Intrathecal** injection 0.5 mg twice weekly for fungal meningitis.

New AMB formulations are for targeted delivery, reduced toxicity and improved tolerability of IV infusion which are: (a) AMB lipid complex (ABCL) with 35% AMB

(b) AMB colloidal dispersion (ABCD) with 50% AMB and (c) Liposomal AMB (small unilamellar vesicles/SUV) with 10% AMB.

ADR:
1. CNS toxicity on intrathecal injection.
2. Anemia due to BMD **(most patient)**.
   Arrhythmia (**"amphoterrible"**) and hypotension.
3. Nephrotoxicity **(most important)**: Azotemia, reduced GFR, acidosis, hypokalemia.
4. Acute reaction due to **cytokinine** release (IL, TNF-α): Aches, nausea, vomiting, dyspnoea, thrombophlebitis, chills and fever lasting 2–5 hrs. Chills and fever are **"shake and bake"**. Hydrocortisone 0.6 mg/kg reduces the reaction.
5. Liver toxicity.

ADR is due to **CANAL** formation

ADR of AMPHOTERICIN B

Azotemia (80%) and anemia, **M**g and K loss in urine, **P**ulmonary stridor, **H**ypoxia and hypotension, **O**ccurrence of headache, **T**ubular acidosis, **E**ncephalopathy. **R**enal damage, **R**eaction of febrile type, **I**ncreased intrarenal vascular resistance, **C**hills, **I**nflammation of vein (phlebitis), **N**ausea, **B**ody weight loss.

U:
1. Topically for oral, vaginal, cutaneous candidiasis and otomacosis.
2. **The most effective drug** for systemic mycosis and **gold standard** of antifungal therapy. **DOC for most systemic fungal infection** (AMB enhances 5-FC penetration into fungus **supradditive action**).
3. **DOC in:**   Candidiasis.   **cAMP**
   Cryptococcosis
   Coccidioidomycosis
   Aspergillosis
   HistoPlasmosis
   Mucormycosis
4. **Intrathecally** for fungal meningitis (drug does not cross BBB).
5. Leishmaniasis: **Reserved drug** for resistant case of kala-azar and mucocutaneous leishmaniasis.
6. Blastomyces

IA:
1. Nephrotoxic drugs (cyclosporin, vancomycin, aminoglycoside) enhance renal impairment caused by AMB.
2. **Rifampin** and **minocycline potentiate AMB**.

Nystatin, hamycin and natamycin are similar to AMB, are used topically.

Griseofulvin: It is obtained from **Penicillium griseofulvum** and its action against dermatophytosis was noticed in **1960**. Active against **most dermatophytes** showing **fungostatic** action. Hence, newly formed keratin is not invaded by fungus (dermatophytes activity concentrate it).

Mech:
1. Interferes with **metaphase** stage of mitosis but does not cause the **arrest like mitotic inhibitor** (colchicine and vinca alkaloid) resulting in **multinucleated** and **stunted hyphae** (disruption of mitosis).
2. Inhibits **microtubular function** and **nucleic acid synthesis.**
3. Gets deposited in **keratin forming cells** of skin, nail and hair.

PK: Deposited in **keratin containing tissue** (skin, nail, hair) and tinea infected cells (ringworm). Metabolism by **methylation.** Excreted in **urine.**
Plasma t½—1 day but presists for weeks in keratin and skin.

ADR: 1. Headache (**commonest**) and confusion. **GRISEOFULVIN**
2. GIT intolerance, Rashes, Gynaecomastia, Impaired work, Syncope, Erythema, OC efficacy reduced due to CYP450 induction, Fatigue, flatulence, Urticaria, Lichen planus, Liver toxicity, Vertigo, Increased porphyria, Neuropathy.
3. Photoallergy
4. Teratogenic and carinogenic

ADR of GRISEOFULVIN
Gut upset, Raised alcohol effect, Increased skin sensitivity, Syncope, Edema, OC efficacy reduced due to CYP450 induction, Fatigue, Urine (albuminuria), Leukopenia, Vertigo, Impaired work, Neuritis.

IA: 1. Intolerance to alcohol
2. Phenobarbitone induces metabolism and reduces oral absorption of griseofulvin (**failure of therapy**).
3. Induces warfarin metabolism.
4. Reduces efficacy of OC.

U: 1. Systemically for dermatophytosis (inhibits growth of dermatophytes and *C. albicans*).
2. Topically in tinea infection, nail, hair and skin infection.
Not effective against Candida, tinea versicolor and deep mycoses.

Flucytosine (5-FC): It is **synthetic** and **narrow** spectrum **fungistatic.**

Spectrum: Cryptococcus
Candida
Aspergillus   **CAT**
Chromoblastomyces
Torula

Mech: 1. **5-FC is taken up by fungal cell** and **converted into**
↓
5-Fluorouracil
↓
5-Fluorodeoxyuridylic acid
↓   (**thymidylate inhibitor**)
Inhibition of **thymidylic** acid (a DNA component).
2. **Mammalian cells** (except some marrows cells—basis of leucopenia and thrombocytopenia) have low capacity to convert 5-FC into 5-fluorouracil.

ADR: 1. Leucopenia, thrombocytopenia and anemia due to BMD.
2. GI intolerance, diarrhoea and enteritis.
3. Liver dysfunction.

PK: Good CSF penetration. **Dose:** 125 mg/kg/day orally. Taken as adjuvant drug.
Usual regimen: AMB (0.3 mg/kg/day) +5-FC (synergistic action).
U:
1. Chromoblastomycosis
2. Deep mycosis
3. Disseminated candidiasis

Azoles (imidazoles and triazoles): Primarily **static**. **Synthetic** broad spectrum antifungal agents. Fluconazole and itraconazole are preferred over KTZ for systemic mycosis.

Coverage: Candida

Resistant **TB**.
MNC = MultiNational Company

Nocardia
Deep Mycosis
Positive and negative **B**acteria
Ringworm and **T**inea versicolor

Mech:
1. Inhibits **ergosterol** synthesis in fungal cell wall.
2. On topical use, damage **cytoplasmic membrane**.
3. Inhibit **fungal CY P450 enzyme lanosterol 14-demethylase** and impair ergosterol (unknown mechanism) though azoles are active against bacteria.

KTZ: **First** orally effective broad spectrum antifungal drug for **deep mycosis** and **dermatophytosis**. More soluble in **gastric acid**. Bound to **albumin** and **RBC**.

Mech: 1. Inhibits **ergosterol** synthesis and damages cell wall.
(KTZ) 2. Inhibits fungal **steroid** synthesis.
3. Testosterone and cortisol synthesis is reduced due to **antiandrogenic** effect.

PK of KTZ: Hepatic metabolism, excreted in urine and faeces.
t½ → 2–6 hrs
Dose: 200 mg OD orally

ADR of KTZ:
1. **Commonest:** Nausea, vomiting, diarrhoea.
2. Alopecia
3. Loss of appetite
4. Headache
5. Rashes
6. Reduced androgen production (gynaecomastia and oligozoosperimia).

ADR of KETOCONAZOLE

Keratin (hair) loss, **E**nzyme (CYP450) inhibitor, **T**estosterone and estradiol loss, **O**ccurrence of hepatotoxicity, **C**ommonest (nausea, anorexia, emesis), **O**vergrowth (gynecomastia), **N**ursing mother to be alerted, **A**llergic rash and pruritis, a**Z**oospermia, **O**verretention of fluid (HTN), **L**oss of Libido and potency, **E**ndocrine (commonest but irregular).

Pharmacology Review

CI of KTZ: Pregnancy and lactation

> **Antiandrogenic drugs**   CCKS
> Cimetidine
> Cyproterone
> KTZ
> Spironolactone

IA of KTZ:
1. Rifampicin and phenytoin induce KTZ metabolism (reduced efficacy of KTZ).
2. Inhibits CY P450 (CYP3A4) and enhances blood level of warfarin, sulfonylurea, phenytoin and cyclosporin.
3. Enhances plasma level of **C**isapride, **A**stemizole, **T**erfenadine leading to tachycardia and fibrillation →**fatal.**   **CAT**
4. H₂ blocker, proton pump inhibitor and antacid reduce oral absorption of KTZ by enhancing pH of stomach.
5. Inhibition of MFO slows drug metabolism.
6. Cortisol and testosterone synthesis is reduced.

U of KTZ:
1. Dermatophytosis (stratum corneum)
2. Monilial vaginitis
3. Systemic mycosis
4. Dermal leishmaniasis and kala-azar
5. **DOC**
   Blastomycosis
   Paracoccidioidomycosis
   Sporotrichosis
   Candidiasis

BPSC = Bihar Public Service Commission

Fluconazole: Water soluble
Wider range than KTZ
Antiandrogenic effect and fungal steroid synthesis are **absent.**

PK: 94% absorbed. Route—oral/IV
Excreted unchanged in urine **(80%).**
t½—28 hrs. **Fungicidal** concentration is attained in saliva, vagina, nail, brain and CSF.

ADR:
1. **Common:** Nausea, vomiting, rashes, headache and abdominal pain.
2. Enhanced hepatic transaminase in AIDS patients.

IA: Enhances plasma level of zidovudine, warfarin, phenytoin and sulfonylureas.

CI: Pregnancy and lactation

U:
1. Candidiasis in both normal and AIDS patient
2. Meiningitis (cryptococcal and coccidioidal)
3. Histoplasmosis
4. Sporotrichosis

Antifungal Agents

Itraconazole: Wider spectrum than KTZ/fluconazole. **Fungistatic** in immunocompromised patient.

Coverage: Mould like Mucor and Aspergillus.

PK: Oral absorption is enhanced by food and gastric acid, and reduced by H_2 blocker and proton pump inhibitor. Accumulated in vaginal mucosa, skin and nail. Hepatic metabolism, faecal excretion, volume of distribution is 10 L/kg, t½—32–64 hrs.

ADR: Tolerated below <200 mg/day. Gastric intolerance at the dose of ≥400 mg/day.
1. Dizziness and headache **DTPH**
2. Raised plasma Transaminase
3. Pruritis
4. Hypokalemia

IA:
1. Ventricular arrhythmia with terfenadine, astemizole and cisapride due to inhibition of CYP3A4 by itraconazole.
2. Carbamazepine, rifampin, phenytoin induce its metabolism **(reduced efficacy)**.
3. Phenytoin, digoxin, sulfonylurea and cyclosporin levels are increased.

U:
1. Systemic mycosis
2. Vaginal Candidiasis **Special DOC**
3. Dermatophytosis
4. Onychomycosis
5. Chromomycosis **(DOC)**

Clotrimazole
Coverage:
1. Tinea infection
2. Otomycosis
3. Candidiasis **COTS**
4. Vaginitis
5. Skin infection caused by Corynebacteria.

Econazole: Similar to cotrimazole and effective in superficial layer.
Coverage:
1. Oral thrush
2. Otomycosis
3. Dermatophytosis
4. Vaginitis

Miconazole: Cure rate is >90%
Coverage:
1. Onychomycosis, otomycosis
2. Candidiasis
3. Pityriasis versicolor
4. Tinea

Terbinafine: Fungicidal. It is used orally and topically.

Mech:
1. **Noncompetitive inhibitor of squalene epoxidase** (early step enzyme in ergosterol biosynthesis). Squalene accumulation within fungal cells leads to **cidal** action.
2. Mammalian enzyme is inhibited at **1000 fold** higher concentration of drug.

PK: 75% orally absorbed
≤5% absorbed from unbroken skin. **Lipophilic:** Widely distributed in the body. Concentrated in nail plate, sebum and stratum corneum. Inactivated by metabolism.
Excretion — 80% (renal)
— 20% (faecal)
Elimination t½ — 14 hrs

ADR: 1. **Oral:** Taste disturbance
Gastric upset
Rashes
2. **Topical:** Dryness
Itching
Erythema   **DIE**

U: 1. Tinea pedis.
T. corporis.
T. cruris.   **TOP**
T. capitis.
2. Pityriasis versicolor.
3. Onychomycosis.

Benzoic acid: Fungistatic. Antibacterial action is present.
Mech: **Whitfield's ointment** = 3% salicylic acid + 5% benzoic acid (keratolytic).
ADR: Irritation and burning
U: Hyperkeratotic lesion

Disease	1st choice (DOC)
1. Candidiasis:	
Disseminated	AMB + 5-FC/FLU
mucocutaneous	FLU/ITR
2. Cryptococcosis	AMB + 5-FC/FLU
3. Histoplasmosis	ITR/KTZ/AMB
4. Coccidioidomycosis	AMB/FLU
5. Blastomycosis	ITR
6. Sporotrichosis (disseminated)	AMB
7. Paracoccidioidomycosis	ITR/KTZ
8. Aspergillosis	AMB
9. Mucormycosis	AMB
10. Chromomycosis	ITR

60 Anthelmintics

Anthelmintics are drugs to kill (**vermicide**) or to expel (**vermifuge**) infesting helminths. **One-third of world's population** harbours helminths. Intestinal nematodes are the **easiest** to treat because drugs are not absorbed into the host.

Classification

Levamisole
Albendazole
Mebendazole, Metronidazole
Praziquantel, Piperazine, Pyrantel pamoate
Niridazole
Thiabendazole, Tetramizole
DEC (diethyl carbamazine citrate)

LAMP. NTD = Neural Tube Defect

Mebendazole: **100%** cure rate in round and hookworm, *Enterobius* and *Trichuris*. 75% cure in tapeworm.

- **Mech:** 1. Blocks **glucose** uptake in the parasite and depletes its glycogen stores.
  2. Binds to **β-tubulin** (a microtubular protein) of microtubules and inhibits its polymerisation. Hence, microtubules are lost.
- **PK:** Minimal intestinal absorption.
  Excretion — 80–90% (faecal)
  — Rest (renal)
- **Dose:** A. **Same** in adult and children >2 yrs
  100 mg BD × 3 days
  B. 50 mg BD × 3 days for children of <2 yrs
  (No fasting/purging is needed)
- **ADR:** 1. GI intolerance, nausea
  2. Expulsion of ascaris from mouth/nose due to starvation.
  3. Granulocytopenia
  4. Allergy   AGE
  5. Alopecia
- **U:** A. DOC in   TECH
  1. Trichuriasis
  2. Enterobius

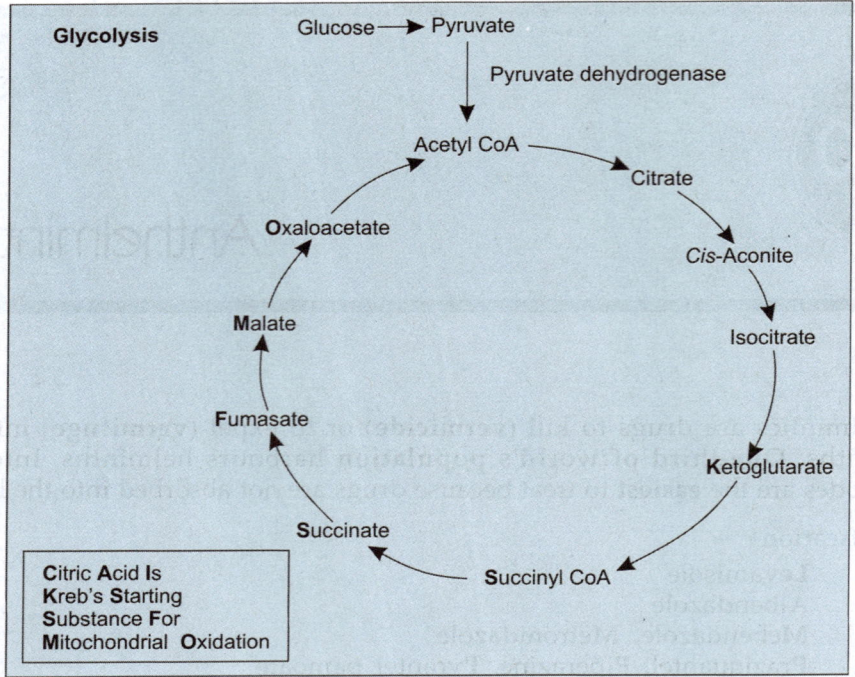

3. Capillaria
4. Hookworm and Hydatid disease

B. Other uses
1. Multiple infestation
2. Roundworm
3. Dracontiasis

Albendazole: Broad spectrum

Mech: Same as mebendazole

PK: Moderate oral absorption.
Fraction absorbed is converted to **sulfoxide metabolite** by first pass metabolism which is active form. Widely distributed, enters brain, renal excretion, t½—8½ hrs.

ADR:
1. Alopecia
2. Jaundice
3. Fever
4. GI intolerance, nausea
5. Dizziness, headache

ADR of ALBENDAZOLE
Abdominal pain, **L**evel of S. transaminase raised, **B**owel dysfunction, **E**mesis and nausea, **N**eutropenia, **D**iarrhoea, **D**rowsiness, **A**lopecia, di**Z**ziness, **O**cular (jaundice due to cholestatis), **L**eukopenia, **E**rythema and edema.

CI: Pregnancy

U:
1. Hookworm ⎫ 400 mg single dose
   Enterobiasis ⎬ for children >2 yrs and adult.
   Ascariasis ⎬ 200 mg single dose
   Trichuris ⎭ for children of 1–2 yrs   **HEAT**
2. **Hydatid disease:** 400 mg BD × 4 weeks.
   Repeat after 3 weeks up to 3 course.
3. **Tapeworm** and **strongyloidosis**
   400 mg OD × 3 days.
   In strongyloidosis, cure rate is **50%**.
   2nd course after 3 weeks cures all patients.
4. **Trichinosis**
5. **Neurocysticercosis (DOC)** 15 mg/kg/day × 30 days.
   Due to the reaction, ocular cysticercosis causes blindness, hence no drug is needed. Albendazole + praziquantel is cheaper regimen **(DOC)**. The inflammatory reaction is due to the release of substances from killed cysticerci.

Thiabendazole was the **first benzimidazole polyanthelmintic** introduced in 1961. Effective against **all species of nematodes** infesting GIT (roundworm, hookworm, Enterobius, Trichuris, Trichinella, Strongyloides).

Mech:
1. Inhibits **egg** development and kills **larvae**. Inhibits dermatophytic fungi (**Antifungal** action). Other actions are:
   Antipyretic
   Analgesic
   Anti-inflammatory
   Scabicidal
2. Mechanism **similar** to mebendazole and effects **T cell function**, inhibits **fumarate reductase** hence microtubule aggregation.

PK: Rapidly absorbed. Can be absorbed from skin. Metabolised by **hydroxylation** and conjugation. Excreted in urine giving **ASPARAGINE like odour to urine**.
Dose: 25 mg/kg/day (tablet must be chewed). Taken after meals.

ADR:
1. **Commonest**
   Nausea, vomiting, giddiness, headache, loss of appetite.
2. **Others**
   A. Loss of alertness (so driving machine operation should be prohibited).
   B. Stevens-Johnson syndrome
   C. Hypersensitivity

CI:
1. Liver and kidney disease
2. Pregnancy

U: **DOC in**
1. Trichinosis
2. Strongyloidosis

3. Cutaneous and visceral leishmaniasis.
   (A **2-day course,** repeated course is given after a gap of 2 days if needed).

DEC: Diethyl carbamazine citrate was developed in **1948.**
The only drug for **filariasis.**
Most effective against microfilariae and **least** effective against adult filaria.

Mech:
1. **Immobilises** microfilariae.
2. Alters Mf membrane so that they are phagocytosed by tissue fixed **monocyte** but not by circulating phagocytes **(most important action).**
3. Effects muscular activity of Mf and adultworms so that they are dislodged.
4. Adult *B. malayi* and *W. bancrofti* worms are also killed on chronic uses.

PK: Absorbed orally. Distributed **all over the body** (volume of distribution 4 L/kg), hepatic metabolism, plasma t½ → 4–12 hrs, excreted in urine **(faster in acidic urine).**

ADR:
1. Nausea, headache, dizziness
2. Loss of appetite, weakness
3. Lymphadenopathy
4. Hypotension
5. Leukocytosis and albuminuria
6. Rashes, pruritis
7. **Mazzotti reaction:** Reaction of skin and eyes in onchocerciasis.

ADR of DIETHYL CARBAMAZINE

Delayed reaction (lymphangitis, swelling), **I**nflamed urea, **E**ncephalitis, **T**ension (BP) decreased, **H**eadache, **Y**ields atrophy of retinal pigment epithelium, **L**ymph node enlarged, **C**ornea (punctate keratitis), **A**norexia, **MAZ**zotti reaction, **I**tching, **N**ausea, **E**mesis.

U:
1. Filariasis: 6 mg/kg/day × 7 days.
   Mf in nodules and hydrocele are not killed.
   Prolonged therapy kills *B. malayi* and *W. bancrofti* **(most cases).**
   Kills Mf of *L. loa* and *O. vulvulus* and adult of *L. loa.*
   Elephantiasis due to chronic obstruction is uneffected.
2. Tropical eosinophilia (4 mg/kg/day)
3. Loiasis
4. Visceral larvae migrans
5. Alternative in onchocerciasis

DEC is DOC in: **L**oiasis   **LFT**
Filariasis
Tropical eosinophilia
visceral **L**arva migrans

Pyrantel pamoate: It is **pyrimidine** derivative. **60%** cure rate.
Mech: 1. **Activation of nicotinic cholinergic receptors in worms.**
↓
Persistant depolarisation
↓
Contracture and **spastic paralysis**
↓
Worms are expelled
2. Has **anticholinesterase** action.
3. Piperazine causes **hyperpolarization** and **flaccid paralysis,** therefore antagonises action of pyrantel.
4. Cholinergic receptors of mammalian skeletal muscle has low affinity for the drug.

PK: 13% oral absorption. Partly metabolised. Renal excretion.
ADR: Free of ADR
1. Tasteless
2. Non-irritant

U: 1. Ascariasis (roundworm)
Ancylostoma (hookworm)
Enterobius (pinworm)
The dose is **15 mg/kg (max 1 gm)** in a single dose.
2. Necator   } 3 days
Strongyloides   course

Piperazine: Developed in 1950. Water soluble. Second choice drug.
Mech: 1. **Blocks neuromuscular transmission in roundworm by antagonising ACh action** and **causing hyperpolarisation**
↓
Flaccid paralysis
↓
Worms expelled alive
2. Antagonises pyrantel, hence not given together.

PK: Orally absorbed, partly hepatic metabolism, renal excretion.
ADR: Free of ADR. **Safe in pregnancy.**
1. Toxic doses cause convulsion and respiratory failure →death.
2. Convulsion and hypotonia.
3. **Worm Wobble** (ataxia of cerebellar type)
4. Nausea, vomiting, GI intolerance, urticaria.

CI: 1. Epilepsy
2. Renal disease

U: 1. Roundworm:
4½ gm OD × 2 days
Child 3/4 gm/yr of age (max. 4½ gm)
Intestinal obstruction occurs due to roundworm relaxation by this drug. Piperazine is **safe in** *Pregnancy* among anthelmintics.
2. Enterobiasis: 2½ gm OD × 7 days (max.).

Tetramisole and Levamisole: Tetramisole was introduced in 1960. Tetramisole is **racemic,** Levamisole is its **Levo isomer** and is **more active.** 70–90% cure rate.

Coverage: Ascariasis
Ancylostomiasis
Strongyloides larvae (but not adult)

Mech:
1. **Stimulates ganglia of worm**
↓
Tonic paralysis
↓
Expulsion of live worm
2. Interferes with carbohydrate metabolism.
3. Levamisole is **immunomodulator** (restores depressed T cell function) hence used as adjunct in malignancy and as a disease modifying drug in RA.

ADR:
1. Abdominal pain, nausea
2. Fatigue, drowsiness
3. Insomnia, giddiness

U: Levamisole in:
1. Mass treatment of roundworm (due to good tolerance and low dose). **>90% cure rate.**
   Dose: 3.5 mg/kg single dose.
2. *A. duodenale* (alternative)
3. Necator
4. RA
5. Adjuvant in malignancy

Niclosamide: Developed in 1960

Coverage: *T. saginata*
T. solium
D. latum
H. nana
Threadworm

Mech:
1. Inhibits oxidative phosphorylation in mitochondria and anaerobic generation of ATP by tapeworm.
Tapeworm is injured by drug/digested in intestine.
2. But digestion of dead segment of *T. solium* causes
↓
Release of larvae from ova
↓
Penetration of larvae into intestinal wall
↓
Visceral cysticercosis

ADR: Tasteless and non-irritating
No systemic toxicity
Safe in pregnancy

U: 1. **Tapeworm:**
   1 gm after breakfast and 1 gm after 1 hr of first dose **(total 2 gm).**
   Total dose for children of 2–6 yrs is **1 gm.**
   After 2 hrs, a saline purge is given to wash off the worm.
   Praziquantel does not digest the worm but kills encysted larvae, hence preferred over niclosamide in *T. solium* (no cysticercosis develops).
2. *H. nana*:
   Dose: 2 gm × 5 days (no purge is needed).

Ivermectin: It is **semisynthetic** drug obtained from *S. avermitilis*.

Mech: Opens **GABA sensitive chloride channel** causing muscle paralysis. Tonic paralysis due to GABA transmission only in the microfilariae.

ADR:
1. Pruritis
2. Giddiness
3. ECG change
4. Reaction due to degradation of Mf.

ADR of IVERMECTIN
Interacts with GABA, **V**ery rarely (prostration, myalgia, arthralgia), **E**dema, **R**aised body temperature, **M**azzotti-like reaction, **E**nlarged lymph node, **C**ardiac dysfunction (low BP), **T**achycardia, **I**tching, **N**ot well known (teratogenicity/carcinogenicity).

U:
1. **DOC** in *O. volvulus* and strongyloidosis.
2. Visceral larva migrans.
3. Alternative drug for single dose treatment of:
   W. bancrofti
   B. malayi
   Ascaris
   Enterobius
   Trichuris
4. **RIVER Blindness (Onchocerciasis) Control Programme (WHO):**
   Reduces Mf count (not adult), suppresses ocular damage and lymphadenopathy, hence replaces DEC for onchocerciasis.

   rIVERmectin → RIVER blindness

   Drugs increasing GABA activity
   Ivermectin
   Valproic acid   IVP
   Progabide   BBB
   BZD
   Barbiturate
   Baclofen

Niridazole (a nitrothiazole)
- **Mech:**
  1. **Same** effect as metronidazole
  2. Inhibits **glucose** uptake by parasites
  3. Has **anti-inflammatory** action
- **PK:** Hepatic metabolism
  Renal and faecal excretion
- **ADR:**
  1. Carcinogenic
  2. CNS and CVS toxicity
- **U:**
  1. Schistosomes
  2. Enterobius
  3. Guinea worm (25 mg/kg/day × 7 days)
  4. Bacteria

ADR of SURAMIN

Skin hypersensitivity, Unusual but the most serious (nausea, emesis, shock, unconciousness), Renal damage, Albuminuria, Most common (coagulopathy) and most serious (polyradiculoneuropathy), Increased (bilirubin, transaminase, creatinine), Neuropathy.

Praziquantel: Wide range activity against Schistosomiasis
  Trematodes
  Cestodes

- **Mech:**
  1. Muscle stimulation and paralysis. **Vacuolization** of cuticle.
  2. Causes leakage of **intracellular Ca^{2+}** from membrane →contracture and paralysis.
  3. At **higher concentration,** vacuolization of **tegment** and release of contents of worms and flukes followed by their destruction by host take place.
- **PK:** Rapidly absorbed from intestines. Undergoes hepatic first pass metabolism **limiting** its systemic bioavailability. Hepatic metabolism. Crosses BBB. Plasma t½—1.5 hr. Renal excretion.
- **ADR:**
  1. Bitter taste; abdominal pain and nausea
  2. Headache, dizziness, sedation
  3. **Reaction** due to degradation of parasites: itching, rash, fever, urticaria and bodyache.
- **IA:**
  1. Phenytoin, carbamazepine and dexamethasone induce praziquantel metabolism.
  2. No interaction with alcohol, tobacco and food.
- **U:** It is **DOC in all trematode except Fasciola hepatica.**
  1. Schistosomes: 70 mg/kg/day
  2. Cestodes
  3. Tapeworm: >90% cure rate
  4. Flukes: 75 mg/kg single dose
  5. Neurocysticercosis: 50 mg/kg/day × 15 day.

Anthelmintic drugs starting with **P** (Pyrantel, Piperazine, Praziquantel) cause **Paralysis.**

Levamisole	Albendazole	Mebendazole	Pyrantel	**LAMP**
100	400	500	600 mg single dose	

Parasites	Treatment of choice
1. **Ascariasis**	(i) **Mebendazole** (100 mg BD for 3 days). (ii) Albendazole (400 mg once), Piperazine (75 mg/kg for 2 days)or pyrantel pamoate (10 mg/kg for 3 days) may be given
2. **Hookworm** (*A. duodenale, Necator americanus*)	(i) **Mebendazole** (100 mg BD for 3 days) (ii) Albendazole (400 mg once),or pyrantel pamoate (10 mg/kg. for 3 days) may be given
3. **Cysticercosis** (*Cysticercus cellulosae*)	(i) **Praziquantel** (50 mg/kg/day in 3 doses for 15 days) (ii) Albendazole (15 mg/kg/day in 3 doses for 8 days) (iii) Surgery
4. **Cutaneous larva migrans** (creeping eruption)	(i) **Thiabendazole** (10% suspension topically or 25 mg/kg for 2–5 days) (ii) Cryotherapy/albendazole
5. **Visceral larva migrans** (toxocariasis)	(i) **Supportive therapy** and **glucocorticoids** (ii) DEC (2 mg/kg TID for 7–10 days)
6. **Anisaklasis**	- **Surgical removal**
7. **Babesiosis**	- **Clindamycin** (1.2 mg BD IV or 600 mg TDS orally for 7 days)
8. **Dracunculiasis** (*D. medinensis*)	(i) Metronidazole (250) mg TDS for 10 days plus worm removal (ii) Thiabendazole, niridazole
9. **Cryptosporidiosis**	**Self-limiting** (no effective therapy available)
10. **Capillariasis** (*Capillaria philippinensis*)	(i) Mebendazole (200 mg BD for 20 days) (ii) Albendazole (iii) Thiabendazole
11. **Balantidiasis** (*Balantidium coli*)	(i) Tetracycline (500 mg 6 hourly) for 20 days) (ii) Metronidazole (750 mg TDS for 5 days)
12. **Trichuriasis** (whipworm)	(i) Mebendazole (100 mg BD for 3 days) (ii) Albendazole (400 mg once)
13. **Trichostrongyliasis**	(i) Pyrantel pamoate (10 mg/kg once) (ii) Mebendazole (iii) Albendazole
14. **Chaga's disease** (*Trypanosoma cruzi*)	(i) Nifurtimox (10 mg/kg/day orally in 4 doses for 4 months) (ii) Benzindazole
15. **Sleeping sickness** (*Trypanosoma brucol gambiense*)	(i) Hemolymphatic stage: Suramin and late stage with CNS-involvement: melarsoprol
16. **Trichomoniasis** (*Trichomonas vaginalis*)	(i) Metronidazole (2 gm once or 250 mg TDS oral for 7 days)/tinidazole
17. **Trichinosis** (*Trichinella spiralis*)	glucocorticoid + albendazole (for Trichuris—albendazole)

(Contd.)

Parasites	Treatment of choice
18. Toxoplasmosis (*Toxoplasma gondii*)	(i) Pyrimethamine (75 mg/day) plus sulfadiazine (2–4 gm/day) (ii) Pyrimethamine + clindamycin
19. Isosporiasis	(i) Cotrimoxazole (ii) Pyrimethamine
20. Gnathostomiasis	– Surgical removal or mebendazole
21. Giardiasis	– Metronidazole (250 mg 6 hourly for 5 days)
22. Enterobiasis (pinworm)	(i) Pyrantel pamoate (ii) Mebendazole/albendazole
23. Hydatid cyst (*Echinococcus granulosis*)	(i) Preoperative albendazole + surgery (ii) Albendazole 400 mg BD for 28 days may be given postoperatively
24. Filariasis	
Wuchereria bancrofti	→Diethyl carbamazine
Brugia malayi	→Diethyl carbamazine
Brugia loa loa	→Diethyl carbamazine
Mansonella ozzarli	→Ivermectin
Mansonella streptocerca	→DEC and (for *M. perstans*-mebendazole)
Onchocerciasis	→Ivermectin
Topical pulmonary eosinophilia	→Diethyl carbamazine (6 mg/kg for 21 days)
25. Strongyloidiasis	(i) Thiabendazole (ii) Ivermectin/albendazole
26. Schistosomiasis	(i) Praziquantel (ii) Oxamniquine
27. Pneumocystic pneumonia	(i) Cotrimoxazole (ii) Pentamidine
28. Tapeworms (Cysticercosis): *D. latum* (fish) *Taenia solium* (pork) *Taenia saginata* (beef) *H. nana* (dwarf) and *H. diminuta*	(i) Praziquantel (ii) Niclosamide
29. FLUKES infection Lung fluke (*P. wetermani*). Intestinal fluke Liver fluke Sheep liver fluke	(i) Praziquantel (ii) Bithionol – Praziquantel (*F. buski*) Praziquantel (*C. sinensis*) Bithionol (*F. hepatica*)
30. Threadworm (*E. vermicularis*)	Albendazole/mebendazole/Pyrantel

Antiviral Drugs

Virus is the ultimate expression of **parasitism** due to both taking nutrition from host and directing metabolic machinery of host to synthesize new virus.

Symptoms appear after viral replication and reach their peak. Hence, therapy should be started in incubation period (**prophylaxis**).

Two types of viruses are

A. **DNA virus**
- Poxvirus
- Parvovirus
- Papovavirus
- Herpes virus
- Hepadna virus
- Adenovirus

P3H2A
= PH 3–2 A
= PH 3–2 Acidic

B. **RNA virus**
- Arbovirus
- Arenavirus
- Bunyavirus
- Filovirus
- Flavivirus
- Orthomyxovirus
- Paramyxovirus
- Picornavirus
- Reovirus
- Retrovirus
- Rhabdovirus
- Togavirus

1. **ROTA**virus Right Out The Anus
   Commonest global cause of infantile gastroenteritis.
2. Naked (non-envoloped) RNA viruses are:
   Calici virus, Picornavirus, Reovirus.   Naked CPR
3. Segmented viruses are: BOARS
   Bunyavirus, Orthomyxovirus, Arenavirus, Reovirus.
4. PicoRNA viruses = small **RNA** viruses are:
   A. Rhinovirus
   B. Hepatitis A virus
   C. Poliovirus
   D. Echovirus
   E. Coxsackie virus

RAPE and (Coxsackie = Co sex →sex) = **RAPE** and **SEX**.
RhiNO has Runny **NO**se.

5. Hepatitis transmission:
   A. Hepatitis A → Asymptomatic usually
   B. Hepatitis B → Blood borne
   C. Hepatitis C → Chronic, Cirrhosis, CA, Carrier
   D. Hepatitis D → Defective, Dependent on HBV
   E. Hepatitis E → Enteric, Expectant mother
   A and E by faecal-oral route
   The **vowels** (A and E) hit the **bowels**

Classification

1. **Antiherpes virus (CMV, HSV)**
   Famciclovir
   Acyclovir   **GIFT For Antiherpes Virus**
   Vidarabine
   Ganciclovir
   Idoxuridine
   Foscarnet
   Trifluridine
   New antiherpes agents — Penciclovir, Valacyclovir,
                            Cidofovir **PCV**

2. **Anti-retrovirus**
   A. Protease inhibitors: **SPRAIN**
      Ritonavir
      Saquinavir
      Indinavir
      Nelfinavir
      Amprenavir and lopinavir
   B. **Reverse transcriptase inhibitor (HIV infection)/RTI**
      (a) Nucleoside RTI: Azidothymidine (AZT)/zidovudine, and Abacavir.
          Stavudine
          Didanosine
          Zalcitabine, Lamivudine   **ADZS (AIDS) Lastly END**
      (b) Non-nucleoside RTI: Nevirapine
                              Delavirdine
                              Efavirenz

3. **Anti-influenza virus**
   Amantadine
   Rimantadine

4. **Nonselective**
   Interferon α
   Ribavirin and lamivudine

Antiviral Drugs

---

1. **ARBO** virus = **AR**thropod **BO**rn virus
2. Mumps virus causes: Meningitis (aseptic)
   Orchitis (testes inflammation)
   Parotitis **MOP**
3. **Measles** Cough
   Coryza **3Cs**
   Conjunctivitis
   Spot (Koplik spot)
   RNA, RTI, Rhazes, Rubeola, Rash, Red spot **6R**
   Measles are caused by Myxovirus.

Acyclovir: It is a **deoxyguanosine** analogue. Requires virus specific enzyme for conversion to active metabolite which inhibits DNA synthesis and viral replication. **Commonest** used antiviral drug. **Order of sensitivity:**
HSV type I (most sensitive) > HSV type II > VZV = EBV.
CMV is not effected.

Mech:
1. Inhibits **viral DNA polymerase** when phosphorylated by **viral thymidine kinase.**
2. Inhibits **DNA synthesis** and **viral replication.**

$$\text{Acyclovir}$$
$$\downarrow \text{ Herpes specific thymidine kinase}$$
$$\text{Acyclovir monophosphate}$$
$$\downarrow \text{ Cellular (host cell) kinase}$$
$$\text{Acyclovir triphosphate}$$
$$\text{(More active on viral DNA polymerase)}$$
$$\downarrow$$
$$\text{Reduced viral DNA polymerase}$$

3. **Acyclovir triphosphate** is **competitive inhibitor** of DNA polymerase of herpes virus. Its incorporation in viral DNA stops DNA lengthening. This terminated DNA **irreversibly** inhibits DNA polymerase. Drug is taken up by **virus infected** cells.

Resistant: It is due to deficiency of virus induced **thymidine kinase**. Resistance to **HSV** is due to mutants deficient in **thymidine kinase activity** and that to **VZV** is due to **reduced affinity** of enzyme for acyclovir.

PK: 20% oral absorption. Widely distributed (attaining CSF concentration which is **50%** of plasma concentration). Penetrates cornea. **80%** excreted unchanged in urine by glomerular filtration and tubular secretion. Plasma t½ →2–3 hrs. Dose reduction is needed in renal dysfunction.

ADR:
1. **IV** →Hypotension, rashes, sweat, emesis
2. **Oral** →CNS effects
3. **Topical** →Stinging and burning sensation
4. **Higher dose:** Hallucination and coma
5. Reduced GFR (**commonest**), Azotemia, Crystalline nephrotoxicit**Y**, Convulsion, Lethargy, Oral (gut upset), Vomiting, Irritation (topical), Rash.

CI: Renal failure

ACYCLOVIR

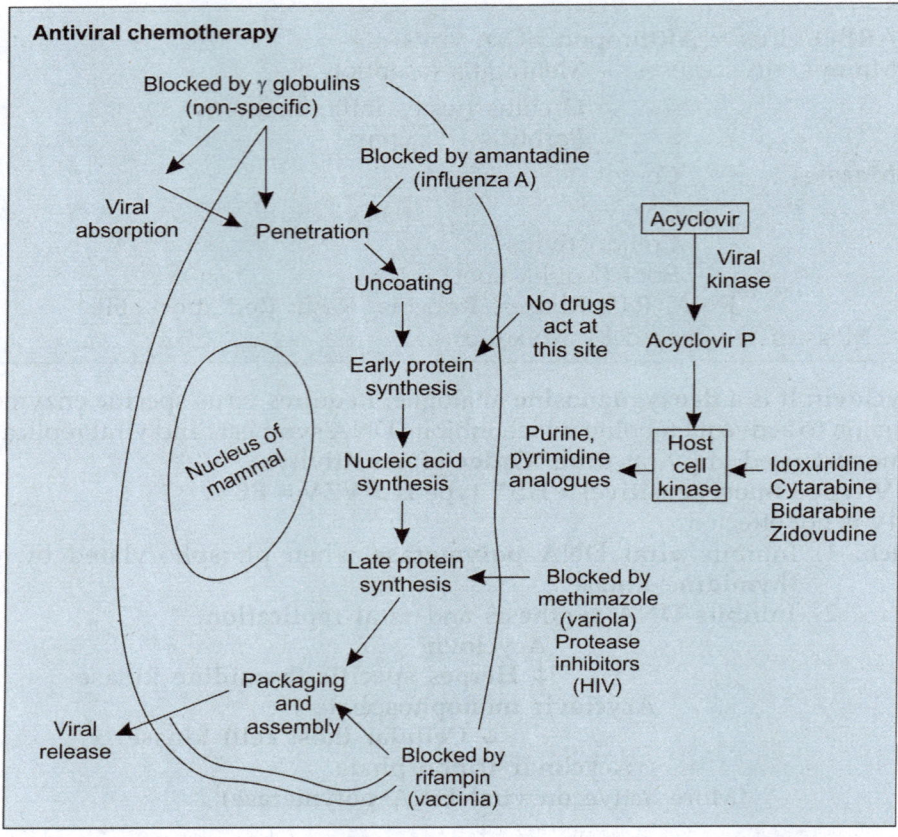

U:
1. **Genital HSV (generally type II) is commonest** indication.
   Route: Oral, local and parenteral
   Dose: Oral—1 gm/day into 5 divided doses × 10 days.
   Recurrent disease
   5 mg/kg IV TDS × 10 days
2. HSV type I:
   A. Mucocutaneous
      Dose: 15 mg/kg/day × 7 days
   B. Encephalitis
      Dose: 10 mg/kg/day
   C. Keratitis.
3. **HZV:** Drug is for severe/immunodeficient case (**DOC**).
   Dose: 5–10 mg/kg/day IV × 7 days

Idoxuridine: It is 5-iodo-2-deoxyuridine (**IUDR**) and **thymidine** analogue. It is the **first** pyrimidine antimetabolite used as antiviral drug.

Mech: Competes with thymidine and gets incorporated in DNA to form **faulty DNA** hence wrong viral protein. Effective against DNA viruses only.

ADR: Bone marrow depression (BMD)
U: 1. HSV: Keratoconjunctivitis and corneal ulcer
      2. Poxvirus

Vidarabine: It is the **first** drug used IV for life-threatening HSV. It is **adenine arabinoside** (an adenine analogue).
Mech: Inhibits **viral DNA polymerase** after phosphorylation.
ADR: 1. Anemia
       2. Thrombocytopenia
       3. Leucopenia
       4. Neurotoxicity
U: DOC in 1. Herpes simplex keratitis
              2. Neonatal herpes simplex
Trifluridine: HSV keratitis is the indication.

Ganciclovir: It is **DHPG** (Dihydroxy-2-propoxy-methylguanine)
Coverage: All herpes virus (HSV, VZV)
            EBV
            CMV (more active than acyclovir)
Mech: **Same** as acyclovir.
PK: Plasma t½ → 2–4 hrs (but t½ of ganciclovir triphosphate inside CMV infected cell is >24 hrs).
Concentration of active inhibitor ganciclovir triphosphate is **more inside** CMV infected cell.
ADR: 1. BMD
       2. Neuropsychiatric disturbances
       3. Nephrotoxic
       4. Thrombocytopenia
U: CMV in immunocompromised patient: 10 mg/kg/day IV prevents blindness in AIDS with CMV retinitis.

Foscarnet: It is pyrophosphate containing compound and is simple straight chain phosphonate.
Coverage: HSV
            HIV
            CMV
Mech: Inhibits **viral DNA polymerase** (that binds to **pyrophosphate** binding site of enzyme) and **reverse transcriptase**. Not require activation by viral kinase.
ADR: 1. Kidney damage
       2. **Convulsion, tremor**
       3. Anemia
       4. Phlebitis
       5. Reduced Ca^{2+}, Mg^{2+}, K^+, P
Route: IV infusion.
U: 1. CMV in AIDS and ganciclovir resistant case. CMV retinitis in AIDS when ganciclovir fails.
       2. Acyclovir resistant HSV type II and VZV in AIDS.

Zidovudine/AZT (azidothymidine): It is **thymidine** analogue

Mech:
1. Zidovudine triphosphate (formed by **phosphorylation** in the body) competitively inhibits viral **reverse transcriptase** (RNA dependent DNA polymerase) of HIV.
2. Zidovudine is **incorporated** into viral DNA and terminates its synthesis. Gets incorporated into growing viral DNA and terminates chain elongation.
3.
Single stranded viral DNA
↓ Reverse transcriptase
Double stranded viral DNA
↓
Integration with host cell DNA
↓
Viral genome and mRNA
↓
Viral regulatory and structural protein
↓

Drugs inhibit new cell infection but no effect on virus directed DNA integrated into host chromosome

Resistance: It is due to **point mutation** altering reverse trancriptase.

PK: Rapid oral absorption, bioavailability **65%, metabolised by hepatic glucuronidation,** t½—1 hr, **20%** renal excretion, plasma protein binding—**30%**. CSF level is 50% of that in plasma, crosses placenta and found in **milk**.

ADR: Anorexia, Zidovudine (high dose) causes Increased blood toxicity, Damage to liver, Oedema, Tumour, Headache, Yet to be known safety in pregnancy (retards growth).
Anaemia and neutropenia (**most important**)
Abdominal pain.
Myalgia, Insomnia, Damaged oesophagus, Increased CPK Neuropathy, Nail pigmentation, Emesis.
Myopathy, convulsion. **AZIDOTHYMIDINE**

AZT = Always Zaps Thrombocytosis

IA:
1. Nephrotoxic and myelosuppressive drugs and probenecid enhance toxicity.
2. Azoles inhibit AZT metabolism
3. Paracetamol enhances AZT toxicity by competing for glucuronidation.

U:
1. AIDS (**DOC**): No cure. Reduces virus titre, neuropathy and Kaposis's lesion and one year mortality among AIDS patient. Slows escalation of ARC to full blown AIDS. Enhances CD_4 cells.
Dose—500 mg/day TDS
2. HIV positive mother for 6 weeks AZT therapy (reduces transmission of HIV to offspring).

Test for HIV:
Western Blot = Confirmatory   WBC
ELISA = Sensitive

Zalcitabine (ddc), stavudine, didanosine: These are **nucleoside** analogues like AZT. Didanosine is **acid labile** and its active form is **dd ATP**.

Mechanism:

1. **Nucleoside analogue**
↓
Intracellular conversion to active triphosphate derivative
↓
Inhibits viral reverse transcriptase
↓
Inhibits proviral DNA of HIV

2. Active against AZT resistant mutant

PK: **All** absorbed orally. Bioavailability of didanosine is low. Plasma t½ of all is **1–3 hrs.**

ADR:
1. Peripheral neuropathy (limb pain and pancreatitis) is the **most important.**
2. GIT intolerance
3. CNS, ocular and cutaneous effects

U:
1. Advanced HIV (AZT + ddc)
2. AZT resistance HIV
3. HIV 1 and 2

Viral RNA entry
↓ Reverse transcriptase
Viral DNA   Protein inhibitors
↓   ↓ (−)
Incorporated into → Precursor ────→ Viral protein
host DNA   polyprotein
↓
Viral RNA

Efavirenz: It is **non-nucleoside reverse transcriptase inhibitor.**

Mech: Reduces viral load and enhances **CD4+** cell count.

PK: Well distributed orally, crosses CNS, **99%** plasma protein bound, t½—40 hrs (hence given OD). **Modest** inducer of CYP450.

ADR:
1. Dizziness, headache
2. Vivid dream   } CNS effects **commonest**
3. Loss of concentration
4. Rash 25% **(second commonest)**

Infection	Drug of choice
1. Primary infection of genital herpes simplex	→ Acyclovir (intravenous) is preferred (Oral preparation may be given to outdoor **patient.** 5% ointment of Acyclovir may be supplanted)
2. For suppression and treatment of recurrent herpes simplex infection	→ Acyclovir (oral)
3. Herpes simplex encephalitis	→ Acyclovir (intravenous) (vidarabine is 2nd drug of choice)

(Contd.)

Infection	Drug of choice
4. Herpes simplex keratitis	→ Trifluorothymidine (IV, topical). (vidarabine topical is second drug of choice)
5. For treatment of mucocutaneous Herpes simplex in immunocompromised patients	→ Acyclovir (IV in severe infection; oral preparation can be given in less severe infection). Topical ointment (5%) may be supplanted
6. Prophylaxis of mucocutaneous Herpes simplex infection in immunocompromised patients.	→ Acyclovir (oral)
7. Prophylaxis and treatment of influenza A	→ Amantadine (oral) (rimantadine may be used)
8. Respiratory syncytial virus	→ Ribavirin (aerosol)
9. Neonatal herpes simplex	→ Vidarabine (IV) (acyclovir has equal efficacy).
10. HIV	→ Zidovudine (oral) (didanosine and zalcitabine may be given orally)
11. Herpes zoster ophthalmicus	→ Acyclovir (oral)
12. Herpes zoster in immunocompetent hosts	→ Acyclovir (oral)
13. Herpes zoster in immunocompromised hosts	→ Acyclovir IV (vidarabine may also be given)
14. Varicella in immunocompetent hosts.	→ Acyclovir (oral)
15. Varicella in immunocompromised hosts	→ Acyclovir (IV)
16. Cytomegalovirus retinitis in immunosuppressed hosts	→ Ganciclovir (IV) (foscarnet IV may be given).
17. Chronic hepatitis (non A, non B/C) and chronic hepatitis B	→ Interferon α 2b (subcutaneous or IM)
18. Condyloma accuminatum	→ Interferon α 2b (or interferon α n3) intralesionally

Retroviral protease inhibitors: Aspartic protease enzyme is for production of **structural protein** and **enzyme** of HIV. This protease acts at **late step** in HIV replication.

Mech:
1. Ritonavir acts by inhibiting **protease** that cleaves viral protein precursor.
2. Act at **late step** of viral cycle effecting both newly and chronically infected cells leading to **immature** viral production and prevention of further round of infection.
3. Reduce **HIV titre** and enhance **CD4 cells.**

Efficacy: Monotherapy < double therapy < triple therapy.

ADR: Most prominant ADR are

PAIRED

1. Paresthesia
2. Asthma
3. Intolerance of GIT
4. Rashes
5. Diabetes Exacerbation
6. Dizziness
7. Headache

Antiviral Drugs

Amantadine: It is a **tricyclic** amine.

Mech:
1. Releases **DA** from intact nerve ending.
2. Acts on RNA virus by preventing **uncoating** of viral nucleic acid → decrease replication of virus. Inhibits influenza A virus replication.
3. **M_2 protein** which acts as ion channel, is the target of action.
4. Promotes presynaptic synthesis and release of DA in brain.
5. Amantadine blocks influenza **A** and rubella **A** and causes problems with the cerebellA.   **4A**
6. Blocks viral penetration/uncoating and may buffer pH of endosome.

Efficacy: Efficacy of amantadine is **lower** than levodopa and **higher** than anticholinergics. Efficacy after months is lost due to tolerance.

Resistance: It is due to **mutation** causing amino acid substitution in **M_2 protein**.

PK: Complete oral absorption, excreted unchanged in urine over 2–3 days. t½—16 hrs. **Dose:** 3 mg/kg/day orally, effects of single dose last 10 hrs.

ADR: More ADR when combined with anticholinergics. **CHINS**
1. Livedo reticularis, ankle edema and peripheral edema are due to CA release causing vasoconstriction.
2. CNS effects: hallucination, loss of mental concentration, dizziness, ataxia.
3. CHD and CHF
4. Postural Hypotension
5. Insomnia
6. Nightmares
7. Slurred speech

ADR of AMANTADINE
Appetite loss, Most common (gut and CNS dysfunction) Arrhythmia, Nervousness, Teratogenic, Antihistaminics/anticholinergics increase neuropathy. Decreased renal function, Insomnia, Neurotoxic, Exacerbation of pre-existing seizures.

CI: Pregnancy
Gastric ulcer   **PGE**
Epilepsy

U:
1. Influenza A_2 (prophylaxis and treatment)
2. Rubella
3. Parkinsonism to supplement levodopa
   Fixed dose—100 mg BD (not titrated according to response).

   Amantadine for influenza **A**

Rimantadine: More potent than amantadine.
Same as amantadine **except** t½—30 hrs. Dose and use same.

Interferon α: It is **LMW glycoprotein cytokines** produced by **host cells** due to viral infection. 3 types of human interferon (α, β, γ) are produced by recombinant DNA technology.

Mechanism

1. Has **antiproliferative, immunomodulator** and **antiviral action**.
2. Acts on tyrosine protein kinase receptors of cell surface
   ↓
   Phosphorylation of cellular protein
   ↓
   Transcription of interferon induced protein
   ↓
   Antiviral effects

Antiviral effects are due to suppression of
   A. Viral penetration
   B. Viral mRNA synthesis
   C. Viral particle assembly
   D. Viral protein synthesis (**most important**)
3. Inhibits **RNA** and **DNA** viruses

PK: Not effective orally
Parenteral route
Interferon—2a is marketed in India as **Reaferon**.

ADR:
1. Myelosuppression (BMD): **Dose limiting**
2. Neurotoxicity
3. Flu-like symptoms (fatigue, aches, anorexia, fever)
4. Hypotension
5. Alopecia   **HALF MAN**
6. Liver dysfunction
7. Arrhythmia

ADR of INTERFERONS
Injection (influenza like syndrome), **N**ausea, **T**olerance, **E**mesis, **R**enal damage, azotemia, **F**ever, **F**atigue, **E**levated liver enzymes and TG, **R**educed WBC, **O**ccurrence of alopecia, **N**eurotoxicity, **S**omnolence.

U:
1. Chronic HBV and HCV
2. Cytopenia
3. Kaposi's sarcoma (AIDS related)
4. Hairy cell leukemia
5. HSV, VZV, CMV in immunocompromised patient
6. Rhinoviral cold (prophylaxis)
7. Condyloma acuminata (papillomavirus)
8. Chronic granulomatous disease: Interferon γ

Ribavirin: Synthetic purine nucleoside analogue. Broad spectrum antiviral activity.
Coverage: Influenza A and B
Respiratory syncytial virus
DNA and double-stranded RNA virus

Mech:
1. Inhibits **guanine nucleotide** synthesis by competitively inhibiting **IMP dehydrogenase.**
2. Mono- and triphosphate derivatives of drug inhibit GTP, viral RNA and DNA synthesis.

PK: Oral bioavailability—**50%**. Partly metabolised and eliminated in a **multiexponential** manner.

ADR:
1. Haemolysis
2. GIT intolerance
3. CNS effects
4. Aerosol causes mucosal irritation and bronchospasm

U:
1. RSV (respiratory syncytical virus): DOC (**Ribavirin**)
2. Herpes virus
3. Acute hepatitis
4. Influenza A and B and measles in immunocompromised patient.

> **RIBAVIR**in: RSV, Influenza B and Arena **VIR**us (Lassa).

Penciclovir: It is **acyclic guanosine** nucleoside derivative active against **HSV type I** and **II and VZV.**

Mech: **Monophosphorylated** by viral thymidine kinase and cellular enzymes form nucleoside triphosphate which inhibits herpes DNA polymerase.

PK: Penciclovir triphosphate has intracellular t½ **20–30 times** longer than acyclovir triphosphate. Negligibly absorbed topically, well tolerated.

Route: Topical only

U: Healing and pain are shortened one-half day in duration, compared to placebo-treated subjects.
1. HSV
2. VZV

Valacyclovir

Mech: **Same** as acyclovir
Plasma t½—2–3 hrs (**same** as acyclovir)

U:
1. HSV
2. VZV
3. CMV

Cidofovir: It is nucleotide analogue of **cytosine** whose phosphorylation is independent of viral enzymes.

Mech: Inhibits viral DNA polymerase

PK: Plasma t½ →2–3 hrs
Intracellular t½ of cidofovir diphosphate is 17–30 hrs.

ADR:
1. Nephrotoxicity
2. Neutropenia
3. Metabolic acidosis
4. Ocular hypotony

CI:
1. Nephrotoxicity
2. Administration with nephrotoxic drugs, including NSAIDs.

U:
1. CMV
2. Virus induced retinitis

Amprenavir: It is protease inhibitor. **Common** ADR of protease inhibitors are:
1. Inhibition of **CYP450** dependent oxidations. Hence, antiarrhythmic, antihistaminic, antimigraine-ergot derivative, BZD, GI prokinetic and antimycobacterial drugs are **contraindicated** with protease inhibitors.
2. **Lypodystrophy** and **hyperglycemia.**

ADR of amprenavir: Nausea, emesis, diarrhoea, rash, paresthesia.

> **ADR** of protease inhibitors **(INDINAVIR):** Increased breast, Nausea, DM, diarrhoea, damaged erythroid stem cells, Increased TG and CHE, Neutral or inhibited CYP450, Abdominal girth (buffalo hump), Vomiting, Intolerance to glucose, Redistributed fat.

Nevirapine: It is **non-nucleoside** reverse transcriptase inhibitor like **delavirdine** and **efavirenz**, and **all are selective noncompetitive** inhibitors of HIV-I reverse transcriptase.

- **Mech:** Reduces viral **RNA** and enhances **CD4+** count. Selectively and noncompetitively inhibits reverse transcriptase of HIV-I.
- **PK:** Well absorbed orally. **Lipophilic** (enters foetus and mother's milk). Crosses CNS. Dependent on metabolism for elimination. Most drug excreted in urine as glucuronide of **hydroxylated metabolites.**
- **ADR:**
  1. **Commonest** →rash, fever, headache, elevated serum transaminase.
  2. Stevens-Johnson syndrome and toxic epidermal necrolysis.
  3. Hepatoxicity.
  4. Induces CYP3A4.

Delavirdine: 98% plasma protein bound. Equally excreted in urine and faeces.
- **ADR:**
  1. **Commonest**—rashes 44%
  2. Dizziness, headache, nausea
- **IA :**
  1. Inhibits metabolism of protease inhibitors
  2. KTZ and fluoxetine enhance its plasma level
  3. Phenytoin, phenobarbital and carbamazepine reduce its plasma level.

Lamivudine: It is deoxycytidine analogue.
- **Mech:** Phosphorylated intracellularly and inhibits **HIV RT** plus **HBV DNA** polymerase. Incorporation into **DNA** causes chain termination. Human **DNA** polymerase is not effected.
- **Resistance:** It is due to point mutation in **RT** and polymerase.
- **PK:** Plasma half-life = 6–9 hrs, intracellular half-life = >12 hrs, excreted unchanged in urine.
- **ADR:** Headache, anorexia, nausea, fatigue, abdominal pain, pancreatitis and neuropathy.
- **U:**
  1. Chronic **HBV** (100 mg OD)
  2. **HIV** (150 mg BD with other drugs)

Famciclovir: It is ester prodrug of guanine nucleoside analogue penciclovir.
- **Mech:** Needs viral thymidine kinase for generation of active **DNA** polymerase inhibition (similar to acyclovir).
- **U:** **Herpes** simplex and **herpes** zoster (**HBV** also).

Depending on infecting bacteria	
Disease or pathogen	*Drug(s) of first choice*
Gram-negative cocci (aerobic):	
1. Gonococcus	Penicillin, ampicillin, tetracycline, ceftriaxone
2. Meningococcus	penicillin
Gram-positive cocci (aerobic):	
1. Pneumococcus	Penicillin
2. Streptococcus, hemolytic A, B, C, D.	Penicillin
3. *Streptococcus viridans*	Penicillin + aminoglycoside
4. Staphylococcus, nonpenicillinase producing	Penicillin
5. Staphylococcus, penicillinase producing	Penicillinase resistant penicillin
6. Staphylococcus, methicillin resistant	Vancomycin
7. Enterococcus	Penicillin + gentamicin
Gram-positive rods (aerobic):	
1. Bacillus (anthrax)	Penicillin BP
2. *Listeria Monocytogenes*	Ampicillin + aminoglycoside MLA
3. Nocardia	Sulfonamide
Gram-negative rods (aerobic):	
1. Coliforms (*E. coli*, Klebsiella, Enterobacter, Serratia, Proteus)	Third generation cephalosporins, aminoglycosides
2. Shigella	Cotrimoxazole
3. Salmonella	Cotrimoxazole, chloramphenicol
4. Brucella	Tetracycline
5. Bordetella	Erythromycin
6. *Yersinia pestis* (plague)	Tetracycline, streptomycin
7. *Vibrio cholerae*	Tetracycline
8. *Pseudomonas aeruginosa*	Aminoglycoside + extended spectrum penicillin
9. Legionella	Erythromycin + rifampicin
10. Haemophilus	Cefuroxime, third generation cephalosporin
11. *Haemophilus ducreyi* (chancroid)	Cotrimoxazole
12. Campylobacter	Erythromycin
Anaerobes	
1. Gram +ve (peptococci, peptostreptococci, clostridia)	Penicillin
2. *Bacteroides fragilis*	Metronidazole
3. Gram −ve other than *B. fragilis* (Fusobacterium).	Penicillin

Depending on infecting bacteria *(Contd.)*	
Disease or pathogen	Drug(s) of first choice
Mycobacteria	
1. *Myc. tuberculosis*	Isoniazid + rifampicin
2. *Myc. leprae*	Dapsone + rifampicin
Spirochetes	
1. Borrelia	Tetracycline
2. Leptospira	Penicillin
3. Treponema (syphilis, yaws)	Penicillin
Mycoplasma pneumonia	Tetracycline, erythromycin
Chlamydia trachomatis	Tetracycline
Rickettsiae	Tetracycline, chloramphenicol

H. Influenzae: Ampicillin is stilll DOC in resistant cases. Chloramphenicol is also added (if resistant to chloramphenicol—cefuroxime or third generation cephalosoprin). DOC in *Mycoplasma pneumoniae* infection in pregnancy—erythromycin. DOC in typhoid (nowadays)—Ciprofloxacin. DOC in lymphogranuloma venereum (caused by Chlamydia)—tetracycline. **Treatment occurs against specific organism infecting individual patient. Prophylaxis is against all organisms causing infection.**

Disease or pathogen	Drug(s) of first choice
Fungi	
1. *Candida albicans*	Amphotericin B
2. *Cryptococcus neoformans*	Amphotericin B + flucytosine.
3. Coccidioidomycosis	Amphotericin B
4. Aspergillosis, mucormycosis	Amphotericin B
5. Histoplasmosis	Amphotericin B
6. **Blastomycosis**	Ketoconazole BSP-KTZ
7. **Sporotrichosis**	Ketoconazole
8. **Paracoccidioidomycosis**	Ketoconazole
Candida albicans	Drug of choice
1. Superficial infections (oral-thrush, vulvovaginitis)	Nystatin
2. Systemic/deep infection	Amphotericin B
3. Chronic mucocutaneous candidiasis	Ketoconazole
DOC for MDR Shigella (resistant to cotrimoxazole) is **nalidixic acid**	

Chemoprophylaxis

Disease or pathogen	Drug(s) of first choice
1. Rheumatic fever Group A Streptococcal	Benzathine Penicillin
2. Meningococcal infection meningitis	Rifampicin—DOC Minocycline Sulfadiazine Sulfisoxazole
3. Tuberculosis	Isoniazid
4. Plague	Tetracycline
5. *H. influenzae*	Rifampicin
6. Syphilis	Benzathine penicillin
7. Gonorrhoea	Penicillin
8. Rickettsial infections	Tetracyclines
9. Malaria	Chloroquine
10. Influenza A	Amantadine
11. Enterotoxigenic *E. coli* (traveller's diarrhoea)	Doxycycline
12. *Pneumocystis carinii*	Cotrimoxazole

Most common cause of traveller's diarrhoea is enterotoxigenic *E. coli*.

Treatment of AIDS:
Dose:
AZT—600 mg BD
Didanosine—300 mg BD

Lamivudine—150 mg BD
Zalcitabine—0.75 mg TDS
Stavudine—40 mg BD

Saquinavir—600 mg TDS
Indinavir—800 mg TDS

Ritonavir—600 mg BD

Nelfinavir—700 mg TDS
Nevirapine—300 mg OD × 2W + 200 mg BD
Delavirdine—400 mg TDS

First line: Didanosine
or Didanosine + AZT
or Lamivudine + AZT
or Zalcitabine + AZT

Second line: **SIR**
Ritonavir/Indinavir or
Saquinavir + **Nucleoside** analogue.
Stavudine + didanosine/ lamivudine.
First line is started when viral load is >5000–10000 and CD4 ≤500/μl.

D
DA
LA
ZA

DDLJ

Viruses are non-living automations that hijack living cells and force cellular machinery to replicate the virus. The best prevention for HIV is Arabian culture and the best culture for HIV is Western culture.

1. CD4 produces IL2 (4 × 2 = 8). IL2 acts on CD8 which synthesises IL1 (8 × 1 = 8).
   CD4 is **HELP**er cells (4 letters)
   CD8 is **SUPPRESS**or cells (8 letters)
   CD4 binds to MCH II = 4 × 2 = 8
   CD8 binds to MCHI = 8 × 1 = 8
2. **CD4 count**
   <500/ml = Anti-HIV started
   <200/ml = Risk of *P. carinii*
   <100/ml = Risk of CMV
   <50/ml = Risk of candidiasis, MIAC
3. **Blots:** Southern = DNA, Northern = RNA and Western = Protein

   SNoW = DRoP

4. C3a, C4a, C5a **A**ctivates **A**cute inflammation (**A**naphylatoxin).
   C3b, C4b **B**inds **B**acteria to macrophages for easy digestion.
   Classical pathway **C**ombines **C**omplexes whereas **A**lternative one **A**ctivates IgA.

Unit 11
Chemotherapy

62. Anticancer Drugs, Immunosuppressants and Gene Therapy

Cells are killed in a **first order manner** (means constant percentage is killed with each course of therapy). **Most anticancer drugs** effect **cell division** and act preferentially on rapidly proliferating cells. Cells in Go (non-dividing) phase survive chemotherapy. Combination therapy is common because each drug is active against tumour, has different mechanism and different toxicity. Time is given for host tissue recovery between treatment cycle.

Aim of therapy
A. To cure/prolonged remission
- Wilms' tumour
- Acute leukemia
- Retinoblastoma — in children **WARE**
- Rhabdomyosarcoma
- Ewing's sarcoma
- Burkitt's lymphoma
- Testicular teratoma
- Mycosis fungoides
- Hodgkin's disease
- Lymphosarcoma
- Choriocarcinoma

B. Palliation (shrinkage of tumour)
- Head and neck cancer
- Breast cancer
- Lung cancer
- Ovarian CA
- Prostatic CA
- Chronic lymphatic leukemia
- Chronic myeloid leukemia
- Non-Hodgkin's lymphoma

> Lung cancer (peripheral bronchogenic) is **"SPHERE"** of complication:
> **S**uperior vena caval syndrome
> **P**ancoast's tumour
> **H**orner's syndrome
> **E**ndocrine (paraneoplastic)
> **R**ecurrent laryngeal symptoms (hoarseness)
> **E**ffusion (pleural/pericardial)

Adjuvant: It is for residual malignant cells after surgery/radiotherapy.

Toxicity: Drugs act on **nucleic acid and their precursors (most important target of action).** Large solid tumour has lower cell division. Anticancer drugs are one of the **most toxic** drugs used in therapy.

They either modify or kill cancer cells.

1. They damage **cells of hair follicles** causing alopecia and dermatitis in skin.

Commonest leukemia by age group			
Age (yrs): <15	15–39	40–59	60+
ALL	AML	AML and CML	CLL

Primary tumours that metastasize to liver:
   Colon 42%, Stomach 23%, Pancreas 21%, Breast 14%, Lung 13%.

> Cancer Sometimes Penetrates Benign Liver

2. They decrease **renewal rate** of mucosal lining causing mucositis (**e.g.** methotrexate, 5-FU and antibiotics). CTZ stimulation causes nausea and vomiting.

    Highly emetogenic drugs are   MAMC Delhi
       Mithramycin
       Actinomycin D
       Mustine
       Cisplatin and Cyclophosphamide
       Dacarbazine

3. Most serious toxicity is **bone marrow depression (BMD)**. BMD is **dose-limiting ADR except** with asparaginase, bleomycin, cisplatin, hormone and vincristine.

    Order of manifestations is—leukopenia > thrombocytopenia > anemia.

4. **Damage to lymphoreticular tissue** causes lymphocytopenia and inhibition of lymphocytic function resulting in reduced humoral and cell mediated immunity. Host defence mechanism is broken down leading to susceptibility to **all infection** specially opportunistic infection.

5. Inhibition of **gonadal cells** and **ovulation** causes impotence and oligozoospermia in male and amernorrhoea in female.

6. All cytotoxic drugs are **teratogenic** because they damage foetus when given to pregnant.

7. **Secondary cancer** (leukemia, lymphomas, histocytic tumour) occurs due to reduced humoral and cell mediated blocking factor against neoplasia.

8. **Hyperuricaemia** occurs due to massive cell destruction.

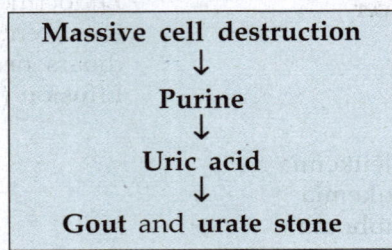

9. Doxorubicin causes cardiomyopathy. Vincristine causes neuropathy. Cyclophosphamide causes cystitis and alopecia.

> A. **Cellular component synthesis:-** G_2 : Mitosis
> M : Mitotic phase
> G_1 : Enzyme synthesis
> S : DNA replication
> B. **Cell cycle specific drugs (for high growth fraction malignancies)**
> Antimetabolite, bleomycin, vinca alkaloid and etoposide.
> C. **Cell cycle nonspecifc drugs** (for both low and high growth fraction malignancies) alkylating agents, antibiotic, nitrosoureas, cisplatin. **Cell cycle nonspecific drugs** kill both resting and dividing cells. All antibiotics except bleomycin are cell cycle nonspecific.
> **Cell cycle specific drugs** kill only dividing cell and they are:
> 1. G_1 : Vinblastine
> 2. S : Mtx, 6-TG, 6-MP, hydroxyurea, cytarabine, mitomycin C, doxorubicin, daunorubicin.
> 3. G_2 : Daunorubicin, bleomycin, etoposide
> 4. M : Vincristine, vinblastine, paclitaxel

Classification
I. Cytotoxic drugs
1. **Antimetabolite**
   A. Folate antagonist:
   Methotrexate (Mtx, amethopterin).
   B. Purine antagonist:
   6-Mercaptopurine (6-MP)
   6-Thioguanine (6-TG)
   Azathioprine
   C. Pyrimidine antagonist:
   5-Fluorouracil (5-FU)
   Ftorafur
   Cytarabine (cytosine arabinoside)
   D. Newer drugs—capecitabine, gemcitabine.
2. **Antibiotics**   **BMD**
   Bleomycin
   Mitomycin C
   Mithramycin (plicamycin)
   Mitoxantrone
   Doxorubicin (epirubicin and idarubicin also)
   Dactinomycin
   Daunorubicin
3. **Microtubule inhibitors**
   A. Vinca alkaloids
   Vincristine (oncovin)
   Vinblastine, venorelbine

B. **Taxanes**
      Paclitaxel
      Docetaxel
4. **Alkylating agents**
   A. **Nitrogen mustards**   MIC
      Ifosfamide
      Cyclophosphamide
      Chlorambucil
      Melphalan
      Mechlorethamine (mustine HCl)
   B. **Nitrosoureas**
      Semustine (methyl-CCNU)
      Carmustine (BCNU)
      Lomustine (CCNU)
      Streptozocin
   C. Triazine—dacarbazine (DTIC)
   D. Ethyl enimine—thio-TEPA
   E. Alkyl sulfonate—busulfan
5. **Others:** Etoposide
              Procarbazine
              Cisplatin
              Carboplatin
              Hydroxyurea
              Interferons, amifostine, anastrozole, letrozole
              L-asparaginase
6. **Camptothecin analogues**
   Topotecan, irinotecan.
II. **Drugs altering hormonal milieu**
    Estrogen
    Antiestrogen (tamoxifen)
    Progestin
    Androgen (testosterone and fluoxymesterone)
    Glucocorticoid (prednisolone)

Alkylating agents: Have actions of **nonspecific** type on cell cycle phase causing **mutagenicity, teratogenicity** and **carcinogenicity. Carbonium ion** intermediates formed by these agents (cytotoxic and radiomimetic) transfer alkyl group mainly to position **7 of guanine risidues** of DNA forming covalent bond, leading to malfunction of DNA.

Cyclophosphamide: It is one of the **most popular** anticancer drugs covalently X-linked (interstrand) DNA at **guanine N-7.**

   Mech: 1. Has anti-tumour action and immunosuppressant property due to **aldophosphamide** and **phosphoramide mustard metabolites.**
           2. Cyclophosphamide (prodrug)
                        ↓
              Hydroxy cyclophosphamide and **phosphoramide mustard**
                         (active metabolites)

3. **Cyclophosphamide and ifosfamide induce P450**
   ↓
   Active phosphoramide mustard
   DNA
   ↓
   Alkylated DNA

PK: Hepatic metabolism, crosses BBB
Dose: A. 3 mg/kg/day **oral**
B. 12 mg/kg/week **IV**

ADR of CYCLOPHOSPHAMIDE

Chemical irritation due to acrolein Yields cystitis.
Cardiomyopathy, **L**eukopenia, **O**ccurrence of cystitis (10%), **P**ulmonary fibrosis.
Haemorrhagic cystitis due to **Acrolein** (prevented by Mensa). **VO**miting, **S**paring of **P**latelets, **H**ormone (SIADH), **A**lopecia, **M**yelosuppression, **I**ntoxication of water, **D**amage to mucosa and **E**pithelium.

U:
1. **B**one marrow transplantation
2. **RA** (third line drug)
3. **I**diopathic thrombocytopenic purpura
4. **N**on-Hodgkin's lymphoma
5. **B**reast and ovarian **CA**   **BRAIN on CAPS**
6. **P**emphigus (maintenance therapy)
7. **SLE** (maintenance therapy)

Mustine HCl (mechlorethamine): It is the **first** nitrogen mustard and is highly reactive and local vesicant (can be given by **IV route** only). Only IV route is preferred.

Dose—0.4 mg/kg/every 2 days
Mech: Nitrogen mustard forms a very reactive **immonium intermediate** which attacks nucleophilic group (**guanine**) leading to:
A. DNA cross-linking
B. Base linking to same DNA strand and to water.

Resistance: Resistance of nitrogen mustard is due to **reduced drug uptake** by cancer cell and increased rate of **DNA repair**.

ADR: **Acute** effects are:
1. Nausea
2. Vomiting
3. Haemodynamic changes

Ifosfamide: It is congener of cyclophosphamide.
ADR:
1. Haemorrhagic cystitis: Treated by Mensa (**SH-compound**) to prevent cystitis which inactivates vesicotoxic metabolites of ifosfamide and cyclophosphamide. **Mensa** is excreted in urine.
2. Emesis and alopecia lesser than cyclophosphamide.

U:
1. **L**ymphoma
2. **O**steogenic sarcoma   **LOC**
3. **C**arcinoma of head, neck, breast, bronchi, bladder and testes.

Chlorambucil: Slowest acting alkylating agent.
Mech: Acts on lymphoid and myeloid tissues.

ADR of CHLORAMBUCIL

Least toxic. Cessation of menses, Hepatotoxic, Leukemia, Other cancer also, Rash, Azoospermia, Moderate depression of peripheral Blood count, Unusual dermatitis, Convulsion (seizures), Intolerance to gut, Lung fibrosis.

U: **DOC** for maintenance therapy in CLL, Hodgkin's disease.

Melphalan:	**ADR:**	BMD (**most important**)
Complications:		Infection, diarrhoea, pancreatitis
	U:	Multiple myeloma

ADR of BUSULFAN: **B**MD, **U**ric acid raised, **S**terility, **U**nusual GIT disturbance, **L**ittle effect on lymphoid tissue, **F**ibrosis of lung, **A**bnormal skin colour (pigmentation), e**N**docrine insufficiency (adrenal).
        1. **Hyperuricaemia (common)**
        2. Pulmonary fibrosis (**specific**)
        3. Addison's like feature, gynaecomastia, sterility
U: CML (granulocyte precursors are **most sensitive**)
        Dose: 4 mg/day orally

Nitrosoureas: These are **lipid soluble** and cross BBB
Mech: Antitumour action is present
ADR:
    1. Optic nerve damage
    2. Cerebral edema
    3. Nephrotoxic
    4. Nausea, vomiting, ataxia, dizziness
    5. BMD
    6. Visceral fibrosis
U:
    1. Brain tumour
    2. Meningeal leukemia

Streptozocin: Accumulates in β-cells of pancreas
ADR: Insulin shock
U: Insulinomas

Dacarbazine (DTIC): The only alkylating agent having primary inhibiting action on **RNA** and **protein** synthesis. All others effect **DNA**. It is activated in liver.
U: Malignant melanoma (**most important**)
        Dose: 3.5 mg/kg/day × 10 days

Antimetabolites: These are **S-phase specific** and are analogue to **DNA/ coenzyme** component.
    Mech: They **competitively** inhibit normal substrate utilization or get incorporated forming dysfunctional macromolecules.

Methotrexate: It is one of the **oldest** anti-cancer drug.

Mech:
1. Inhibits **DHFRase** (dihydrofolate reductase) leading to reduced dTMP resulting in reduced DNA and protein.

$$DHFA \xrightarrow{DHFRase} THFA$$
$$\Theta \uparrow$$
$$Mtx$$

2. Kills cells in **S-phase** (DNA synthesis phase).
3. Has **50,000 times** higher affinity for enzyme than normal substrate, hence inhibition is **pseudoirreversible**.
4. Inhibits DNA somewhat RNA and protein synthesis.
5. Reduces **CMI** and **cytokine** production.
6. Has **anti-inflammatory** effect.
7. **Highest** activity occurs with thymidine derivative and normal RNA + protein.

Resistance: It is due to:
1. Enhanced DHFRase
2. Reduced affinity of enzyme for Mtx.
3. Reduced active transport of Mtx into cancer cell.

PK: 50% plasma protein bound, absorbed orally, excreted unchanged in urine, aspirin and sulfonamide reduce renal tubular secretion of Mtx.

ADR:
1. Bone marrow toxicities. Toxicity is reduced by **folinic acid/ leucovorin** treatment. Leucovorin is citrovorum factor which is directly converted into **tetrahydrofolate**. Thymidine also **counteracts** Mtx toxicity.
2. Desquamation and bleeding

Folinic acid (leucovorin)
↓
N^5N^{10} methylene-FH_4
↓
Bypasses inhibited reductase

ADR of METHOTREXATE: Mucositis, Elevated liver enzyme, Toxicity of marrow, Hepatic fibrosis, Oral Mtx →portal fibrosis, Thrombocytopenia maximum in 10 days and Reverse thereafter. Epithelial damage of gut, X-ray lung Abnormal (pneumonitis), Toxic to Embryo.

IA: Sulfonamide, phenylbutazone, dicumarol and salicylates enhance toxicity by displacing Mtx from protein binding site.

U:
1. Abortion, ectopic pregnancy
2. RA: Beneficial effect is due to inhibition of cytokine production, CMI reaction and chemotaxis.
3. Choriocarcinoma
4. ALL, CA breast, CA testes
5. Immunosuppressive therapy
6. Psoriasis (non-cancerous disease)
7. **DOC** in autoimmune disease:
   Chronic active **H**epatitis
   Uveitis   **HUMP**
   Myasthenia gravis
   Pemphigus

Mercaptopurine (6-MP) and thioguanine (6-TG)
6-TG is **not substrate of xanthene oxidase.**
Mech: 1. 6-TG → Monoribonucleotide
↓ (−)
Inosine monophosphate ⇄ Adenine and guanine nucleotides
2. 6-MP → Thioinosine monophosphate
↓
Inhibition of amidotranferase
(which leads to reduced purine synthesis)
↑
6-TG → Thioguanine monophosphate
↓
Deoxythioguanine triphosphate
↓
Incorporated into tumour cell DNA

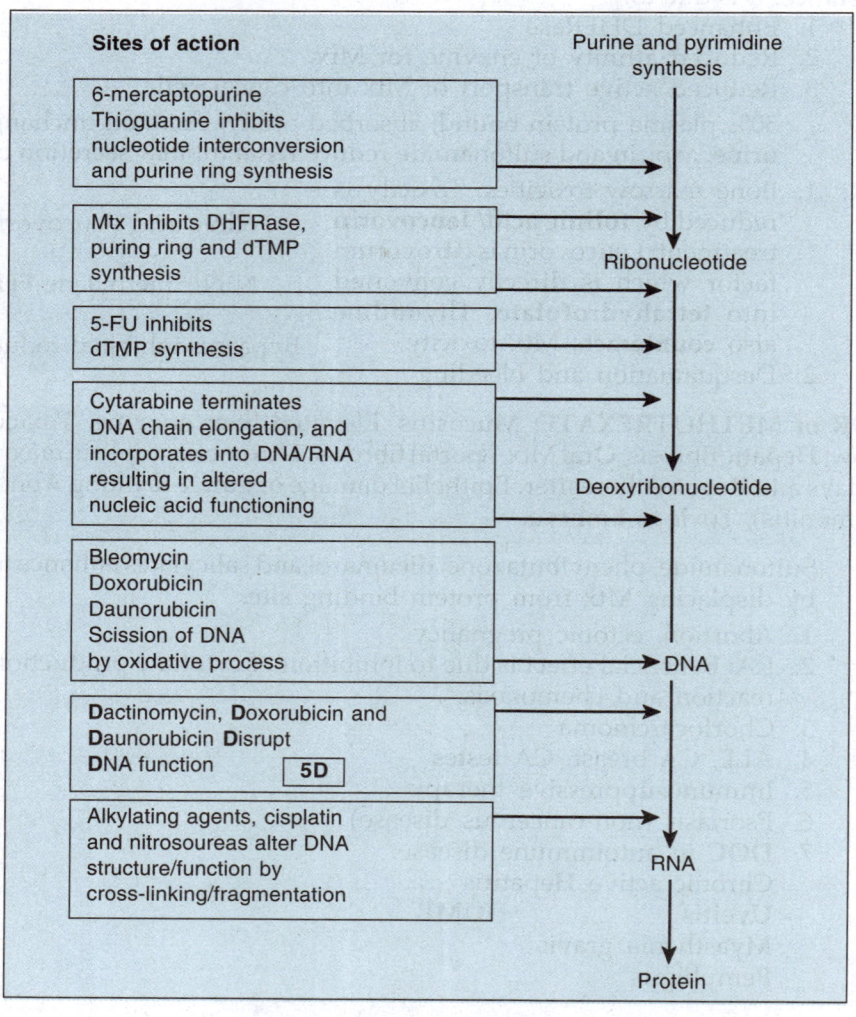

3. **Xanthene oxidase metabolises 6-MP (but not 6-TG) and azathioprine. allopurinol inhibits xanthene oxidase.**
ADR: 1. **BMD**
2. Hyperuricaemia
U: Dose—6-MP 2.5 mg/kg/day and 6-TG 2 mg/kg/day.
1. Choriocarcinoma
2. 6-MP in ALL

Azathioprine: It is antimetabolite derivative of 6-MP.
Mech: 1. Reduces CMI and inhibits T-lymphocyte.
2. **More immunosuppressant** than antitumour action.
3. Interferes with metabolism and synthesis of nucleic acid.
PK: Absorbed orally
Dose: 4 mg/kg/day

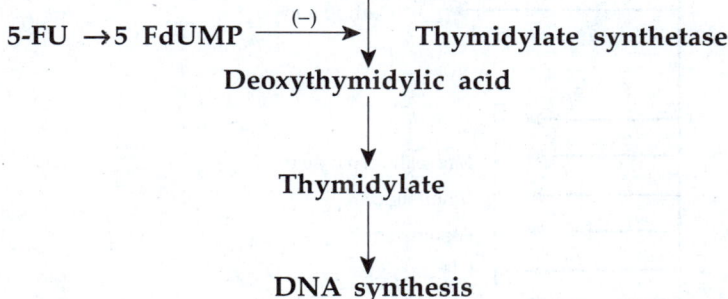

Azathioprine and 6-MP — xanthene oxidase → metabolites.
So dose should be reduced to ¼ if allopurinol is given concurrently.
U: 1. As immunosuppressant in organ transplantation and RA.
2. Graft rejection (**most important**)

Pyrimidine analogues: Possess antifungal, antipsoriatic and antineoplastic activities.

5-FU: It is converted to 5 FdUMP (5-fluoro-2-deoxyuridine monophosphate) which complexes folic acid and inhibits thymidylate synthetase.
Mech: 1.
          Deoxyuridilic acid

5-FU → 5 FdUMP ──(−)──▶ Thymidylate synthetase

         Deoxythymidylic acid

           Thymidylate

          DNA synthesis

2. Effect is enhanced by **leucovorin** and reversed by thymidine.
3. Inhibition of thymidylate synthetase reduces dTMP.
4. Drug is incorporated into **nucleic acid** and produces toxicity which is not reversible by leucovorin but partially reversed by thymidine. 5 FdUMP competes with dUMP for **thymidylate synthetase.**

ADR of FLUOROURACIL: Fulminant diarrhoea, Loss of hair Unusually (phototoxicity), Rash, On CNS (cerebellar syndrome), Ulcer of gut mucosa, myelosuppression (Overdose), Rarely angina, Anorexia and nausea (earliest), Continuous Infusion Leads to shock and death.
U: 1. Rule of **5** for **5**-FU = **5**-FU 500 mg **5** days/month for **5** cycle in, **5** solid tumour (breast, colon, urinary bladder, liver, pancreas, stomach).
2. Solar keratosis   **SCAM**
3. Cutaneous basal cell CA

4. All adenocarcinoma (DOC): Solid tumour, BCC.
5. Mycosis fungoides.

Cytarabine: Acts on S-phase.
Mech:
$$\text{Phosphorylation of drug}$$
$$\downarrow$$
$$\text{Triphosphate of cytarabine}$$
$$\downarrow$$
$$\text{Inhibition of DNA polymerase and inhibition of cytidilic acid}$$
$$\downarrow$$
$$\text{Inhibition of DNA synthesis}$$

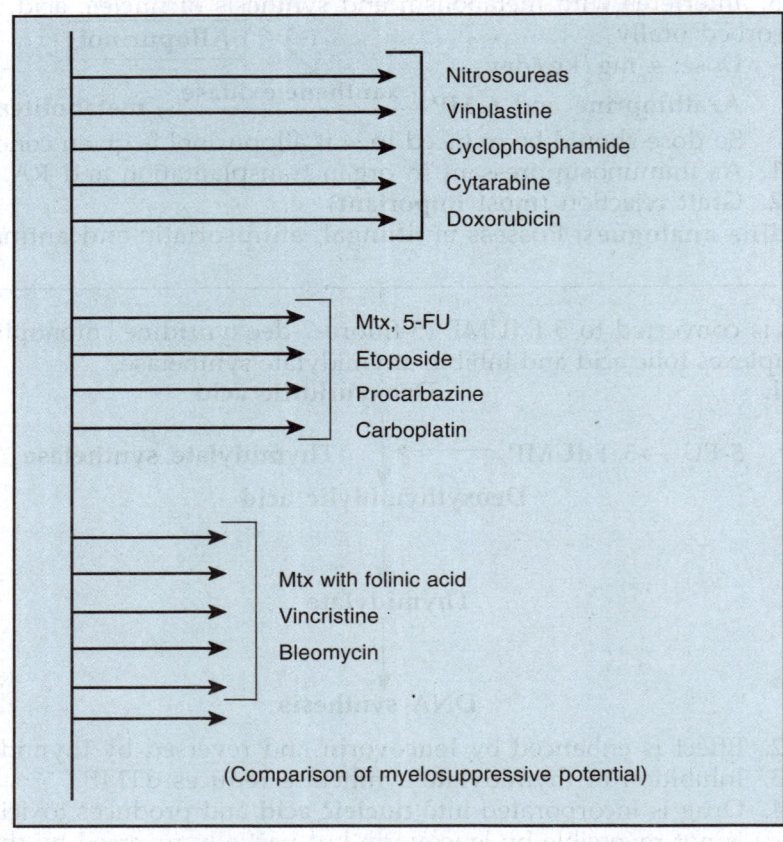

(Comparison of myelosuppressive potential)

U:
1. Hodgkin's disease.
2. ALL
3. Non-Hodgkin's lymphoma.

Ftorafur: It is congener of 5-FU
U: Dose—1 gm/day orally
1. Breast cancer
2. GIT cancer

Vinca alkaloids: These are obtained from **Vinka rosea (Periwinkle plant)**. Cell cycle specific (kill cells in **M-phase**). They are part of **MOPP** regimen.

Mech: Bind to **tubulin** and inhibit their polymerisation causing mitotic spindle disruption (**metaphase arrest**).

> **Vinca Checks MicroTubular Growth**
> Vincristine and Vinblastine
> Colchicine
> Mebendazole
> Taxol (antibreast CA), Thiabendazole
> Griseofulvin

ADR:
1. Vincristine:
   A. BMD
   B. Paralytic ileus
   C. Alopecia
   D. Neurotoxicity (dose limiting step): Peripheral neuropathy
2. Vinblastine:
   A. BMD more than vincristine

> **VinBLASTine BLASTS Bone marrow**

U:
1. Vincristine (rapidly acting):
   A. Wilms' tumour
   B. Hodgkin's disease
   C. ALL   **Largest WHALE**
   D. Lymphosarcoma
   E. Ewing's sarcoma
   F. Lung CA
2. Vinblastine:
   A. Hodgkin's disease
   B. Testicular CA

Paclitaxel: It is **texane** obtained from Western Yew tree bark.

Mech:
1. Mechanism is **opposite** to that of vinca alkaloid (enhances tubulin polymerization).
2. Inhibits normal dynamic reorganisation of microtubular network. Abnormal arrays/microtubular bundles are produced throughout the cell cycle.
3. Taxol/Texane binds to tubulin and hyperstabilise polymerised microtubules so that mitotic spindle cannot breakdown (**anaphase-arrest**).

ADR:
1. Myelosuppression
2. "**Stocking** and **Glove neuropathy**"
3. Cardiotoxicity

U:
1. Lung cancer
2. Prostatic cancer
3. Head and neck cancer
4. Metastatic ovarian and breast CA in relapse cases.

Docetaxel: Mech. and other properties same as paclitaxel.
ADR: 1. Neutropenia
2. Neuropathy
U: 1. Metastatic CA breast (DOC)
2. Ovarian cancer
3. Pancreatic cancer

Etoposide: It is **semisynthetic** derivative of podophyllotoxin (a plant glycoside). eTOPoside inhibits TOPoisomerase II, affects TOP of the head causing alopecia, is used in TOP CA (Testicular, Oat cell, Prostate).
Mech: 1. Arrests cells in G_2 **phase** and causes DNA break due to DNA **topoisomerase II stimulation** leading to DNA degradation.
2. Topoisomerase II stimulation results in breakdown of DNA strand. Cells are arrested in late **S or G_2 phase**.
ADR: 1. Leukopenia
2. Alopecia   **LAG**
3. GIT intolerance.
U: 1. Testicular tumour
2. Lung cancer
3. Hodgkin's lymphoma
4. CA bladder

Actinomycin D/dactinomycin: All antibiotics of anticancer values **intercalate** between DNA strands and interfere with its template function.
Mech: 1. Cytotoxic at **all phase** of cell cycle and is not proliferation dependent.
2. Reduces DNA dependent **RNA polymerase** activity resulting in reduced RNA synthesis.
Resistance: It is due to reduced drug entry into cell.

Cytotoxic drugs with high potential to cause **vomiting: CADMiuM**
   Cisplatin—Most important.
   Cyclophosphamide
   Actinomycin D
   Dacarbazine, Mustine, Mithramycin.

Drug of choice to treat vomiting due to cancer chemotherapy is Metoclopramide.
Recent drug which may become DOC to treat vomiting due to chemotherapy—ondansetron (5-HT3 antagonist).
Cytotoxic drug causing **haemorrhagic pancreatitis**—L-asparaginase.
ADR: 1. Stomatitis
2. Alopecia   **SAVE Blood**
3. Vomiting
4. Erythema
5. BMD
6. Skin desquamation
U: 1. Wilms' tumour
2. Rhabdomyosarcoma
3. Mtx resistant choriocarcinoma

Daunorubicin (rubidomycin)/doxorubicin (adriamycin): They are **anthracycline antibiotics**.
Mech: 1.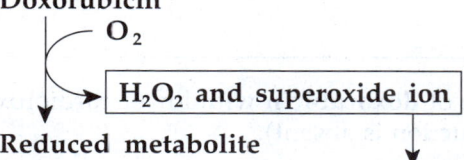
Doxorubicin → Reduced metabolite (+ O₂) → H₂O₂ and superoxide ion → Single strand breaks in DNA

2. Cause breaks in DNA strand due to **quinone type free radical generation** and **topoisomerase II stimulation (in S-phase)** but toxicity occurs in G_2 phase. **Maximum** action in S-phase.
3. Mutagenic and carcinogenic activities are present.
4. **Noncovalently** intercalate into DNA to reduce replication and transcription and to generate **free radical.**

ADR: 1. **A**lopecia   **ABCs**
2. **B**MD
3. Cumulative **C**ardiotoxicity due to superoxide anion.
4. Stomatitis

Bleomycin: It is a **mixture** of glycopeptide antibiotics.
Mech: 1. Chelates Cu/Fe
↓
Superoxide ions intercalate between DNA strands
↓
Causes chain scission and inhibits repair
2. Induces DNA fragmentation

Bleomycin is **B**lowing machine for DNA to **B**reak into **B**its.

ADR: 1. BMD
2. Pulmonary fibrosis
3. Mucocutaneous toxicity
4. Myelosuppression
U: 1. **T**esticular tumour
2. **S**quamous cell CA   **TSH**
3. **H**odgkin's lymphoma

Plicamycin: Same as actinomycin D in mechanism. But it reduces **serum Ca^{2+}** and is highly toxic.
U: 1. Testicular cancer (embryonal)
2. Disseminated cancer
3. Hypercalcemia

Mitomycin C: It is highly toxic
Mech: After intracellular transformation, it acts as **alkylating agent** and kills cells in G_1-M phase.
ADR: 1. BMD

        2. GI intolerance
U: 1. CA cervix
        2. CA bladder
        3. GIT cancer

Mitoxantrone: It is analogue of **doxorubicin** with lower cardiotoxicity (because quinone type free radical production is absent).
ADR: 1. BMD
        2. Mucosal inflammation
        3. Cardiotoxicity
U: 1. Acute non-haemolytic leukemia
        2. Non-Hodgkin's lymphoma — ANC C (see) Breast
        3. CML
        4. CA Breast

L-asparaginase: It is obtained from *E. coli*. It is an **enzyme**. This anticancer drug causes **no BMD**.
Mech: 1. **Leukemia cells are deficient in L-asparagine synthetase, hence depend on L-asparagine supply from the medium. Drug also metabolises asparagine and glutamine.**
        2. L-asparagine
           ↓ L-asparaginase
           L-aspartic acid
           ↓
           Cell death
ADR: 1. Liver damage
        2. CNS effects
        3. Allergy
        4. Haemorrhagic pancreatitis
U: 1. ALL
        2. When other drugs are failed to induce remission (ineffective in solid tumour).

Cisplatin: It is a **platinum** coordination complex hydrolysed **intracellularly** to a reactive moiety which binds mainly to N^7 **of guanine** residue of DNA.
Cisplatin or *Cis*-Diamminedichloroplatinum (II) is a coordination complex that hijacks cancerous cells and forces cellular machinery to denaturate DNA by losing two chloride ions only, just as America captured Iraq and forced Iraqis to leave oil for the **development of Iraq**, by losing outdated American weapons only.

It is a water-soluble square planar coordination complex containing a central platinum atom surrounded by two chloride atoms on one side and two ammonia groups on the other in **the *Cis* configuration, the two chloride atoms are on one side and the two ammonia groups on the other**. In 1965, Rosenberg was the first to identify by serendipitous observation that neutral platinum complex (radiomimetic) inhibits division and induces filamentous growth of *E. coli* when a current was passed between platinum electrodes. **It also possesses radiomimetic property.**

Mech: Though exact mechanism of action is unknown, it seems that it enters the cells by diffusion where chloride ions dissociate leaving a reactive diamine platinum complex which **reacts with water and then** binds DNA through both intrastrand and interstrand cross-links, thus inhibiting DNA replication and transcription and leads to breaks and miscoding of DNA to kill cells in all stages of the cell cycle. **It also reacts with SH group of proteins.**
1. Drugs are hydrolysed **intracellularly** to a reactive moiety which binds mainly to N^7 of guanine residue of DNA.
2. Reacts with **SH group** in protein and has **radiomimetic** effects.

PK: Plasma protein bound, enters tissue, excreted unchanged in **urine**. A little enters brain, t½—72 hrs.

Its clearance from plasma is biphasic with a half-life of minutes for first phase and days for second phase. It is excreted in the unchanged form by kidney with a half-life of 3 days.

It has poor penetration in CNS.

ADR:
1. Hyperuricaemia
2. Renal failure (**most important** and **maximum**)
3. Emetic (**most emetic** anticancer drug)
4. Neuropathy   **HR END**
5. Deafness

Side effects of **CISPLATIN** are: Carcinogenic and cardiopathy (tachycardia, hypotension), Increased urate level in plasma, Suppression of bone marrow, Peripheral neuropathy, Loss of hearing, Anaphylaxis, Tetany due to loss of calcium and magnesium, Increased frequency of seizures, Nephrotic (the commonest side effect treated by saline infusion).

U:
1. Metastatic testicular and ovarian CA.
2. CA lung

It is mainly used in solid tumour of ovaries and testes, the dose is 20 mg/m² per day for 5 days.

Procarbazine:

Mech: Depolymerises **DNA**, causes chromosomal damage and inhibits nucleic acid synthesis.
Mutagenic and carcinogenic action present.

ADR:
1. Dermatitis
2. Emesis   **DELTA**
3. Leucopenia
4. Thrombocytopenia
5. Alcohol produces hot flushing

IA:
1. It is **weak MAO inhibitor.**
2. Alcohol + Procarbazine show **disulfiram** like reaction and hot flushing.

U:
1. Component of MOPP regimen for Hodgkin's lymphoma.
2. Non-Hodgkin's lymphoma.
3. Oat cell CA of lung. Dose—3 mg/kg/day.

Hydroxyurea

Mech: 1. **Inhibits ribonucleoside diphosphate reductase.**

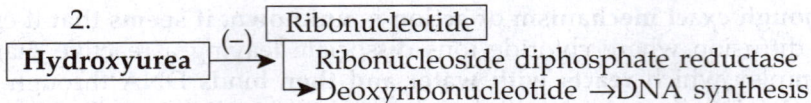

ADR: BMD
U: 1. CML
2. Polycythemia vera

Carboplatin: It is a second generation **platinum** compound. Thrombocytopenia and less often leukopenia are **dose limiting.**

PK: t½—5 hrs
Excreted in urine
ADR: 1. Nephro-, neuro-, ototoxicity
2. Thrombocytopenia (dose limiting)
U: 1. Lung cancer
2. Ovarian CA
3. Seminoma
4. Squamous cell CA of head and neck.

LOSS

Capecitabine: It is antimetabolite. Cell cycle specific (**S-phase**). It is **novel oral fluoropyrimidine carbamate** approved in 1999 for metastatic breast CA resistant to first line drug.

Mech: Same as 5-FU

Capecitabine
↓ Carboxyl esterase
5-DFCR (5-deoxy-5-fluorocytidine)
↓ Deaminase
5-DFUR (5-deoxy-5-fluorouridine)
↓ Thymidine phosphorylase
5-FU

PK: Well absorbed orally. Extensively metabolised to 5-FU but eventually biotransformed into **α-fluoro-β-alanine.** Renal elimination
ADR: Same as 5-FU
1. GIT: Diarrhoea, nausea, vomiting, necrotising enterocolitis, hyperbilirubinemia
2. **Palmar–plantar erythrodysesthesia**
CI: 1. Pregnant and lactating mother
2. Hepatic/renal impairment
U: 1. CA breast
2. Colorectal cancer

Gemcitabine: It is analogue of **nucleoside deoxycytidine,** its chemical structure is dFdc (2, 2-difluorodeoxycytidine).

Mech: 1. **Gemcitabine (dFdc)**
↓ Deoxycytidine kinase
dFdCTP (dFdc triphosphate)
↓
Inhibits DNA synthesis
2. **Inhibits ribonucleotide reductase**

Resistant: It is due to its inability to be converted to **nucleotide.** The tumour cell produces more **endogenous deoxycytidine** that competes for kinase, thereby **bypassing** inhibition.

PK: Route—IV

Deaminated to difluorodeoxyuridine which is not cytotoxic and is excreted in urine.

ADR:
1. Nausea, vomiting
2. Elevation of proteinuria, hematuria and serum transaminase.
3. Alopecia   NEAR M
4. Rash
5. Myelosuppression (**dose limiting**)

U:
1. DOC in adenocarcinoma of pancreas
2. Other tumours also

Irinotecan and topotecan: These are **semisynthetic** derivatives of earlier drug **camptothecin.** Topotecan has complicated multiring structure **containg lactone ring** that is essential for activity. Both obtained from Chinese tree.

Mech:
1. Inhibit **topoisomerase I** (torsion strain in DNA is not relieved) →single strand breaks in DNA without its resealing during replication →cell cycle arrest at G_2 phase.
2. Prevent **reannealing** of single strand break. Irinotecan also inhibits ACh E.
3. Damages double-stranded DNA during DNA synthesis, such breaks do not undergo **repair** resulting in cytotoxicity.

PK: Route—IV infusion 30 min × 5 days. **Hydrolysis** of lactone ring destroys drug's activity. 30% renal excretion. Irinotecan (prodrug) is decarboxylated in liver to active metabolite.

ADR:
A. **Topotecan**
1. BMD (**commonest**)   BAD ACh E
2. Alopecia, anorexia
3. Diarrhoea, nausea, vomiting
4. Headache, abdominal pain

B. **Irinotecan**
1. Haemorrhage, Thrombocytopenia, Neutropenia
2. Diarrhoea (dose limiting)

HTN Decreases

U: Metastatic ovarian cancer; CA lung, cervix and colorectum.
Dose: 1.5 mg/m² IV over 30 min daily for 5 days (topotecan).
125 mg/m² IV weekly over 90 min for 1 month (irinotecan).

Pulmonary infiltration inducing drugs: BAN ME
Bleomycin/Busulfan/BcNU
Azathioprine/Amiodarone/Acyclovir
Nitrofurantoin
MEthotrexate/MElphalan/MEthysergide

Idarubicin: It is a newly introduced anthracycline with general properties similar to doxorubicin. Route is IV.

Epirubicin: Structurally related to doxorubicin and similarly effective in breast cancer.

Vinorelbine: It is semisynthetic vinca alkaloid and causes metaphase arrest. Route is 30 mg/m^2 over 10 min IV/week.

ADR: BMD, gut upset, alopecia.

U: Lung, blood, airway, breast cancers and Kaposi's sarcoma.

Amifostine: It is organic thiophosphate cytoprotective agent and diphosphorylated into active free thiol metabolites that can reduce the toxic effect of cisplatin.

PK: Half-life <1 min and elimination half-life = 8 min.

U: Renal toxicity (910 mg/m^2 once a day IV before 30 min of chemotherapy).

Anastrozole and letrozole: They are nonsteroidal aromatase inhibitor alternative to tamoxifen.

Combination therapy
1. **MOPP** = Mechlorethamine + Oncovin (vincristine) + procarbazine + prednisolone.
   U: Hodgkin's lymphoma
2. **VAMP** = Vincristine + Mtx + 6-MP + prednisolone.
   U: Acute leukemia
3. **COAP** = Cyclophosphamide + oncovin + arac (cytarabine) + prednisolone
4. **POMP** = Prednisolone + oncovin + Mtx + purinethol (6-MP).
5. **CART** = Cytarabine + asparaginase + rubidomycin + 6-TG.
6. **BACOP** = Bleomycin + adriamycin + cyclophosphamide + oncovin + prednisolone.

Malignancy	Drugs of choice	Other drugs
1. Acute leukemias	VAMP combination, daunorubicin, 6-TG, cytarabine	Cyclophosphamide, L-asparaginase, doxorubicin, cytarabine
2. Chr. lymphatic leukemia	Chlorambucil, cyclophosphamide, prednisolone	
3. CML	Busulfan, mitoxantrone	6-MP, 6-TG, hydroxyurea, cyclophosphamide, melphalan
4. Hodgkin's disease	MOPP, vinblastine, cyclophosphamide	Bleomycin, carmustine, lomustine, doxorubicin, decarbazine, cytarabine.
5. Lymphosarcoma	Cyclophosphamide, chlorambucil, vincristine	Prednisolone, doxorubicin vinblastine,
6. Multiple myeloma	Melphalan, prednisolone, cyclophosphamide	Carmustine, doxorubicin, chlorambucil, vincristine

(Contd.)

Malignancy	Drugs of choice	Other drugs
7. Ewing's sarcoma cyclophosphamide	Doxorubicin, vincristine, actinomycin D,	Carmustine, daunorubicin
8. Burkitt's lymphoma	Cyclophosphamide	Carmustine, Mtx
9. Wilms' tumour	Actinomycin D, vincristine	Cyclophosphamide, doxorubicin
10. Choriocarcinoma	Mtx actinomycin D	6-MP, chlorambucil, vinblastine
11. Prostate carcinoma	Estrogens (orchiectomy)	Cyproterone, cyclophosphamide
12. Breast carcinoma	Tamoxifen, Mtx, 5-FU, vincristine, paclitaxel, estrogens/androgens, CMF regimen	Prednisolone, cyclophosphamide, mitoxantrone
13. Ovarian carcinoma	Melphalan, chlorambucil cyclophosphamide, doxorubicin, paclitaxel	Cisplatin, 5-FU, Mtx, Vincristine, carboplatin
14. Ca endometrium	Progestin,	Doxorubicin
15. Testicular tumour	Melphalan, chlorambucil, Mtx, bleomycin, cisplatin, carboplatin	Actinomycin D, ifosamide, vinblastine, etoposide, mithramycin
16. Cancer lung (small cell)	Cyclophosphamide, vincristine, doxorubicin	Mustine HCl, carbopaltin, Mtx, lomustine, etoposide, procarbazine
17. Carcinoma, cervix	Mitomycin C, Mtx	Cyclophosphamide, bleomycin, cisplatin
18. Carcinoma bladder	Doxorubicin, cisplatin, thiotepa, etoposide	5-FU, ifosfamide, mitomycin C
19. Osteogenic sarcoma	Mtx with rescue, doxorubicin, vincristine	Cisplatin, ifosfamide, melphalan
20. ALL (induction of remission)	Vincristine + prednisolone	
21. ALL (remission maintenance)	Cyclophosphamide, Mtx, 6-MP	
22. AML	Doxorubicin, cytarabine,	
23. CA thyroid	^{131}I, doxorubicin	
24. CA stomach and pancreas	5-FU, mitomycin, doxorubicin	
25. CA colon	5-FU	
26. Malignant myeloma	Vindesine	
27. Adenocarcinoma (CA colon/stomach)	5-FU	

Immunosuppressants

They inhibit cell mediated immunity and humoral **immunity** and are used in **organ transplantation** and **autoimmune disease.**

Drugs are
1. **Specific T cell inhibitors (calcineurin inhibitors)**
   Cyclosporin (**most costly**), tacrolimus and sirolimus.
2. **Cytotoxic drugs**
   Mtx
   Cyclophosphamide
   Chlorambucil
   Azathioprine
   MMF (mycophenolate mofetil)

Immunosuppressive agents with sites of action

Agent	Site	Agent	Site
Prednisolone	2, 6	Cyclophosphamide	2
Cyclosporin	2, 3	Antilymphocytic globulin and monoclonal anti-T cell antibodies	1, 2, 3
Azathioprine	2		
Methotrexate	2		
Dactinomycin	2, 3	$Rh_3(D)$ immunoglobulin	1

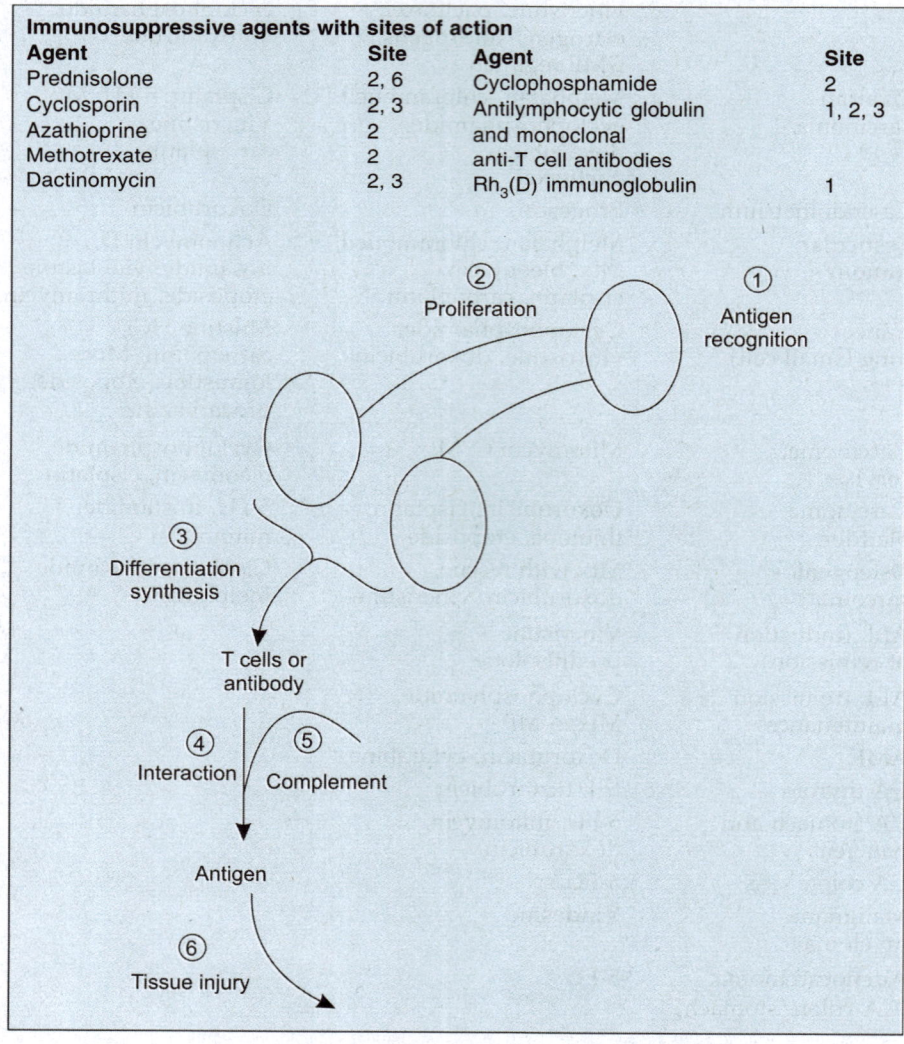

3. **Antibodies**
   ATG (antithymocyte globulin)
   Muromonab CD3
   Rho (D) Ig
4. **Glucocorticoids**

Cyclosporin: It is **the costliest** drug.

Mech: Binds intracellular protein cyclophilin (peptidyl-proline *cis*-trans-isomerase).

$$\downarrow$$

Cyclosporin + cyclophilin complex
$$\downarrow (-)$$
Calcineurin

(Ca^{2+}—calmodulin activated enzyme "serine/threonine phosphatase")

$$NFAT/OAP \xrightarrow{\dfrac{Calcineurin}{(Normally)}} IL\text{-}2,\ TNF\text{-}\alpha,\ GM\text{-}CSF,\ T\text{-}lymphocyte.$$

Normally, T cell R activates calcineurin which activates cytokine gene through **NFAT (nuclear factor of activated T cells)** and **OAP (octamer activating protein)** resulting in transcription of cytokine genes and production of cytokines. Drug inhibits calcineurin.

PK: Accumulates in **WBC** and **RBC,** hepatic metabolism, excreted in bile, t½—6 hrs.

ADR:
1. Nephrotoxic
2. Hepatotoxic
3. Lymphoma
4. Hirsutism
5. Viral infection

IA: All nephrotoxic drugs (AMB, aminoglycoside, vancomycin) enhance its toxicity. KTZ and erythromycin inhibits its metabolism. Cyclosporin A is **best immunosuppressant** but nephrotoxic.

U:
1. Graft rejection (**most effective**)
2. Autoimmune disease—2nd line

Tacrolimus (FK 506): 100 times more potent than cyclosporin. Its t½ is 18 hrs.
Route: Oral/IV
Mech: Same as cyclosporin
ADR : Same as cyclosporin
U: Same as cyclosporin (sirolimus in liver disease)

MMF: It is prodrug of **mycophenolic acid** that inhibits inosine monophosphate dehydrogenase responsible for guanosine nucleotide synthesis in T and B cells.

Mech:
1. Inhibits inosine monophosphate dehydrogenase.
2. Inhibits **lymphocyte proliferation,** antibody production and CMI.

ADR:
1. Diarrhoea
2. Vomiting

Muromonab CD3: It is a **murine monoclonal Ab** against CD3 glycoprotein located on T_H cell near T cell receptor.

Mech: Ab + CD3 Ag obstructs binding of **MHC II—Ag** to T cell receptor. Immunity due to T cell is prevented

ADR:
1. **Cytokine release syndrome** with flu-like symptoms.
2. Infection (meningitis)

U:
1. Organ transplantation
2. Steroid resistant graft rejection reaction

ATG: It is a **polyclonal Ab from horse**

Mech: Binds to **T-lymphocytes** and depletes them

ADR:
1. Serum sickness
2. Anaphylaxis

U: Acute allograft rejection

Anti-D Ig: It is a **human Ig** against **Rh(D) Ag**

U:
1. Rho-D negative mother to check abortion
2. DU negative mother to check abortion
3. Rh haemolytic disease

CI:
1. Infant
2. Rho-D +ve
3. DU +ve

Three regimens for organ transplantation

1. **Induction regimen (DOC) is the commonest regimen**
   Cyclosporin + prednisolone + azathioprine with/without ATG/ muromonab CD3.
2. **Maintenance regimen**
   A. Cyclosporin + prednisolone + azathioprine **(DOC)**
   B. Cyclophosphamide + MMF + chlorambucil **(second line if first line fails)**.
3. **Antirejection therapy: Methylprednisolone/muromonab CD3/ATG.**

Common ADR of immunosuppressant therpy is

A. Opportunistic infection
B. Bacterial, fungal and viral infection
C. Malignancies

A. **FC fragments of Ab**   5C
   Constant. Carboxy terminal. Carbohydrate side chain; Complement binding (IgG + IgM only).
B. **T cell glycoprotein:** Helper T cell has **CD4** which binds to **Class II MHC** on Ag presenting cells. Cytotoxic T cell has **CD8** which binds to **Class I MHC** on viral infected cell.

$$CD4 \times MHC\ II = 8 = CD8 \times MHC\ I$$

Gene therapy: It is the replacement of defective **genes** by functional genes in target cells.

Approaches of gene therapy
A. Gene modification: Correction of defective gene sequence or its removal.
B. Gene transfer: Introduction of gene without removal or alteration of existing gene.

Methods of gene transfer
1. **Physical** method by microinjection
2. **Chemical** method by liposomal delivery
3. **Biological** method by fusion of recipient cell with bacteria and virus. **Commonest viral vectors (retrovirus most popular): gag, pol, env** genes of virus are removed by genes to be transferred. Retroviral vectors infect host cells inserting desired DNA into random site subsequently expressing transferred genes. Gene is transferred into **somatic** cells (fibroblast, stem cell, hepatocyte, myocyte) by *ex vivo/in vivo* **(retrovirus) techniques.**

U:
1. Cystic fibrosis: **CFTR** (cystic fibrosis transport regulatory) gene into respiratory epithelial cell to regulate chloride channel.
2. GH gene in GH deficiency
3. SCID (severe combined immunodeficiency disease) gene for **adenosine deaminase.**
4. LDL receptor gene into hepatocyte in familial hypercholesterolemia.
5. Lesch-Nyhan syndrome (severe neuropsychiatric disorder): It is corrected by **hypoxanthine phosphoribosyl transferase** gene introduction.
6. Parkinsonism: It is corrected by introduction of gene for **tyrosine hydroxylase** to augment DA production in basal gangila.
7. Gaucher's and Alzheimer's disease and Huntington's chorea.
8. Head injury, multiple sclerosis: Nerve growth factor gene.
9. Duchenne muscular dystrophy: Muscle dystropin gene.
10. HTN: Human tissue kallikrein gene
11. Grafted coronary vessels restenosis is corrected by introduction of genes inhibiting **Intimal cell growth.**
12. Anaemia: Erythropoietin gene
13. Sickle cell anaemia: Beta/delta sickle cell inhibitor **hybrid gene.**
14. Haemophilia: Factor VIII gene
15. IDDM: **Insulin-I gene into liver**
16. **HIV infection: HIV envelop glycoprotein gene to augment immunity.**
17. Malaria: Multicomponent nacked malaria DNA (vaccine)
18. Influenza: Nacked influenza virus DNA (vaccine)
19. Cancer: a. TNF-α and IL-2 gene
  b. Suppressor gene
  c. Promotor antisense gene
  d. Multidrug resistant gene into bone marrow cells so that myelosuppression by drugs may be limited.

1. **P**aclitaxel and **G**emcitabine are **R**adiosensitizers.
   PG is Radiosensitive

   Radioprotectives are Amifostine, Pentoxyphylline, ZnO **RAPZ**
2. Radiosensitive tumors are **WELMS**: **W**ilms tumor, **E**wing's sarcoma, **L**ymphoma, **M**ultiple myeloma, **S**eminoma.
3. **T**esticular tumour (seminoma), **R**habdomyosarcoma, **E**wing's tumor and **A**cute lymphoma (ALL and AML) are cured when **TREA**ted by chemotherapy.
4. True killer of cells (killer of all phases of cell cycle) are Nitrosoureas (**SE-MUSTI**ne, **CARMUSTI**ne and **LOMUSTI**ne).

   (Tere Naam ... **SE CAR LO MUSTI**)

Unit 12
Drugs for Community Medicine

63. Anaemia

Anaemia is present when there is a decrease in the level of Hb in the blood below the reference level for the age and sex of the individual.

Symptoms and signs of anaemia

Symptoms	Signs
Fatigue	Pallor
Faintness	Tachycardia
Headache	Systolic flow murmur
Palpitations	Cardiac failure
Angina of effort	Koilonychia
Breathlessness	Jaundice

Classification of anaemia

Anaemias are of three major types
1. Hypochromic microcytic with a low MCV: Iron deficiency anaemia.
2. Normochromic normocytic with a normal MCV.
3. Macrocytic with a high MCV: Vitamin B_{12} and folate deficiency anaemia.

Hematinics: Hematinics are the agents that cause stimulation of haemopoiesis (increase RBC or Hb content of RBC or both) which results in correction of anaemia. Important haematinics are:
1. Iron
2. Vitamin B_{12}
3. Folic acid

Hematinics	Clinical use
Iron	Iron deficiency anaemia
Vitamin B_{12}	Megaloblastic anaemia
Folic acid	Folate deficiency anaemia (megaloblastic)
Iron (the body content of iron):	

Pharmacology Review

	Male (mg/kg of body weight)	Female
Essential iron		
Haemoglobin	31	28
Myoglobin and enzymes	6	5
Storage iron		
Ferritin, hemosiderin	13	4
Total	50	37

Haemoglobin contains 2/3 of total iron. Diet (average Western) contains 15–20 mg iron per day. Only 10% dietary iron is absorbed (0.5–1.0 mg per day). Anaemic person absorbs about 20–30% of dietary iron. Average menstrual loss: 30 mg per period.

Source and daily iron requirements: Iron requirements are determined by obligatory physiological losses and the needs impose by growth. The total daily requirement be considered in the context of dietary iron available for absorption.

Source	Daily dietary requirements
Animal source	Children : 10–15 mg
liver, meat, egg	Adult male : 5–10 mg
Plant source	Adult female : 15–18 mg
Green leafy vegetables,	Pregnant women : 30–60 mg
green banana, cereals,	Lactating mother : 30–60 mg
peas, lentils.	**(Most iron in food is ferric iron)**

As iron deficiency develops, storage iron decreases and then disappears; next, serum ferritin decreases; and the serum iron decreases and iron binding capacity (transferrin) increases resulting in a decrease in iron binding saturation. Thereafter anaemia begins to develop. So one of the **most sensitive** ways to detect early iron deficiency is to examine bone marrow stained to detect the presence or absence of storage iron.

Iron absorption: Site of absorption is duodenum and upper jejunum.

Iron is absorbed in the GIT in the form of ferrous iron. So, all ferric iron must be converted to ferrous iron for absorption in the GIT.

Absorption of iron is a two-stage process

Firstly; Active transport: Rapid absorption of iron takes place at the brush border of the intestinal epithelium by active transport mechanism.

Secondly; in the mucosal cells, ferrous iron is oxidized to ferric iron. Ferric iron then binds with **transferrin (beta-globulin).** Then transferrin bound iron transfer from the interior of the cells into the plasma, or stored as ferritin in the mucosal cells.

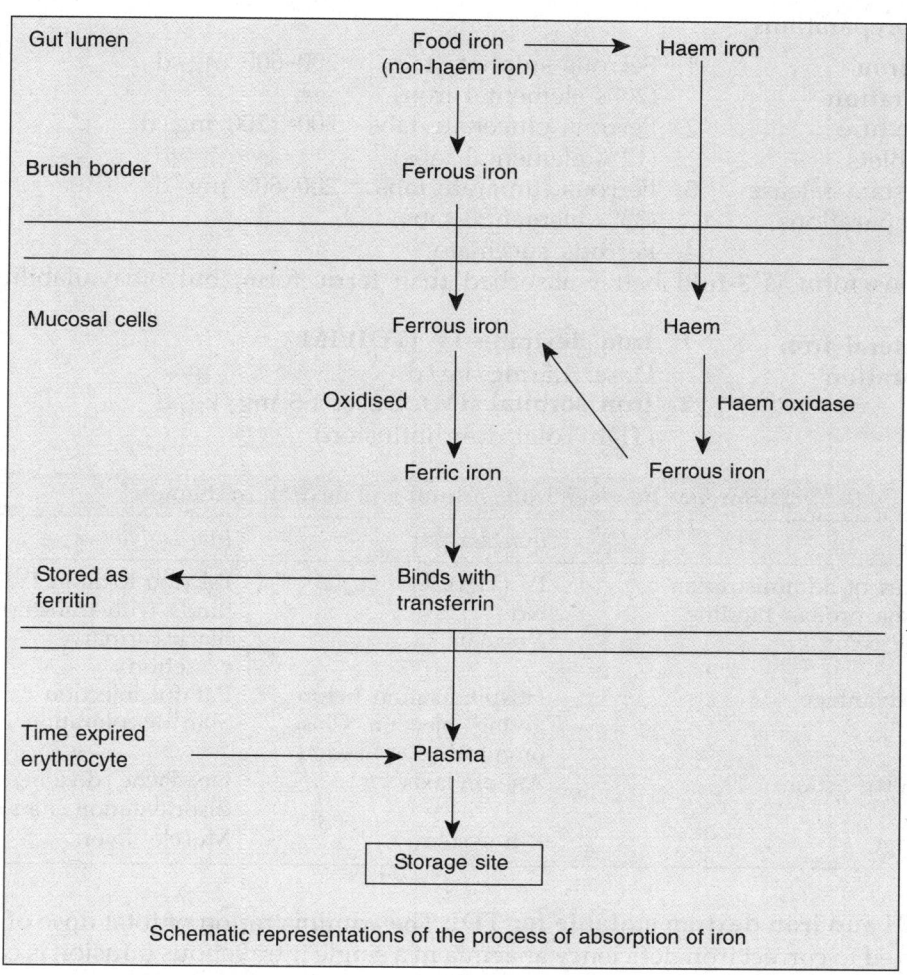

Schematic representations of the process of absorption of iron

Factors influencing absorption of iron	
Absorption increases in	*Absorption decreases in*
Ferrous iron	Ferric iron
Haem iron	Non-haem iron
Fasting condition	Fulled stomach
Increase gastric acidity	Decrease gastric acidity (antacids)
Low iron stores	Iron overload
Ascorbic acid	Phosphate (from insoluble complex with iron)
Alcohol	
Increase erythropoiesis (bleeding, haemolysis, high altitude)	

Iron preparations

Oral iron preparation
— Mixture
— Tablets
— Sustain release preparations

1. Ferrous sulphate tabs 200–600 mg/d (20% elemental iron)
2. Ferrous gluconate tabs 300–1200 mg/d (12% elemental tabs)
3. Ferrous fumarate tabs 200–600 mg/d (33% elemental tabs)
4. Ferrous succinate

(Ferrous form is **3-fold** better absorbed than ferric form; but bioavailability is same).

Parenteral iron preparation

1. **Iron dextran—IV (TDI)/IM** Dose: 1.5 mg/kg/d
2. **Iron sorbital (IM).** Dose: 1.5 mg/kg/d (TDI: Total dose infusion)

Difference between iron sorbitol and dextran in therapy		
Point	Iron dextran	Iron sorbitol
Routes of administration	IV (TDI). IM	IM (too toxic in IV)
Plasma protein binding	No	Binds with transferrin
Urine color	Normal	Black (urinary excretion)
Disadvantage	Hospitalization before giving injection. Close monitoring is needed	Painful injection Skin discoloration
Adverse actions	Anaphylaxis	Headache, dizziness, disorientation, nausea
Storage	R-E system	Muscle, liver

TDI and iron dextran suitable for TDI: The administration of total dose of iron required to correct iron deficiency anaemia in a single intravenous infusion is called **TDI**. It provides enough iron to correct anemia and replenishes iron stores on a single occasion (to avoid intermittent IV injection).

Utilisable iron is released over month from stores.
TDI eliminates the local pain and tissue staining.

Iron sorbital unsuitable for TDI: Iron sorbital is bound to transferrin and not stored in R-E system. So if TDI is given, rapid saturation of transferrin occurs and there would be very high free iron levels in the blood which is too toxic for patient.

Indications of oral iron therapy

1. Iron deficiency anaemia
2. **Prophylatic use:** Pregnancy, menstruation, early infancy, blood donors.
3. Chronic blood loss
4. Glossitis
5. Stomatitis

The response to iron therapy can be evaluated with the reticulocyte production index and the rate of rise in the levels of haemoglobin or the haematocrit. An average increment of Hb of 2 g per litre per day is observed with the usual therapeutic dose

(4–7 days after beginning of therapy). Treatment with oral iron should be continued for 3–6 months for correction of anaemia as well as to replenish iron stores. The haemoglobin level should increase significantly in 2–4 weeks and should reach normal levels **(men = 14–18 g/dl; women= 12–16 g/dl) in 1–3 months.**

Indications of parenteral iron therapy
1. Patients with documented iron deficiency unable to tolerate or absorb oral iron (malabsorption syndrome, sprue).
2. Patients with extensive chronic blood loss who cannot be maintained with oral iron alone. **This includes:** Postgastrectomy conditions, small bowel resection, inflammatory bowel disease (small gut), chronic bleeding from nonresectable lesion.

Calculation of total required parenteral iron
The total amount of parenteral iron required to correct iron deficiency anaemia and to replenish iron store in a 70 kg adult can be calculated as follows:

> **Grams of iron required = 0.25 (normal Hb minus patient's Hb).**

Method of parenteral iron (iron dextran) therapy: At first, entire calculated dose of iron is mixed with several hundred ml of normal saline. First inject the injection of **0.5 ml of iron dextran over a period of 5 minutes;** the patient is then observed for 1 hour for signs and symptoms of anaphylaxis. Then administer the total dose in a **sigle intravenous infusion over 1–2 hours** (total dose infusion). Intravenous administration eliminates the local pain and tissue staining that often occur with the total intramuscular route.

Adverse effects of iron therapy
Oral preparations
Gastrointestinal upsets: Nausea, heart burn, upper abdominal discomfort, diarrhoea, constipation, haemochromatosis (rare).

Parenteral preparations: Local discomfort, discoloration of skin, headache, fever, arthralgia, lymphadenopathy, anaphylactic reaction (rare but fatal).

Advantages of parenteral iron over oral iron
Although the rate of response of parenteral iron therapy is similar to that which follows usual oral doses, the following advantages of parenteral iron therapy are notable:
1. The response to parenteral iron is faster than that to oral iron.
2. Iron stores may be created rapidly with parenteral iron.

Iron poisoning
Caused by long continued use of large amount of iron. Children are more susceptible (tablets of most iron preparations are attractive to children because they are coloured and sugar-coated). **Usual fatal dose: 2–10 gm** (as few as ten tablets can be lethal in young children).

Clinical course of typical case of acute oral iron poisoning has *four phases*	
First stage (0.5–1 hr after ingestion)	— Abdominal pain, vomiting — Bloody diarrhoea — Acidosis — Cardiovascular collapse — Coma Death in 4–6 hrs in 20% case
Second stage (80% cases)	— Period of improvement lasting 8–16 hrs which may be permanent or which may pass into 3rd stage
Third stage	— Cardiovascular collapse — Convulsions — Coma Death in about 24 hrs of ingestion
Fourth stage	— Gastrointestinal obstruction from scaring

Management of iron poisoning: First aid—raw egg, milk (binds with iron). Chelation therapy (immediately). Chelating agent: **Desferrioxamine**. Iron + desferrioxamine →ferrioxamine (unabsorbable).

	Mode of treatment
Iron chelating agent	Desferrioxamine IM or IV (continuous infusion).
Gastric lavage/emesis	Done by NaHCO$_3$ or phosphate solution Water should contain 2 g desferrioxamine per litre. After emptying the stomach, 10 g desferrioxamine in 50–100 ml water should be left in stomach. It is not absorbed.
Correction of water and electrolyte imbalance	Dextrose saline/normal saline
Supportive treatment	For convulsion, shock

Chronic iron toxicity: It may result from:
1. Grossly excessive parenteral iron therapy.
2. Repeated blood transfusion to treat haemolytic anaemia (one unit of blood contains 250 mg of iron).
3. Deposition of excess iron in heart, liver, pancreas and other organs leads to haemosiderosis and hemochromatosis.

Treatment
1. **Desferrioxamine:** Subcutaneous infusion 12 hrs nocturnal on 5 night/week.
2. Oral ascorbic acid increases the availability of free iron for chelation.
3. Large intake of tea (tannins).
4. **Phlebotomy (venesection):** Chronic iron overload in the absence of anaemia is most efficiently treated by intermittent phlebotomy. One unit of blood (containing 250 mg of iron) can be removed per week or so untill all of the excess iron is removed.

Desferrioxamine

1.
> It is an iron chelating agent
> Iron + desferrioxamine
> ↓
> Ferrioxamine
> (nonabsorbable)
> ↓
> Excreted in bile and faeces

2. Not absorbed from the gut
3. **Indication**
   — Acute iron toxicity
   — Diagnosis and treatment of chronic iron toxicity
   — Ocular siderosis (topical formulation)
4. **Iron chelating capicity**
   100 mg desferrioxamine chelates 8.5 mg iron.
   (e.g. 10 tablets of ferrous sulphate or gluconate).

Drug interactions	
Interaction	Possible cause
Iron + tetracycline/methyldopa/ciprofloxacin decreases iron absorption	Iron chelates in the gut with these agents (chemical antagonism)
Iron + antacid reduces bioavailability of iron	Antacids may interfere with the absorption of iron

1. Diagnosis of iron deficiency anemia:
   Hb   = <10 gm%
   RBC   = <4 × 10^6/dl
   PCV   = <30%
   MCH   = <25 pg
   MCHC   = <34% (the most sensitive index)
   MCV   = <75 µm^3
   Serum ferritin = <10 mg/L (the single most sensitive tool for iron status)
2. Hb = >11 gm% normal
      = 8–11 gm% mild anemia
      = 5–8 gm% moderate anemia
      = <5 gm% severe anaemia.
3. Commonest cause of anaemia = Nutritional deficiency.

64. Poisoning and Antidotes

Introduction

Toxicology: Toxicology deals with study of adverse or poisonous effect of drugs, toxins and their management.

Toxicokinetics: The term *toxicokinetics* denotes the absorption, distribution, excretion and metabolism of toxins, toxic doses of therapeutic agents and their metabolites.

Toxicodynamics: *Toxicodynamics* denotes the injurious effects of toxins, toxic doses of therapeutic agents and their metabolites on vital function.

Principles of treatment of the poisoned patient

The initial management of a patient with seizures or otherwise altered mental status should follow the same approach regardless of the poison involved.

I. Initial supportive measure: ABCDs measure

- A : Airway
- B : Breathing
- C : Circulation
- D : Dextrose

Airway : Airway should be cleared of vomitus/any other obstruction.
Keep the patient in lateral decubitus position
Establish an endotracheal tube if needed

Breathing : Adequacy of breathing should be assessed by observation.
Measure arterial blood gases
Establish artificial respiration if needed

Circulation : Measure pulse rate, blood pressure, urine output
An intravenous line should be placed
Blood sample collection for routine determinations and serum glucose.

Dextrose : Give **IV dextrose (50 ml of 50% dextrose) routinely** because patients comatosed from hypoglycaemia are rapidly and irreversibly losing brain cells.

II. History, physical examination and laboratory procedure to identify the specific poison.

III. Decontamination involves removing toxins from the skin or GIT:

Poisoning and Antidotes

A. Skin (to prevent percutaneous absorption)
- Remove the patient from toxic environment
- Remove contaminated clothings
- Wash skin with copious water and soap

B. Gastrointestinal tract
- Gastric lavage
- **Emesis** by ipecac syrup (children: 10–15 ml)
- Activated charcoal, cathartics or whole bowel irrigation.
  (Gastric lavage and emesis are **contraindicated for corrosive poisons** when there is a risk of perforation of the gut.)

IV. Use specific antidotes (see below)

V. **Acceleration of elimination of poison by**

A. Alteration of urine pH
Alkalinization: In acidic drug poisoning (aspirin, barbiturates)
Acidification: In alkaline drug poisoning (amphetamine, quinidine)

B. Dialysis:
Hemodialysis, peritoneal dialysis, hemoperfusion as required.

Specific antidotes: Specific antidotes reduce or abolish the effects of poisons through a variety of mechanism, which may be categorised as follows:

1. On receptors which may be blocked, stimulated or bypassed.
2. On **enzyme** which may be inhibited or reactivated.
3. By **displacement** from tissue binding sites.
4. By **replenishment** of an essential substance.
5. By **binding** to the poison (chelation).

Chelating agents: Chelating agents act by incorporation with heavy metals to form an insoluble, stable, biologically inert complexes that are excreted in the urine.

Chelating agents are
1. **Dimercaprol (BAL: British Anti-Lewisite)**
2. **Desferrioxamine**
3. **Sodium calcium edetate (calcium EDTA** = ethylenediamine-tetra-acetic acid).
4. **Dicobalt edetate**
5. **Unithiol and penicillamine**

Dimercaprol (BAL): Developed in World War II. Chelates metal ions (arsenic, copper, Bi, Sb, Ni, gold, lead, inorganic mercury). Dimercaprol provides—SH group which combines with metal ions to form harmless compound, is excreted in the urine (metal ions bind with SH group of essential enzymes in the body and thus inactivate them). (See flow chart on mechanism of action on BAL):

Uses of BAL
1. Poisoning by **As, Hb, Au, Bi, Ni, Sb**
   Dose: 5 mg/kg stat followed by 2–5 mg/kg 6 hourly for 2 days then once a day for 10 days.
2. Adjuvant to calcium disodium edetate in **lead poisoning.**
3. Adjuvant to penicillamine in **Cu poisoning** and **Wilson's disease.**
   Dose: 300 mg/day for 10 days every second month.

Mechanism of action on BAL

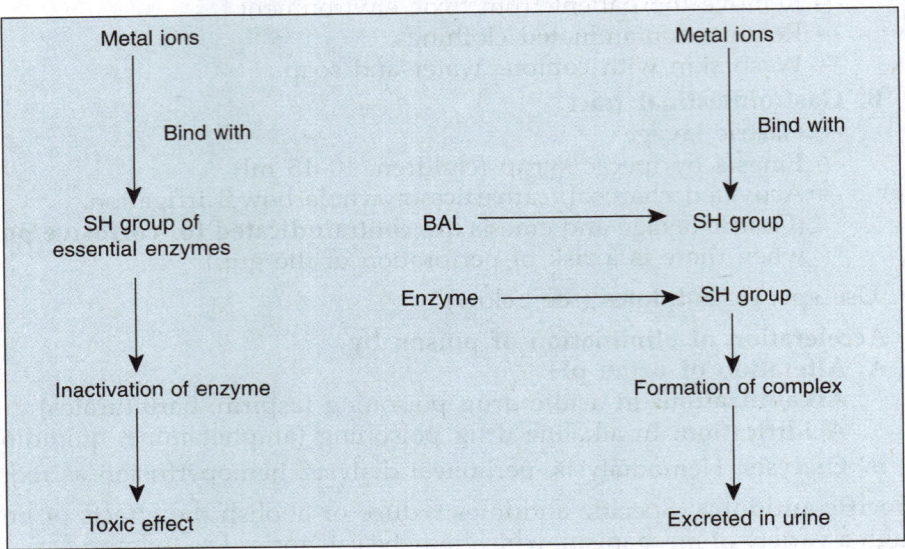

Adverse effect of dimercaprol
1. Nausea and vomiting
2. Lacrymation
3. Salivation
4. Paraesthesia
5. Muscular aches
6. Urticarial rashes
7. Tachycardia.
8. Overbreathing, convulsions, coma (gross overdose)

CI: Fe and Cd poisoning (BAL-Fe and BAL-Cd complexes are toxic)

Use: **BALHANGC**
Bi
As
Lead
Hg
Antimony
Ni
Gold
Cu

Calcium EDTA: It is **Ca disodium edetate (Ca Na$_2$ EDTA).**

Used as antidote of lead poisoning. Its effectiveness is due to its capacity to exchange, in Pb poisoning, Ca for Pb. Pb chelate is excreted in the urine, leaving behind a harmless amount of calcium. Effective in **Pb, Zn, Cd, Mn, Cu.**

Adverse effects: Hypotension, sneezing, lacrimation, muscle pains, nasal stuffiness, renal damage (**most important**), anaphylactoid reaction.

Antidotes, indications, mode of actions		
Antidotes	Indications	Mode of actions
Atropine	Organophosphorus, insecticides (OPC poisoning)	Blocks muscarinic receptors
Naloxane	Opioids (morphine)	Competes for opioid receptors
Flumazenil	Benzodiazepines (diazepam)	Competes for benzodiazepine R

Poisoning and Antidotes

Antidotes, indications, mode of actions *(Contd.)*		
Antidotes	*Indications*	*Mode of actions*
Neostigmine	Antimuscarinic drug	Inhibits acetylcholinesterase
Pralidoxime (2-PAM)	OPC poisoning	Reactivates cholinesterase
Phytomenadione (vitamin K_1)	Warfarin overdose	Replenishes vitamin K
Acetylcysteine	Paracetamol Carbon tetrachloride	Replenishes depleted glutathione stores
Desferrioaxime	Iron toxicity	Chelates ferrous iron
Penicillamine	Copper, gold, lead, mercury, zinc	Chelates metal ions
Dimercaprol (BAL)	Arsenic, lead, mercury	Chelates metal ions
Ca^{++} EDTA	Lead poisoning	Exchanges calcium for Pb.
Oxygen	Carbon monoxide	Competitively displaces CO from binding sites of Hb
Protamine	Heparin overdose	Binds ionically to neutralize

PK of Ca Na_2 EDTA: Ionised. Distributed extracellularly. Excreted in urine by glomerular filtration (t½ ≤1 hr.). Not absorbed from GIT due to ionisation (given parenterally). IM is painful (IV is preferred).

Uses of EDTA

1. Pb poisoning (**most important** indication): 1 gm diluted in 250 ml saline/glucose solution and infused IV over 1 hr twice daily for 4 days. Renal Pb excretion reduces quickly. Second dose after 6 days is given for Pb to redistribute extracellularly.
2. Fe, Zn, Cu, Mn and radioactive metal poisoning (but not Hg poisoning as it is bound to tissues).

Penicillamine

Penicillamine is **dimethyl cystein**e, obtained as degradation product of **penicillin**. It chelates **Cu, Hg, Pb, Zn**. The **d-isomer** is used therapeutically. **L-isomer** and racemate produce optic neuritis.

PK: Absorbed orally, slowly metabolised in the body, excreted in urine and faeces.

ADR: Dermatological, renal, haematological, and collagen tissue toxicities are prominent.

U: 1. **Wilson's disease/hepatocellular degeneration** is due to genetic deficiency of ceruloplasmin which normally binds and disposes off Cu from the body.

Uses	
1. EDTA	2. Penicillamine
Mercury	Mercury
Iron	Gold
Cu	Cu
Cd	Cd
Pb	Pb
Zn	Zn
MIC CPZ	MG CPZ

Dose: 1 gm 1 hr before/2 hrs after meal.
2. Chronic Pb poisoning (as adjuvant)
3. Hg poisoning
4. Cu poisoning (DOC)
5. Cystinuria and cystine stone
6. Scleroderma

Specific antidotes

Toxin	Antidotes/treatment
1. Acetaminophen	1. N-acetylcysteine
2. Anticholinesterases, organophosphates	2. Atropine, pralidoxime
3. Iron salts	3. Desferrioxamine
4. Methanol, ethylene glycol (antifreeze)	4. Ethanol, dialysis
5. Lead	5. Ca EDTA, dimercaprol
6. Arsenic, mercury, gold	6. Dimercaprol (BAL), succimer
7. Copper, arsenic, lead, gold	7. Penicillamine
8. Antimuscarinic, anticholinergic agents	8. Physostigmine salicylate
9. Cyanide	9. Nitrite, hydroxycobalamin
10. Salicylates	10. Alkalinize urine, dialysis
11. Heparin	11. Protamine
12. Methemoglobinemia	12. Methylene blue
13. Opioids	13. Naloxone
14. Benzodiazepines	14. Flumazenil
15. Tricyclic antidepressant arrhythmias	15. $NaHCO_3$ (nonspecific)
16. Warfarin	16. Vitamin K, FFP
17. Carbon monoxide	17. 100% O_2, hyperbaric O_2
18. Digitalis	18. Stop digitalis, normalize K^+, lidocaine, anti-dig Fab fragments
19. β-blockers	19. Glucagon
20. t-PA, streptokinase	20. Aminocaproic acid
21. PCP	21. Nasogastric suction

Lead poisoning

Lead **L**ines on gingivae and on **e**piphyses of long bones on X-ray. **E**ncephalopathy and **E**rythrocyte basophilic stippling. **A**bdominal colic and sideroblastic **A**nemia. **D**rops: Wrist and foot drop. **D**imercaprol and **E**DTA as first line of treatment.

LEAD
High-risk in houses with chipped paint

Urine pH and drug elimination: Weak acids (phenobarbital, methotrexate, aspirin) →alkalinize urine to increase clearance. Weak bases (amphetamine) → acidify urine to increase clearance.

Drugs reactions	Causal agents
1. Pulmonary fibrosis	1. Bleomycin, amiodarone
2. Hepatitis	2. Isoniazid (INH)
3. Focal to massive hepatic necrosis	3. Halothane, valproic acid
4. Anaphylaxis	4. Penicillin
5. SLE-like syndrome	5. Hydralazine, procainamide, INH
6. Blood dyscrasias	6. Ibuprofen, quinidine, methyldopa, chemotherapy
7. Hemolysis in G6PD deficient patients	7. Sulfonamides, INH, aspirin, ibuprofen, primaquine
8. Breast and endometrial cancer	8. Estrogens
9. Thrombotic complications	9. Oral contraceptives (e.g. estrogens and progestin)
10. Adrenocortical insufficiency	10. Glucocorticoids (HPA axis suppression)
11. Photosensitivity reactions	11. Tetracyclines, amiodarone
12. Gynecomastia	12. Cimetidine, ketoconazole, spironolactone
13. Induce (↑) P450 system	13. Barbiturates, phenytoin, carbamazepine, rifampin
14. Inhibit (↓) P450 system	14. Cimetidine, ketoconazole, itraconazole
15. Tubulointerstitial nephritis	15. Sulfonamides
16. Teratogenic effects	16. Ethanol, lithium, warfarin, valproic acid, thalidomide, isotretinoin, androgens
17. Carcinogenic effects	17. Alfatoxin, vinyl chloride, coaltar, tobacco smoke
18. Mutagenic effects	18. Alfatoxin, cancer chemotherapy
19. Hot flushes	19. Tamoxifen
20. Cutaneous flushing	20. Niacin, CCB, adenosine, vancomycin
21. Cardiac toxicity	21. Doxorubicin (adriamycin)
22. Agranulocytosis	22. Clozapine, carbamazepine
23. Stevens-Johnson syndrome	23. Ethosuximide, sulfonamides
24. Cinchonism	24. Quinidine, quinine
25. Tendonitis, tendon rupture	25. Fluoroquinolones
26. Disulfiram-like reaction	26. Metronidazole, cephalosporins, procarbazine

Coma treatment

Airway (protect)
Breathing (assist)
Circulation (assist)
Dextrose (thiamine, naloxone IV also)

ABCD (in that order)

Rule out: IT'S COMA

Infection (lumbar puncture)
Trauma (bleeding, consider CT scan)
Seizure
Carbon monoxide (give O_2)
Overdose/Opioids (give naloxone)
Metabolic (hypo-/hyperthermia, hypo-/hyperglycemia, thiamine deficiency).
Alcohol (check serum osmolarity)

Drugs visible on roentgenogram

Chloral hydrate,
Heavy metals,
Iodides, and
Phenothiaxines   CHIP

Vaccines, Serum, Immunoglobulins and Immunopharmacology

Immunity and immunization

Immunity: Ability of the body to resist infection is called immunity. Immunity is usually induced by having been exposed to the antigenic marker on an organism that invades the body, or by having been immunized with a vaccine that has the capability of stimulating production of specific antibodies.

Immunization: The process of creating immunity to a specific disease in an individual is called immunization.

There are two types of immunization.
1. Active immunization
2. Passive immunization

Active immunization: Active immunization means administration of antigens to the host to induce formation of antibodies that provides immunity. Active immunization can only be achieved by vaccines. These include:

1. Live attenuated vaccines
2. Killed or inactivated vaccines
3. Toxoid (microbial toxin preparation)
4. Recombinant vaccines

Preparation available for active immunization

Live vaccines: Oral polio (sabin) vaccine (OPV), measles, mumps, rubella, BCG (tuberculosis), typhoid, yellow fever.

Killed vaccines (killed organism): Hepatitis A, pertussis, influenza, cholera, rabies, meningococci (group A and C), pneumococcal.

Toxoids: Diphtheria, tetanus

Recombinant vaccines: Hepatitis B

Passive immunization: Passive immunization means transfer of immunity to host using preformed immunological effectors (antibody).

| Passive immunization procedures with antisera ||
Disease	Passive immunization (antisera)
Diphtheria	A dose of 500–1,000 of IU of diphtheria antitoxin is given intramuscularly to susceptible contacts immediately after exposure. Protection does not last more than 2–3 weeks.
Tetanus	The usual prophylactic dose is 1,500 units of horse ATS given subcutaneously or intramuscularly, soon after injury.
Gas gangrene	A polyvalent antitoxin is used. A patient who has sustained a wound possibly contaminated with spores of gas gangrene should receive a dose of 10,000 IU of *Cl. perfringens*, *Cl. welchii* antitoxin, 5,000 units of *Cl. septicum* antitoxin and 10,000 units of *Cl. oedematiens* antitoxin, intramuscularly, or in urgent cases intravenously.
Rabies	Antirabies serum in a dose of 40 IU per kg of body weight should be given intramuscularly within 72 hours and preferably within 24 hours of exposure. A part of antiserum applied locally to the wound.
Botulism	When botulism is suspected, 10,000 units of polyvalent antitoxin is recommended every 3 to 4 hours.

| Appropriate uses for human immunoglobulin in the prevention and treatment of disease |||||
Agents/condition	Target population	Preparation (1)	Dose (2)	Status (3)
Hepatitis A	Family contacts Institutional outbreaks	IG	(0.02 mg/kg of body weight) (3.2–8.0 mg/kg of body weight	Recommended for prevention
	Travellers exposed to unhygienic conditions in tropical or developing countries	IG	(0.02 ml/kg of body weight) (3.2–8.0 mg/kg of body weight) every 4 months	
Hepatitis non-A, non-B	Percutaneous or mucosal exposure	IG	(0.05 ml/kg of body weight) (8 mg/kg of body weight)	Optional for prevention
Hepatitis B	Percutaneous or mucosal exposure	HBIG	0.05–0.07 mg/kg of body weight (8–11 mg/kg of body weight) Repeat after one month	Recommended for prevention
	Newborns of mothers with HBsAg	HBIG	0.05 ml (8 mg) at birth, 3, and 6 months	Recommended for prevention
	Sexual contacts of acute hepatitis B patients	HBIG	0.5 ml/kg of body weight (8 mg/kg of body weight)	Optional for prevention

Appropriate uses for human immunoglobulin in the prevention and treatment of disease (Contd.)

Agents/condition	Target population	Preparation (1)	Dose (2)	Status (3)
Rubella	Women exposed during early pregnancy	IG	Repeat after one month 20 ml	Optional for prevention
Varicella-zoster	Immunosuppressed contacts of acute cases or newborn contacts	VZIG	15–25 units/kg body weight; minimum 125 units	Recommended for prevention
Measles (rubeola)	Infants less than 1-year-old or immunosuppressed contacts of acute cases exposed less than 6 days previously	IG	0.25 ml/kg body weight or 0.5 ml/kg of body weight if immunosuppressed	Recommended for prevention
Rabies	Subjects exposed to rabid animals	RIG	20 IU/kg of body weight	Recommended for prevention
Tetanus	Following significant exposure if unimmunized or incompletely immunized person or immediatey on diagnosis of disease	TIG	250 units for prophylaxis, 3000–6000 units for therapy	Recommended for prevention or treatment
RH isoimmunization	Rh(D)-negative mother on delivery of Rh-positive infant, or after uncompleted pregnancy with Rh-positive father, or after transfusion of Rh-positive blood to Rh-negative mother	RhIG	1 vial (200–300 µg) per 15 ml of (+) blood exposure	Recommended for prevention

1. **IG** = immune globulin (human); **HBIG** = hepatitis B immune globulin **VZIG** = varicella-zoster immune globulin; **RIG** = rabies immune globulin; **TIG** = tetanus immune globulin; **RhIG** = rhesus factor immune globulin.
   Hyperimmune immunoglobulins have also been used in prophylaxis of mumps and prophylaxis and treatment of pertussis and diphtheria; there are no conclusive data available, and no recommendations can be given.
2. Dose based on intramuscular administration of 16.5% solution.
3. Of limited availability at the present time.

Passive immunization is useful
1. For individuals unable to form antibodies (e.g. congenital agammaglobulinemia).
2. For prevention of disease when time does not permit active immunization (e.g. postexposure).

3. For treatment of certain diseases normally prevented by immunization (e.g. tetanus).
4. For treatment of conditions for which active immunization is unavailable or impractical (e.g. snake-bite).

Passive immunizing agents are
— Purified serum (sera)
— Immunoglobulins (purified gammaglobulin)

Examples of passive immunization available

Infection	Antibody	Indication
Bacterial		
Tetanus	Human tetanus immunoglobulin	Prevention and treatment
Diphtheria	Horse serum	Prevention and treatment
Botulism	Horse serum	Treatment
Viral		
Hepatitis A	Human tetanus immunoglobulin	Prevention
Measles	Human normal immunoglobulin	Prevention
Rubella	Human normal immunoglobulin	Prevention
Hepatitis B	Human hepatitis B immunoglobulin	Prevention
VZV	Human varicella-zoster immunoglobulin	Prevention
Rabies	Human rabies immunoglobulin	Prevention

Active immunization vs passive immunization

Active immunization	Passive immunization
1. Primary immunization	1. For prevention and treatment (prophylactic)
2. Long-lasting immunoglobulin	2. Short-lasting immunity
3. Immunizing agents: Vaccines	3. Immunizing agents: Serum, immunoglobulins
4. Host resistance is better (i.e. higher level of antibody at the time of exposure)	4. Host resistance is comparatively less
5. Suitable for mass immunization	5. Not suitable for mass immunization
6. Procedures need not be repeated as frequently	6. Repeated and frequent doses are required
7. Associated with complications — Allergy — Nonspecific toxic reactions	7. Hypersensitivity reactions may occur

Contraindications of immunization
1. Hypersensitivity to components
2. Mild respiratory infections
3. Diarrhoea
4. Immunosuppressed patient

5. Patient with corticosteroid therapy
6. Encephalopathy
7. Convulsions

NATIONAL IMMUNIZATION SCHEDULE

a. **For infants**
   - At birth (for institutional deliveries) — BCG and OPV-O dose
   - At 6 weeks — BCG (if not given at birth)
     — DPT-1 and OPV-1.
   - At 10 weeks — DPT-2 and OPV-2
   - At 14 weeks — DPT-3 and OPV-3
   - At 9 months — Measles
b. At 6–24 months — DPT and OPV
c. At 5–6 years — DT—the second dose of DT should be given at an interval of 1 month if there is no clear history or documented evidence of previous immunization with DPT.
d. At 10 and at 16 years — Tetanus toxoid—the second dose of TT vaccine should be given at an interval of one month if there is no clear history or documented evidence of previous immunization with DPT, DT or TT vaccines
e. **For pregnant women**
   - Early in pregnancy — TT-1 or booster
   - One month after TT-1 — TT-2

Note: (i) Interval between 2 doses should not be less than one month.
(ii) Minor cough, colds and mild fever are not a contraindication to vaccination.
(iii) In some states hepatitis B vaccine is given as routine immunization.

Vaccines: Vaccines are antigenic materials consisting of the whole microorganisms or one of its products (exotoxin). Vaccines bridge the disciplines of microbiology, infectious disease, immunology and immunopharmacology.

Vaccines are of 2 types: 1. Live attenuated, 2. Killed (by heat/chemical).

Live attenuated vaccine: Vaccine contains live virus or bacteria having no virulence (capacity to produce infection).

Immunizing agents
A. **Vaccines**
   a. **Live attenuated vaccines**
      1. **Bacteria:** BCG, typhoids oral, plague.
      2. **Viral:** Oral polio, yellow fever, measles, rubella, mumps, influenza
      3. **Rickettsial:** Epi. typhus

b. **Killed/inactivated vaccines**
      1. **Bacteria:** Typhoid, cholera, pertussis, plague, CS meningitis.
      2. **Viral:** Rabies, Salk (polio), influenza, hepatits B, Japanese encephalitis, KFD.
   c. **Toxoid:** 1. **Bacteria:** Diphtheria, tetanus.
B. **Immunoglobulins**
   a. **Human Ig**
      1. **Human normal Ig:** Hepatitis A, measles, rabies, tetanus, mumps.
      2. **Human specific Ig:** Hepatitis B, varicella, diphtheria.
   b. **Non-human (antisera):**
      1. **Bacterial:** Diphtheria, tetanus, gas gangrene, botulism.
      2. **Viral:** Rabies.

Killed vaccine: Vaccine contains killed microorganisms (killed by heat or chemical).

Toxoids: Toxoids are modified (detoxification) bacterial exotoxins having no toxicity (to host) but retaining their antigenicity.

ANTISERA: "Antisera" antibodies derived from immune animal serum. Antisera are purified and concentrated preparations of serum of animal (horses) actively immunized against a specific antigen. Risk of hypersensitivity reactions is more. Half-life in humans is not so longer (5–7 days or less). Larger doses are required to provide therapeutic concentrations.

Antisnake venom serum polyvalent: It is available as **purified, enzyme refined and concentrated EQUINE GLOBULINS** in lyophilized vial with 10 ml distilled water. After reconstitution, each ml neutralises:

| 0.6CR | SIXER |

A. **0.6** mg of standard **Cobra/Russel's viper** venom.
B. 0.45 mg of standard krait/saw scaled viper venom.
Dose: 20 ml IV (1 ml/min injection) repeated 1–6 hourly interval till symptoms disappear (**max 300 ml**). **Sensitivity test** for anaphylactic shock to serum is done, if possible, otherwise **adrenaline** is injected concurrently. Antihistaminic and glucocorticoid may be given prophylactically.

Examples of antisera
   ATS : Tetanus antitoxin
   ADS : Diphtheria antitoxin
   ARS : Antirabies serum
   AGS : Anti-gas gangrene serum

Immunoglobulins: Immunoglobulins are purified gamma globulin derived from human serum. Avoid risk of hypersensitivity reactions. Have a much longer half-life in humans (about 23 days for IgG antibodies). Smaller doses are required to provide therapeutic concentrations.

Examples

Tetanus	:	Human tetanus immunoglobulins
Hepatitis B	:	Human hepatitis B immunoglobulins
Rabies	:	Human rabies immunoglobulins
Rh incompatibility	:	Anti-D gammaglobulins

Desired properties of an ideal immunoglobulin: Production of prolonged immunity with a minimum of immunizations.
Absence of toxicity. Prevention of the carrier state.
Complete prevention of disease
Suitable for mass immunization
Cheap and easy to administer

Immunopharmacology

Immunomodulating agents: Immunomodulating agents can be used to increase immunoresponsiveness of patients who have either selective or generalized immunodeficiency.

Name of the immunomodulating agents: BCG (Bacille Calmette Guérin), levamisole, isoprinosine, thymosin.

Uses of immunomodulating agents
1. Immunodeficiency disorders
2. Chronic infectious diseases
3. Cancer

Immunosuppressant drugs: Drugs that modify the immune status (suppression of immunity) are as follows:
1. Cyclosporin
2. Glucocorticoids
3. **Cytotoxic agents:** Azathioprine, cyclophosphamide
4. **Immunoglobulins (Ig):** Anti-lymphocyte Ig, normal human Ig.

Clinical uses of immunosuppressive agents

Disease	Drugs of choice
(A) Autoimmune	
1. Idiopathic thrombocytopenic purpura	Prednisolone Vincristine Azathioprine
2. Autoimmune hemolytic anaemia	Prednisone Cyclophosphamide Mercaptopurine
3. Acute glomerulonephritis	Prednisone Mercaptopurine Cyclophosphamide
4. Systemic lupus erythematosus Rheumatoid arthritis Chronic active hepatitis Inflammatory bowel disease	Prednisone Cyclophosphamide Azathioprine Cyclosporin
5. Acquired factor XIII Ab	Cyclophosphamide + factor XIII

Clinical uses of immunosuppressive agents (Contd.)

Disease	Drugs of choice
(B) Isoimmune	
1. Hemolytic anaemia of the newborn	Rho (D) immunoglobulins
2. Organ transplantation	Cyclosporin
(a) Heart	Azathioprine
(b) Kidney	Prednisone, Ab
(c) Liver	Cyclosporin
	Prednisone
(d) Bone marrow	Cyclosporin
	Cyclophosphamide
	Methotrexate
	Prednisone

Dermatologic Pharmacology

Human skin is a simple three layered structure which provides a complex series of diffusion barriers. Influx of drugs and drug vehicles through these barriers is the basis of pharmacokinetic analysis of dermatologic therapy. Major variables that determine pharmacologic response to drugs applied to the skin include the following:

1. **Regional variation in drug penetration**
   Low: Palm and sole
   Moderate: Face, axilla, scalp
   High: Scrotum, vulva
2. **Concentration gradient:** Increasing the concentration gradient increases mass of drug transferred per unit time. Thus, resistance to topical corticosteroids can sometimes be overcome by use of higher concentration of drug.
3. **Dosing schedule:** The skin acts as reservoir for many drugs. As a result, the **"local half-life"** may be long enough to permit once daily application of drugs with short **systemic half lives.**
4. **Vehicles and occlusion:** An appropriate vehicle maximizes the ability of the drug to penetrate the outer layer of the skin. Occlusion (application of a plastic wrap to hold the drug and its vehicle in close contact with the skin) is extremely effective in maximizing absorption of many drugs.

Dermatologic vehicles: Dermatologic vehicles are pharmacologically inert substance which incorporates with active ingradients (active drug) and thus facilitates cutaneous application.

Considerations in selection of vehicles

1. The solubility of the active agents in the vehicle.
2. The rate of release of the agent from the vehicle.
3. The ability of the vehicle to hydrate stratum corneum, thus enhancing penetration.
4. The stability of the active agent in the vehicle.
5. Interaction of the active agents, vehicle and stratum corneum.

Various dermatologic formulations: Depending upon the vehicles, dermatologic formulations may be classified as: Tinctures, wet dressings, lotions, creams, ointment, gel, powder, paste, aerosols.

Most modern dermatologic formulations are washable hydrophilic oil-in-water emulsions.

Topical antibacterial agents
Indications
1. Preventing infections in clean wounds
2. Early treatment of infected wounds
3. Infected dermatoses
4. Acne vulgaris
5. Management of burn

Topical antifungal agents
1. Topical antifungal azoles: Clotrimazole, miconazole, oxiconazole, econazole, sulconazole, ketoconazole.
2. Tolnaftate
3. Haloprogin
4. Nystatin
5. Amphotericin B

Acne vulgaris is the **commonest** skin disease in adolescent

Causes are:

Androgenic stimulation
↓
Production of sebum from sebaceous follicles of face and neck
↓
Colonisation by bacteria and yeast
(*P. acne, P. ovale, S. epidermidis*)
↓
Fatty acid production by bacterial lipase
↓
Irritation of follicular ducts
↓
Retention of secretion and **hyperkeratosis**
↓
Comedones formation and **rupture into dermis**
↓
Inflammation and **pustulation**

Treatment:
1. Benzoyl peroxide (commonest drug for acne)
$$\downarrow H_2O$$
$$O_2$$
↓
O_2 kills bacteria
2. Retinoic acid
3. Antibiotics

Dermatologic Pharmacology

Antibiotics	Organism/uses
1. Bacitracin (ointment) with neomycin	Streptococci, pneumococci, staphylococci, anaerobic cocci, Neisseria, *Clostridium tetani, C. diphtheriae*
2. Gentamicin (ointment, cream)	*E. coli*, proteus, Klebsiella, Enterobacter, Pseudomonas
3. Neomycin (ointment, powder)	Staphylococci hemolytic, streptococci
4. Polymyxin B (ointment, solutions)	Pseudomonas, *E. coli*, Enterobacter, Klebsiella
5. Silver sulfadiazine (ointment)	Used in burn
6. Tetracycline (cream)	Acne vulgaris
7. Metronidazole (gel)	Acne rosacea
8. Clindamycin (gel)	Acne
9. Erythromycin	Acne

Indications of topical antifungal agents
1. Ringworm infections (teniasis)
2. Oropharyngeal candidiasis
3. Cutaneous candidiasis:
   a. Paronychia and intertriginous candidiasis
   b. Vulvovaginal candidiasis
4. Seborrheic dermatitis

Pharmacological formulations (topical)	
Formulations	Uses
Clotrimazole Miconazole (cream, lotion, vaginal cream, tab)	Taeniasis Vulvovaginal candidiasis
Ketoconazole (cream, shampoo)	Taeniasis (cream) Candidiasis (cream) Oropharyngeal candidiasis (drop)
Nystatin (tab, oral drop, vaginal tab)	Vulvovaginal candidiasis Oropharyngeal candidiasis (drop)
Antifungal (clotrimazole) + Steroid (beta-methasone)	For rapid improvement than an antifungal agent alone

Scabies

Scabies is an ectoparasitic infection of the skin caused by **female *Sarcoptes scabiei*,** the first disease of man with known cause (1687) caused by *S. scabiei/Acarus scabiei/* itchmite/visible arthropod, is characterized by:
— Papulovesicular eruptions
— Severe itching (nocturnal itching more)
— Pustule formation (secondarily infected) and papules
— Later eczematization

Scabicidal drugs: Benzyl benzoate lotion, tetraethyl monosulfiram, unguintum sulfaris, crotamiton oil, permethrin, lindane (hexachlorocyclohexane).

Pharmacological action and adverse effects
1. **Benzyl benzoate:** Scabicide, pediculicide, non-toxic after topical application.
2. **Crotamiton:** Scabicide, antipruritic.
   Adverse effects: Hypersensitivity, primary irritation.
3. **Permethrin:** Neurotoxic to *Sarcoptes scabiei*, *Pediculus humanis*.
   Adverse reactions: Transient burning, pruritus.

Treatment of scabies
1. Treatment of secondary infection (if any) with appropriate antibiotics.
2. Antipruritic agent: antihistaminics
3. Scabicidal drugs (any one):
   a. **Benzyl-benzoate lotion (BBL)—25%**
      Three consecutive days application (from the neck down)
   b. **Tetraethyl monosulfiram (tetmosol)**
      Application after bath (3 consecutive days)
   c. **Permethrin (5% cream)**
      Single application, left on for 8–12 hours, and then washed off.
   d. **Crotamiton oil**
      Two applications to the entire body at 24 hours intervals, with a cleansing bath 48 hours after the last application.
4. Wash (boiling) all clothes (sophisticated clothings keep separate *in a polythene bag for life cycle time (2–3 weeks) of Sarcoptes scabiei.*
5. Treatment of the family members.

TOPICAL STEROIDS

Pharmacological actions of topical steroids
1. Anti-inflammatory action.
2. Antimitotic action is to reduce epidermal cell division (effective in psoriasis).

Classification of topical steroids
According to their therapeutic potency (e.g. efficacy), topical steroids are classified as follows:
- **A. Very potent (highest efficacy)**
  Clobetasol (0.05%)
  Diflorasone (0.05%)
  Betamethasone (0.05%)
- **B. Potent (high efficacy)**
  Beclomethasone (0.025%)
  Desoximetasone (0.025%)
  Triamcinolone (0.5%)
  Fluocinolone (0.2%)
- **C. Moderately potent (intermediate efficacy)**
  Hydrocortisone (0.2%)
  Triamcinolone (0.1%)
  Desoximetasone (0.05%)

Fluticasone (0.05%)
Fluocinolone (0.025%)
D. Mildly potent (low efficacy)
Hydrocortisone (0.1–2.5%)
Methylprednisolone (0.25%)
Dexamethasone (0.1%)
Triamcinolone (0.025%)

Indications of topical steroids
1. Dermatitis and eczema
2. Psoriasis (genitalia, face, palms and soles)
3. Lichen simplex chronicus
4. Pemphigus
5. Acne
6. Pruritus ani
7. Sarcoidosis

Adverse effects of topical steroids
1. **Short-term use:** Spread of infection
2. **Local effects (long-term use)**
   — Atrophy of the skin (**"cigarette paper"** appearance of skin)
   — Steroid rosacea
   — Perioral dermatitis
   — Hypopigmentation
   — Local hirsutism and allergic contact dermatitis
3. **Systemic effects:** From systemic absorption when topical steroids are used in large body surface area for prolonged time.

Keratolytic agents: Keratolytic agents are used to destroy unwanted tissue, including warts and corns. **These are** salicyclic acid, silver nitrate sticks, trichloroacetic acid, resorsinol, propylene glycol, urea.

Salicyclic acid: White powder: Soluble in alcohol, little in water.

Absorption: Percutaneously
Mechanism of action of salicylic acid

Salicylic acid
↓
Solubilizes cell surface protein
↓
Keeps the stratum corneum intact
↓
Desquamation of keratotic debris

(overview of the mechanism of action of salicylic acid)
Therapeutic uses: For keratolytic action (Salicylic acid: 3 to 6%)
For tissue destruction (salicylic acid: >6%)

Adverse effects of salicylic acid
1. **Hypersensitivity reactions:** Urticaria, anaphylactic shock, erythema multiforme.

2. **Ulceration** (if high concentration is used)
3. **Salicylism:** Due to systemic absorption.

Topical acne preparations

Retinoic acid (retin A cream): Increased epidermal cell turnover. Reduced sebum formation and keratinization. Expulsion of open comedones. Transformation of closed comedones into open ones. Used in acne vulgaris.

Benzyl peroxide: Comedolytic action (unlocks the pilosebaceous duct)
Mild keratolytic action. Used in acne vulgaris

Antibiotic tetracycline (cream): Inhibits the *Corynebacterium acne*. Used in acne vulgaris.

Antiseborrheic agents

Selenium sulphide shampoo
Chloroxine shampoo
Ketoconazole shampoo
Coaltar shampoo
Zinc pyrithione shampoo

Sunscreens and sunshades: Protection of the skin from ultraviolet radiation is effected by sunscreens and sunshades.

Sunscreens: Absorb ultraviolet light
— p-aminobenzoic acid (PABA)
— Benzophenones
— Dibenzoylmethanes

Most sunscreens absorb ultraviolet light in beta-ultraviolet (UVB) wavelength range from **280 to 320 nm** which is the range responsible for erythema and tanning associated with sun exposure.

Sunshades: Reflect light. These are inert minerals such as titanium dioxide, zinc oxide and calamine.

Photosensitive drugs: Drug photosensitivity means an adverse effect occurs as a result of drug plus light. There are two forms of photosensitivity:
1. **Phototoxicity:** This is, like drug toxicity, a normal effect of too high a dose of UVB in a subject who has been exposed to the drugs.
2. **Photoallergy:** This is, like drug allergy. Photoallergy due to drugs is the result of a photochemical reaction caused by UVA by which the drug combines with tissue protein to form an antigen.

Photosensitive drugs	
Systemic drugs	*Topical drugs*
Sulfonamides	Deodorant substance
Tetracycline	Halogenated salicylanilides
Griseofulvin and amiodarone	Para-aminobenzoic acid
Nalidixic acid and piroxicam	Coaltar derivatives

Drugs causing rash

Acne: Corticosteroids, androgens.
Toxic erythema: Sulfonamides, ampicillin, sulfonylureas, frusemide, thiazide.
Erythema multiforme (SJ syndrome): NSAIDs, phenytoin, sulfonamides, barbiturates.
Eczema: Penicillins, phenothiazines
Purpura: Thiazides, sulfonamides, sulfonylureas, phenylbutazones, quinine.
Lupus erythema: Isoniazid, phenytoin, hydralazine
Urticaria: Penicillins, enalapril, NSAIDs
Pruritus: Rifampicin, phenothiazine, OCP
Pigmentation: OCP, phenothiazine, chloroquine
Toxic epidermal necrolysis (TEN): Phenytoin, sulfonamides, penicillins, NSAIDs.
Tar compounds: Coaltar is the principal byproduct of the destructive distillation of bituminous coal.

Pharmacological value of tar

Mildly antiseptic
Antipruritic
Modifies keratinization
Uses of tar: Coaltar is used in chronic condition with parakeratosis:
1. Psoriasis
2. Dermatitis (chronic lichenified dermatitis)
3. Lichen simplex chronicus

Adverse effects of tar

1. Irritant folliculitis
2. Phototoxicity
3. Allergic contact dermatitis

Melanising agents: They cause repigmentation of vitiliginous area of skin and enhanced sensitising to solar radiation.
Drugs are: Psoralen (obtained from Amm; majus fruit)
Methoxsalen
Trioxsalen
Synthetic psoralen
PUVA (photochemotherapy)

Mech: They sensitise skin →erythema, inflammation and pigmentation. PUVA is DNA synthesis inhibitor and transfers melanosomes from melanocyte to epidermal cells.
PK: $t½ = 1$ hr
Methoxsalen is more absorbed.
Dose: Oral 20 mg on alternate day and topical.
ADR:
1. Mottling
2. Erythema
3. Burn and blister

U:
1. Psoriasis (PUVA)
2. Vitiligo
3. Lichen planus
4. Urticaria pigmentosa

5. Atopic dermatitis
6. Cutaneous T cell lymphoma

Emolients: They soothe and soften skin, e.g. vegetative oil, petroleum product
Demelanising agents: Hydroquinone (weak)
Monobenzone (strong)
Azelaic acid
Demulcents: These are inert substance to inflamed mucosa and skin. They are glycerine, propylene, glycol and methyl cellulose.

Astringents: Effect superficial layer only by precipitating proteins without penetration into cells.
Drugs are: Minerals (alum, ZnO, etc.), tannic acid and alcohol (for bedsore at 50–90% concentration but irritating to raw surface).
Tannic acid and tannin: Obtained from nutgalls of oak and found in tea, betel nut and catechu.
Mech: Denaturate proteins →protein tennate
U: 1. Bleeding gums and piles
2. Alkaloidal poisoning

Irritants and counter irritants

Mech: Irritant stimulates sensory nerve endings, induces inflammation, produces cooling sensation, pricking, tingling, numbness, vasodilation and warmth.
Rubefacient is irritant causing hyperemia. **Vasicant** increases capillary permeability and collection of fluid under epidermis (vesicles).
Counter-irritant relieves pain and inflammation.
Cutaneous sensation is localised. Deeper sensation is **Diffused**. Spinal segment modulates afferent impulse from surface and deeper organs conducting it from surface to higher centres. Cutaneous impulse of counter irritant obscures the deeper sensation. Irritation produces vasodilation in both skin and deeper organs, thus increases blood supply and reduces pain and inflammation.

Counter-irritants are
1. Volatile/essential oils of clone, turpentine and eucalyptus.
2. **Stearoptenes: Camphor** of C. camphora relieves itching.
3. Mustard seeds contain **sinigrin** (glycoside) and myrosin (enzyme). Seeds + water → myrosin hydrolyses sinigrin to release allyl isothiocyanate (irritant). Used as
   a. Rubefacient and counter-irritant.
   b. Emetic.
4. **Capsicum** gives **capsaicin** which depletes afferent nerve endings of transmitter substance P to relieve neuralgia.
5. **Canthridin** increases vascularity of scalp →↑ hair growth.
6. Wintergreen oil and alcohol.

67 Vitamins

Vitamins: Energise body. Categorised as essential nutrients–**micronutrients**. Vitamins are **organic** substance in food which are **noncalorigenic** and required in small amount but cannot be synthesized in adequate quantities in the body. Not yield energy but enable the body to use other nutrients.

Name of vitamins

Recommended name	Alternative name
Vitamin A	Retinol
Thiamine	Vitamin B_1
Riboflavin	Vitamin B_2
Pyridoxine	Vitamin B_6
Vitamin B_{12}	Cyanocobalamin
Niacin	Nicotinic acid, nicotinamide/vitamin B_3
Folate	Folacin
Pentothenate	Vitamin B_5
Biotin	—
Vitamin C	Ascorbic acid
Vitamin D	D_2 and D_3/calciferol
Vitamin E	α-Tocopherol
Vitamin K	Vitamin K_1

B_1 – The
B_2 – Rich
B_3 – Never
B_5 – Pay
B_6 –
B_{12} – Cash

ADR is **most serious** with overdose of vitamin **A, B_6, D**.

Classification of vitamins: Vitamers (analogy-isomers) = different chemical forms and precursor of a vitamin.

According to their **solubility** in the water and fat, vitamins are classified into **two main groups**
1. Fat soluble vitamin: Vitamin A, D, E, K (**cumulative toxicity**)
2. **W**ater soluble vitamins (excreted → no **toxicity**)
   a. Vitamin **B** complex
   b. Vitamin **C**   WBC

Vitamin A

Other name: **Retinol, anti-infective vitamin**

Vitamin A exists in **two forms**
1. Animal food, as retinol **(pre-formed)**
2. Vegetables, as β-carotene **(pro-vitamin)**

Cheapest source of vitamin A—green leafy vegetables. β-carotene = **most** important with the **highest** vitamin A activity. Carotenes in small intestine form vitamin A. Retinol (vitamin A_1) is **unsaturated alcohol** having **"ionone"** ring. **Dehydroretinol (vitamin A_2)** is found in fresh water fishes. **Carotenoids** are pigments of green plant. β-carotene is **the most important carotenoid.** One molecule of β-carotene splits into 2 molecules of **retinol.**

Normal diet gives **50% retinol esters** and **50% carotenoids.**

1 μg retinol = **3.3 IU** vitamin A activity.

1 retinol equivalent = **6 μg** of dietary carotene (due to incomplete use of pro-vitamin). β-carotene is **antioxidant** and **scavanger** for free radicals.

Sources of vitamin A	
Retinol	β-carotene
Liver	Dark green leafy vegetables
Egg yolk	Yellow and red fruits
Cod liver oil	Red palm oil
Milk butter	Carrot—**Richest** source of **Carotene**

The richest natural source of retinol—fish liver oil.

Functions of vitamin A
1. Maintains normal epithelia
2. Forms retinal photochemicals (rhodopsin)
3. Anti-infective; enhances immune function
4. Anti-carcinogenic for epithelium
5. Helps in skeletal growth

Pharmacological preparations

Retinol (for prevention and treatment of deficiency):
— Retin A cream (topical use)
— Cap. retinal forte (oral)
Etretinate (effective in psoriasis)
Tretinoin (acne preparation)
Isotretinoin (acne preparation)

200,000 units of vitamin A + 30 units of vitamin E, the latter is added for **better absorption** of vitamin A.

Indication of vitamin A

I. **Replacement therapy**

Age <1 year with eye change:	2 cap. 1st day
	2 cap. 2nd day
	2 cap. after 2 weeks
Age >1 year with eye change:	4 cap. 1st day
	4 cap. 2nd day
	4 cap. after 14 days
No eye change:	Single dose
(IM given in diarrhoea/vomiting)	

Distribution of vitamin A capsules should be done to the communities with low vitamin A status, one cap. every 6 months up to 6 years of age, started after 6 months of age.

II. Pharmacotherapy
Skin diseases (acne, psoriasis, ichthyosis) → retinoic acid.

III. Prophylaxis
(infancy, pregnancy, lactation, steatorrhoea, hepatobiliary disease). Fortified dalda/milk. Dose: 4000 IU/day.

IV. Xerophthalmia prophylaxis

- — Birth
  ½ lakh IU single dose orally
- — ½ yr
  1 lakh IU single dose orally
- — 1 yr
  2 lakh IU orally/6 monthly
- — 6 yrs

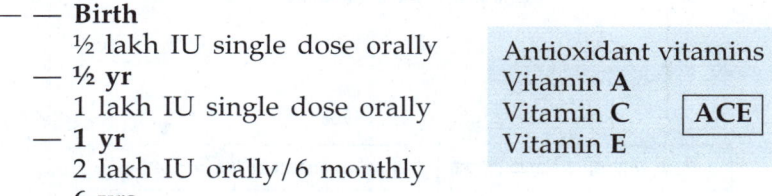

Antioxidant vitamins
Vitamin A
Vitamin C   ACE
Vitamin E

Lactating mother—2 lakh IU (single dose orally at delivery or during next 2 months).

Daily intake of vitamin A recommended by ICMR (1989)			
	Group	Retinol or (mcg)	β-carotene (mcg)
Adults:	Men	600	2400
	Women	600	2400
	Pregnancy	600	2400
	Lactation	950	3800
Infants:	0 to 12 months	350	1200
Children:	1 to 6 years	400	1600
	7 to 12 years	600	2400
Adolescents:	13 to 19 years	600	2400

Absorption and fate of vitamin A: Liver stores vitamin A in the form of retinol palmitate (**retinyl ester**) to meet the needs for 6–9 months. Retinol palmitate is hydrolysed in intestine to retinol. **Retinol + bile→lacteals.** Retinol ester circulates in the form of chylomicrones and is stored in liver cells. Free retinol released from hepatocytes combines with retinol binding protein (RBP, a plasmaglobulin) and is transported to target cells. In target cells, it is bound to **CRBP** (cellular retinol binding protein). Small amount conjugated with **glucuronic acid** → excreted in bile → enterohepatic circulation → water soluble metabolites excreted in urine and faeces.

Retinyl palmitate →retinol (+ bile) → lacteal →liver (+ RBP) →targets cells (CRBP)

Physiological role and action
A. Visual cycle: Retinal is component of light sensitive pigment **rhodopsin** (synthesized by **rods** during dark adaptation). Rhodopsin in dimlight splits into its **component** → nerve impulse through G-protein (transducin).

Iodopsin is a similar pigment synthesized in **cones** for vision in bright light, colour vision and primary dark adaptation. Effects of vitamin A deficiency → **rods > cones** → irreversible change with night blindness on chronic deficiency. *II-cis* **retinal dehyde** is initial part of photoreceptor complex in rods and cones.

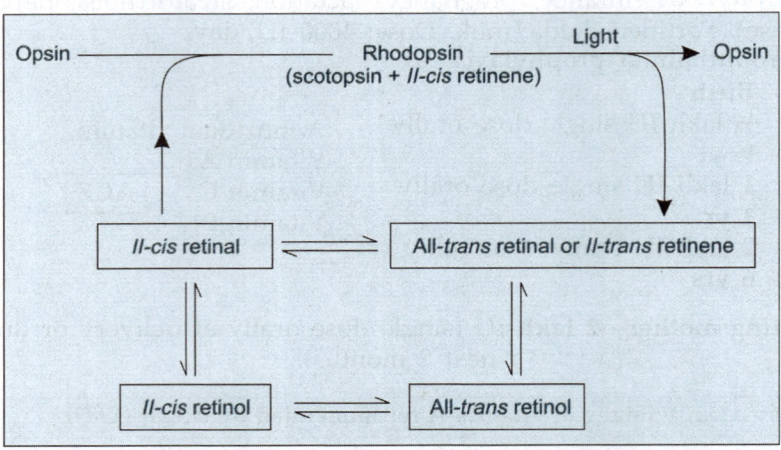

B. **Epithelial tissue:** Promotes differentiation and mucus secretion, maintains epithelia all over the body, inhibits keratinization, enhances immunity, retards epithelial malignancy, helps in bone growth.
C. Retinol maintains spermatogenesis and foetal development, accumulates in last trimester of pregnancy (hence low level in preterm baby). Vitamin A enhances lymphocyte proliferation, Ab response and killer cell function.

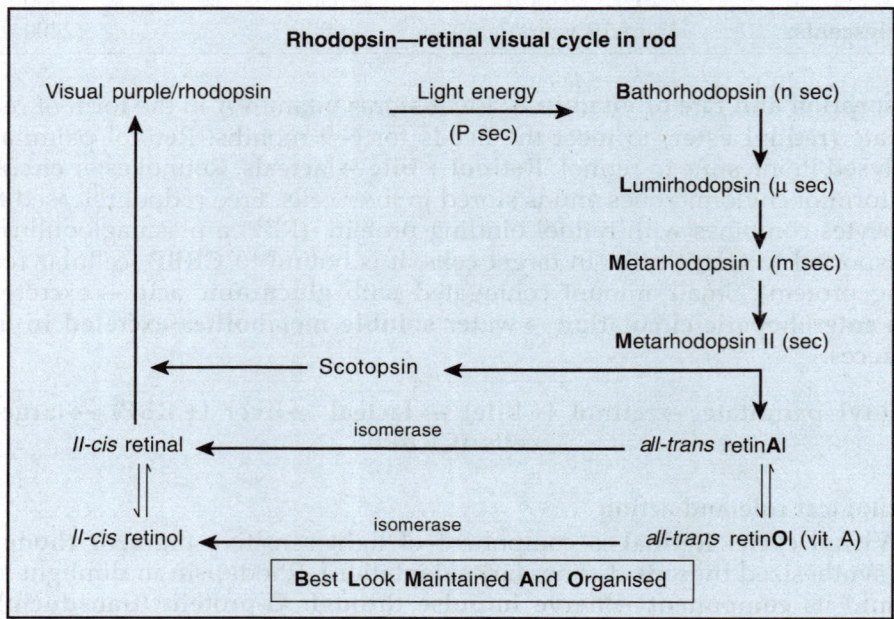

Vitamins

Vitamin A deficiency

On the world scale, vitamin A deficiency causes **5,00,000 new cases of blindness per yr** in young children, **mostly in Asia.**

Signs and symptoms

1. Xerophthalmia: **WHO classification (1982)**

Primary signs

X1A	—	Conjunctival xerosis **(first sign/the earliest sign)**
X1B	—	Bitot's spots
X2	—	Corneal xerosis/corneal dryness
X3A	—	Corneal ulcer/keratomalacia (less than 1/3 cornea)/corneal liquefaction.
X3B	—	Corneal ulcer/keratomalacia (more than 1/3 cornea)/irreversible process.

Secondary signs

XS	—	Corneal Scar
XF	—	Xerophthalmic Fundus
XN	—	Nyctalopia/Night blindness **(the earliest symptom, the most characteristic)**

Xerophthalmia is acute/subacute/chronic → serum level of retinol (<12 µg/dl)
2. Reproduction: Abortion, sterility due to faulty spermatogenesis.
3. Urinary stone formation: Due to shadded epithelia of ureter acting as nidus.
4. Skin: Phrynoderma (dry and rough toad-like skin with papules), hyperkeratinisation, atrophy of sweat gland.
5. Growth: Retarded growth, impaired special senses, foetal malformation.
   X-ray, USG

PEM + Vitamin A deficiency are together in most children. **All carotenoids** including **lycopene and lutein** with/without vitamin A activity are **antioxidants.**

IA:
1. **Vitamin E** promotes storage and use of retinol and reduces its toxicity.
2. **Neomycin** → steatorrhoea → ↓ vitamin A absorption.
3. **Liquid paraffin** causes vitamin A deficiency on chronic use.

Hypervitaminosis A: Toxic dose = 1 lakh daily for months.

Toxicity (manifestations)   **ABCDEFGHIJ**
Appetite loss
Bleeding
Bone and joint pain
Chronic liver failure
Dermatitis, disorder of sleep, dizziness
Erythema, Exfoliation, Edema
Foetal damage
GIT (nausea, vomiting)
Hair loss, Headache, Hypoplastic anaemia
Irritability
Intracranial tension raised + anterior fontanel bulges

called pseudotumor cerebri syndrome
Joint pain.
(The most serious ADR: Liver damage, teratogenicity, hyperostosis).

Acute poisoning: Single ingestion (>1 million IU)/polar bear liver consumption (30,000 IU/gm liver).

ADR: Nausea, headache, ↑ ICT, skin desquamation.
Saturated RBP → ↑ retinol esters in circulation in free form →tissue damage due to surfactant property, hepatomegaly.

No hypervitaminosis with **excess carotenoid occurs** because conversion to retinol has ceiling effect (but may colour plasma and skin).

Treatment: 1. Stop vitamin A use
2. Vitamin E

Retinoic acid (vitamin A acid): It has vitamin **A activity in epithelial tissue** to promote growth (inactive in eye and reproductive organs).

CRABP (cellular retinoic acid binding protein) is different from **CRBP,** is present in skin and other tissue but not in **retina** (hence no participation in visual cycle).

Mechanism: Comedolytic. Inhibits **sebaceous** glands. Enhances lysis of **keratinocytes** and prevents **horny** cells from binding to each other.

Stimulates **epidermal** cell turnover → **peeling.**

Prevents **photoaging of** skin. Induces epithelial cell differentiation by binding to **nuclear receptors** which turn on responsive genes.

ADR: 1. Irritation of skin, stinging, feeling of warmth.
2. Redness, edema, crusting.
3. In vitamin A deficiency, **mucus** secreting cells are replaced by **keratin** producing cells.

PK: Not stored. Rapidly metabolised and excreted in **bile** and **urine.**

U: 1. Acne: All-*trans* retinoic acid (tretinoin) used topically.
13-Cis retinoic acid (isotretinoin) used orally.
2. Arrest **dry scaly surface, mottling, wrinkles, rough** and **leathery texture,** sagging of **loose skin.**

Vitamin D/kidney hormone: It is the collective name of **antirachitic** substances synthesised in the body, activated by UV radiation and also found in the food.

Common types
1. D_1 (mixture of antirachitic substances)
2. D_2/Calciferol (found in irradiated food—yeast, fungi, milk): Ergocalciferol/D_2/calciferol is of **plant** origin.
3. D_3/Cholecalciferol: Animal origin, **most important** vitamin D, synthesised in the skin by photoactivation (UV rays). **Preformed** and found in fats and liver. Vitamin D is stored largely in **fat depots.** Vitamin D is a **pro-hormone.** It is a member of **steroid derivatives.** The main precursor substrate of vitamin D is **cholesterol.**

Dietary sources of vitamin D: Fish liver oil, e.g. cod liver oil, **Halibat liver oil (richest source** 500–10000 μg/100 gm liver), fatty fish, egg yolk, liver, butter, human milk (vitamin D **sulfate).**

D_2 and D_3 are **equally** effective in the body but calcitriol is more significant physiologically and is released by liver into the blood which binds to **globulin**. The **rate limiting step** is **final hydroxylation** in the kidney. Vitamin D is **hormone** because it is synthesised in the **body**, transported by **blood**, acts on **specific** receptors after activation, regulated by **feedback inhibition** due to its active form itself, and plasma Ca^{++} level.

Ergosterol has extra double bond between C_{22-23} and **methyl group at C_{24}**.

Vitamin D_3 is **absorbed better** than vitamin D_2. **Alfacalcidol** is **prodrug 1-α-OHD_3** that is rapidly hydroxylated in liver to **1, 25-$(OH)_2$ D_3 (active)**.

Exposure to UV rays is **critical**. It is filtered off by **air pollution. Dark skinned** races (negroes) cause **95%** UV rays to be filtered off due to black skin **(disadvantage)**. Hence dark skin (and older also) synthesise **less vitamin D** in the skin. Sunlight exposure is needed for **5 min**/day for synthesis of vitamin D.

Functions of vitamin D: (A) Calcitriol enhances Ca^{2+} and PO_4^{3-} absorption from intestine by enhancing synthesis of **"Ca binding protein (CaBP)/Calcibindin"**.

Like steroid hormones, it acts at **cytoplasmic R** → translocated to nucleus → ↑ **mRNA** → protein synthesis regulation.

The most sensitive physiological action of 1,25-dihydroxy vitamin D is to enhance intestinal absorption of Ca^{2+}.

(B) **Calcitriol** enhances Ca^{++} and PO_4^{3-} reabsorption from bone by **osteoclast precursor** in bone remodeling unit (but mature osteoclast lacks vitamin D R).

(C) Calcitriol enhances Ca^{++} and PO_4^{3-} reabsorption from **PCT** but in **hypervitaminosis** D, Ca^{2+} is excreted in urine. It also acts on **skeletal muscle, epidermal** cell, **neuronal** and **immunological cells**.

Functions of vitamin D

Calcitriol (1, 25-$(OH)_2$ D_3) is the active metabolite of vitamin D. There are three principal sites of action of vitamin D: **Intestine, bone and kidney**. It maintains the calcium homeostasis in the body.

Intestine: Increased calcium and phosphate absorption by calcitriol.

Kidney: Decreased calcium and phosphate excretion by 25-(OH) D_3 and 1, 25-$(OH)_2$ D_3.

Bone: Increased calcium and phosphate resorption by 1, 25-$(OH)_2$ D_3. Bone formation may be increased by 24, 25-$(OH)_2$ D_3. Affects **collogen** maturation.

Net effects on serum levels: Both serum calcium and phosphate are increased.

(D) **Vitamin D deficiency** →↑ osteoblastic activity →↑ serum alkaline phosphatase

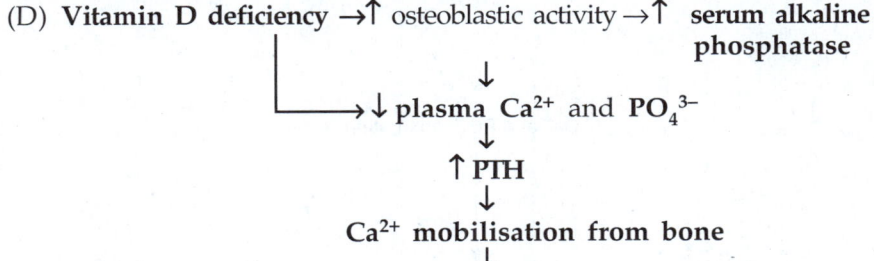

Rickets in children and osteomalacia in adults
(Commonest outcome of vitamin D deficiency).

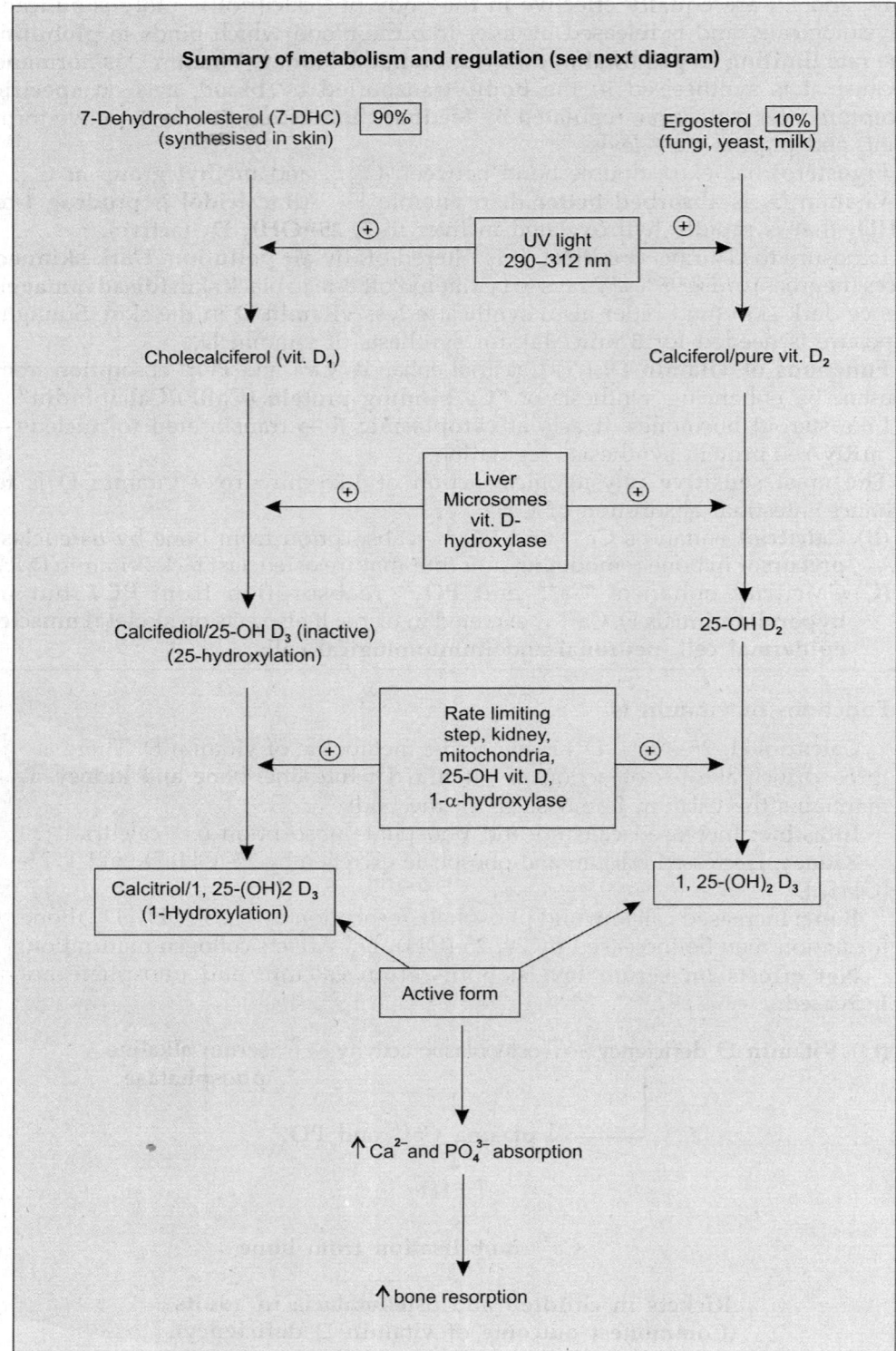

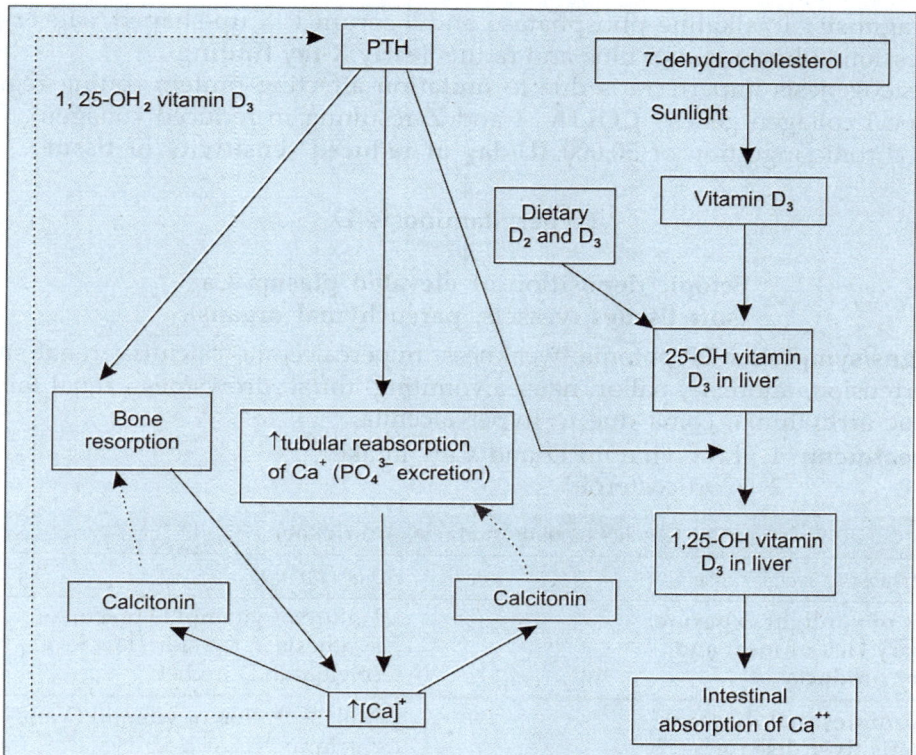

But **organic matrix (osteoid)** is normal in these conditions. Osteoid is **abnormal** in **osteoporosis**. In rickets, incomplete proliferation, degeneration and calcification occur. Calcification of osteoid tissue is irregular and incomplete resulting in **rarefied bone shaft**.

Clinical features of vitamin D deficiency

> A Big Craziness: Ki - Ki - Kiran, Tum Meri Ho Sirf Meri

1. Anterior fontanelle (delayed closure)
2. Bossing of frontal/parietal bone after 6 months.
3. Craniotabes is the **earliest** feature of ricket (unossified area in skull→**Cracking feeling/feeling of Ping-Pong ball** being compressed and released). Coxavera.
4. Knee and wrist broadening—**most** prominent (due to widened epiphyses of long bone in 6–9 months). Scoliosis, lordosis, **Kyphosis**.
5. Deformed long bones of leg due to weight → Knock-Knees/bow-legs.
6. Teeth eruption is delayed
7. Muscle hypotonia →Pot-belly abdomen
8. Harrison's groove/sulcus (horizontal depression along the lower border of chest corresponding to insertion of diaphragm).
9. Pigeon breast (forward projection of Sternum). Rachitic rosary (prominent osteochondral junction on anterior chest wall).
10. Most characteristic sign is bony changes.

(**Commonest** differential diagnosis of osteomalacia in adult is osteoporosis)

Diagnosis: ↑ alkaline phosphatase and ↓ serum P. Cup-shaped/saucer like depression in lower end of ulna and radius **(early X-ray finding).**

(Osteogenesis imperfecta is due to **mutation** affecting protein coding regions of type I collagen genes—**COLIA I and Z** resulting in reduced collagen).

E. chronic ingestion of **50,000 IU/day or reduced sensitivity of tissue.**

↓

Hypervitaminosis D

↓

Ectopic deposition of elevated plasma Ca^{2+}
(soft tissues, vessels, parenchymal organs).

Signs/symptoms: Hypotonia, weakness, hypercalcemia, calciuria, renal stone, hypertension, anorexia, pallor, nausea, vomiting, thirst, drowsiness, renal failure, cardiac arrhythmia, coma due to hypercalcemia.

Treatment: 1. Low vitamin D and Ca^{2+} intake
2. Corticosteroid

Causes of osteomalacia and rickets	
Predisposing factor/cause	*Mechanism*
Lack of sunlight exposure; dietary lack of meat and dairy products	Failure of vitamin D precursor synthesis in the skin/low levels of vitamin D in diet
Gastrointestinal disease/chronic liver disease	Malabsorption of vitamin D and calcium
Aluminium toxicity/bisphosphonate	Direct inhibition of bone mineralisation
Chronic renal failure	Reduced conversion of $25\text{-}(OH) D_3$ to $1, 25\text{-}(OH)_2 D_3$
Vitamin D dependent rickets type I (autosomal recessive) (commonest cause—malnutrition)	Mutation in renal 1-α-hydroxylase which convert $25 (OH) D_3$ to $1, 25\text{-}(OH)_2 D_3$. Low vitamin D level
Vitamin D dependent rickets type II (autosomal recessive)	Mutation in vitamin D receptor. Low phosphate level
Hypophosphataemic rickets (X-linked dominant)	Inherited defect in renal tubular phosphate reabsorption leading to **hypophosphataemia**
Hypophosphatasia (autosomal recessive)	Defect/mutation in bone alkaline phosphatase which normally degrades inhibitors of bone mineralisation at the calcification front

PK: Well absorbed orally in the presence of **bile salt. Malabsorption** and **steatorrhoea** reduce its absorption. **Hydroxylated** in liver, excreted in **bile.** t½ of different forms = **1–18 days.** 25-OH D3 has the **longest** t½.

Uses

1. **Nutritional vitamin D deficiency:**
   Prophylaxis — 400 IU/day and
   Cure   — 3000–4000 IU day

> Types of rickets:
> Type I (decreased vit. D)
> Type II (decreased phosphate level).

Safety margin between normal dose and toxic dose is **narrow**.

Daily dose: 100 IU — Adult
200 IU — Child
400 IU — Mother (lactating and pregnat)
(1 IU = 0.025 µg calciferol).

Fortified milk with vitamin D_2 is given. Periodic dosing and education are **the most practical approach** in developing countries.

2. Metabolic Rickets in ½–2 yrs children.
   a. **Vit. D resistant** rickets (Ca^{2+} PO_4^{3-} metabolism deranged).
   b. **Vit. D dependent rickets** (genetic disorders due to deficiency of renal hydroxylating mechanism which converts 25-OH D_3 → calcitriol).
   c. **Renal rickets** (conversion of 25-OH D_3 into calcitriol inhibited).
      Treatment: Alphacalcidol/calcitriol (DHT also given in renal rickets).
3. Senile/postmenopausal Osteoporosis.
4. Hypoparathyroidism: Calcitriol/alphacalcidol/dihydrotachysterol are **most effective**.
5. Fanconi syndrome ($\downarrow PO_4^{3-}$): Vitamin D enhances PO_4^{3-} level.
6. **P**soriasis
7. Intestinal **O**steodystrophy
8. Bone pain and muscle weakness (**F**atigue)
9. Hypocalcemia

> **POOR** **N**utrition **H**aving **F**atigue

Alphacalcidol is I-α-OH D_3 **(prodrug)** which is rapidly hydroxylated in the liver to 1, 25-$(OH)_2$ D_3/calcitriol, it needs **no hydroxylation.**

DHT (Dihydrotachysterol) is synthetic analogue of vitamin D and directly mobilises Ca^{2+} from bone. **Dose:** 0.25–0.50 mg/day.

IA:
1. **Phenytoin** and **phenobarbitone** reduce responsiveness to target tissue to calcitriol.
2. **Cholestyramine** and **liquid paraffin** reduce vitamin D absorption.

Pharmacological preparations of vitamin D	
Generic name	*Chemical name*
Cholecalciferol (tab)	Vitamin D_3
Calcipotriol (topical vit D_3)	
Ergocalciferol (tab, cap, inj.)	Vitamin D_2
Calcitriol (cap, inj.)	1, 25-$(OH)_2$ D_3
Calciferol (tab, cap)	25-$(OH)_2$ D_3
Calcifediol (cap)	24, 25-$(OH)_2$ D_3

Indication of vitamin D
1. Prevention and treatment of rickets
2. Osteomalacia and osteoporosis
3. Psoriasis (calcipotriol)
4. Treatment of hypocalcaemia
5. Intestinal osteodystrophy
6. Muscle weakness and bone pain

Vitamin K: It is needed for clotting factor synthesis. Has a basic **naphthoquinone** structure with or without side chain at position **3**.

Vitamin	Side chain	Source
K_1 (phytonadione/phylloquinone)	Phytyl	Plant (leafy veg)
K_2 (menaquinone)	Prenyl	Intestinal bacteria
K_3 (menadione or acetomenaphthone)	No side chain	Synthetic

(Water soluble K_3—menadione sodium bisulfite/diphosphate)

Cow's milk: 60 µg/L milk vitamin K
Human milk: 15 µg/L milk vitamin K
Daily dose for adult = 50–100 µg/day (0.03 µg/kg). Vitamin K is stored in liver.
Actions: Acts as a cofactor in the synthesis of clotting factor **II, VII, IX and X** by liver.
$$II, X$$
Vitamin K dependent change in these factors (**Y carboxylation** of glutamate residues of these zymogen proteins) confers on them the capacity to bind Ca^{2+} and to get bound to phospholipid surfaces for coagulation cascade. Synthesises amino acid **Y-carboxyglutamic(gla)**—part of clotting factors II, VII IX and X.

Vitamin K, a strong oxidant increases heamolysis and blocks **Y proteins** necessary for bilirubin uptake by the cells.

Vitamin K deficiency: Causes—liver disease, obstructive jaundice, malabsorption, altered intestinal flora by antibiotic and deficient diet.

Manifestations: Bleeding (**most important**) due to deficient clotting factor in blood leading to haematuria (**first appears**), epistaxis, ecchymoses.

Absorption: It requires bile salts to be absorbed from the intestine. Vitamin K is necessary for the final stages of the synthesis of the coagulation proteins, factor II (prothrombin) VII, IX and X in the liver.

Deficiency of vitamin K arises from
1. **Bile** failing to enter the intestine, e.g. obstructive jaundice and biliary fistula.
2. Certain malabsorption syndromes, e.g. sprue.
3. Reduced alimentary tract **flora**, e.g. in newborn infants and rarely after broad spectrum antimicrobials.

Vitamin K toxicity: On IV injection, it causes flushing, dyspnoea, angina, hypotension and haemolysis (kernicterus).
It is probably due to emulsified injection.

U: Prophylaxis and treatment of bleeding due to **clotting factor deficiency** in:
— **Deficient vitamin K:** 5–10 mg/day oral/parenteral
— **Warfarin** overdose (K_1-DOC →acts **most** rapidly)
— **Chronic liver disease** (prolongs prothrombin time)
— **Obstructive jaundice** (IM route): 10 mg/day
— **Premature infants** (hypoprothrombinaemia)
— **Malabsorption** syndrome (hypoprothrombinaemia): 10 mg/day I
— **Aspirin overdose** (hypoprothrombinaemia)
— **Newborn** due to low level of clotting factors and lack of intestinal flora. K_3 contraindicated due to **haemolysis** in neonates and G6PD deficient person →kernicterus due to ↑ bilirubin and inhibition of glucuronidation of bilirubin.
— **Antibiotic use.**

Vitamin E (tocopherol)

Source: Wheat germ oil (**richest source**), cereal, nut, spinach, egg yolk.

Chemistry: d-isomer more potent than l-isomer. α-tocopherol is **the most potent** and **abundant.** 1 mg alpha tocopherol = 1.49 mg vitamin E. **Daily dose:** 10 mg.

Fate: Absorbed from GIT. Circulates in plasma with β-lipoprotein, stored in tissues, excreted in bile and urine.

Action: Antioxidant (protects unsaturated lipid and coenzyme Q).

Deficiency symptoms

1. Sterility
2. Nerve degeneration
3. Degeneration of skeletal muscle and heart
4. Anaemia

U:
1. Supplement dose (20 mg/day)
2. G6PD deficiency (100 mg/day)
3. Acanthocytosis (100 mg/week IM)
4. With vitamin A (reduces toxicity and enhances absorption of vitamin A)
5. Retrolental fibroplasia (100 mg/kg/day)
6. **Claudication** and muscle cramp (500 mg/day)

Toxicity (due to large doses)

1. Impaired wound healing
2. Creatinuria
3. Abdominal cramp
4. Lethargy
5. Loose motion

Riboflavin (B_2): It is yellow **flavone** compound.
    Source — Milk, egg liver, green leaf.
    Fate — Absorbed and phosphorylated in GIT.

Riboflavin phosphate: (FMN—flavin mononucleotide) is formed in other tissue.

Action: FMN and FAD (flavin mononucleotide) are coenzymes for flavoprotein of oxidation–reduction reaction. Riboflavin and thiamine are **devoid of pharmacological action.**

Deficiency symptoms
1. Sore and raw tongue
2. Mouth ulcer
3. Vascular cornea
4. Dry skin, alopecia, anaemia
5. Neuropathy

U: Ariboflavinosis (2–20 mg/day oral/parenteral)

VITAMIN B COMPLEX

Thiamine B_1: Indications
1. Oral: Nutritional supplement
2. Parenteral (IV or IM):   IV: Wernicke-Korsakoff syndrome
   IM: Wet-beriberi (diagnostic purpose)

Pyridoxine B_6: Indications
1. To prevent peripheral neuritis (antituberculous drug INH causes peripheral neuritis).
2. Radiation sickness
3. Hyperemesis gravidarum
4. Premenstrual tension
5. Sideroblastic anaemia

Vitamin B_{12} (hydroxy-/cynocobalamin)

Vitamin B_{12} (extrinsic factor) is necessary for nuclear maturation and DNA synthesis. Its deficiency leads to megaloblastic anaemia characterized by the presence in the bone marrow of erythroblast with delayed nuclear maturation because of defective DNA synthesis (megaloblast).

Sources of vitamin B_{12}: Synthesized by certain microorganism, the vitamin is not synthesized by animals or plants. The chief dietary source of vitamin B_{12} is microbially derived vitamin B_{12} in meat (especially liver) fish, egg and milk.

The average daily diet contains 5–30 μg of vitamin B_{12} of which 2–3 μg is absorbed.

Site of store: Liver (2–3 mg per day). **Normal daily requirement:** 2 mg.

It would take about 5 years for all the stored vitamin B_{12} to be exhausted and for megaloblastic anaemia to develop if B_{12} absorption stopped.

Vitamin B_{12} deficiency: Causes
1. Lack of intrinsic factor (pernicious anaemia)
2. Disease affecting distal ileum:
   a. Malabsorption syndrome
   b. Inflammatory bowel disease
   c. Small bowel resection
   d. Fish tapeworm infestations
3. Partial or total gastrectomy

Effects
1. Megaloblastic anaemia is due to impaired DNA synthesis, inhibition of normal mitosis and abnormal maturation and function of the cell produced.
2. Peripheral neuropathy

Absorption of vitamin B_{12}
Site of absorption: Distal ileum

Vitamin B_{12} is liberated from protein complexes in food by gastric enzymes. Vitamin B_{12} then binds to **vitamin B_{12} binding protein "intrinsic factor"**. Intrinsic factor is a **glycoprotein** that is secreted by **gastric parietal cells** with H^+ ions. Intrinsic factor carries vitamin B_{12} to the specific receptors on the surface of the distal ileum where it is absorbed.

$$\text{Vitamin } B_{12} + \text{intrinsic factor}$$
$$\downarrow$$
$$\text{Vitamin } B_{12} \text{ intrinsic factor complex}$$
$$\downarrow$$
$$\text{Binds with specific R on the distal ileum}$$
$$\downarrow$$
$$\text{Absorption of vitamin } B_{12}$$
$$\text{(intrinsic factor remains in the lumen)}$$
$$\downarrow$$
$$\text{Vitamin } B_{12} \text{ binds with transcobalamin II}$$
$$\downarrow$$
$$\text{Transcobalamin II carries vitamin } B_{12} \text{ to the bone marrow and other tissue. [In the plasma, vitamin } B_{12} \text{ binds with tanscobalamin I and III.]}$$

Function of vitamin B_{12}
Vitamin B_{12} is required for two enzymatic reactions:
1. Methylation of homocysteine to methionine by methyltetrahydrofolate.
2. Isomerization of methylmalonyl-CoA to succinyl-CoA.

Discussion of the next diagram
a. Conversion of methyltetrahydrofolate **(methyl FH_4)** to tetrahydrofolate **(FH_4)** by vitamin B_{12}.
b. Methyl FH_4 donates methyl group to vitamin B_{12} (methyl B_{12}).
c. From methyl B_{12}, methyl group is transferred to homocysteine to form methionine.
d. Methionine donates formate to FH_4 to form **Formyl FH_4**.
e. Formation of folate polyglutamate from formyl FH_4 by polyglutamation.
f. Folate polyglutamate acts as cofactor in the synthesis of purine and pyrimidine (DNA base).

Role of vitamin B_{12} in megaloblastic anaemia
The underlying pathology in megaloblastic anaemia are:
1. Impaired DNA synthesis
2. Diminished cell division (mitosis) in the face of continued RNA and protein synthesis. This leads to production of large cells that have a **high RNA : DNA ratio**.

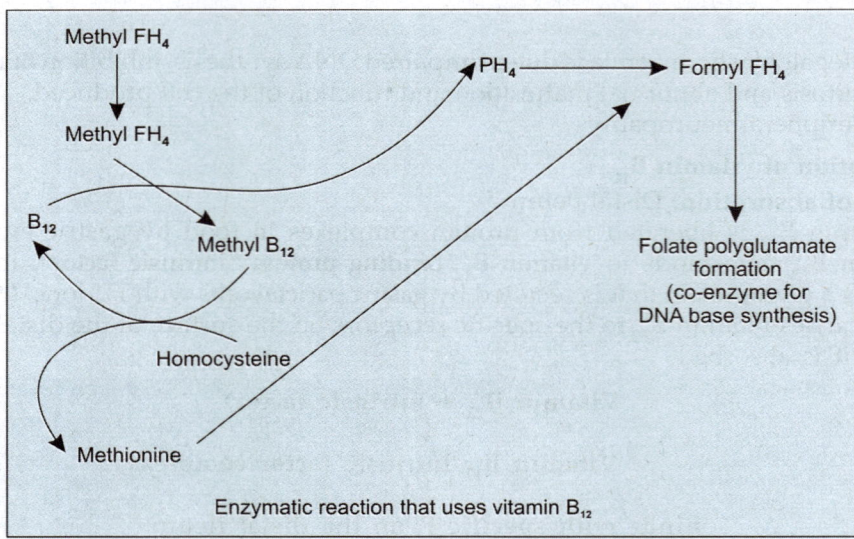

Enzymatic reaction that uses vitamin B_{12}

Parenteral vitamin B_{12} causes
1. Vitamin B_{12} is involved in the enzymatic reactions for synthesis of DNA.
2. It normalizes the RNA : DNA ratio
3. Normalizes the cell division (mitosis)
4. Bone marrow usually returns to normal within 48 hours.
5. **Reticulocytosis** begins on the 2nd or 3rd day and is usually maximal by the 5–10 days.
6. Hemoglobin begins to increase in the 1st week and returns to normal by 1–2 months.
7. Correction of anaemia.

Indications of vitamin B_{12}
1. To treat pernicious anaemia and other causes of vitamin B_{12} deficiency.
2. After total gastrectomy.

Contraindication: Undiagnosed anaemia.

Pharmacological preparations of vitamin B_{12}

Available for therapeutic use: Cyanocobalamin, hydroxycobalamin.

Active form of vitamin B_{12} is **methylcobalamin and deoxyadenosylcobalamin**. **Cyanocobalamin** and **hydroxycobalamin** must be converted into above active forms.

Routes: Parenteral (IM): hydroxycobalamin = 1000 μg/ml and oral (cyanocobalamin) = 1000 μg tablets.

Dose: To replenish body stores

Hydroxycobalamin IM injection 100–1000 μg daily or every other day for 1–2 weeks.

Maintenance dose (lifelong): Hydroxycobalamin (IM): 100–1000 mg once a month for life.

Folic acid/vitamin M/Wills' factor (first name)
Folic acid is formed from three building blocks
Pteridine (similar to xanthopterin) + PABA + glutamic acid.
It is not present in nature but is the parent compound of folates.
Source of folates: Liver, nuts, green vegetables, cereals, yeast, fruits.

Functions of folic acid (coined by Mitchell means "from leaf")
1. Folates are essential for DNA synthesis in that they are cofactors in the synthesis of purines and pyrimidines.
2. Folate cofactor is necessary in the synthesis of thymidylic acid and essential precursor of DNA.

Causes of folate deficiency (total body store of FA = 5–10 mg)
I. **Nutritional (major cause)**
   Poor intake (old age, starvation, anorexia).
   Gastrointestinal disease (partial gastrectomy, coeliac disease, Crohn's disease).
II. **Poor utilization**
   Physiological: Pregnancy, starvation, prematurity.
   Pathological:
   — Haemolytic disease with excess red cell production.
   — Malignant disease with increased cell turnover.
   — Inflammatory disease
III. **Malabsorption syndrome**
IV. **Antifolate drugs**   **STAMP**
   Sulfonamides
   Trimethoprim
   Anticonvulsants and OC impair absorption
   Methotrexate
   Pyrimethamine

Effects of deficiency of folic acid (pteroylglutamic entration acid/PGA)
1. Megaloblastic anaemia
2. Neural tube defect (spina bifida) in foetus of a pregnant lady.

Pharmacokinetics of folic acid (plasma concentration = 4–20 ng/ml)
Routes of administration	: Oral/parenteral
Absorption	: From proximal jejunum
Distribution	: Widely distributed
Daily requirements	: 60–100 µg
Site of stores	: Liver and other tissues

Since body stores of folates are relatively low and daily requirements are high, folic acid deficiency and megaloblastic anaemia can develop within 1–6 months after the intake of folic acid stopped.

Indications of folic acid (FA)
1. To treat megaloblastic anaemia due to folate deficiency.
2. Pregnant women (if there is a risk of birth defect)
3. Premature infants

4. Patient with haemolytic anaemia
5. Liver disease
6. Chronic skin disease
7. Renal dialysis
8. With anticonvulsant drugs

> Daily requirement:
> Pure FA <0.1 mg/day
> Dietary FA 0.2 mg/day
> Pregnancy 0.8 mg/day

Pharmacological preparations
Synthetic folic acid is available for administration.
Oral: Tablet folacin
Parenteral: Injection

Niacin: Indications
1. Treatment of pellagra
2. Hyperlipidaemia (niacin decreases **VLDL, LDL** levels in the plasma, reduces FFA and lypolysis).
3. Familial dysbetalipoproteinemia

Adverse effects of niacin
a. Cutaneous vasodilatation: Flushing
b. Itching (pruritus)
c. Rashes, dry skin
d. Hepatotoxicity (rarely)
e. Dyspepsia, diarrhoea
f. Hyperpigmentation of skin
g. Gout
h. DM
i. Jaundice

CI: Pregnancy and children

Vitamin C (ascorbic acid)

Sources of vitamin C: Amlaki, cabagge, guavas, potatoes, green peppers, cauliflowers, orange and citrus fruits, tomatto.

Functions of vitamin C
1. Synthesis of collagen (helps in wound healing)
2. Antioxidant agent

Indication of vitamin C
1. Prevention and treatment of scurvy
2. Urinary acidification
3. Methemoglobinaemia
4. Coryza
5. Postoperative patient

Neonatal vitamin toxicities
Hypervitaminosis A = Anomalies (teratogenic)
Hypervitaminosis E = Enterocolitis (necrotising)
Hypervitaminosis K = Kernicterus (hemolysis)

Hypervitaminosis D causes SARCOIDOSIS, which manifests as:
Schaumann calcification, **A**steroid bodies, **R**espiratory/**R**enal complication, **C**a^{++} increased, **O**cular lesion, **I**g mediated noncaseating granuloma, **D**I, **O**steopathy, **S**ubcutaneous nodule, **I**L-1/interstitial lung fibrosis, **S**eventh CN palsy.

Vitamin	Chemical form	Thermostability	Daily allowance (adult males)
A	**Retinol (A_1)** Dehydroretinol (A_2) β-carotene (pro-vit)	Stable in absence of air	**Fat soluble vitamins** 1000 μg (4000 IU)
D	Calciferol (D_2) Cholecalciferol (D_3) Calcitriol	Stable	5 μg (200 IU) 1 μg
E	α-tocopherol	Stable (air and UV light decompose)	10 mg
K	Phytonadione (K_1) (phylloquinone) Menaquinones (K_2) Menadione (K_3) Acetomenaphthone	Stable, decomposed by light	50–100 μg
B_1	Thiamine	Relatively labile	**Water soluble vitamin** 1.5 mg
B_2	Riboflavin	Relatively stable	1.7 mg
B_3	Nicotinic acid } Nicotinamide } Tryptophan (pro-vit)	Stable Niacin	20 mg
B_6	Pyridoxine Pyridoxal Pyridoxamine	Stable in absence of air	2 mg
	Pantothenic acid	Labile	4–7 mg
	Biotin	Stable	0.1–0.2 mg
	Folic acid Folinic acid	Labile	0.2 mg
B_{12}	Cyanocobalamin Hydroxocobalamin	Stable	2 μg
C	Ascorbic acid	Labile in solution	60 mg

Folinic acid/leucovorin calcium/citrovorum factor/5-formyl THFA

It is a congener of **folic acid** with (-CHO) radical at position 5 (N^5) of pteridine ring (5-formyl derivative of THFA). Folic acid is pteridine ring linked by **methylene bridge** to PABA which is joined by amide linkage to glutamic acid. THFA mediates **one carbon** transfer reaction as an adduct.

U: 1. Folinic acid is used to circumvent inhibition of DHFRase as a part of high dose methotrexate, to potentiate 5-FU and as antidote in **folate antagonist toxicity** (pyrimethamine and trimethoprim). Folinic acid is active coenzyme form which needs no reduction by DHFRase before it can act. Methotrexate (DHFRase inhibitor) toxicity is, therefore, antagonised by folinic acid but not by folic acid.
2. Folinic acid is more expensive, hence not used in folate deficiency, but exception is megaloblastic anemia with congenital DHFRase deficiency.

CI: Folic acid is not used in pernicious anemia or other megaloblastic anemia secondary to cyanocobalamin deficiency. Just as is seen with FA, use of leucovorin can result in an apparent response of hematopoietic system, but neurological damage may occur or progress if already present. FA does not present neurological defect of cyanocobalamin deficiency and its high dose counteracts **antiepileptic drug** action (phenytoin, primidone) leading to more seizures. **Alcohol** impairs methyl-THFA release from liver.

Ethionamide, **C**ycloserine, **H**ydralazine, **I**NH, **P**enicillamine **S**upplements vitamin B_6.   **Eat CHIPS**

Unit 13

Classification of Drugs and Adverse Drug Reactions

68 Classification of Drugs (COD)

CHOLINERGIC AGONISTS

1. **Directly acting**
   a. Esters
      - **Be**thanechol
      - **Ca**rbachol
      - **Me**thacholine
      - **A**cetylcholine (ACh)   **BCAME**
   b. **A**lkaloids
      - **A**recoline
      - **L**obeline
      - **M**uscarine
      - **N**icotine
      - **O**xotremorine
      - **P**ilocarpine   **LMNOP**

2. **Indirectly acting/ anticholinesterase**
   (reversible and irreversible)
   Reversible
   - **R**ivastigmine   **sin (PAP) END**
   - **P**hysostigmine
   - **A**mbenonium
   - **P**yridostigmine
   - **E**drophonium
   - **N**eostigmine (eserine)
   - **D**emecarium, donepezil

   Irreversible
   - **T**abun, sarin, soman (nerve gas for chemical warfare)
   - **I**soflurophate
   - **M**alathion
   - **E**chothiophate
   - **P**arathion   **TIME Please**

   Reactivator of acetylcholinesterase
   - Pralidoxime
   - Obidoxime

ANTICHOLINERGIC DRUGS

1. **Natural alkaloids**
   - Atropine
   - Hyoscine (scopolamine)
2. **Semisynthetic derivatives**
   - Homatropine
   - Homatropine methyl bromide
   - Hyoscine butyl bromide
   - Ipratropium bromide
   - Tiotropium bromide
3. **Synthetic compound**
   a. **Mydriatics**
      - Cyclopentolate
      - Tropicamide
   b. **Antisecretory-antispasmodics**
      i. **Quarternary compounds**
         - Propantheline
         - Oxyphenonium
         - Clidinium
         - Penthienate
         - Pipenzolate methyl bromide
         - Mepenzolate methyl bromide

- Isopropamide
- Glycopyrrolate

ii. **Tertiary amines**
- Dicyclomine
- Pirenzepine
- Telenzepine   **DPT**

iii. **Antiparkinsonians**
- Trihexyphenidyl (benzhexol)
- Procyclidine, biperiden
- Benztropine
- Cycrimine
- Ethopropazine

Drugs acting on autonomic ganglia

Ganglia has adrenergic R, dopaminergic R, peptidergic R, cholinergic (N_N and M_1) R.

Classification

Ganglionic stimulants

1. **Nicotinic agonist (selective)**
   - Nicotine **(small dose)**
   - Lobeline
   - DMPP
   - TMA (tetramethyl ammonium)
2. **Muscarinic agonist (nonselective)**
   - ACh
   - Pilocarpine
   - Carbachol
   - Anti-ChE   **A CAP**

ADRENERGIC DRUGS

1. **Direct sympathomimetics (bind and activate R)**
   - Apraclonidine
   - Phenylephrine
   - Methoxamine
   - Salbutamol
   - Brimonidine
   - Ritodrine
   - Adrenaline
   - Isoprenaline
   - NA   **APM'S BRAIN**
2. **Indirect sympathomimetics**
   - Tyramine (releases NA to act on R)
3. **Mixed action sympathomimetics**
   - Metaraminol
   - Amphetamine
   - Mephentermine
   - Ephedrine   **MAME**

THERAPEUTIC CLASSIFICATION OF ADRENERGIC DRUGS

1. **Pressure agents**
   - Noradrenaline
   - Ephedrine
   - Dopamine
   - Phenylephrine
   - Methoxamine
   - Metaraminol
   - Mephentermine
2. **Bronchodilators**
   - Isoprenaline
   - Albuterol/salbutamol
   - Metaproterenol/orciprenaline
   - Formeterol
   - Adrenaline
   - Salmeterol
   - Terbutaline   **I AM FAST**
3. **CNS stimulants**
   - Methamphetamine
   - Amphetamine
   - Dexamphetamine
   - Ephedrine   **MADE**
4. **Uterine Relaxant and vasodilators**
   - Salbutamol
   - Isoxsuprine   **SIT**
   - Terbutaline
   - Ritodrine
5. **Cardiac stimulants**
   - Isoprenaline
   - Dobutamine
   - Ephedrine
   - Adrenaline   **IDEA**
6. **Nasal decongestants**
   - Ephedrine
   - Pseudoephedrine
   - Phenyl propanolamine
   - Phenylephrine
   - Naphazoline
   - Oxymetazoline
   - Xylometazoline   **NOX**
7. **Anorectics**
   - Fenfluramine
   - Mazindol

- Dexfenfluramine
- SIBUtramine

          For My Darling SIBU

Selective β_2 Stimulants
- Terbutaline
- Orciprenaline (β_2: β_1 least selective)
- Salbutamol (β_2: β_1 highest, 10 times)
- Salmeterol   TOSS

α blockers
1. **Equilibrium type (competitive/reversible)**

   A. **Selective**

      a. α_1
   - Doxazosin
   - Prazosin
   - Terazosin
   - Trimazosin

      b. α_2
   - Roumolscine
   - Yohimbine

   B. **Nonselective**
   - Ergotamine
   - Ergotoxine
   - Dihydroergotoxine
   - Dihydroergotamine
   - Tolazoline
   - Phentolamine
   - Ketanserin
   - Chlorpromazine

2. **Nonequilibrium type (irreversible)**
   - Phenoxybenzamine
   - Dibenamine

β blockers
1. **Selective (β_2)**
   Butoxamine
   ICI 118551

2. **Cardioselective (β_1)**
   - Bisoprolol
   - Celiprolol
   - Metoprolol
   - Atenolol
   - Acebutolol
   - Betaxolol
   - Esmolol   A to M = B CAME

3. **Nonselective** (β_1 and β_2)

   a. **Without intrinsic** sympathomimetic activity ($\beta_1 = \beta_2$)
   - Propranolol
   - Nadolol
   - Timolol
   - Sotalol   NTPs

   b. **With intrinsic** sympathomimetic activity:
   - Alprenolol
   - Pindolol
   - Oxprenolol   A Postal Order

   c. **α and β blockers**
   - Labetalol
   - Dilevalol
   - Carvedilol   DLC

4. **Newer drugs**
   - Selective β_1 blocker (nabivolol) and
   - α_1 + β blockers (medroxalol and bucindolol)

β blockers with
- **Shortest t½** : Esmolol (10 min)
- **Longest t½** : Nadolol (14–24 hrs)
- **Highest bioavailability** : Pindolol (90%)
- **Lowest bioavailability** : Alprenolol (10%)
- **Maximum LA property** Propranolol

α + β blocker
- **Labetalol**

Selective α_{1A} blocker
- **Tamsulosin**

Muscle relaxants
1. **Peripherally acting**

   a. **Directly acting**
   - Quinine
   - Dantroline sodium

b. **Neuromuscular blockers**
  A. **Depolarising blockers**
    - Succinylcholine (SCh, suxamethonium)
    - Decamethonium (C-10)
  B. **Nondepolarising (competitive) blockers**
  Short-acting
  - Mivacurium
  Intermediate acting
  - Vecuronium
  - Rocuronium
  - Atracurium
  Long-acting
  - Pancuronium
  - Pipecuronium
  - Doxacurium
  - d-tubocurarine
  - Gallamine triethiodide
  - Cisatracurium
  - Rapacuronium
2. **Centrally acting**
  a. **BZD** and cyclobenzaprine
  b. **GABA** derivative
    - Baclofen
  c. **Mephenesin** group
    - Mephenesin
    - Methocarbamol
    - Carisoprodol
    - Chlorzoxazone
    - Chlormezanone
  d. Central α_2 agonist
    - Tizanidine

Muscle relaxation potentiating agents
- Aminoglycosides   **ATP ABC**
- Tetracycline
- Polypeptide antibiotic
- Antiarrhythmic
- Beta blocker
- Calcium channel blocker

ANAESTHESIA
Amide linked LA
    AmiDe LA has Double i in name
1. **Long-acting**
  - Etidocaine
  - Bupivacaine
  - Ropivacaine
  - Dibucaine (**longest**-acting LA)
2. **Intermediate-acting**
  - Lidocaine
  - Mepivacaine
  - Prilocaine
3. **Ester-linked LA**
  - Cocaine
  - Procaine
  - Tetracaine
  - Benzocaine
  - Chloroprocaine (**shortest**-acting LA)

Functional classification of LA
Injectable
1. **Low potency and short duration**
  - Procaine
  - Chloroprocaine
2. **Intermediate potency and duration**
  - Lidocaine (lignocaine)
  - Prilocaine
3. **High potency and long duration**
  - Amethocaine (tetracaine)
  - Ropivacaine   **A Red Blood Cell**
  - Bupivacaine
  - Cinchocaine (dibucaine)

Surface anaesthesia
1. **Soluble**
  - Tetracaine
  - Lidocaine
  - Cocaine   **TLC**
2. **Insoluble**
  - Benzocaine   **BOB**
  - Oxethazaine
  - Butamben (butylaminobenzoate)

General anaesthesia
Inhalational
1. **Gas**
  - N_2O (nitrous oxide)
2. **Liquid**
  - Ether
  - Halothane

- Sevoflurane   SIDE
- Isoflurane
- Desflurane
- Enflurane

Intravenous
1. **Inducing agents**
   - Thiopentone sodium
   - Methohexitone sodium
   - Etomidate
   - Propofol   TEMP
2. **Slower-acting drugs**

BZD
- Diazepam
- Lorazepam
- Midazolam

Dissociative anaesthesia
- Ketamine

Neurolept analgesia
- Fentanyl + droperidol

Arrhythmia causing GA
- Halothane
- $CHCl_3$
- Methoxyflurane
- Trilene
- Cyclopropane

DAY CARE GA

For maintenance
- Desflurane
- Isoflurane, and
- Sevoflurane

For induction
- Thiopentone
- Etomidate
- Methohexitone
- Propofol

For analgesia
- afEntanil
- Remifentanil   DISTEMPER

Sedatives and hypnotics

1. **Classification of barbiturates**
   A. **Long-acting barbiturates** (8 hrs or more)
      a. Phenobarbitone
      b. Mephobarbitone

   B. **Intermediate acting barbiturates** (4–8 hrs)
      a. Pentobarbitone
      b. Amylobarbitone
      c. Butobarbitone
   C. **Short-acting barbiturates** (<4 hrs)
      a. Secobarbitone
      b. Hexobarbitone
   D. **Ultrashort acting barbiturates**
      a. Thiopentone
      b. Methohexitone

2. **Classification of BZD (benzodiazepine) based on use**

   Hypnotics
   - Temazepam
   - Triazolam
   - Midazolam
   - Nitrazepam   To This Mid-Night
   - Flurazepam   Famous Film: **Darr**
   - Flunitrazepam
   - Diazepam
   - Estazolam

   Antianxiety
   - Alprazolam   A COLD
   - Chlordiazepoxide
   - Oxazepam
   - Lorazepam
   - Diazepam

   Anticonvulsant
   - Diazepam
   - Clonazepam
   - Clobazepam

3. **Newer non-BZD hypnotic**
   - Zopiclone
   - Zolpidem

4. **Others**
   - Opioids   ON CHD
   - Some Neuroleptic
   - Some anti-Cholinergic
   - Some anti-Histaminic, and
   - Anti-Depressant have sedative action

BZD CLASSIFICATION (BASED ON DURATION OF ACTION)
1. **Long-acting**
   - Diazepam
   - Nitrazepam

- Flurazepam
- Prazepam
- Chlorazepate
- Chlordiazepoxide
2. **Short-acting**
    - Temazepam
    - Oxazepam
    - Triazolam
    - Alprazolam
    - Lorazepam   TOTAL

ANTIEPILEPTICS
Oxazolidinediones
- Trimethadone

Hydantoin
- Phenytoin
- Mephenytoin

Iminostilbene
- Oxcarbazepine
- CBZ (carbamazepine)

Succinimide
- Ethosuximide
- Phensuximide

Aliphatic carboxylic acid
- Valproic acid/sodium valproate

BZD
- Diazepam
- Clonazepam
- Clobazepam

Barbiturates
- Phenobarbitone
- Mephobarbitone

Deoxybarbiturates
- Primidone

Newer drugs   LPG FTV
- Lamotrigine
- Levetiracetam
- Progabide
- Gabapentin
- Felbamate
- Topiramate
- Tiagabine
- Vigabatrin

Others
- Phenacemide
- Acetazolamide

ALCOHOLIC BEVERAGES
1. **Malted liquor**
    - 3–6% alcohol produced by germinated **cereal** fermentation
2. **Wines:** 9–22% alcohol, produced by **fruit** fermentation
    - **All alcohol fermented**
      — dry wine
    - **Some left**
      — sweet wine
3. **Spirit**
    - 40–55% alcohol
    - Fermentation → distillation → spirit formation
    - **Proof spirit**
      — explosive
    - **Rectified spirit**
      — 90% W/W ethanol
    - **Absolute alcohol**
      — 99% W/W ethanol
    - **100% proof spirit** is 49.29% W/W or 57.1% V/V alcohol

Drugs causing disulfiram like reaction
- Anti-**A**moebic (metronidazole)
- Anti-**B**iotic (chloramphenicol, furoxone, cephalosporin)
- Anti-**C**ancer (procarbazine)
- Anti-**D**iabetic (oral hypoglycaemic, e.g. chlorpropamide)
- Anti-**E**pileptic (phenytoin)
- Anti-**F**ungal (griseofulvin)
                                   ABCDEF

Aldehyde dehydrogenase is inhibited by:
- **C**ephalosporins
- **O**ral hypoglycaemic
- **M**etronidazole   Ald. COM

ANTIPSYCHOTIC DRUGS
1. **Butyrophenones**   BOAT in Pond
    - Droperidol
    - Haloperidol
    - Penfluridol   DTPH =
    - Trifluperidol   Dil To Pagal Hai
2. **Others**
    - Molindone
    - Reserpine

- Pimozide
- Sulpiride
- Loxapine   MRP—Six Lacs

3. Atypical
   - Clozapine
   - Olanzapine
   - REsperidone   CORE

4. Thioxanthenes
   - Chlorprothixene
   - Flupenthixol
       CFT = Complement
   - Thiothixene   Fixation Test

5. Phenothiazines
   - Chlorpromazine
   - Aliphatic side chain
   - Triflupromazine   CAT

   PiperiDine side chain
   - ThioriDazine

   Piperazine side chain
   - Trifluoperazine
   - Thioproperazine, and
   - Fluphenazine

     Fertilization of Two ova in Two different cycles (superfeTation)

ANXIOLYTIC DRUGS

1. BZD
2. β blocker
3. Azapirone
   - Buspirone
   - Ipsapirone
   - Gepirone   BIG
4. Other sedatives
   - Meprobamate
   - Hydroxyzine

DRUGS FOR AFFECTIVE DISORDERS

1. Antimanic (mood stabilizer): Li_2CO_3
2. Antidepressant: TCA, MAO inhibitors

MAO inhibitors

A. Isoenzyme selective
   1. MOA-A: Clorgiline, Moclobemide MCA
   2. MOA-B: Selegiline (deprenyl)

B. Nonselective
   1. Hydrazine: Isocarboxazid, Phenelzine   HIP
   2. Nonhydrazine: Tranylcypromine

TCA (TRICYCLIC AND RELATED ANTIDEPRESSANT)

1. Nonselective (NA: 5-HT) RI
   - Amitriptyline
   - Doxepin
   - Dothiepin
   - Imipramine
   - Clomipramine
   - Trimipramine

     Never ADD ICT (hypotension)

2. PreDominantly NA (NA >5-HT) reuptake inhibitors
   - Proptriptyline
   - Desipramine
   - Nortriptyline
   - Amoxapine

3. **Selective 5-HT reuptake inhibitors (SSRI)**
   - Fluoxetine
   - Fluvoxamine
   - Paroxetine
   - Sertraline
   - Citalopram

     Firstline For Prophylaxis + Severe Case

4. **Atypical**
   - Mianserin
   - Bupropion
   - Congener of trazodone (nefazodone)
   - Amineptine
   - Trazodone
   - Mianserin
   - Tianeptine
   - Venlafaxine

     Monica + Bill Clinton AT MTV

5. **Newer compound**
   - Maprotiline (DA R inhibitor)

Toxic value for most commonly monitored drugs (Magic of 2)

- Digitalis (0.5–1.5)   = Toxicity (2)
- Dilantin/phenytoin (10–20)   = Toxicity (20)

- Lithium (0.6–1.2) = Toxicity (2)
- Jogger/stimulant drugs (Theophylline) (10–20) = Toxicity (20)

Dilwale Dulhenia Le Jayenge = DDLJ

DRUGS OF ABUSE
Hallucinogens
- PCP
- LSD
- $^9\Delta$THC
- Dronabinol

Cannabinoids
- **Bhang** (dried leaves) acts slowly
- **Ganja** (dried female influorescence) is smoked and acts instantaneously
- **Charas/Hashish** (dried resinous extract from flowering tops and leaves) is the **most potent** and smoked with tobacco
- **Dronabinol:** (a $^9\Delta$THC) is **antiemetic** used in cancer

CNS Stimulants
1. **Convulsants**
   - Strychnine
   - Picrotoxin
   - Bicuculline
   - PTZ (pentylene tetrazol)
2. **Psychostimulants**
   - Cocaine
   - Amphetamine
   - Methylphenidate, Methylxanthine
   - Pemoline   CAMP
3. **Analeptics**
   - Doxapram
   - Nikethamide
   - Ethyl, and
   - Propyl butamide

ANALGESICS
1. Opioid/narcotic/morphine like
2. Non-opioid/non-narcotic/antipyretic/anti-inflammatory analgesics

Opioid analgesics
Phenanthrene derivatives
- **Morphine** = 10% opium
- **Codeine** = 1% opium

Benzo-iso-quinoline derivative
- **Papaverine**
- **Noscapine**

Classification (based on origin)
1. **Natural opium alkaloid**
   - Morphine
   - Codeine
2. **Semisynthetic opiates**
   - Pholcodeine
   - Oxycodone
   - Hydromorphone
   - Oxymorphone
   - Hydrocodone
   - Oxycodone
   - Heroin (diacetyl-morphine)
3. **Synthetic**
   - Pethidine (meperidine)
   - Methadone
   - Tramadol
   - Fentanyl
   - Ethoheptazone
   - Dextropropoxyphene
   - Alfentanil
   - Remifentanil
   - Sufentanil
   - Dipipanone
   - Levorphanol
   - Dextromoramide

Classification (based on function)
1. **Strong stimulant**
   - Morphine
   - Heroin
   - Fentanyl
   - Methadone
   - Meperidine
   - Sufentanil
2. **Moderate agonists**
   - Codeine
   - Propoxyphene

3. **Mixed agonist-antagonists** (activate some R and block others)
   - Nalorphine
   - Nalbuphine*
   - Pentazocine
   - Levallorphan*
   - Butorphanol
   - Buprenorphine

   (*Not used as analgesic)

4. **Pure antagonist**
   - Nalmefene (nonhepatotoxic, longer-acting, high oral bioavailability)

5. Antagonist
   - Naloxone (**competitive** inhibitor of opioid)
   - Naltrexone (**17 times** more potent than naloxone)

Antiparkinsonian drugs

1. Drugs affecting **dopaminergic** system
   a. **Dopaminergic agonists**
      - Bromocriptine
      - Lisurgide
      - Pergolide
      - Piribedil
      - Ropinirole
      - Pramipexole
   b. **Peripheral carboxylase inhibitors**
      - Carbidopa
      - Benserazide
   c. **DA precursor**
      - Levodopa (L-dopa)
   d. **Facilitate dopaminergic transmission**
      - Amantadine
      - Selegiline (deprenyl)
   e. **COMT inhibitors**
      - Tolcapone, and
      - Entacapone

2. Drugs affecting brain **cholinergic** system
   a. **Antihistaminics**
      - Orphenadrine
      - Promethazine
   b. **Central anticholinergics**
      - Biperiden
      - Benztropine
      - Benzhexol (trihexyphenidyl)
      - Cycrimine
      - Ethopropazine
      - Procyclidine

Direct D aergic agonists
1. **Aporphines** (related to apomorphine)
   - Piribedil
2. **Ergolines** (synthetic ergot derivates)
   - Bromocriptine
   - Pergolide
   - Lisurgide

DRUGS FOR RA

1. **DMDs**
   - d-penicillamine
   - Sulfasalazine
   - Chloroquine/hydroxychloroquine
   - Gold
   - Immunosuppressant (Mtx, cyclosporin, azathioprine, chlorambucil, cyclophosphamide)
   - Infliximab and leflunomide (newer drugs)

2. **NSAID**

   Compounds of gold
   1. **Aurothiomalate sodium** (gold sodium thiomalate) has **50% gold** and is **water soluble. Starting dose:** 10 mg IM/week up to 50 mg IM/week (max. total dose 1 gm). **Maintenance dose:** 50 mg IM/month.
   2. **Auranorfin (orally)** is orally active, has **29% gold**. Plasma gold level and efficacy is lower than gold sodium thiomalate and is less toxic.
   3. **Aurothioglucose** (IM).

DRUGS FOR GOUT

A. **Acute gout**
   - NSAID
   - Corticosteroid
   - Colchicine

B. **Chronic gout/hyperuricemia**
   - Synthesis inhibitor (allopurinol)
   - Uricosurics (probenecid and sulfinpyrazone)
   Aspirin is **contraindicated** in gout because it reduces renal clearance of uric acid and enhances hyperuricemia.

NSAIDs

A. **Selective COX-2 inhibitors**
   1. Celecoxib
   2. Rofecoxib
   3. Valdecoxib
B. **Analgesic and anti-inflammatory (selective for COX-1)**
   1. **Salicylates**
      - **B**enorylate
      - **A**spirin
      - **D**iflunisal, and
      - **S**alicylamide   **BADS**
   2. **Propionic acid derivatives**
      - **K**etoprofen
      - **N**aproxen
      - **I**buprofen
      - **F**lurbiprofen
      - **FE**noprofen   **KNIFE**
   3. **Oxicam derivatives**
      - **P**iroxicam
      - **M**eloxicam
      - **T**enoxicam   **PMT**
   4. **Pyrazolone derivatives**
      - Phenylbutazone
      - Oxyphenbutazone (active metabolite)
   5. **Indole derivatives**
      - Indomethacin, sulindac
   6. **Sulfonanilide derivative**
      - Nimesulide
   7. **Alkanones**
      - Nabumetone
   8. **Pyrrolo-pyrrole derivative**
      - Ketorolac
   9. **Anthranilic acid derivative**
      - Mephenamic acid
   10. **Arylacetic acid derivatives**
      - Diclofenac
      - Tolmetin

C. **Analgesic but poor anti-inflammatory (selective for COX-1)**
   1. **Para-aminophenol derivative**
      - Paracetamol (acetaminophen)
   2. **Pyrazolone derivatives**
      - Propiphenazone, and
      - Metamizol (dipyrone)
   3. **Benzoxazocine derivative**
      - Nefopam

STEROID HORMONES

1. Estrogen
2. Antiestrogen
3. Progesterone
4. Antiprogestin
5. Androgen
6. Antiandrogen
7. Corticosteroid
8. Inhibitors of adrenocorticoid biosynthesis:
   - Spironolactone
   - KTZ
   - Mifepristone
   - Metyrapone
   - Aminoglutethimide

PREPARATION OF GnRH

- Gonadorelin (induces FSH and LH release)
- Leuprolide (Lessens FSH and LH release)

Superactive GnRH

- Buserelin
- Goserelin
- Histrelin
- Nafarelin
- Leuprolide

Androgens

Synthetic androgen (orally active)
- Methyltestosterone
- Fluoxymesterone

Anabolic steroids

- **S**tanozolol
- **E**thyl **E**strenol

- Methandienone
- Oxandrolone
- Oxymetholone
- Nandrolone   **SEE MOON**

Impeded androgens/antiandrogens
- Danazol
- Leuprolide
- Cyproterone acetate
- Flutamide
- Finasteride   **DLC Film**

Estrogens
Natural estrogens
- Estradiol

Synthetic estrogens
1. **Steroidal**
   - Ethinyl estradiol
   - Mestranol
   - Tibolone
2. **Non-steroidal**
   - *Oral*—diethylstilbestrol (stilbestrol)
   - *Topical*—dienesterol, hexesterol

ANTIESTROGENS
- Clomiphene citrate
- Tamoxifen citrate
- Aromatase inhibitors (anastrozole, letrozole)
- Chlormadinone acetate
- Raloxifene
- Ormeloxifene
- Chlormadinone acetate has antiestrogenic and progestational action

Antiestrogen/SERM (selective estrogen receptor modulator) has estrogenic and antiestrogenic effect. First SERM is tamoxifen.

SYNTHETIC PROGESTIN
A. **19-Nortestosterone derivatives (18 C)**
   - Northindrone (northisterone)
   - Norethynodrel
   - Ethynodiol diacetate
   - Lynestrenol (ethinyl estrenol)
   - Allylestrenol
   - Norgestrel (gonane)
   - Newer compounds (desogestrel and norgestimate are prodrugs; gestodene)

B. **Progesterone derivatives (21 C)**
   - Megesterol acetate
   - Medroxyprogesterone acetate
   - Chlormadinone acetate
   - Hydroxyprogesterone caproate
   - Dydrogesterone
   - Newer compounds (norgestrel acetate)

C. **Antiprogestin**
   - Mifepristone

FEMALE CONTRACEPTIVES
Two types
- Oral
- Injectable

Oral contraceptives (OC)
1. **Phased regimen:** It is to reduce total steroid dose →E + P. Estrogen (E) **constant** + progestin (P) increases **gradually.**
2. **Minipill (luteal supplements):** Only low dose progestin (P) has **96–98%** efficacy. It reduces implantation of fertilized ovum.
3. **Postcoital (morning after) pills (E/E/+/P):** High dose estrogen for a few days → discontinued →bleeding →/dislodge implanted blastocyst.
       Estrogen (stilbestrol 25 mg/ethinyl estradiol 2.5 mg BD for 5 days) or ethinylestradiol 0.1 mg + levonorgestrel 1 mg BD starting within 3 days of intercourse. Efficacy is 90–95% and it is used in rape, etc.
4. **Combined pill:** Most efficaceous **(98–99.9%)** and most popular. Estrogen (ethinylestradiol/mestranol) + **progestin** (19-nortestosterone—has potent antiovulatory action).

OC PREPARATIONS

	Progestin	+ Estrogen
Post-coital pill	1. Levonorgestrel 2. XXXXXXXXX	+ Elhinylestradiol Diethylstilbestrol
Minipill	1. Norethindrone 2. Norgestrel	XXXXXXXXXX XXXXXXXXXX
Phased pill	1. Norethindrone 2. Levonorgestrel	+ Ethinylestradiol + Elthinylestradiol
Combined pill	1. Ethynodiol diacetate 2. Lynestrenol 3. Noregestrel 4. Levonorgestrel 5. Desogestrel	+ Mestranol + " + " + " + "

Oral contraceptive pills (OCPs)
1. **4 types**
   a. Only progestin pill (minipill)
   b. Combined pill
   c. Phasic pill and post-coital pill
   d. Sequential pill
2. **Mechanism of action**
   - Ovulation inhibition
   - Cervical mucus thickening
   - Prevention of implantation
   - Suppression of contraction

MALE CONTRACEPTIVES

1. Androgen and antiandrogen.
2. Estrogen and progestin suppress Gn (feminization occurs).
3. Superactive GnRH analogues (inhibit Gn release and testosterone secretion).
4. Cytotoxic drugs (cadmium, indoles, nitrofurans) suppress spermatogenesis but toxic and also cause irreversible action.
5. **Gossypol** is a non-steroidal compound obtained from cotton seed (China) and has no hormonal/antihormonal activity.

UTERINE STIMULANT (ABORTIFACIENTS/ECBOLICS/OXYTOCICS)

Drugs acting on uterus effect endometrium (estrogen and progestin—most important) and myometrium.

TocoLytics (reduce uterine motility)
Tone Lytics
1. Progesterone
2. Adrenergic agonists
3. Alcohol ($CH_3 CH_2 OH$)
4. CCB
5. $MgSO_4$
6. PG synthesis inhibitors, ritodrine

Progesterone And Abortion Cure Madam's Pain

UTERINE RELAXANTS/STIMULANTS

1. **Hormones:** Oxytocin (pitocin and syntocinon are synthetic oxytocin)
2. **PGs:** PGE_2, $PGF_2\alpha$, Misoprostol, 15-methyl $PGF_2\alpha$
3. **Ergot alkaloids:** Methylergometrine, ergometrine (ergonovine)
4. **Others:** Quinine, ethacridine

DRUGS FOR THYROID GLANDS

Thyroid inhibitors/antithyroid drugs (They lower the functional capacity of hyperactive glands)

1. **Goitrogens**
   a. **Ionic inhibitors/iodide trapping inhibitors**
      - Thiocyanates (—SCN)

- Perchlorates (—ClO_4)
- Nitrates (—NO_3^-)

b. **Synthesis inhibitors/thioamide/ antithyroid drugs by convention**
  - Propylthiouracil (PTU)
  - Carbimazole
  - Methimazole (active metabolite of carbimazole)

2. **TH release inhibitors**
   - NaI
   - KI
   - I_2
   - Organic iodide

3. **Thyroid tissue destroyer**
   - Radioactive iodide (^{123}I, ^{125}I, ^{131}I)

Other drugs
1. Li → inhibits TH release
2. Amiodarone → inhibits peripheral conversion from T_4 to T_3.
3. Sulfonamide and para-aminosalicylic acid inhibit T_4 iodination and coupling reaction.
4. CBZ, rifampin, phenytoin and phenobarbitone induce metabolic degradation of TH.

DRUGS FOR CALCIUM METABOLISM

1. **Bisphosphonates** (analogues of pyrophosphate)
   - Pamidronate sodium
   - Etidronate sodium
   - Alendronate   **PEA**
   - Gasidronate
   - Ibandronate
   - Risedronate   **GIRLS ~ GIRTZ**
   - Tiludronate
   - Zolendronate

2. **Hormones**
   - Parathormone (PTH)
   - Calcitonin
   - Calcitriol (active form of vitamin D)

CORTICOSTEROIDS

A. **Glucocorticoids** (**most** potent anti-inflammatory drugs)
   1. **Short-acting** (dose: 20 mg; biological t½—<12 hrs)
      - Cortisone
      - Hydrocortisone (cortisol)
   2. **Intermediate acting** (biological t½—<12–24 hrs; dose: 4 mg)
      - Prednisone
      - Prednisolone
      - Methylprednisolone
      - Triamcinolone
   3. **Long-acting** (biological t½— >24 hrs; dose: 1–2 mg)
      - Paramethasone
      - Dexamethasone
      - Betamethasone (highest glucocorticoid activity)

B. **Mineralocorticoids** (↓H⁺ ↓K⁺ ↑Na⁺)
   - Aldosterone (not used clinically)
   - Fludrocortisone (dose: 0.2 mg)
   - Desoxycorticosterone acetate (DOCA; dose: 2.5 mg)

GLUCOCORTICOID ANTAGONISTS

1. **Mitotaneb**
2. **Amphenone-B** inhibits 11-, 17-, and 21-hydroxylase
3. **Metyrapone** inhibits 11-hydroxylase. It is the common drug in assessing adrenal function.
4. **Aminoglutethimide.**
5. **Mifepristone/Ru-486** is glucocorticoid receptor antagonist, and mifepristone is antiprogestin.
6. **Ketoconazole** inhibits 11β- and 17-hydroxylase (steroidogenic enzyme).

ORAL HYPOGLYCAEMIC DRUGS

Sulfonylurea
1. First generation   **TACT**
   - **T**olazomide
   - **A**cetohexamide
   - **C**hlorpropamide
   - **T**olbutamide

2. **Second generation**
   - Glipizide
   - Gliclazide
   - Glibenclamide (glyburide)
   - Glimepiride

Biguanides
- Phenformin
- Metformin

Thiazolidinediones
- Troglitazone
- Pioglitazone
- Rosiglitazone   TPR
- Thiaglitazone (banned)

Meglitinide analogues
- Repaglinide
- Nateglinide

α-glucosidase inhibitor
- Acarbose
- Miglitol (similar to acarbose)

Others
- Guargum

DIGITALIS

Important digitalis	Source
(Cardiac glycosides)	
Digitoxin	Digitalis purpurea (leaf)
Digoxin	D. lanata (leaf)
Gitoxin	D. lanata, and D. purpurea (leaf)
Quabain	Strophanthus gratus (seed)
(Strophanthin-G)	
Strophanthin-K	Strophanthus kombe (seed)
Lanatoside-C	Semisynthetic

Drugs for CHF treatment
1. **6Ds**
   - **D**igitalis
   - **D**iuretic
   - **V**aso**d**ilator
   - **D**A
   - **D**obutamine

- PDE inhibitor (bipyridine, dipyridamole, methylxanthine)
2. **Bipyridines (PDE III inhibitor)**
   - Amrinone
   - Milrinone

ANTIARRHYTHMIC DRUGS

1. Class I   : Na⁺ channel blocker
2. Class II   : β blocker
3. Class III   : K⁺ channel blocker
4. Class IV A   : Ca²⁺ channel blocker (CCB)
   Class IV B   : K⁺ channel opener
                   —ATP
                   —Adenosine
5. Others   : Digoxin
                   Atropine
                   Isoprenaline
                   Mg²⁺ and K⁺

ANTIANGINAL DRUGS
- β blocker
- CCB
- Nitrates
- K⁺ channel opener
- Others: Dipyridamole, lidoflazine, oxyphedrine

Antihypertensive drugs   **ABCD**
1. **A**CE inhibitors
2. **A**ngiotensin (AT1) antagonist (losartan)
3. α **b**locker
4. β **b**locker
5. α + β **b**locker (labetalol)
6. **C**CB
7. **C**entral sympatholytics: Clonidine, methyldopa
8. **D**iuretics
9. **V**aso**d**ilator
10. **G**anglionic blockers: Pentolinium, trimethaphan
11. 5-HT antagonist (ketanserin)
12. **A**drenergic neurone blockers: Reserpine, guanethidine

Classification of Drugs (COD)

A. **Class I: Na⁺ channel blockers (membrane stabilising agents)**
   1. **Class IA:** Quinidine
      Procainamide
      Disopyramide
      Moricizine
      Queen Pe Dil Mera
   2. **Class IB:** Lidocaine
      Lo Phir Mein Tera
      Phenytoin
      Mexiletine
      Tocainide
   3. **Class IC:** Propafenone
      Flecainide
      Encainide
      Moricizine
      Indecainide
B. **Class III: K⁺ channel blockers** (Agents widening AP/prolonging repolarisation and ERP)
   - Amiodarone
   - Bretylium
   - Sotalol
C. **CCB**
   1. Phenyl alkylamine
      - Verapamil (hydrophilic)
   2. Benzothiazepine
      - Diltiazem (hydrophilic)
   3. Dihydropyridine (DHP)—lipophilic
      - Felodipine
      - Amlodipine   FAIL
      - Isradipine   NNNN
      - Lacidipine
      - Nicardipine
      - Nemodipine
      - Nitrendipine
      - Nifedipine
D. **K⁺ channel openers**
   - Nicorandil
   - Adenosine
   - Diazoxide   NAD
   - Cromakalim   CAMP
   - ATP
   - Minoxidil
   - Pinacidil
E. **ACE inhibitors**
   - Captopril
   - Enalapril
   - Ramipril
   - Perindopril
   - Benazepril
   - Lisinopril
F. **Nitrates**
   1. **Short-acting**
      - Glyceryl trinitrate (GTN, nitroglycerine)
      - Isosorbide dinitrate (sublingually)
   2. **Long-acting**
      - Isosorbide mononitrate
      - Isosorbide dinitrate
      - Erythrityl tetranitrate
      - Penta erythritol tetranitrate

Class channel effects	
IA	Na⁺ channel inhibition + dissociation time constant from channel (10 sec) + ↑ AP
I B	Na⁺ channel inhibition + dissociation time constant from channel (0.5 sec) + ↓ AP
IC	Na⁺ channel inhibition + dissociation time constant (20 sec) + slow conduction in His–Purkinje tissue
II	Suppress phase 4 depolarisation
III	Repolarise K⁺ current + ↑ ERP by increasing AP
IV A	Ca²⁺ channel inhibition
IV B	K⁺ channel open (hyperpolarisation)

DIURETICS
(net loss of Na⁺ and water in urine)

1. **High efficacy diuretics (inhibitors of Na⁺-K⁺-2Cl⁻ cotransport)**
   a. **Sulphamoyl derivatives**
      - Furosemide
      - Bumetanide
      - Piretanide
   b. **Phenoxyacetic acid derivative**
      - Ethacrynic acid
   c. **Organomercurials**
      - Mersalyl
2. **Medium efficacy diuretics (inhibitors of Na⁺-Cl⁻ symport)**

a. **Benzothiadiazines (thiazides)**
  - Chlorothiazide
  - Hydrochlorothiazide
  - Polythiazide
  - Cyclopenthiazide
  - Benzthiazide
  - Hydroflumethiazide
  - Bendroflumethiazide
  - Clopamide
b. **Thiazide like (related heterocyclics)**
  - Chlorthalidone
  - Metolazone
  - Xipamide
  - Indapamide

3. **Weak/adjuvant diuretics**
   a. **Carbonic anhydrase inhibitors**
     - Acetazolamide
     - Ethoxzolamide
     - *Topical ($\downarrow$ IOP)*: Brinzolamide, dorzolamide
   b. **Potassium sparing diuretics**
     i. **Aldosterone antagonist**
       - Spironolactone
     ii. **Directly acting (inhibitors of renal epithelial Na$^+$ channel)**
       - Triamterene
       - Amiloride   **K$^+$ STAys**
   c. **Xanthines**
     - Theophylline (renal adenosine A1 blocker)
   d. **Osmotic diuretics**
     - Mannitol
     - Isosorbide
     - Glycerol
   e. **Acidifying or alkalinizing salts**
     - Ammonium chloride
     - Potassium citrate
     - Potassium acetate
   f. **Action on renin-AT system**
     - NSAIDs, and
     - ACE inhibitor
   g. **Uricosuric diuretics**
     - Tienilic acid
     - Indacrinone

Diuretic efficacy: Loop > thiazide > K$^+$ sparing diuretics

ANTIDIURETICS
(reduce urine volume specially in DI)
- ADH/vasopressin, desmopressin, lypressin, terlipressin
- Thiazide—amiloride
- Others—clofibrate, carbamazepine, chlorpropamide

ACE INHIBITORS (ACE I)
Teprotide (first ACE inhibitor) was synthesized from **BPF** (bradykinin potentiating factor) of **pituitary viper venom**
- **Bena**zepril
- **Capto**pril
- **Perindo**pril   Marketed in India
- **Enala**pril   **B**lood **C**ell **PER L**akh
- **Rami**pril
- **Lisino**pril
- **Quin**april
- **Cilaz**april   Not Marketed in India
- **Zofen**opril   **Quin-Cilaz-**
- **Fosino**pril   **Zofen-Fosin**

ANGIOTENSIN II ANTAGONISTS
- **I**rbesartan
- **T**elmisartan
- **C**andesartan
- **Z**olasartan
- **L**osartan
- **O**lmesartan
- **V**alsartan
- **E**prosartan

ITCZ LOVE ~ IT'S LOVE

ANTIHISTAMINICS
A. **H$_1$ blockers (competitive blockers)**
  a. **First generation**
    1. **Highly sedative**
       - Diphenhydramine*
       - Dimenhydrinate*
       - Hydroxyzine*
       - Promethazine
       - Doxylamine

2. **Moderately sedative**
   - Meclizine*
   - Buclizine
   - Trimeprazine
   - Pheniramine
   - Antazoline
   - Cyproheptadine
   (4* drugs are for treatment of motion sickness)
3. **Mild sedative**
   - Chlorpheniramine
   - Cyclizine
   - Clemastine
   - Dimethindene
   - Methdilazine
   - Mepyramine (pyrilamine)
   - Mebhydroline
   - Triprolidine
   b. **Second generation**
   1. **Antivertigo drug**
      - Cinnarizine
   2. **Non-sedating antiallergics**
      - Tarfenadine   Least sedative
      - Astemizole   Least sedative
      - Cetirizine
      - Azelastine
      - Loratadine
      - Desloratadine
      - Mizolastine
      - Ebastine

B. **H_2 blockers**
(First H_2 blocker **Burimamide** was developed by **Black** in 1972)
   - Cimetidine
   - Ranitidine
   - Famotidine
   - Roxatidine
   - Nizatidine
   - Loxatidine

C. **H_2 agonist**
   - Betazole (enhances gastric secretion)

D. **H_3 blocker:** Thioperamide (no clinical use)

ANTIVERTIGO DRUGS

A. **Vasodilator**
   - Nicotinic acid

B. **Diuretics**
   - Loops
   - Thiazide, and
   - Acetazolamide

C. **Anxiolytic** and **antidepressant** (modify sensation of vertigo)
   - Diazepam
   - Amitriptyline

D. **Corticosteroid** (reduces intralabyrinthine edema due to viral infection)

E. **Labyrinthine suppressants** (suppress end organ receptors/inhibit central cholinergic pathway in vestibular nuclei):
   1. **Anticholinergics**
      - Atropine
      - Hyoscine
   2. **Antihistaminic with anticholinergic actions**
      - Cinnarizine
      - Cyclizine
      - Promethazine
      - Dimenhydrinate
      - Diphenhydramine
   3. **Antiemetic phenothiazines**
      - Thiethyle perazine
   4. **Prochlorperazine** (perenterally, **the most effective** drug for controlling vertigo and vomiting)

DRUGS EFFECTING 5-HT SYSTEM

1. **5-HT precursor:** Tryptophan enhances 5-HT.
2. **Synthesis inhibitor:** PCPA (P-chlorophenylalanine) inhibits tryptophan hydroxylase (**rate limiting step**) and reduces 5-HT level.
3. **Uptake inhibitor:** TCA inhibits 5-HT and NA uptake.
4. **Storage inhibitor:** Reserpine inhibits 5-HT and NA uptake into storage granule → depletion of **all monoamines.** Fenfluramine releases 5-HT.
5. **Degradation inhibitor:** MAO inhibitors prevent degradation of 5-HT.
6. **Neuronal degeneration:** 5, 6-dihydroxytryptamine destroys 5-HT neurones.

7. **5-HT R agonists**
   A. **LSD** (potent hallucinogen, non-selective 5-HT agonist) stimulates $5\text{-}HT_{1A}$ on raphe cell body, and $5\text{-}HT_{2A}$, $5\text{-}HT_{2C}$ and $5\text{-}HT_{5-7}$ in brain.
   B. **Azapirones** (non-sedative anti-anxiety) is partial agonist of $5\text{-}HT_{1A}R$.
   C. **Sumatriptan**
   D. **Cisapride** and **renzapride** are prokinetic drugs, enhance GIT motility and are $5\text{-}HT_4$ agonist.
   E. **Trazodone** →active metabolite—mCPP (m-chlorophenyl piperazine).
   mCPP is $5\text{-}HT_{1B}$, $5\text{-}HT_{2A}/5\text{-}HT_{2C}$ agonist in brain.

5-HT BLOCKERS

A. **Nonselective/partial agonist**
   1. **Ergot derivaties:** LSD, L-bromo LSD, ergotamine, methysergide
   2. **α blocker:** Phenoxybenzamine
   3. **Antihistaminic:** Cyproheptadine, cinnarizine
   4. **CPZ**
   5. **Morphine**
B. **Clinically used drugs**
                               PCM ROCK
   - Pizotifin (pizotyline)
   - Cyproheptadine
   - Methysergide
   - Risperidone
   - GranisetrOn
   - Clozapine
   Ketanserin and ritanserin

PG ANALOGUES

- PGE_1 (misoprostol, rioprostil and alprostadil)
- PGE_2 (dinoprostone and enprostil)
- $PGF_2\alpha$ (dinoprost)
- PGI_2 (epoprostenol)
- 15-methyl $PGF_2\alpha$ (carboprost)

COAGULANTS

1. **Fresh whole blood/plasma**
2. **Vit. K**
   a. K_1: Phytonadione or phylloquinone (obtained from plant, fat soluble)
   b. K_2: Menaquinone (obtained from bacteria)
   c. K_3 (synthetic, fat and water soluble)
      Fat soluble
      — Menadione, acetomenaphthone
      Water soluble
      — Menadione sodium bisulfite
      — Menadione sodium diphosphate
3. **Others**　　　　　　　　　**FRAME**
   - Fibrinogen
   - Rutin
   - Antihaemophilic factor
   - Adrenochrome
   - MonosemicarbazonE

SCLEROSING AGENTS

Cause irritation, inflammation, coagulation and fibrosis on injection into piles/varicose vein mass

1. **Phenol (5%)** in almond/peanut oil
2. **Ethanolamine oleate** (5% in 25% glycerine and 2% benzyl alcohol)
3. **Sodium tetradecyl sulfate** (5% in 2% benzyl alcohol)
4. **Quinine** (12.5%) + **urethane** (6.25%)

LOCAL HAEMOSTATICS (STYPTICS)

*Substances used to stop bleeding locally particularly from oozing surface that **must never be injected.***

A. **Thrombin:** Dry powder/solution applied on bleeding surface. Used in **skin grafting, neurosurgery** and **haemophilia.**
B. **Fibrin:** Used as **sheet/foam** on bleeding surface.
C. **Gelatin foam:** Sponging gelatin of various shapes used in **wound packing.**
D. **Astringent:** Used for bleeding gums/piles.

E. Vasoconstrictors
F. **Russel viper venom:** Acts as **thromboplastin,** applied locally, used to stop external bleeding in haemophilia.

ANTICOAGULANTS

Used *in vitro*
1. **Heparin**—1.5 U/ml
2. **Ca^{2+} complexing agents**
   Sodium Edetate—2 mg/ml
   →for Investigation
   Sodium Citrate—5 mg/ml
   →for Transfusion
   Sodium Oxalate—10 mg/ml
   →for Investigation
       "C, T = Consonants"
       "E, I, O = Vowels"

Used *in vivo*   DR. END HAD A WEB
1. **Heparin**
2. **LMW heparin**
   - Danaproid   (MW 2000–9000)
   - Reviparin
   - Enoxaprin   (MW 2000–9000)
   - Nadoparin   DR. END
   - Dalteparin
3. **Heparinoids**
   - Heparan sulfate   HAD
   - Ancrod
   - Dextran sulfate, lepirudin
4. **Oral anticoagulants**
   A. **Indandione** derivatives:
      - Phenindione
   B. **Coumarin** derivatives:
      - Acenocoumarol (nicoumalone)
      - Warfarin sodium
      - Ethyl biscoumacetate   **A WEB**
      - Bishydroxycoumarin (dicoumarol)
   C. **Hirulog** and **hirudin** (newer agents being tested)
5. **Heparin antagonist:** Protamine sulfate
6. **Warfarin antagonist:** Phytonadione (vitamin K)
   Specific antidote of oral anticoagulants: Vitamin K$_1$

FIBRINOLYTICS

1. **Activators**
   i. **Extrinsic** (available in India)
      - Urokinase   USA
      - Streptokinase
      - Alteplase (rt-PA)
   ii. **Intrinsic**
      - t-PA
      - Factor XIIa
      - Kallikrein
2. **Inhibitors**
   i. **Extrinsic**
      - Tranexaemic acid
      - EACA
      - Aprotinin   TEA
   ii. **Intrinsic**
      - α_2 antiplasmin
      - α_2 macroglobulin
3. **Plasmin blocker**
   - Aminocaproic acid (antidote for fibrinolytics)

NEWER FIBRINOLYTICS

1. **Anistreplase**
2. **Saruplase:** Recombinant human single chain urokinase type plasminogen activator, fibrin selective, non-pyrogenic, non-antigenic.
3. **Reteplase:** Non-glycosylated mutant of alteplase, 5 times more potent.

ANTIPLATELET DRUGS

A. **Antithrombolytic/antiplatelet agents**
   - Ticlopidine and clopidogrel
   - Dipyridamole and dazoxiben
   - Sulfinpyrazone
   - Daxtran-40
   - Clofibrate
   - NSAID (aspirin)
   - Monoclonal antibodies
   - Peptides (recombinant and synthesized)

- Analogues of leech anticoagulant peptide hirudin
- **Newer drugs:** Tirofiban, Eptifibatide, Abciximab   **TEA**

B. **Thrombin inhibitor:** Lepirudin

HYPOLIPIDEMIC DRUGS

1. **HMG-CoA reductase inhibitors (statin)**
   - Fluvastatin
   - Lovastatin   **FLAPS**
   - Atorvastatin
   - Pravastatin
   - Simvastatin
2. **VLDL production** and **lipolysis inhibitors**
   - Nicotinic acid (niacin/vit B_3)
3. **Antioxidant**
   - Probucol
4. **Fibric acid (isobutyric acid) derivatives**
   - Bezafibrate
   - Clofibrate   **BCG Failure**
   - Gemfibrozil
   - Fenofibrate
5. **Resins**
   - Colestipol
   - Cholestyramine
6. **Others**
   - Neomycin
   - Gugulipid

PLASMA EXPANDERS

- Dextran
- Human albumin
- PVP (polyvinyl pyrrolidone)
- HES (hetastarch/hydroxyethyl starch)
- Polygeline (degraded gelatin polymer)

DRUGS FOR GIT

A. **Drugs for reduction of gastric acid secretion**
   1. **PG analogues**   **REM**
      - Rioprostil
      - Enprostil
      - Misoprostol
   2. **Proton Pump inhibitors**
      - Panto**prazole**
      - Rabe**prazole**
      - Ome**prazole**
      - Lanso**prazole**
      - Esome**prazole**   **ROLE**
   3. **H_2 antihistaminics/H_2 blockers/H_2 antagonists (reversible blockers)**
      - **RANI**tidine
          RANI RUKJA NAJA
      - **ROXA**tidine
      - **NIZA**tidine
      - Cime**tidine**
      - Famo**tidine**
      - Loxa**tidine**
      (Except loxatidine and nizatidine, all are available in India).
   4. **Anticholinergic**   **TOP**
      - Trimipramine, doxepin
      - Oxyphenonium
      - Pirenzepine, propantheline

B. **Ulcer protective**
   - Sucralfate
   - CBS (colloidal bismuth subcitrate)

C. **Ulcer healing drugs**
   - Cabenoxolone sodium
   - Deglycyrrhizinised liquorice

D. **Antacid (neutralization of gastric acid)**
   a. **Systemic**
      - $NaHCO_3$
      - Sodium citrate
   b. **Nonsystemic**
      - $Mg(OH)_2$
      - $Mg\,CO_3$
      - $Al(OH)_3$ gel
      - $CaCO_3$
      - Mg trisilicate
      - Magaldrate

Anti-*H. pylori* drugs
- Clarithromycin
- Amoxycillin

- Tetracycline
- Tinidazole
- Metronidazole

EMETICS

A. **Acting on CTZ:** Apomorphine
B. **Acting on CTZ** and **reflexly:** Ipecacuanha
C. **In emergency such as poisoning:** Powdered mustard suspension

ANTIEMETICS

1. **Anticholinergics:** Hyoscine, dicyclomine
2. H_1 **blocker:** Promethazine
3. **Neuroleptic:** CPZ, prochlorperazine, haloperidol, thiethylperazine.
4. **Prokinetics**
   - Metoclopramide
   - Domperidone
   - Cisapride, mosapride

   MD Cardiology
5. **5-HT$_3$ blockers**
   - Granisetron
   - Ondansetron   GOT
   - Trapisetron
6. **Adjuvant antiemetics**
   - BZD   BDC
   - Dexamethasone
   - Cannabinoids

CARMINATIVE

*Promotes **expulsion of gases** from GIT leading to warmth and comfort in epigastrium.*
- **NaHCO$_3$: 1 gm** (range 0.6–1.5 gm)
- Tincture ginger: **1 ml**
- Tincture cardamom CO: **1 ml**
- Oil of dil: **0.1 ml** →0.1 = oil
- Oil of peppermint: **0.1 ml** →0.1 = oil

BITTERS

Promote gastric secretion causing increase appetite.
A. **Simple bitters**
   1. Chirata
   2. Ethylalcohol
   3. Picrorrhiza
   4. Tincture gentian
B. **Aromatic bitter:** Orange peel (as tincture aurantil 2–4 ml)

Digestant
Promotes food digestion, and is used in pancreatic insufficiency.
1. HCl (used in **achlorhydria**) 10 ml of 10% HCl in 200 ml H$_2$O
2. Pepsin used in **gastric achylia**
3. Papain of **row papaya**
4. Pancreatin
5. **Diastase** and **takadiastase** (amylolytic enzyme of *Aspergillus oryzae*)

GALLSTONE DISSOLVING DRUGS

- **Ursodiol,** and
- **Chenodiol**

LAXATIVES

(Purgatives/cathartics/aperients)
Drugs in: = Low dose act as Laxative
= High dose act as purgative
1. **Stool softener**
   - DOSS (docusates)
2. **Lubricant**
   - Liquid paraffin
3. **Osmotic purgative**
   - MgSO$_4$
   - Mg(OH)$_2$
   - Na$_2$SO$_4$
   - Na$_3$PO$_4$
   - Sodium potassium tartrate
   - Lactulose
4. **Bulk forming**
   - Dietary fibre (bran)
   - Ispaghula
   - Methylcellulose
   - Psyllium/plantago
5. **Stimulant (contact) purgatives**
   - Castor oil
   - **Diphenyl methane:** Bisacodyl, phenolphthalein
   - **Anthraquinones/emodins**
     Senna, caseara

COMPOSITION OF IVF (DHAKA FLUID)

NaCl	— 5 gm	= 85 mM
KCl	— 1 gm	= 13 mM in 1 L of H_2O/ 5% glucose solution
$NaHCO_3$	— 4 gm	= 48 mM
This gives	— Na^+	= 133 mM "+ →13"
	— K^+	= 13 mM "– →8"
	— Cl^-	= 98 mM
	— HCO_3^-	= 48 mM

ALTERNATIVELY (IVF)

Ringer lactase recommended by WHO-1991 gives

Na^+	= 130 mM
K^+	= 4 mM
Cl^-	= 109 mM
Lactate	= 28 mM

ORT (oral rehydration therapy)

Mild	= 5–7.5% fluid loss of body weight
Moderate	= 7.5–10% fluid loss of body weight
Severe	= >10% fluid loss of body weight

Excess glucose facilitates Na^+ absorption.

Principles of ORS (oral rehydration salt/solution)
1. Should be **isotonic**
2. **Molar ratio of glucose/Na^+ should be higher**
3. **K^+ and HCO_3^- provided,** make up the losses

Universal formula of WHO (ORS)

NaCl	= 3.5 gm
Citrate	= 2.9 gm
KCl	= 1.5 gm in 1 L of water
Glucose	= 20 gm
This gives	Na^+ = 90 mM
	K^+ = 20 mM
	Cl^- = 80 mM
	Citrate = 30 mM
	Glucose = 110 mM

ORS recommended by WHO causes **periorbital edema** due to **excess Na^+ absorption.**

Electrolyte composition of diarrhoea

Diarrhoeas	Na^+	Cl^-	K^+	HCO_3^-
Cholera (adult)	140	104	13	44
Cholera (infant, children)	88	86	30	32
ETEC	53	24	37	18
Rotavirus	37	22	38	06

Non-specific anti-diarrhoeal agents
A. **Absorbants**
   Ispaghula
   Psyllium, and
   Methylcellulose
B. **Antisecretory**
   Bismuth subsalicylate
   Atropine
   Mesalazine
   Sulfasalazine   BAMS = O
   Octreotide
C. **Antimotility**
   Diphenoxylate-atropine
   Loperamide
   Codeine   DLC

DRUGS FOR RESPIRATORY SYSTEM

1. **Mucokinetic (expectorant)**
   A. **Directly acting:** Na/K citrate/acetate, KI, Guaiacol, guaiphenesin (glyceryl guaiacolate), balsam of tolu, vasaka, terpin hydrate.
   B. **Reflexly acting:** KI, NH_4Cl ($(NH_4)_2CO_3$), ipecac (ipecacuanha).
   C. **Mucolytics:** Acetyl cysteine, Ambroxol, Bromhexine, and Carbocysteine
      ABC
2. **Antitussives (cough centre suppressants)**
   A. **Opioid:** Codeine, pholcodeine, morphine and ethylmorphine.
   B. **Nonopioid**
      Pipazethate

Oxeladin **POND**
Noscapine
Dextromethorphan, carbetapentane, chlophedianol
C. **Antihistaminics:** Chlorpheniramine, diphenhydramine, promethazine.
3. **Pharyngeal demulcents:** Lozenges, linctuses, liquorice, glycerine.
4. **Antibiotics**

DRUGS FOR ASTHMA
1. **Bronchodilators**
   A. **Anticholinergic**
   B. **Sympathomimetics**
                     TEA IS FOR BOSS
   - Terbutaline
   - Ephedrine
   - Adrenaline
   - **IS**oprenaline
   - **FOR**moterol
   - **B**ambuterol
   - Orciprenaline
   - Salmeterol
   - Salbutamol

   C. **Methylxanthines**
   - Theophylline
   - Aminophylline
   - Theophylline ethanolate
   - Choline theophylline, and
   - Hydroxyethyl theophylline
2. **Corticosteroids**
   A. **Systemic**
   - Prednisolone

   B. **Inhalational**
   - Beclomethasone dipropionate
   - Budesonide
   - Flunisolide
   - Fluticasone propionate
   - Triamcinolone acetomide
3. **Mast cell stabilisers**
   - Ketotifen
   - Nedocromil
   - Sodium cromoglycate
4. **Anti-LT** (anti-**LUK**otrienes**)**
   - Zileuton (inhibits LOX **hence** no LT formation)
- Zafir**LUK**ast (inhibits LT R)
- Monte**LUK**ast, and
- Cina**LUK**ast

Methylxanthines are **methylated xanthine alkaloids,** consumed as **beverages.**
- Theophylline
- Theobromine
- Caffeine

CLASSIFICATION OF ANTIBIOTICS
I. **Based on mechanism of action**
   1. **Cell wall synthesis inhibitors**
      - Ristocetin   **RBC, PVC**
      - Bactericin
      - Cephalosporin
      - Penicillin
      - Vancomycin
      - Cyclosporin
   2. **Causing cell membrane leakage**
      A. **Polypeptide**
      - Polymixin   **PCB**
      - Cilastin
      - Bacitracin

      B. **Polyenes**
      - AMB
      - Nystatin
      - Hamycin

      C. **Imidazole—not antibiotic**
   3. **Protein synthesis inhibitors**
      30s inhibitors
      - **A**minoglycoside (bactericidal)
      - **T**etracycline (bacterostatic)

      50s inhibitors
      - **C**hloramphenicol (bacterostatic)
      - **E**rythromycin (bacterostatic)
      - **L**incomycin (bacterostatic)
      - C**L**indamycin (bacterostatic)
      Streptogramins
          Buy **AT 30** and **CELLS** at **50**
   4. **Interfering with DNA synthesis**
      - Zidovudine   **ZIA**
      - Idoxuridine
      - Acyclovir

5. **Interfering with DNA function**   MNR
   - Metronidazole
   - Norfloxacin
   - Rifampicin (inhibits DNA dependent RNA polymerase)
6. **DNA gyrase inhibitors**
   - Quinolone
7. **Misreading of m-RNA code**
   - Aminoglycoside
8. **Interfering intermediate metabolism**   PEST
   - PAS and pyrimethamine
   - Ethambutol
   - Sulfone and sulfonamide
   - Trimethoprim

II. **Based on chemical structures**
   1. **Aminoglycoside:** Streptomycin
   2. **Macrolide:** Erythromycin
   3. **Nitrobenzene:** Chloramphenicol
   4. **Nitrofurans:** Ntirofurantoin
   5. **Nitroimidazole:** Metronidazole
   6. **Imidazole derivative:** KTZ
   7. **Nicotinic acid derivative:** INH, pyrazinamide
   8. **Diaminopyrimidine** Trimethoprim
   9. **Quinolones:** Ciprofloxacin, gatifloxacin
   10. **Polypeptides:** Polymyxin B
   11. **Tetracycline:** Oxytetracycline
   12. **β-lactam antibiotics:** Penicillin
   13. **Sulfonamide:** Dapsone, sulfadiazine
   14. **Polyene:** AMB
   15. Others: Rifampicin, clindamycin, vancomycin, ethambutol and griseofulvin

III. **Based on type of action**
   Bacteriostatic   CL TENSE
   - Chloramphenicol
   - Lincomycin
   - Tetracycline
   - Erythromycin (at low dose)
   - Nitrofurans (at low dose)
   - Sulfonamide (at low dose)
   - Ethambutol
   Bactericidal
   - Penicillin
   - Cephalosporin
   - Ciprofloxacin
   - Vancomycin
   - Polypeptide
   - Aminoglycoside
   - Cotrimoxazole
   - INH
   - Rifampicin
   - Nalidixic acid

IV. **Spectrum of activity**
   Broad spectrum
   - Tetracycline
   - Chloramphenicol
   Narrow spectrum
   - Penicillin G
   - Erythromycin
   - Streptomycin
   - Cephalosporin

V. **Based on source**
   A. **Fungi**
      - Penicillin
      - Cephalosporin
      - Griseofulvin
   B. **Actinomycetes**   PACT
      - Polyene
      - Aminogylcoside and macrolide
      - Chloramphenicol
      - Tetracycline
   C. **Bacterial**   BACTerial
      - Bacitracin and polymyxin B
      - Aztreonam
      - Colistin
      - Tyrothricin
   D. **DNA recombinant technology**
      - Chloramphenicol

All **AMAs** are contraindicated in pregnancy due to risk to foetus. However, some **safe AMAs are**
   - Miconazole
      MEN = Not Contraindicated in Pregnancy
   - Erythromycin
   - Nitrofurantoin
   - Nystatin
   - Cephalosporin
   - Penicillin

Drugs used without dose reduction in renal failure are
   - Doxycycline   DR
   - Rifampicin

β-LACTAM ANTIBIOTICS
1. **Penicillin**
2. **Cephalosporin**
   Both of the above antibiotics are destroyed by **β-lactamase (penicillinase** and **cephalosporinase)** of bacteria.
3. **Carbapenems** and **monobactam** (parenterally).

PENICILLIN
A. **Acid resistant**   A CAP For DON
   - **A**moxycillin
   - **C**loxacillin
   - **A**mpicillin
   - **P**enicillin V (phenoxy methyl Pn)
   - **F**lucloxacillin
   - **D**icloxacillin
   - **O**xacillin
   - **N**afcillin

B. **Penicillinase resistant**
                          MCQ For DON
   - **M**ethicillin
   - **C**loxacillin
   - **Q**uinacillin
   - **F**lucloxacillin
   - **D**icloxacillin
   - **O**xacillin
   - **N**afcillin

C. **β-lactamase inhibitors**
   - Sulbactam, and
   - Clavulanic acid

D. **Antistaphylococcal Pn/β-lactamase resistant**
   - Cloxacillin
   - Flucloxacillin, and
   - Methicillin

E. **Extended spectrum Pn**
   1. **Aminopenicillin**
      - Ampicillin
      - Amoxycillin, and
      - Bacampicillin
   2. **Antipseudomonal**
      a. **Carboxy Pn**
         - Carbenicillin
         - Carbenicillin indanyl
         - Carbenicillin phenyl (carfecillin)
         - Ticarcillin
      b. **Ureido Pn**
         - Mezlocillin
         - Azlocillin, and
         - Piperacillin
   3. **For Gram –ve except *P. aeruginosa***
      - Mecillinam (amdinocillin)

CEPHALOSPORIN
First generation
A. **Parenteral**
   - Cephalothin
   - Cephaloridine
   - Cefazolin
   - Cephapirin

B. **Oral**
   - Cephalexin
   - Cephradine
   - Cefadroxil

Second generation
A. **Parenteral**
   - **Cefo**tetan
   - **Cefo**xitin   2 Cefu
   - **Cefo**nicid
   - **Cefo**ranide and cefmetazole
   - **Cefu**roxime   4 Cefo
   - **Cefa**mandole   2 Cefa

B. **Oral**
   - **Cefu**roxime axetil
   - **Cefa**clor
   - **Cefp**rozil
   - **Lora**carbef

Third generation
A. **Parenteral**   Cefta
   - **Cefta**zimide   2 Cefti
   - **Cefti**zoxime   Ceftri
   - **Ceftri**axone   2 Cefo
   - **Cefo**taxime
   - **Cefo**perazone   Cefi

B. **Oral**
- **Cefi**xime
- Cefpodoxime, and
- **Cefti**buten

Fourth generation
Parenteral
- Cefepime
- Cefpirome

TETRACYCLINES

Group I (Low potency)
- **C**hlortetracycline   COT
- **O**xytetracycline
- **T**etracycline

Group II (intermediate potency)
- Demeclocycline
- Methacycline
- Lymecycline

Group III (highest potency)
- Doxycycline
- Minocycline

AMINOGLYCOSIDES
- **F**ramycetin and kanamycin
- **A**mikacin, neomycin and netilmicin
- **T**obramycin, gentamicin
- **S**isomycin   FATS

MACROLIDES
Clarithromycin
Azithromycin   CARES
Roxithromycin
Erythromycin, and
Spiramycin

OTHER ANTIBIOTICS
- Clindamycin and lincomycin
- Glycopeptide: Vancomycin and teicoplanin
- Spectinomycin
- Fusidic acid and linezolid
- Polypeptide antibiotics
- Urinary antiseptic and streptogramins

POLYPEPTIDE ANTIBIOTICS
- Polymyxin B and polymyxin E
- Colistin
- Bacitracin
- Tyrothricin

URINARY ANTISEPTICS
- Nalidixic acid
- Nitrofurantoin
- Phenazopyridine, and
- Methenamine

STREPTOGRAMINS
- Dalfopristin/quinapristin

DRUGS FOR CHRONIC AND RECURRENT UTI
- Sulfonamide
- Cotrimoxazole
- Trimethoprim
- Nitrofurantoin
- Ampicillin
- Cephalexin
- Norfloxacin
- FQ (for complicated cases)
- Gentamicin (effective against **most** urinary pathogen)

SULPHONAMIDES
A. **Highly absorbed**
  1. **Short-acting (4–8 hrs)**
     - Sulfadiazine
     - Sulfamethizole
     - Sulfasomidine
     - Sulfasoxazole
  2. **Intermediate-acting (8–16 hrs)**
     - Sulfaphenazole
     - Sulfamethoxazole
  3. Long-acting (1–7 days)
     - Sulfamethoxypyridazine
     - Sulfadimethoxine
  4. Ultralong-acting (>1 week)
     - Sulfadoxine
     - Sulfamethopyrazine
B. **Poorly absorbed**
   - Succinylsulfathiazole
   - Phthalylsulfathiazole
C. **Special purpose**
   - Mafenide (burn)

- Sulfasalazine (RA and ulcerative colitis)
- Silver sulfadiazine (topical)
- Sulfacetamide sodium (eye drop)

COMBINATIONS
- **Cotrimoxazole** = Trimethoprim + Sulfamethoxazole
- **Cotrimazine** = Trimethoprim + sulfadiazine

FLUOROQUINOLONES
A. **First generation**
   - Pefloxacin
   - Ofloxacin   PONC~PONS
   - Norfloxacin
   - Ciprofloxacin
B. **Second generation**
   - Fleroxacin
   - Amifloxacin   FALSe
   - Lomefloxacin
   - Sparfloxacin
C. **Newer FQs**
   - Moxifloxacin   Must Get TLC
   - Gatifloxacin
   - Trovafloxacin
   - Levofloxacin
   - Clinafloxacin
   - Grepafloxacin

ANTITUBERCULAR DRUGS
A. **First line drugs** (high efficacy with low toxicity):
   - **Pyrazinamide (Z)**
   - **Ethambutol* (E)**   PERIS
   - **Rifampin (R)**
   - **Isoniazid (INH)**/iso nicotinic acid hydrazide (H)
   - **Streptomycin* (S)**
   (*supplementary drugs)
B. **Second line drugs** (low efficacy and high toxicity):
   - Amikacin, azithromycin
                               A ROCK
   - Rifabutin
   - Ofloxacin
   - Ciprofloxacin, capreomycin, clarithromycin
   - Kanamycin

Tuberculostatic
- PAS (para-aminobenzoic acid)   **PET**
- Ethambutol
- Thiacetazone
- Ethionamide
- Cycloserine

ANTILEPROSY DRUGS
A. **Sulfones**
   - Dapsone (DDS)
   - Acedapsone (DA-DDS)
   - Solapsone
   - Sulfadoxine
B. **Phenazine derivatives**
   - Clofazimine
C. **Antitubercular drugs**
   - Rifampin
   - Ethionamide
   - Thiacetazone
D. **Antibiotics**
   - Clarithromycin
   - Ofloxacin
   - Minocycline

ANTIMALARIAL DRUGS
                     ABC Quinine /TDS

1. **4-Aminoquinoline** : Chloroquine, amodiaquine
2. **8-Aminoquinoline** : Primaquine, bulaquine
3. **Acridine** : Mepacrine (quinacrine, atabrine)
4. **Biguanides** : Chloroguanide (proguanil)
5. **Cinchona alkaloid** : Quinine
6. **Quinoline–methanol** : Mefloquine
7. **Diaminopyrimidines** : Pyrimethamine Trimethoprim
8. **Sulfonamide and sulfone** : DDS, : sulfadoxine, sulfamethopyrazine

9. Tetracycline : Tetracycline, doxycycline
10. Newer drugs : Halofantrine, pyronardine, artemisinin (artesunate, artemether and arteether), atovaquone

ANTIAMOEBIC DRUGS
1. **Tissue amoebicides**
   A. **For both intestinal and extraintestinal amoebiasis**
      a. Nitroimidazole
         - Tinidazole
         - Nimorazole   **TN MOSS**
         - Metronidazole
         - Ornidazole
         - Secnidazole
         - Satranidazole
      b. **Alkaloid**
         - Emetine
         - Dehydroemetine
   B. **For extraintestinal amoebiasis**
      - Chloroquine
2. **Luminal amoebiasis**
   A. **Amide**
      - Diloxanide furoate
   B. **8-hydroxyquinolines**
      - Quiniodochlor (clioquinol, iodochlorohydroxyquin)
      - Diiodohydroxyquin (iodoquinol)
   C. **Antibiotic**
      - Tetracycline

ANTIFUNGAL DRUGS
1. **Antimetabolite**
   - Flucytosine
2. **Allylamine**
   - Terbinafine
3. **Antibiotics**
   A. **Polyenes**
      - AMB
      - Nystatin
      - Hamycin
      - Natamycin (pimaricin)
   B. **Heterocyclic benzofuran**
      - Griseofulvin
4. **Azoles**
   A. **Imidazoles**
      a. **Topical**
         - KTZ
         - Clotrimazole   **K COMES**
         - Oxiconazole
         - Meconazole
         - Econazole
         - Sulconazole
      b. **Systemic**
         - KTZ (ketoconazole)
   B. **Triazole**
      a. **Topical**
         - Terconazole
      b. **Systemic**
         - Fluconazole, and
         - Itraconazole
5. **Other topical agents**
   - Naftifine
   - Tolnaftate
   - Undecylenic acid
   - Ciclopirox olamine
                  Never ToUCH B
   - Haloprogrin
   - Benzoic acid

ANTIHELMINTIC DRUGS
- Levamisole
- Albendazole
- Mebendazole, Metronidazole
- Praziquantel, Piperazine, Pyrantel pamoate
- Niridazole
- Thiabendazole, Tetramizole
- DEC (diethyl carbamazine citrate)
   LAMP–NTD = Neural Tube Defect

ANTIVIRAL DRUGS
1. **Antiherpes virus (CMV, HSV)**
   - Ganciclovir
   - Idoxuridine

- Foscarnet
- Trifluridine
- Famciclovir
    GIFT For Antiherpes Virus
- Acyclovir
- Vidarabine

New antiherpes agents
- Penciclovir
- Valacyclovir   PVC
- Cidofovir

2. **Anti-retrovirus**
   A. **Protease inhibitors**
   - Ritonavir (PI)
   - Nelfinavir (PI)
   - Atazanavir (PI)
   - Fosamprenavir (PI)
   - Amprenavir (PI)
   - Indinavir (PI)
   - Lopinavir (PI)
   - Saquinavir (PI)
       RNA FAILS (to be formed)
   B. **Reverse transcriptase inhibitor/ RTI**
   a. **Nucleoside RTI**
   - Lamivudine (NRTI)
   - Emtricitabine (NRTI)
   - Tenofovir (nucleotide RTI)
   - Abacavir (NRTI)
   - Didanosine (NRTI)
   - Zalcitabine (NRTI)
   - Zidovudine (NRTI)
   - Stavudine (NRTI)
   b. **Non-nucleoside RTI**
   - Efavirenz (NNRTI)
   - Nevirapine (NNRTI)
   - Delavirdine (NNRTI)
       LET ADZZS (AIDS) END
   c. **FUsion Inhibitor**
   - EnFUvirtide

3. **Anti-influenza virus**
   - Amantadine
   - Rimantadine

4. **Non-selective**
   - Interferon α
   - Ribavirin, and
   - Lamivudine

ANTICANCER DRUGS

I. **Cytotoxic drugs**
   1. **Antimetabolites**
      A. Folate antagonist
      - Methotrexate (Mtx, amethopterin)
      B. Purine antagonists
      - 6-mercaptopurine (6-MP)
      - 6-thioguanine (6-TG)
      - Azathioprine
      C. Pyrimidine antagonists
      - 5-fluorouracil (5-FU)
      - Ftorafur
      - Cytarabine (cytosine arabinoside)
      D. Newer drugs
      - Capecitabine
      - Gemcitabine
   2. **Antibiotics**   BMD
      - Bleomycin
      - Mitomycin C
      - Mithramycin (plicamycin)
      - Mitoxantrone
      - Doxorubicin (epirubicin and idarubicin also)
      - Dactinomycin
      - Daunorubicin
   3. **Microtubule inhibitors**
      A. Vinca alkaloids
      - Vincristine (oncovin)
      - Vinblastine
      - Venorelbine
      B. Taxanes
      - Paclitaxel
      - Docetaxel
   4. **Alkylating agents**
      A. Nitrogen mustards: MIC
      - Melphalan
      - Mechlorethamine (mustine HCl)
      - Ifosfamide
      - Cyclophosphamide
      - Chlorambucil
      B. Nitrosoureas
      - Semustine (methyl-CCNU)
      - Carmustine (BCNU)
      - Lomustine (CCNU)
      - Streptozocin

- C. Triazine
  - Dacarabazine (DTIC)
- D. Ethyl enimine
  - Thio-TEPA
- E. Alkyl sulfonate
  - Busulfan
5. **Others**
   - Etoposide
   - Procarbazine
   - Cisplatin
   - Carboplatin
   - Hydroxyurea
   - Interferons
   - Amifostine
   - Anastrozole
   - Letrozole
   - L-asparaginase
6. **Camptothecin analogues**
   - Topotecan
   - Irinotecan
II. **Drugs altering hormonal milieu**
   - Estrogen
   - Antiestrogen (tamoxifen)
   - Progestin
   - Androgen (testosterone and fluoxymesterone)
   - Glucocorticoid (prednisolone)

IMMUNOSUPPRESSANTS
1. **Specific T cell inhibitors (calcineurin inhibitors)**
   - Cyclosporin (**most costly**)
   - Tacrolimus, and
   - Sirolimus
2. **Cytotoxic drugs**
   - Mtx
   - Cyclophosphamide
   - Chlorambucil
   - Azathioprine
   - MMF (mycophenolate mofetil)
3. **Antibodies**
   - ATG (antithymocyte globulin)
   - Muromonab CD3
   - Rho (D) Ig

HAEMATINICS
- Iron
- Vitamin B_{12}
- Folic acid

IMMUNITY AND IMMUNISATION
Active immunisation
- Live attenuated vaccines
- Killed or inactivated vaccines
- Toxoid (microbial toxin preparation)
- Recombinant vaccines

Preparation available for active immunisation

Live vaccines
- Oral polio (sabin) vaccine (OPV)
- Measles
- Mumps
- Rubella
- BCG (tuberculosis)
- Typhoid
- Yellow fever

Killed vaccines (killed organism)
- Hepatitis A
- Pertussis
- Influenza
- Cholera
- Rabies
- Meningococci (group A and C)
- Pneumococcal

Toxoids
- Diphtheria
- Tetanus

Recombinant vaccines
- Hepatitis B

Passive immunising agents
- Purified serum (sera)
- Immunoglobulins (purified gamma globulin)

Contraindications of immunisation
- Hypersensitivity to components
- Mild respiratory infections
- Diarrhoea
- Immunosuppressed patient
- Patient with corticosteroid therapy
- Encephalopathy
- Convulsion

IMMUNISING AGENTS
A. **Vaccines**
   a. **Live attenuated vaccines**

1. **Bacteria:** BCG, typhoids oral, plague
2. **Viral:** Oral polio, yellow fever, measles, rubella, mumps, influenza
3. **Rickettsial:** Epi. typhus

b. **Killed/inactivated vaccines**
1. **Bacteria:** Typhoid, cholera, pertussis, plague, CS meningitis
2. **Viral:** Rabies, Salk (polio), influenza, hepatitis B, Japanese encephalitis, KFD

c. **Toxoid**
1. **Bacteria:** Diphtheria, tetanus

B. **Immunoglobulins**
a. **Human Ig**
1. **Human normal Ig:** Hepatitis A, measles, rabies, tetanus, mumps
2. **Human specific Ig:** Hepatitis B, varicella, diphtheria

b. **Non-human (antisera)**
1. **Bacterial:** Diphtheria, tetanus, gas gangrene, botulism
2. **Viral:** Rabies

NATIONAL IMMUNISATION SCHEDULE

A. **FOR INFANTS**
At birth (for institutional deliveries)
- BCG and OPV—O dose

At 6 weeks
- BCG (if not given at birth)
- DPT-1 and OPV-1

At 10 weeks
- DPT-2 and OPV-2

At 14 weeks
- DPT-3 and OPV-3

At 9 months
- Measles

B. **AT 6–24 MONTHS**
- DPT and OPV

C. **AT 5–6 YEARS**
- DT—second dose of DT should be given at an interval of 1 month if there is no clear history or documented evidence of previous immunisation with DPT.

D. **AT 10 AND AT 16 YEARS**
- Tetanus toxoid: The second dose of TT vaccine should be given at an interval of one month if there is no clear history or documented evidence of previous immunisation with DPT, DT or TT vaccines

E. **FOR PREGNANT WOMEN**
Early in pregnancy
- TT-1 or booster

One month after TT-1
- TT-2

Note
i. Interval between 2 doses should not be less than one month.
ii. Minor cough, cold and mild fever are not a contraindication to vaccination.
iii. In some states, hepatitis B vaccine is given as routine immunisation.

ANTISERA

"Antisera" antibodies derived from immune animal serum. Antisera are purified and concentrated preparations of serum of animal (horses) actively immunised against a specific antigen. Risk of hypersensitivity reactions is more. Half-life in humans is not so longer (5–7 days or less).

Examples of antisera

ATS : Tetanus antitoxin
ADS : Diphtheria antitoxin
ARS : Antirabies serum
AGS : Anti-gas gangrene serum

Immunoglobulins: Immunoglobulins are purified gammaglobulin derived from human serum. Avoid risk of hypersensitivity reactions. Have a much longer half-life in humans (about 23 days for IgG antibodies). Smaller doses are required to provide therapeutic concentrations.

Examples
Tetanus : Human tetanus immunoglobulins

Hepatitis B	: Human hepatitis B immunoglobulins
Rabies	: Human rabies immunoglobulins
Rh incompatibility	: Anti-D gamma globulins

ANTISNAKE VENOM SERUM POLYVALENT

It is available as **purified, enzyme refined and concentrated equine globulins** in lyophilized vial with 10/ml distilled water. After reconstitution, each ml neutralises:

A. **0.6 mg** of standard Cobra/Russel's viper venom   "**6CR = SIXER**"
B. **0.45 mg** of standard krait/saw scaled viper venom.

Dose: 20 ml IV (1 ml/min injection) repeated 1–6 hourly interval till symptoms disappear (**max 300 ml**). **Sensitivity test** for anaphylactic shock to serum is done, if possible, otherwise **adrenaline** is injected concurrently.

IMMUNOPHARMACOLOGY
Immunomodulating agents
- BCG (bacille Calmette-Guérin)
- Levamisole
- Isoprinosine
- Thymosin

Uses of immunomodulating agents
- Immunodeficiency disorders
- Chronic infectious diseases
- Cancer

Immunosuppressant drugs
- Cyclosporin
- Glucocorticoids
- **Cytotoxics:** Azathioprine, cyclophosphamide
- **Ig:** Antilymphocyte Ig, normal human Ig

TOPICAL STEROIDS
A. **Very potent (highest efficacy)**
   - Clobetasol (0.05%)
   - Diflorasone (0.05%)
   - Betamethasone (0.05%)

B. **Potent (high efficacy)**
   - Beclomethasone (0.025%)
   - Desoximetasone (0.025%)
   - Triamcinolone (0.5%)
   - Fluocinolone (0.2%)

C. **Moderately potent (intermediate efficacy)**
   - Hydrocortisone (0.2%)
   - Triamcinolone (0.1%)
   - Desoximetasone (0.05%)
   - Fluticasone (0.05%)
   - Fluocinolone (0.025%)

D. **Mildly potent (low efficacy)**
   - Hydrocortisone (0.1–2.5%)
   - Methylprednisolone (0.25%)
   - Dexamethasone (0.1%)
   - Triamcinolone (0.025%)

Keratolytic agents
- Salicyclic acid
- Silver nitrate sticks
- Trichloroacetic acid
- Resorcinol
- Propylene glycol
- Urea

Topical acne preparations
- Retinoic acid (retina cream)
- Benzyl peroxide
- Tetracycline (cream)

Antiseborrheic agents
- Selenium sulphide shampoo
- Chloroxine shampoo
- Ketoconazole shampoo
- Coal tar shampoo
- Zinc pyrithione shampoo

Sunscreens
Absorb ultraviolet light
- p-aminobenzoic acid (PABA)
- Benzophenones
- Dibenzoylmethanes

Sunshades
Reflect light
- Titanium dioxide
- Zinc oxide and
- Calamine

PHOTOSENSITIVE DRUGS
Systemic drugs
- Sulfonamides
- Tetracycline
- Griseofulvin and amiodarone
- Nalidixic acid and piroxicam

Topical drugs
- Deodorant substance
- Halogenated salicylanilides
- Para-aminobenzoic acid
- Coaltar derivatives

MELANISING AGENTS
- Psoralen (obtained from Amm; majus fruit)
- Methoxsalen
- Trioxsalen
- Synthetic psoralen
- PUVA (photochemotherapy)

EMOLIENTS
- Vegetative oil
- Petroleum product

DEMELANISING AGENTS
- Hydroquinone (weak)
- Monobenzone (strong)
- Azelaic acid

DEMULCENTS
- Glycerine
- Propylene
- Glycol, and
- Methyl cellulose

ASTRINGENTS
- Minerals (alum, ZnO, etc.)
- Tannic acid, and
- Alcohol (for bedsore at 50–90% concentration but irritating to raw surface)

NAMES OF VITAMINS

Recommended name	Alternative name
Vitamin A	Retinol
Thiamine	Vitamin B_1
Riboflavin	Vitamin B_2
Niacin	Nicotinic acid, nicotinamide/ vitamin B_3
Vitamin B_{12}	Cyanocobalamin
Pentothenate	Vitamin B_5
Pyridoxine	Vitamin B_6
Folate	Folacin
Biotin	XXXXXXXXXXXX
Vitamin C	Ascorbic acid
Vitamin D	D_2 and D_3 / calciferol
Vitamin E	α-tocopherol
Vitamin K	Vitamin K_1

"The Rich Never Pre-Pays Cash"

Classification of vitamins
1. Fat soluble vitamin: Vitamins A, D, E, K (**cumulative toxicity**)
2. Water soluble vitamins (excreted → no **toxicity**)
   a. Vitamin **B** complex
   b. Vitamin **C**
   WBC

VITAMIN D/KIDNEY HORMONE
1. D_1 **(mixture of antirachitic substances).**
2. D_2**/calciferol (found in irradiated food-yeast, fungi, milk):** Ergocalciferol/D_2/calciferol is of **plant** origin.
3. D_3**/cholecalciferol: Animal** origin, **most important** vitamin D, synthesised in the skin by photoactivation (UV rays). **Preformed** and found in fats and liver. Vit. D is stored largely in **fat depots**. Vitamin D is a **pro-hormone.** It is a member of **steroid derivatives.** The main precursor substrate of vitamin D is **cholesterol.**

Adverse Drug Reactions (ADR)

MULTISYSTEM MANIFESTATIONS
1. **Anaphylaxis**   **ACID SLIPS**
   - ACE inhibitors and dialysis
   - Cephalosporin
   - Insulin, intravenous Ig, iodinated drug
   - Dextran, demeclocycline
   - Streptomycin
   - Lidocaine
   - Iron dextran
   - Procaine, penicillin
   - Sulfobromophthalein
2. **Angioedema**
   - ACE inhibitors
   - Penicillin
3. **Drug-induced lupus erythematosus**
   - Methyldopa
   - Cephalosporin
   - Quinidine   **MCQ – IT IS A BPH**
   - INH
   - Thiouracil
   - Iodides
   - Sulfonamides
   - Acebutolol, asparaginase
   - Bleomycin, barbiturates
   - Procainamide, phenytoin, phenolphthalein
   - Hydralazine
4. **Fever**   **IN CAPS**
   - Intravenous Ig
   - Novobiocin
   - Carbenicillin
   - AMB, aminosalicylic acid
   - Pamidronate, penicillin
   - Streptokinase
5. **Hyperpyrexia:** Antipsychotics
6. **Neuroleptic:** Antidopaminergics
7. **Serum sickness**
   - Penicillin   **PASS**
   - Aspirin
   - Streptokinase
   - Streptomycin, sulfonamide
8. **Vasculitis**   **PAST**
   - Penicillin, phenytoin (hydantoin), propylthiouracil
   - Allopurinol, aminopenicillin
   - Sulfonamide
   - Thiazides

ENDOCRINE MANIFESTATIONS
1. **Addisonian-like syndrome:** Busulfan, etomidate, KTZ
2. **Galactorrhea (may also cause amenorrhoea)**
   - TCA
   - Methyldopa, metoclopramide
   - Phenothiazine
   - Domperidone
   - Reserpine   **Treat Me Please DR**
3. **Gynaecomastia**
   - Griseofulvin
   - Yeast removing drug (KTZ)
   - HYdantoin
   - Nifedipine and other CCB
   - Alkylating agents
   - Ethionamide

- Cimetidine, clomiphene, cardiac glycoside
- OC constituent (estrogen)
- Methyldopa and marijuana
- Alcohol
- Spironolactone
- Testosterone
- Inhibitor of 5-alpha reductase (finasteride), INH
- Alkaloid of sarpgandha (reserpine)

GYNAECOMASTIA

4. **Sexual dysfunction**
   a. **Impaired ejaculation**
      - Guanethidine
      - Thioridazine
      - Bethanidine
      - Debrisoquin

      Guess True Birth Day

   b. **Decreased libido and impotence**
      - Tranquilizers   The **LIBIDOS**
      - **LI**thium
      - **B**eta blockers
      - **I**nhibitor of adrenergic outflow in brainstem (clonidine, methyldopa)
      - **D**iuretics
      - **O**ral contraceptive (OC)
      - **S**edatives

   c. **Priapism:** Trazodone
   d. **Impairment of spermatogenesis/oogenesis:** Cytotoxic drugs

5. **Thyroid dysfunction (disorders causing abnormal results on thyroid function tests)**
   - Acetazolamide

   ABCD IS A PLOT
   - Bromosulfophthalein
   - Chlorpropamide, clofibrate, colestipol, nicotinic acid
   - Dimercaprol
   - Iodides
   - Sulfonamides, salt of gold
   - Amiodarone
   - Phenytoin, phenylbutazone, phenothiazine, phenindione
   - Lithium
- Oral contraceptive
- Tolbutamide

6. **Vaginal carcinoma:** Diethylstilbestrol (if given to mother)

METABOLIC MANIFESTATIONS

1. **Hyperbilirubinemia:** Novobiocin, rifampin
2. **HypErcalcemia**   **ACTED**
   - **A**ntacids with absorbable alkali
   - **C**alcitonin
   - **T**hiazide
   - **(D) V**itamin D
3. **HypErglycemia**

   NOT FEED Glucose PACK
   - Niacin
   - Oral contraceptive
   - Thiazide
   - Furosemide
   - Ethacrynic acid
   - Encainide
   - Diazoxide
   - GH, glucocorticoids
   - Phenytoin, pentamidine
   - Asparaginase
   - Clorthalidone
   - K sparing diuretic (triamterene) reduces glucose tolerance

4. **Hypoglycemia**

   IQ = O Presents hypoglycemia
   - Insulin
   - Quinine, quinidine
   - Oral hypoglycemics
   - Pentamidine

5. **Hypokalemia**

   MOST ACID Gets Life
   - Mineralocorticoids and some glucocorticoids
   - Osmotic diuretics
   - Sympathomimetic agents
   - Tetracycline, theophylline
   - AMB, alkali induced alkalosis
   - Carbenoxolone, corticosteroids, cyanocobalamin
   - Insulin
   - Diuretics
   - Gentamicin
   - Laxatives

6. **Hyperkalemia**

   PLANTS Cause Heart Death
   - Pentamidine, potassium preparation (of salt/drugs)
   - Lithium
   - ACE inhibitors, amiloride
   - NSAID
   - Triamterene, trimethoprim
   - Spironolactone, succinylcholine
   - Cyclosporin, cytotoxics
   - Heparin
   - Digitalis overdose

7. **Hyperuricemia**

   Too Pretty FACE
   - Thiazide
   - Pyrazinamide
   - Fructose
   - Aspirin (low dose), hyperalimentation
   - Cytotoxic, cyclosporin, chlorthalidone
   - Ethacrynic acid

8. **Hyponatremia**

   a. **Dilutional**   A Cubic VOID
   - Antipsychotics
   - Carbamazepine, chlorpropamide, cyclophosphamide
   - Vincristine
   - Octreotide
   - Intravenous Ig
   - Diuretics, desmopressin

   b. **Salt-wasting**   MEDicine
   - Mannitol
   - Enemas
   - Diuretics

9. **Metabolic acidosis**   SPASM
   - Salicylates
   - Phenformin, paraldehyde (degraded)
   - Acetazolamide
   - Spironolactone
   - Metformin

10. **Porphyria exacerbation**

    BCG SPERM
    - Barbiturate
    - Chlordiazepoxide, chlorpropamide, OC
    - Glutethimide, griseofulvin
    - Sulfonamide
    - Phenytoin
    - Estrogen
    - Rifampin
    - Meprobamate

DERMATOLOGICAL MANIFESTATIONS

1. **Acne**   TO BIGS
   - Troxidone
   - Oral contraceptive
   - Bromides
   - INH, iodides
   - Glucocorticoids
   - Steroids (anabolic and androgenic)

2. **Alopecia**
   - Fluconazole
   - Dactinomycin
   - Etoposide and other cytotoxics
   - Vitamin A (retinoid)
   - Drug withdrawal (OC)
   - Albendazole
   - Specific suppressor of acute gout (colchicine)
   - Beta blocker
   - Stabilizer of mood (Li)
   - Anticoagulant oral (heparin), and Parenteral (warfarin)
   - Ethionamide
   - Suppressor of viral protein synthesis (interferon) and antithyroid drugs

   Film **DEVDAS**

   Bapu ne kaha gaun chhoddo
   Sab ne kaha ghar chhoddo
   Aapne kaha Paro ko chhoddo
   Paro ne kaha Sharab chhoddo
   Ek din aisabhi aaiga jab
   Sablog Kaheinge is duniya ko chhoddo

   Drugs causing **ALOPECIA**
   - Antithyroid
   - Lithium
   - OC withdrawal
   - Phenytoin
   - Ethionamide
   - Cytotoxics

- Interferon
- Anticoagulants and albendazole

3. **Eczema**   **TLC**
   - Topical LA, topical antihistaminic, topical antimicrobial
   - Lanolin
   - Captopril, cream and lotion preservatives

4. **Erythema multiforme/Stevens–Johnson syndrome/toxic epidermal necrolysis PSVT CLEANS** Broadened **QT** Interval
   - Phenytoin, Pn, Phenolphthalein, phenylbutazone, piroxicam
   - Salicylates, sulfonamide
   - Valproic acid
   - Thiazides, tocainide
   - Carbamazepine, cephalosporin, chlorpropamide, codeine
   - Lamotrigine
   - Ethosuximide
   - Allopurinol, Aminopenicillin
   - Nalidixic acid
   - Sulfones
   - Barbiturates
   - Quinolones
   - Tetracyclines
   - Imidazole, iodides

5. **Erythema nodosum**
   - Penicillin   **PONS**
   - Oral contraceptive
   - N (nodosum)
   - Sulfonamide

6. **Exfoliative dermatitis**
       BSP = **B**hartiya **S**amajwadi **P**arty
   - Barbiturates
   - Salt of gold
   - Penicillin, phenytoin, phenylbutazone

7. **Fixed drug eruption**
          BPSC = **B**ihar **P**ublic **S**ervice **C**ommission
   - Barbiturates
   - Phenylbutazone, phenolphthalein, penile ulcer by foscarnet
   - Sulfonamide, salicylates
   - Captopril, quinine

8. **Hyperpigmentation**   **BCG OPV**
   - Bleomycin, busulfan
   - Chloroquine and other antimalarial
   - Gold salt
   - Oral contraceptive
   - Phenothiazine
   - Vitamin A (hypervitaminosis)

9. **Hypertrichosis**   **PCM**
   - Phenytoin
   - Cyclosporin
   - Minoxidil

10. **Lichenoid eruptions**   **CAMP**
    - Chlorpropamide
    - Aminosalicylic acid, antimalarials, gold salt
    - Methyldopa
    - Phenothiazine

11. **Nail changes**
    - Tetracycline
    - Penicillamine
    - Retinoids
    TPR = **T**otal **P**eripheral **R**esistance

12. **Photodermatitis**
    Photodermatitis Generously Causes SOFT Skin's Necrosis
    - Phenothiazines
    - Griseofulvin
    - Captopril, chlordiazepoxide
    - Sulfonamide
    - Oral contraceptive
    - Furosemide
    - Tetracycline particularly dimeclocycline, thiazide
    - Sulfonylureas
    - NSAID, nalidixic acid

13. **Purpura (also see thrombocytopenia)**
    - Indapamide
    - Methyldopa
    - Phenytoin
    - Barbiturates
    - Allopurinol, ampicillin, aspirin
    - Glucocorticoids
                                IMPortant **BAG**

14. **Raynaud's disease /digital necrosis**
    - Beta blocker, bleomycin
    - Ergot Alkaloid   **BEAR**

15. **Skin necrosis:** Warfarin
16. **Urticaria**
    - Barbiturates   **BIG PACES**
    - Intravenous Ig
    - Ganciclovir
    - Penicillin
    - Aspirin
    - Captopril
    - Enalapril
    - Sulfonamide

HAEMATOLOGIC MANIFESTATIONS

1. **Agranulocytosis**
               IT'S SGOT + cAMP
    - Indomethacin
    - Ticlopidine
    - Sulfonamide and chloramphenicol
    - SMX + TMP (cotrimoxazole)
    - Gold salt
    - Oxyphenbutazone
    - Tolbutamide, TCA
    - Cytotoxics, captopril, carbimazole, cefotaxime, clozapine
    - Aprindine
    - Methimazole
    - Phenothiazine, phenylbutazone, propylthiouracil

2. **Clotting and bleeding abnormalities/ hypothrombinemia**
    - Ketorolac
    - Piperacillin
    - Mezlocillin, moxalactam
    - Cefoperazone, cefamandole
    - Sodium valproate
            Kindly Pay My Cash Sir

3. **Eosinophilia**
    - Methotrexate
    - Aminosalicylic acid
    - Nitrofurantoin
    - Sulfonamide
    - L-tryptophan
    - Imipramine
    - Chlorpropamide
    - Erythromycin estolate
    - Procarbazine
       MAN'S LICE Produces Eosinophilia

4. **Haemolytic anemia**
               A MILD Changed QRS Complex Is Produced
    - Aminosalicylic acid
    - Methotrexate
    - Insulin
    - Levodopa
    - DDS
    - Cephalosporin
    - Quinidine
    - Rifampin
    - Sulfonamide
    - CPZ
    - Isoniazid
    - Penicillin, phenacetin, procainamide

5. **Haemolytic anemia in G6PD deficiency**
    - First quinolone (nalidixic acid)
    - DDS
    - Oldest NSAID (aspirin)
    - Nitrofurantoin
    - Aminosalicylic acid
    - Phenacetin
    - Antimalarial (primaquine)
    - Procainamide
    - K (vitamin K and C)
    - Quinidine
    - Probenecid
    - Sulphonamide
    - Cotrimoxazole
    - Chloramphenicol

Film DON
Aare bhang ka rang jama ho chakachak
Phir lo pan chabai
Aare aisan jhatka lage jiya pe
Puner janam hoi jai
Khaike pan banaraswala
Qhul jai bande aqal ka tala
Phirto aisa kare kamal
Sidhi karde sabki chaal
Chaura ganga kinare wala
Chaura ganga kinare wala

6. **Leukocytosis:** Glucocorticoids, lithium
7. **Lymphadenopathy:** Primidone, phenytoin
8. **Megaloblastic anemia**
   Causes For Pollar = NOT
   - Cotrimoxazole
   - Folate antagonist
   - Phenobarbital, phenytoin, primidone
   - Nitrous oxide (chronic exposure)
   - Oral contraceptive
   - Triamterene, trimethoprim
9. **Pancytopenia (aplastic anemia)**
   MOST PACQ (PACK)
   - Mepacrine, mephenytoin
   - Oxyphenbutazone
   - Sulfonamide
   - Thiouracil, trimethadione
   - Phenylbutazone, phenytoin, potassium perchlorate
   - AZT
   - Carbamazepine, carbimazole, chloramphenicol
   - Quinacrine
10. **Pure red cell aplasia**   PICA
    - Phenytoin
    - INH
    - Chlorpropamide
    - Azathioprine
11. **Thrombocytopenia (see also pancytopenia)**
    - Methyldopa, moxalactam
    - Chlorthalidone, chlorpropamide, cotrimoxazole
    - Quinine, quinidine
    - Furosemide

    MCQ: Find Thrombocytopenia ON ACIDIC PH
    - Thiazides, ticarcillin
    - Oxyphenbutazone
    - Novobiocin
    - Acetazolamide, aspirin and gold salt
    - Carbamazepine
- INH
- Digitoxin
- Indomethacin
- Carbenicillin
- Phenylbutazone, phenytoin and other hydantoin
- Heparin

CARDIOVASCULAR MANIFESTATIONS

1. **Acute chest pain (non-ischaemic):** Bleomycin
2. **Angina exacerbation**
   SHAME ON Vasoconstriction
   - Sumatriptan
   - Hydralazine
   - Alpha and beta blocker
   - Methysergide, minoxidil
   - Excessive thyroxine
   - Oxytocin
   - Nifedipine
   - Vasopressin
3. **Cardiopathy**
   LEADS Pathy
   - Lithium
   - Emetine
   - Adriamycin
   - Daunorubicin
   - Sulfonamides, sympathomimetics
   - Phenothiazines
4. **Arrhythmias**
   Class – LKG →A, B, C, D, E—PSVT
   - Cisapride
   - Lithium
   - Ketanserin
   - Gaunethidine
   - Adriamycin
   - Beta blocker
   - Cholinesterase inhibitors
   - Digitalis, daunorubicin
   - Erythromycin, emetine
   - Papaverine, Pentamidine, probucol, phenothiazine
   - Sympathomimetics
   - Verapamil
   - Terfenadine, theophylline, TH, TCA

5. **AV Block**   **CMV**
   - Clonidine
   - Methyldopa
   - Verapamil
6. **Hypertension**   **MOST Can Not Go**
   - MAO inhibitors with sympathomimetics
   - Oral contraceptive
   - Sympathomimetics
   - TCA with sympathomimetics
   - Clonidine withdrawal, cyclosporin, corticotropin
   - NSAIDs (some)
   - Glucocorticoids
7. **Pericarditis**
   - Hydralazine   **HEMP**
   - Emetine
   - Methysergide
   - Procainamide
8. **Pericardial Effusion:** Minoxidil
                                                   PEM
9. **Thromboembolism:** Oral contraceptive
10. **Hypotension**   **ACID LMNOPQ**
    - Amiodarone (perioperative)
    - Calcium channel blockers, citrated blood
    - IL-2
    - Diuretics
    - Levodopa
    - Morphine
    - Nitroglycerin
    - hypOtension
    - Protamine, phenothiazines
    - Quinidine
11. **Fluid retention/CHF/edema**
    - Beta blocker
    - Edema
    - Steroid
    - Triterpenoid derivative (carbenoxolone)
    - Minoxidil, mannitol
    - Estrogen   **BEST MEDICine**
    - Diazoxide
    - Indomethacin
    - Calcium channel blockers

RESPIRATORY MANIFESTATIONS

1. **Airway obstruction (bronchospasm, asthma: See also anaphylaxis)**
   - Beta blockers   **BC PAST**
   - Cephalosporin
   - Penicillin
   - Aspirin, indomethacin and other NSAIDs
   - Streptomycin
   - Tartrazine (drug with yellow dye)
2. **Cough**   **GOD IS Right**
   - Guanethidine
   - Oral contraceptive
   - Decongestant abuse
   - ISoproterenol
   - Reserpine
3. **Pulmonary edema**   **IMPortant CH**
   - IL-2
   - Methadone
   - Propoxyphene
   - Contrast media
   - Heroin, hydrochlorthiazide
4. **Pulmonary HTN:** Fenfluramine
5. **Pulmonary infiltrates**
                              ABC Shows MPGN
   - Acyclovir, amiodarone, azathioprine
   - Bleomycin, busulfan, BCNU (carmustine)
   - Cyclophosphamide, chlorambucil
   - Sulfonamides
   - Melphalan, methotrexate, methysergide, mitomycin C
   - Procarbazine
   - Gold
   - Nitrofurantoin
6. **Respiratory depression**
                                      AT SHOP
   - Aminoglycoside
   - Trimethaphan
   - Sedatives
   - Hypnotics
   - Opiates
   - Polymyxins

GIT MANIFESTATIONS

1. **Cholestatic hepatitis**
                                        MOON FACE
   - Methimazole
   - Oral contraceptive

- gOld salt, phenOthiazine
- Nitrofurantoin
- Flucloxacillin
- Androgen, acetohexamide, anabolic steroid
- Chlorpropamide, clavulanic acid/amoxicillin, cyclosporin
- Erythromycin estolate

2. **CONSTIPATION or ileus**
   - CCB, CaCO$_3$
   - Opiates
   - Nicotine at large dose (other ganglionic blocker also)
   - Sedatives
   - TCA
   - Ion exchange resins
   - Phenothiazine
   - Aluminium hydroxide
   - Two (II) gp element (barium sulfate)
   - Iron (ferrous sulfate)
   - Oxyphenonium and other anticholinergics
   - INhibitor of thyroid and histamine

3. **Diarrhoea/colitis**
   - Gatifloxacin
   - Inhibitor of NA release (guanethidine), lactose excipients
   - Ticlopidine
   - Clindamycin and its congener lincomycin, cocaine, colchicine
   - Reserpine
   - Antibiotic (broad spectrum)
   - Mg in antacid
   - Purgatives
   - Sympatholytic (central)—methyldopa
   - Misoprostol
   - Digitalis

   GIT CRAMPS, Means Diarrhoea

4. **Diffuse hepatocellular damage**
   - Felbamate
   - Salicylates, sulfonamide
   - Tacrine, tetracycline, trazodone
   - KTZ
   - Halothane
   - Rifampin
   - Carbenicillin, cyclophosphamide
   - Verapamil, valproic acid
   - DDS, diclofenac
   - INH
   - Erythromycin
   - Glyburide
   - Methimazole, MAO inhibitors
   - AZT, acetaminophen, acebutolol, allopurinol, amiodarone, ASA, aprindine
   - Sodium valproate

   Film: Sholey — Tera Kya Hoga Re Calya

   Veeru–(DIEing) Gaunwalo Mera Akhri Salam
   - Labetalol, lovastatin **LMNOPQ**
   - Methotrexate, methoxyflurane, methyldopa
   - Niacin, nifedipine, nitrofurantoin
   - Oxyphenisatin
   - Phenytoin and other hydantoin, pyridium, propylthiouracil, propoxyphene
   - Quinidine

5. **Gallstone/biliary pseudolithiasis:** Ceftriaxone

6. **Intestinal ulceration:** Solid KCl preparation

7. a. **Malabsorption**
   - Aminosalicylic acid, antibiotic (broad spectrum)
   - Phenobarbital, phenytoin
   - Neomycin
   - Cytotoxic drugs, colestipol, cholestyramine
   - Primidone

   b. **Nausea/vomiting**

   A PNC Patient LEFT OPD
   - Levodopa
   - Estrogen
   - Ferrous sulfate
   - Tetracycline, theophylline
   - Opiates
   - Potassium chloride
   - Digitalis

8. **Dental discolouration:** Tetracycline
9. **Dry mouth**   **CALM**
   - Clonidine
   - Anticholinergics, antidepressant (TCA)
   - Levodopa
   - Methyldopa
10. **Gingival hyperplasia:** Calcium antagonist, cyclosporine, phenytoin
11. **Salivary gland swelling**   **BCG (IP)**
    - Bretylium, bethanidine
    - Clonidine
    - Guanethidine
    - Iodides
    - Phenylbutazone
12. **Taste disturbances**   **PLAB, GRAM**
    - Penicillamine
    - Lithium
    - Acetazolamide
    - Biguanide
    - Griseofulvin
    - Rifampin
    - ACE inhibitors
    - Metronidazole
13. **Peptic ulceration/haemorrhage**   **RANGE**
    - Reserpine (large doses)
    - Aspirin
    - NSAIDs
    - Glucocorticoids
    - Ethacrynic acid
14. **Pancreatitis**   **MOST OPV FADES**
    - Mercaptopurine
    - Opiate
    - Sulfonamide
    - Thiazide
    - Oral contraceptive
    - Pentamidine
    - Valproic acid
    - Furosemide
    - Asparaginase, azathioprine
    - Didanosine
    - Estrogen, ethacrynic acid
    - Steroid (glucocorticoids)

RENAL MANIFESTATIONS

1. **Bladder dysfunction/incontinence**   **MDAT**
   - MAO inhibitors
   - Disopyramide
   - Anticholinergics
   - TCA, terazosin and prazosin
2. **Calculi:** Acetazolamide, vitamin D
3. **Hemorrhagic cystitis:** Cyclophosphamide
4. **Concentrating defect with polyuria/nephrogenic DI**
   - Methoxyflurane, lithium   **MD**
   - Demeclocycline, vitamin D
5. **Interstitial nephritis**
   - Penicillin, phenindione
   - Allopurinol
   - Rifampin
   - Thiazides
           PARTS–Causes For Nephritis
   - Sulfonamide
   - Ciprofloxacin, cephalosporin
   - Furosemide
   - NSAIDs
6. **Nephropathies:** Analgesics
7. **Nephrotic syndrome**
   - Salt of gold   **Serum CPK**
   - Captopril
   - Penicillamine, phenindione, probenecid
   - Ketoprofen
8. **Renal tubular acidosis:** Degraded tetracycline, acetazolamide, AMB
9. **Obstructive uropathy**
   a. **Extrarenal:** Methysergide
   b. **Intrarenal**   **MAMC**
   - Metyrosine
   - Acyclovir
   - Methotrexate
   - Cytotoxic drugs
10. **Renal dysfunction**
    - Cyclosporin
    - ACE inhibitors
    - NSAIDs
    - Pentamidine
    - Triamterene
                      CAN Produce Trouble

Adverse Drug Reactions (ADR)

11. **Tubular necrosis** **IT'S CRAMP**
    - Intravenous Ig
    - Tetracycline
    - Sulfonamide
    - Cyclosporin, colistin, cephaloridine
    - Radioiodinated contrast medium
    - AMB, aminoglycoside
    - Methoxyflurane
    - Polymyxins

NEUROLOGICAL MANIFESTATIONS

1. **Aseptic meningitis:** IV Ig.
2. **CNS/vasculitis/cerebral hemorrhage:** Phenylpropanolamine
3. **Exacerbation of myasthenia**
    - Aminoglycoside   **ADP**
    - D-penicillamine
    - Polymyxins
4. **Extrapyramidal effects**
    - Contraceptive (oral)
    - Butyrophenone
    - Sympatholytic (methyldopa)
    - TCA
    - Other neuroleptic (reserpine)
    - Phenothiazines
    - Metoclopramide
    - Parkinsonian drug (levodopa)
    - Droperidol
      CBS TOP Most **P**ublishers & **D**istributors
5. **Headache**   **BE HIGH**
    - Bromide
    - Ergotamine (withdrawal)
    - Hydralazine
    - Indomethacin, IV Ig
    - Glyceryl trinitrate
    - H (headache)
6. **Pseudotumour cerebri/intracranial HTN**   **GOAT**
    - Glucocorticoid, mineralocorticoid
    - Oral contraceptive
    - Amiodarone, vitamin A (hypervitaminosis A)
    - Tetracycline
7. **Sleep disorders:** Lovastatin
8. **Stroke:** Cocaine, oral contraceptive
9. **Tremor:** Beta agonists
10. **Peripheral neuropathy**
    PVST AND ECG Change **H**aving **MI**
    - Phenytoin, perhexiline, phenelzine, polymyxin, procarbazine
    - Streptomycin
    - Vincristine
    - TCA, tolbutamide
    - Amiodarone
    - Nitrofurantoin, nalidixic acid
    - Disopyramide, demeclocycline
    - Ethambutol, Ethionamide
    - Colistin, cisplatin, clioquinol, clofibrate
    - Glutethimide
    - Chloramphenicol, chloroquine, chlorpropamide
    - Hydralazine
    - Metronidazole, mustine, methysergide
    - INH
11. **Seizures**   **TALL MAN IS VIP**
    - TCA, theophylline
    - Amphetamine
    - Lithium
    - Lidocaine
    - Meperidine
    - Analeptics
    - Nalidixic acid
    - **IS**oniazid
    - Vincristine
    - Imipenem
    - Physostigmine, penicillin, phenothiazines

OCULAR MANIFESTATIONS

1. **Cataract**   **BCG P**roduces cataract
    - Busulfan
    - Chlorambucil
    - Glucocorticoids
    - Phenothiazines
2. **Colour vision alteration**
    The **M**an **S**ee **B**eauty **D**efectively
    - Thiazide, troxidone
    - Methaqualone
    - Streptomycin, sulfonamide
    - Barbiturates
    - Digitalis

3. **Corneal edema:** Oral contraceptive
4. **Eye pain:** Nifedipine
5. **Retinopathy:** Chloroquine, phenothiazine
6. **Glaucoma**   **SIM**
   - Sympathomimetics
   - Ipratropium bromide
   - Mydriatics
7. **Corneal opacities**   **Drug MIC**
   - **D** vitamin D
   - Mepacrine
   - Indomethacin
   - Chloroquine
8. **Optic neuritis**   **CASE–PQ Interval**
   - Chloramphenicol, clioquinol
   - Aminosalicylic acid
   - Streptomycin
   - Ethambutol
   - Penicillamine, phenothiazine, phenylbutazone
   - Quinine
   - INH

EAR MANIFESTATIONS

1. **Deafness**   **ABCDEF IN MCQ**
   - Aspirin, aminoglycoside
   - Bleomycin
   - Chloroquine, cisplatin
   - Desferrioxamine
   - Erythromycin, ethacrynic acid
   - Furosemide
   - Interferon
   - Nortriptyline
   - Mustine
   - Cisplatin
   - Quinine
2. **Vestibular disorders:** Aminoglycoside, mustine, quinine

MUSCULOSKELETAL MANIFESTATIONS

1. **Bone disorders**
   a. **Osteoporosis:** Heparin, glucocorticoids
   b. **Gout (see hyperuricemia)**
   c. **Osteomalacia:** Aluminium hydroxide, anticonvulsant, glutethimide

2. **Myopathy/myalgia**   **CICAGO**
   - **CI**metidine
   - **C**arbenoxolone, chloroquine, clofibrate
   - **A**MB
   - **G**lucocorticoids
   - **O**ral contraceptive
3. **Rhabdomyolysis:** Gemfibrozil, lovastatin
4. **Tendon rupture:** Quinolones

PSYCHIATRIC MANIFESTATIONS

1. **Sleep disturbances**   **MLAs**
   - **M**AO inhibitors
   - **L**evodopa
   - **A**norexiants
   - **S**ympathomimetics
2. a. **Delirious/confusional states**
   - Cardiac glycoside (digitalis)
   - Methyldopa, drug (ranitidine)
   - Amantadine
   - Bromides, aminophylline
   - Ulcer reducing anticholinergic and antidepressants, antiparkinsonian (levodopa)
   - Phenothiazines and penicillin
   - Hydrazide (INH)
   - Cimetidine
   - Hypnotics and sedative
   - Glucocorticoids, vigabatrin

   > Chahe jo koi tumhe dilse
   > Milta hai wo bari mushkilse
   > Aisajo koi kahein hai
   > Bas wo sabse hasein hai
   > Us hath ko tum tham lo
   > Phirye meherbaan KHNH
   > Har ghari badal rahi hai roop zindagi
   > Chaun hai kahin kabhi hai dhoop zindagi
   > Harpal yahan jee bhar jiyo
   > Go hai sama KHNH

2. b. **Depression**
   - **L**evodopa
            Let **A** Beautiful Chance Go
   - **A**mphetamine withdrawal
   - **B**eta blockers

Adverse Drug Reactions (ADR)

- Centrally acting antihypertensives (clonidine, methyldopa, reserpine)
- Glucocorticoids

3. **Drowsiness**

   The Maieusiophobia (fear of pregnancy)
   Comes After Romance
   - TCA
   - Major tranquilizers, methyldopa
   - Clonidine
   - Antihistaminics, anxiolytics
   - Reserpine

4. **Hallucinatory states**
   Let Me Not Preface A Bad Time
   - Levodopa
   - Meperidine
   - Narcotics
   - Pentazocine
   - Amantadine
   - Beta blockers
   - TCA

5. **Hypomania/mania/excited reactions**
   - TCA
   - Glucocorticoids
   - Fentanyl
   - Opioid
     The Golden Fact Of A Life Is—Wines
   - Amphetamine
   - Levodopa
   - Inhibitors of MAO
   - Wines
   - Ulcer reducing agents (ranitidine)
   - Sympathomimetics

6. **Schizophrenic-like/paranoid reactions**
   - Levodopa, lysergic acid
   - Amphetamines
   - TCA   Look At Money Bags
   - MAO inhibitors
   - Bromides

7. **Hypersexuality:** Antiparkinsonian drugs

8. **Memory loss:** Triazolam

AGRANULOCYTOSIS causing drugs
- Antithyroid drugs (propylthiouracil, carbimazole, methimazole), ACE inhibitors
- Gold salts like sodium aurothiomalate
- Radioactive elements like ^{131}I
- Alkylating agents
- Nitrogen mustards like mechlorethamine
- Urethane (obsolete)
- Largactil (chlorpromazine)
- Oxyphenbutazone/phenylbutazone
- Chloramphenicol and clozapine
- Cyclophosphamide
- Yellow drug, i.e. mepacrine (obsolete)
- Thioureas, tricyclic antidepressants
- Oxazolidine/phenytoin
- Sulphonamides like cotrimoxazole
- Indomethacin
- Sulfones, sulfonylureas (Ist generation)

Drugs causing SLE
- Antiarrhythmic (procainamide, quinidine)
- Beta blocker   ABCDEFGHI
- Contraceptive pills
- D-penicillamine
- Ethosuximide
- F (Ph) enytoin
- Gestational antihypertensive (methyldopa)
- Hydralazine
- INH and interferon

TERATOGENIC drugs
- Thalidomide
- Epileptic drugs
- Retinoid
- ACE inhibitors
- Third element (lithium)
- OC
- Griseofulvin

Pharmacology Review

Biochemical mechanisms of sexual dysfunction	
Dopamine agonists	Enhance sexual functioning
Dopamine antagonists	Impair sexual functioning
SSRIs	Diminish sexual functioning
Serotonin antagonists	Improve sexual functioning
Alpha-2 receptor antagonists	Aids in arousal and orgasm by increasing norepinephrine
Nitric oxide	Leads to engorgement of erectile tissue in men, increases blood flow in men, increases blood flow to clitoris and vulva

Sexual side effects of specific psychotropic drugs	
Drug	*Sexual side effects*
Tricyclic anti-depressants	High incidence of sexual side effects (clomipramine had highest frequency of incidence)
SSRIs (citalopram, escitalopram, fluoxetine, fluvoxamine, paroxetine, sertraline)	High incidence of sexual side effects
MAOIs (isocarboxazid, phenelzine, tranylcypromine)	High incidence of sexual dysfunction
MAOIs (nefazodone, mirtazapine)	Low incidence of sexual dysfunction

Medications of offset sexual side effects of antidepressants			
Agent	*Mechanism*	*Initial dosage*	*Risks*
Bupropion	Increases dopaminergic tone	75 mg qd 1–2 h PTSA (prior to sexual activity)	Hypertension, increases seizure risk
Methylphenidate	Increases dopaminergic tone	5–10 mg qd or PTSA	Overstimulation, potential abuse
Cyproheptadine	Antagonizes 5-HT receptors	4–12 mg qd or PTSA	Sedation, dry mouth, may decrease anti-depressant effect
Yohimbine	Increases norepinephrine outflow	5.4–10.8 mg qd or PTSA	Increases anxiety, hypertension; not studied in women
Sildenafil	Increases nitric oxide	50 mg PTSA	Hypotension, other cardiovascular side effects
Bethanechol	Increases cholinergic tone	25–50 mg qd or PTSA	Diarrhoea, autonomic side effects

- Ergot
- NSAID
- Iodine
- Clindamycin and cyclophosphamide

GA causing

1. ↑ *IOT is*
   - Cyclopropane
   - SCh
   - N₂O, And
   - KEtamine

2. ↑ *ICT is*
   - SCh
   - N₂O, And
   - KEtamine with Halothane

   C SNAKE, SNAKE with Hood

3. ↓ *IOT is*
   - Halothane   **HMT**
   - Morphine
   - Thiopentone

4. ↓ *ICT is*
   - Droperidol
   - Thiopentone
   - Propofol
   - AltHesin   **DTPH**

- Penicillin
- Aspirin
- Imipramine
- Nematodes, and
- Sulfonamide

cause Loeffler's syndrome
                                  PAINS

- Penicillin
- Amiodarone
- Dextran 70, and
- Cocaine

cause hemoptysis
        PADC ~ PADS are needed in bleeding

Unit 14
Newer Drugs and Drugs of Choice

70 Newer Drugs and their Uses

Cinacalcet (calciuric)
- Secondary hyperparathyroidism in CRF

Tiotropin bromide (anticholinergic)
- Bronchospasm (COPD, chronic bronchitis, emphysema)

Duloxetine (SSRI/SNRI)
- Major depressive disorder

Acamprosate (NMDA antagonist)
- Maintenance of abstinence from alcohol

Cetuximab (EGFR/HER 1 antagonist)
- Colorectal cancer

Pegaptinib (VEGF antagonist)
- Age related macular degeneration

PreGABAlin (GABA antagonist)
- Neuralgia

Orlistat (GI lipase inhibitor)
- Antiobesity

Gefitinib and erlotinib (tyrosine kinase inhibitor)
- Non-small cell CA of lung

Pemetrexed (folate enzyme antagonist)
- Malignant pleural mesothelioma

Bevacixumab (anti-VEGF Ab)
- Metastatic colorectal CA

Eplerenone (selective aldosterone antagonist) and Eplerenone (aldosterone antagonist)
- Hypertension

Treprostinil (prostacycline analogue)
- Pulmonary arterial hypertension

Botulinum toxin type A (inhibits ACh release)
- Strabismus
- Blepharospasm
- Cervical dystonia
- Hemifacial spasm
- Glabellar lines (cosmetic use) in adults

Urofollitropin (human FSH)
- Ovulation induction

Imatinib mesylate (tyrosine kinase inhibitor)
- Inoperable/metastatic malignant GIT stromal tumors
- CML

Nitazoxanide (antiprotozoal agent)
- Cryptosporidium parvum

Nitisinone (hydroxyphenyl dioxygenase inhibitor)
- Hereditary tyrosinemia type 1

Peginterferon alfa-2a
- Chronic hepatitis C

Tegaserod (5-HT_4 antagonist)
- Irritable bowel syndrome with constipation

Voriconazole (antifungal)
- Acute invasive aspergillosis
- *Scedosporium apiospermum*
- Fusarium

Adefovir (anti-HBV)
- Active HBV infection

Fulvestrant (ER antagonist)
- Hormone receptor positive metastatic breast cancer

Aripiprazole (D_1 partial agonist)
- Schizophrenia
- Anxiety

Ecitalopram (SSRI)
- Major depressive disorder

Interferon beta-1a
- Relapsing multiple sclerosis

Atomoxetine (SNRI)
- Attention deficit hyperkinetic disorder

Sodium oxybate (neurotransmitter)
- Cataplexy with narcolepsy

Ziprasidone (D_2 and $5-HT_2A$ antagonist)
- Acute schizophrenia

Adalimumab (IgG_1 Ab)
- Structural damage in RA

Omalizumab (IgE Ab-inhibits mast cell activation and release)
- Asthma

Etanercept
- Psoriatic arthropathy
- Rheumatoid arthritis

Alefacept (fusion protein-reduces lymphocyte count)
- Chronic plaque psoriasis

Rosuvastatin (statin)
- Hypercholesterolemia

Laronidase (recombinant enzyme)
- Mucopolysaccharidosis I

Acalsidase beta (recombinant enzyme)
- Fabry's disease

Pegvisomant (GH receptor antagonist)
- Acromegaly

Alpha 1 proteinase inhibitor
- Alph 1 proteinase inhibitor deficiency

Vardenafil and tadalafil (PD_5 inhibitors)
- Erectile dysfunction

Enfuvertide (fusion inhibitor)
- Anti-HIV drug

Bortezomib (proteosome inhibitor)
- Multiple myeloma

Memantine (NMDA receptor antagonist); donapezil and galantamine (anti-AChE)
- Moderate to severe dementia in Alzheimer's disease

Letrozole (aromatase inhibitor)
- Locally advanced/metastatic breast cancer

Somatropin (recombinant GH)
- Growth failure in small for gestational age

Nesiritide (ANP analogue)
- CHF

Trovaprost (PG analogue)
- Open angle glaucoma/ocular HTN

Mesalamine (anti-inflammatory)
- Active ulcerative proctitis

Zoledronic acid (bisphosphonate)
- Hypercalcemia of malignancy

Sultroban (TXA_2 antagonist)
- Thromboembolic disorder/pulmonary HTN

Pranlukast, montelukast, zafirlukast (LT receptor antagonist)
- Asthma

Amifostine (SH donating agent)
- To reduce anticancers toxicity

Miltifosine (SH donating agent)
- Leishmaniasis (most effective agent so far)

Ibutilide/dofetilide (K⁺ channel openers)
- Atrial arrhythmia

Licofelone (LOX and COX inhibitor)
- NSAID for arthritis

Levobupivacaine (local anaesthetic)
- Obstetrical anaesthesia

Ecitalopram (SSRI)
- Depression (most specific anti-depressant)

Lumefantrine (antimalarial)
- Severe malaria/MDR

Fluticasone (inhalational corticosteroid)
- Bronchial asthma

Bambuterol (beta-2 agonist)
- Asthma (longest action)

Zaleplon/zolpidem (BZD₁ agonists)
- Hypnosis

Topiramate/lamotrigine/zonisamide (Na⁺ channel blockers)
- Antiepileptic, neuropathic pain

Felbamate (increases GABA, decreases glutamate)
- Lenox-Gestaut syndrome

Oxcarbazepine (Na⁺ channel blockers)
- Antiepileptic

Fosphenytoin (inhibits depolarization shift)
- Antiepileptic status

Tolcapone and entacapone (COMT inhibitors); ropinirole (D₂ agonist) and pramipixole (D₃ agonist); rasigiline (neuroprotective)
- Parkinson's disease

Ostelmavir and rimantidine (antiviral)
- Influenza A₂

Sertindole (antipsychotic)
- Schizophrenia

Tirofiban (GP IIa/IIIb inhibitor)
- Unstable angina/PTCA

Argotroban (thrombin inhibitor)
- Heparin induced thrombocytopenia

Oprelvekin (haematopoietic stimulant)
- Bone marrow suppression

Atomoxetine (reuptake inhibitor)
- ADHD

Dezocine (opioid)
- Pain

Dipivefrine (adrenaline prodrug)
- Glaucoma

Tazoretene (retinoic acid analogue)
- Psoriasis

Trientine (cupper chelator)
- Wilson's disease

Cilostazole (antiplatelet)
- Intermittent claudication

Colesvelam (bile acid binding resin)
- Hyperlipidemia

Eflornithine (facial growth inhibitor)
- Hirsutism

Rituximab (anti-CD20)
- Multiple myeloma

Exenatide (glucagon like peptide-1 analogue)
- Antidiabetic

Mecasermin (IGF like analogue)
- GH deficiency

Tipranivir (protease inhibitor)
- Anti-HIV

Entecavir (anti-HBV)
- Active/acute HBV infection

Ibandronate (bisphosphonate)
- Postmenopausal osteoporosis

Remelteon (melatonin receptor agonist)
- Narcolepsy

Natalizumab (monoclonal Ab)
- Multiple sclerosis

Azacytidine (antipyrimidine)
- Myelodysplastic syndrome

Rifaximin (antibiotic)
- Travellers diarrhoea

Anastrozole

It is a non-steroid aromatase inhibitor (1 mg dose reduces oestradiol by 70% within 24 hours and 80% within 14 days). In estrogen receptor positive breast cancer, it reduces relative risk by 22%.

Well absorbed orally, 40% bound to plasma protein. Hepatic metabolism, elimination half-life = 50 hrs in post-menopausal woman. Used in advanced breast cancer in postmenopausal woman (dose 1 mg/d). Contraindicated in hypersensitivity and pregnancy. Hot flushes, vaginal dryness and bleeding, hair thinning, arthralgia, rash, asthenia and gut upset are ADR.

Zaleplon

It is non-BZD hypnotic and binds to brain omega-1 receptor situated on alpha subunit of $GABA_A$ receptor complex. Complete oral absorption and significant presystemic circulation. Amnesia, paresthesia, somnolence, myalgia are ADR. Pregnancy and lactation contraindicated. Rifampin reduces and cimetidine increases zaleplon level. Used in insomnia (10–15 mg).

Siledin (100 mg TDS) is used in stress and headache.

Analgin

It is a pyrazolone derivative with a potent analgesic and antipyretic actions and weak anti-inflammatory action. ADR is hypotension and hypersensitivity reaction. CI is porphyria, shock, hypersensitivity and pregnancy. Used in pain and fever (dose = 500 mg TDS).

Divalproex

It is for epilepsies (petitmal, grand mal, myoclonic), mania and migraine. ADR is alopecia, rash, oedema, hepatitis.

Ropinirole

It is antiparkinsonian drug and non-ergoline DA agonist. Well absorbed orally. ADR is dyskinesia, asthenia and somnolence and diltiazem increase drug level.

Leavulose + glucose + phosphoric acid

They relieve nausea by local action on hyperactive wall of GIT and reduces smooth muscle contraction. It contains glucose + fructose (CI: DM and hereditary fructose intolerance).

Pyritinol

It enhances cholinergic transmission and improves cerebral microcirculation in ischaemic area. Rash, gut upset and excitement are ADR. CI: RA and hypersensitivity. Used in organic brain syndrome, head injury and encephalitis.

Nimodipine

It is Ca channel antagonist, enters brain and inhibits Ca entry in nerves and smooth muscle cells. Used in ischaemic neurological deficit. CCB, caffeine and phenytoin increase its level.

Sulbutiamine

It binds RAS (body's energy regulator) and exerts procholinergic action on CNS. Used in asthenia (400 mg OD).

Levobunolol

It is potent non-selective beta blockers for COA glaucoma.

Latanoprost (PG analogue)

It increases uveoscleral outflow and is used in open angle glaucoma.

Nabivolol

It is a competitive and selective beta-1 antagonist releasing NO. Extensively metabolised to active hydroxy metabolites. Headache, visual disturbance, oedema and dyspnoea are ADR. Used in essential HTN (5 mg OD).

Lercanidipine and benidipine (mech. same as CCB). They are used in HTN.

Lidoflazine, trimetazidine, oxyfedrine and dilazep

They are anti-anginal agents. Oxyfedrine improves metabolism of myocardium (hypoxia is tolerated better).

Xanthinol nicotuate
It improves blood flow to periphery and brain (vasodilation).

Nylidrin
It is peripheral vasodilator and is used in PVD and TAO.

Feracrylum
It is local haemostatic and antiseptic agent and forms a complex with albumin.

Polidocanol
It is sclerosing agent for bleeding oesophageal varices.

Cilostazol
It reversibly inhibits platelet aggregation and is used in intermittent claudication.

Flavonoids, diosmins, Ca dobesilate
They strengthen venous tone to reduce venous stasis and distension and normalise capillary permeability.

Tamsulosin
It is antagonist of alpha-1 receptor in prostate and is used in BPH.

Mebeverine
It effects colonic muscle activity and is used in irritable colon syndrome.

Drotaverine
It is spasmolytic drug, inhibits PDE IV and corrects cAMP and Ca imbalance thereby relieves smooth muscle spasm. Used in colics, post MTP, D/ and/C, cholelithiasis, etc. Dose is 40–80 mg TDS.

Valethamate
It acts similar to atropine and is used in colics.

Tegaserod
It is a novel selective 5-HT_4 receptor partial agonist stimulating small bowel and colonic motility to normalise GI function. Renal disease and bowel obstruction are CI. Used in IBS. Dose is 6 mg BD before meals × 36 days.

Danthron
It is stimulant laxative increasing motility of colon.

Mesterolone
It is a type of androgen causing frequent erection and priapism (ADR) and is used in hypogonadism.

Spirulina
It is a blue green algae having excellent nutrient composition and antioxidant properties (only source of superoxide dismutase besides highest natural protein 65%, richest source of betacarotene). Iron from spirulina (phycocyanin) is 60% better absorbed. Carbohydrate is 15% and fat is 5%. Dose: 1 gm BD × 60 days then 500 mg × 60 days.

Omega-3 fatty acid (eicosapentaenoic/docosahexaenoic acid)
It increases the stability and integrity of cells and lowers TG in normal persons. It is used in CAD and atherosclerosis.

Levetiracetam
It is adjunctive therapy for partial seizures. Somnolence, asthenia and dizziness are ADR.

Adapalene
It is synthetic retinoic acid analogue (naphthoic acid derivative) for acne vulgaris. It prevents microcomedone formation. Stinging of skin, erythema, scaling and acne flares are ADR.

Aldesleukin
It is IL-2 for metastatic RCC and melanoma, given by slow IV/SC. Capillary leak syndrome, anemia, tachycardia, hypothyroidism are ADR.

Amifostine (antineoplastic adjunct)
It is prodrug metabolised to active free thiol, and reduces cisplatin-induced nephrotoxicity. Given by IV infusion over 15 minutes, 30 minutes prior to cisplatin.

Bicalutamide
It is non-steroidal competitive anti-androgen for advanced prostatic carcinoma.

Brimonidine
It is selective α_2 agonist, decreases aqueous humor production, increases outflow and is used in OA glaucoma or ocular HTN.

Becaplermin
It is rhPDGF-BB and the first drug for diabetic ulcers, used topically.

Cidofovir
It inhibits viral DNA polymerase, and is used in CMV retinitis in AIDS. Renal damage, neutropenia and ocular hypotony are ADR.

Deferiprone
It is orally active iron chelating agent for thalassemia, iron poisoning and hemosiderosis. Neutropenia, agranulocytosis and SLE are ADR.

Denileukin Difititox
It is cytotoxic protein (amino acid sequences for diphtheria toxia and IL-2). It has cytocidal action of diphtheria toxin to cells expressing IL-2 receptor (mycosis fungoides).

Dexrazoxane
It is cyclic derivative of EDTA which prevents anthracycline-induced cardiomyopathy.

Cilostazol
It is PDE III inhibitor (dilates arteries) and is used in intermittent claudication.

Ibutilide
It is class III antiarrhythmic (converts atrial flutter or fibrillation to sinus rhythm).

Orlistat
It inhibits intestinal lipase (no fat digestion and absorption) and is used for weight loss.

Molgramostim
It is granulocyte macrophage colony-stimulating factor.

Porfimer
It is antineoplastic agent formed of oligomers of 8 porphyrin rings. It is photosensitizing agent (uses light of 630 nm wavelength to cause cellular death). It is used in esophageal cancer.

Riluzole/benzothiazole
It presynaptically inhibits glutamate release in CNS and postsynaptically interferes with the effects of excitatory amino acids. It is used in amyotrophic lateral sclerosis (ALS).

Tizanidine
It is α_2 agonist and inhibits α_2 R presynaptic motor nerve to reduce spasticity.

71. Drugs of Choice (DOC)

GYNECOLOGICAL DRUGS OF CHOICE (DOC)

Maintenance of DUB patients
- Medroxyprogesterone acetate

Intractable cases of DUB
- Danazole
- GnRH analogue (buserelin, goserelin)

Mood change in premenstrual tension
- SSRIs

Prevention of dysmenorrhoea
- OCPs

Vulvovaginal candidiasis in pregnancy
- Clotrimazole 1% locally

Cervical cancer
- Cisplatin

Endometrial cancer
- Medroxyprogesterone acetate

Ovarian cancer
- Cisplatin

Reduction of vascularity in fibroid uterus before surgery
- GnRH analogue (buserelin, goserelin)

DOC IN PREGNANCY

Acne
- *Topical*—benzylbenzoate
- *Oral*—erythromycin

Allergic rhinitis
- *Topical*—corticosteroids/sodium-chromoglycate/nasal decongestants
- *Systemic*—antihistaminics

Anemia due to B_{12} deficiency
- Cyanocobalamin

Anemia due to iron deficiency
- Ferrous sulphate

Anemia due to folate deficiency
- Folic acid

Sickle cell anemia
- *Prophylaxis of infection*—penicillin
- *Crises stage*—morphine

Anticoagulant
- Heparin (**WAR**Farin causes **WAR** against **F**oetus in first trimester)

Antiplatelet
- Aspirin

Arrhythmia
- Quinidine/digoxin

Anxiety
- Benzodiazepines

Asthma
- *Inhalational*—corticosteroids/mast cell stabilizer ipratropium/beta-2 agonists
- *Systemic*—theophylline
- *Emergency*—Epinephrine

Mania
- Lithium

Myasthenia gravis
- Pyridostigmine

Nausea/vomiting
- Metoclopramide (3rd trimester only)/Meclizine

- Cyclizine/Chlorpromazine
- Hydroxyzine + B_6
- Prochlorperazine

MCH in Pregnancy

Analgesics
- *Somatic pain*—aspirin/paracetamol
- *Severe pain*—morphine/codeine/pethidine

Worm infestation
- Piperazine/Pyrantel pamoate in Pregnancy

Pruritus
- *Topical*—moisturising cream/lotion
- *Systemic*—older antihistaminics

Psoriasis
- *Topical*—salicylic acid/corticosteroid/kalamine lotion

Reflux esophagitis
- Alginate + antacids (small and frequent meal also)

Rheumatoid arthritis
- Aspirin

Rosacea
- NSAIDs

Seizures
- *Acute control*—benzodiazepines
- *Maintenance*—phenobarbitone

Schizophrenia
- Phenothiazines (chlorpromazine/haloperidol)

Seborrheic dermatitis
- Salicylic acid/Selenium sulphide

SLE
- *Initially*—corticosteroids
- *After first trimester*—azathioprine

Trigeminal neuralgia
- TCA/carbamazepine

Superficial thrombophlebitis
- Aspirin

Deep vein thrombosis
- *First trimester*—heparin
- *Later*—warfarin

UTI during pregnancy
- Ampicillin/nitrofurantoin

Chloroquine resistant malaria
- Mefloquine

MDR or cerebral malaria
- Quinine

Gonorrhoea
- Penicillin/ceftriaxone

Amoebiasis
- Metronidazole (CI in first trimester)

Amoebiasis in first trimester
- Furazolidone

Cholera
- Furazolidone

Typhoid fever
- Ampicillin/ceftriaxone

Acute lower UTI (cystitis)
- Fosphomycin single dose

Shigella dysentery
- Ampicillin

Toxoplasmosis
- Spiramicin

Hyperthyroidism
- Propylthiouracil

Hypothyroidism
- Levothyroxine

Anaerobic infection
- *First trimester*—clindamycin/penicillin
- *Later*—metronidazole

Tuberculosis
- Rifampicin + INH

Cholestasis
- Cholestyramine

DOC IN NEUROLOGICAL DISORDERS

Alzheimer's disease
- Donepezil   Deep Tendon Reflex
- Tacrine
- Rivastigmine
- Galantamine

Amyotrophic lateral sclerosis
- Baclofen

Idiopathic facial nerve palsy (Bell's palsy)
- Acyclovir + corticosteroids

Hemifacial/clonic facial spasm
- Botulinum toxin (injected into affected muscles)

Coital/exercise induced cephalgia
- *Acute attack*—NSAIDs
- *Prophylaxis*—Propranolol

Drug induced hyperexcitability, febrile seizure, picrotoxin and strychnine poisoning, convulsion due to tetanus and lidocaine, emergence delirium due to ketamine, tardive dyskinesia
- Diazepam

Sedation and hypnosis in porphyrias
- Benzodiazepines

Endoscopy and colonoscopy (short procedures)
- Midazolam

Hemolytic anemia, jaundice in newborn, epilepsy due to febrile seizure, epilepsy during pregnancy, epilepsy in children, hypnosedative withdrawal
- Phenobarbitone (commonest used barbiturate)

Hypnosis in elderly
- Zolpidem (safest hypnosis in elderly)

Refractory convulsion
- Paraldehyde

Delirium tremens
- Thiamine + clomethiazole/chlordiazepoxide

Primary generalized tonic-clonic (grand mal)
- Valproate, lamotrigine

Partial and secondary generalized tonic-clonic seizures
- Carbamazepine, phenytoin, lamotrigine, valproate

Absence seizures
- Ethosuximide (valproate also)
  A and **E** are vowels

Atypical absence, atonic, myoclonic, GTCS, akinetic, mixed
- Valproate (broadest spectrum-releases GABA)

Partial epilepsy (simple/complex also called psychomotor)
- Carbamazepine/iminostilbine

Infantile spasm
- ACTH/prednisolone

Status epilepticus, febrile seizures
- Diazepam (10 mg IV/rectally)

Status epilepticus in partial/generalized seizures
- *Acute*—lorazepam/diazepam
- *Maintenance*—phenytoin

Status absence/prolonged absence
- Dizepam/lorazepam

Lennox-Gastaut syndrome
- Felbamate (hepatitis and bone marrow depression are MC ADR)

West syndrome
- ACTH/clonazepam

Chorea in Huntington's disease
- Haloperidol

Guillain-Barré syndrome
- Ig (IV)

Huntington's disease
- *Chorea*—DA depletors (tetrabenazine) and antidopaminergics (haloperidol and sulpiride)
- *Mood stabilization*—carbamazepine
- *Depression*—fluoxetine
- *Psychosis*—clozapine

Lambert-Eaton syndrome
- 3, 4-diaminopyridine

Meniere's disease
- Vestibular sedatives (cinnarizine, betahistine, prochlorperazine)

Migraine
- *Mild to moderate*—NSAIDs (aspirin, paracetamol) and anti-emetics (metoclopramide, domperidone)
- *Severe*—sumatriptan/zolmitriptan (5-HT$_1$D agonists)
- *Prophylaxis*—propranolol/metoprolol

Migrainous neuralgia (cluster headache)
- *Acute attack*—sumatriptan
- *Prophylaxis*—verapamil

Motor neuron disease
- Riluzole (glutamate antagonist)

Myotonia
- Phenytoin/diazepam

Rhinorrhoea
- Fexofenadine/citrizine (most sedative)/Loratidine (Least sedative)

Multiple sclerosis
- *Acute relapse*—methyl prednisolone 1 gm IV × 3 days
- *Prevention of prolapse*—azathioprine, immunomodulators (interferon beta 1a/b, glatiramer)

Myasthenia gravis
- Pyridostigmine + corticosteroids + azathioprine

Narcolepsy
- Modafinil 200–400 mg/day

Parkinson's disease (PD)
- Levodopa (most effective but for bradykinesia) + carbidopa (peripheral decarboxylase inhibitor)

Motor fluctuation due to levodopa
- Amantadine

PD with high incidence of motor ADR
- Ropinirole/pramipexole

Advanced PD
- COMT inhibitors (tolcapine/entacapine)

Drug-induced PD
- Benzhexol/trihexyphenydyl

Psychosis in PD
- Quitiapine

Depression in PD
- SSRIs

Parkinson's induced by antidopaminergic drugs
- Anticholinergics (benztropine, orphenadrine, trihexyphenydyl)

Periodic limb movements
- Levodopa

Ekbom's syndrome (restless leg syndrome)
- Clonazepam

Trigeminal neuralgia
- Carbamazepine/gabapentin/pregabalin

UMN spastic/neurogenic/hypertonic bladder
- Tolterodine/oxybutynin

Wernicke-Korsakoff disease
- Vitamins IV in high doses followed by thiamine orally

Sedation and hypnosis in severe hepatic failure
- Lorazepam/oxazepam

Selective antianxiety without sedation
- Buspirone

To reduce preanesthetic anxiety
- Lorazepam

Borderline personality disorder
- Thiothixene

DOC IN PSYCHIATRICS

Alcohol withdrawal
- Chlordiazepoxide (clomethiazole) + thiamine 50 mg IV

Alcohol craving
- Naltrexone

Relapse of alcoholism
- Acamprosate (NMDA receptor antagonist)

Methyl alcohol and ethylene glycol poisoning
- Fomepizole / 4-methyl pyrrazole (alcohol dehydrogenase inhibitor)

Alcohol detoxification
- Disulfiram (aldehyde dehydrogenase inhibitor) and carbamazepine

Anxiety disorders
- *Generalised*—alprazolam / diazepam
- *Panic*—fluoxetine
- *Maintenace*—buspirone
- Chil**D** (preoperatively)—**D**iphenhydramine / **D**imenhydrinate

Mixed anxiety and depressive disorders
- Alprazolam

Chronic low grade anxiety
- Chlordiazepoxide

Anorexia nervosa
- Imipramine

Attention deficit hyperactive disorder
- Dexamphetamine / methylphenidate

Bipolar disorders (manic depressive psychosis)
- *Acute manic* episodes—lithium
- *Depressive episodes*—fluoxetine, imipramine

Maintenance of mania, schizoeffective disorders, unipolar mood disorders (prophylaxis), neutropenia in Felty's syndrome, cyclical vomiting
- Lithium

Nonpsychotic unipolar depression (trichotillomania)
- SSRIs

For reducing excitement in
1. Acute mania
2. Acute agitation
3. Acute schizophrenia
4. Chorea
5. Delirium
6. Gilles de la Taurette's syndrome
7. Tics
- Haloperidol (*most potent, no hypotension, metabolized by Hoffmann's elimination*)

Prophylaxis of bipolar disorders
- *Slow cycling disorder (1–3 episodes/ year)*—lithium
- *Rapid cycling disorder (>3 episodes/ year)*—valproate / carbamazepine
- *Lithium and carbamazepine refractory cases*—valproate

Bulimia nervosa
- Fluoxetine

Depressive disorders
- *Mild to moderate, defaulters*—fluoxetine
- *Severe*—imipramine
- *Severe refractory*—moclobemide (MAO-A inhibitors)
- *Atypical*—tranylcypromine (MAO-AI)
- *Atypical depression with phobic neurosis*—phenelzine (MAO-AI)
- *Retarded depression*—trazadone (atypical antidepressant)
- *Psychotic depression*—loxapine (amoxapine precursor)

Insomnia, drug induced hyperexcitability, sedation and hypnosis in porphyrias
- Diazepam

Melancholia
- TCA

Nocturnal enuresis
- Imipramine, trimipramine

Obsessive compulsive neurosis (OCN)
- Clomipramine

OCD
- SSRIs / clomipramine (TCA*)*

Opioid withdrawal
- Methadone

Psychosis/schizophrenia
- *Agitative and violent*—chlorpromazine
- *Withdrawn and apathic*—triflupromazine
- *Negative symptoms, EPS and resistant cases*—clozapine
- *Prophylaxis in relapse and remitting*—penfluridol

Drugs of Choice (DOC)

Extrapyramidal symptoms (EPS)
- Thioridazine

Smoking cessation
- Bupropion

Chronic pain
- TCAs

Peripheral neuropathy
- Lamotrigine

Panic disorder and agoraphobia
- Alprazolam

Sleep walking
- Carbamazepine

Heat stroke, hiccups
- Chlorpromazine

Serotonin syndrome
- Cyproheptadine

Premenstrual tension, kleptomania, cyclothymia, dysthymia, body dysmorphic disorder, seasonal affective disorder, post-traumatic stress disorder
- SSRIs

Phobias other than social phobias
- Peroxetine/venlafexine

DOC AS ANALGESICS

Mild to moderate somatic pain
- NSAIDs

Primary and secondary dysmenorrhoea
- NSAIDs

Osteoarthritis
- Paracetamol

Rheumatoid arthritis
- Aspirin

Closure of PDA, ankylosing spondylitis, Barter syndrome, post-coital headache, acute gout (colchicines preferred)
- Indomethacin

Chronic gout
- Allopurinol

Pain in ulcers, elderly taking concomitant gastrotoxic drugs, NSAID induced ulcers (prevention and treatment)
- PPIs

Ulcer prevention in smokers
- Misoprostol (PGE$_1$)

NSAID for severe pain
- Ketorolac

Chronic cancer pain, pulmonary edema, tetralogy of Fallot, acute MI, pain of terminal illness, sickle cell crises (painful periods), epidural analgesia
- Morphine

Morphine/opioid poisoning
- Naloxone (most potent is naltrexone)

TIVA
- Alfentanil

To reduce sympathetic response to endotracheal intubation
- Sufentanil (most potent opioid)

Pain and fever in routine patients, children, pregnancy, haemophilia, bleeding disorders, bronchial asthma, ulcers, nasal polyps
- Paracetamol

Disease modification in RA/joint diseases
- Methotrexate

Paracetamol poisoning
- Acetylcysteine

Aspirin poisoning
- Vitamin K/fresh frozen plasma

Neuropathic pain
- TCA/lamotrigine/gabapentin/topiramate

Diabetic neuropathy
- TCA/topiramate

Biliary spasm
- Pethidine

Opioid withdrawal
- Methadone/buprenorphine (reduces craving)

Relapse of opioid use
- Buprenorphine

DOC FOR CARDIOVASCULAR DISEASES

Anaphylactic shock
- Adrenaline

Cardiac arrest
- Adrenaline and CPR

Shock with decreased renal output
- DA

Cardiogenic shock
- Dobutamine

Complete heart block
- Isoprenaline

Anorectic
- Fenfluramine (now sibutramine)

Narcolepsy; hyperkinetic child syndrome
- Amphetamine

Diagnosis of pheochromocytoma
- Phentolamine

Prostatic hypertrophy; preoperative control of HTN in pheochromocytoma
- Phenoxybenzamine

Intraoperative control of HTN in pheochromocytoma
- Sodium nitroprusside

Malignant HTN (HTN emergency)
- Labetalol

Chronic HTN
- Prazosin

Arrhythmia in thyrotoxicosis or pheochromocytoma; hypertrophic obstructive cardiomyopathy; prophylaxis of migraine after >4 attacks; tremor:
- Propranolol

Treatment of acute attack of migraine
- Ergotamine

Glaucoma
- Timolol preferred, betaxolol, levobunolol

Stable angina
- *Acute attack*—nitroglycerine (MC sublingual nitrate)
- *Prophylaxis*—beta blockers (reduce mortality), verapamil

Unstable angina
- Heparin + aspirin
- *High risk*—GP IIb/IIIa antagonists (tirofiban)

Prinzmetal/variant angina
- Diltiazem

To reduce mortality in angina
- Beta blockers (the only drug for the same use)

Medically refractory patients
- CABG

Prevention of post-coronary stent thrombosis
- Clopidogrel + aspirin

Medically refractory angina
- Angioplasty

To reduce restenosis and need for revascularization following angioplasty
- Multivitamins (B_6, B_{12}, folic acid)

PTCA
- Abciximab

Biliary sphincter spasm, achalasia cardia, cyanide poisoning
- Nitrates

Microvascular angina (syndrome X)
- CCB

Methaemoglobinemia
- Methylene blue (reducing agent)

PSVT
- Adenosine (shortest acting antiarrhythmic)

Atrial flutter and atrial fibrillation
- Esmolol and cardioversion
- *Acute attack*—ibutilide

Past DOC for atrial flutter
- *Quinidine*

Drugs of Choice (DOC)

Current DOC for atrial flutter/fibrillation
- *Dofetelide/ibutelide (K channel blockers)*

Paradoxical tachycardia
- Digoxin

Hypothermia induced atrial fibrillation
- Bretylium

Maintenance of sinus rhythm
- Amiodarone

Haemodynamically unstable patients
- Cardioversion

Multifocal atrial tachycardia
- Verapamil

Ventricular fibrillation
- Electrical defibrillation/lidocaine

Ventricular extrasystole
- *After acute MI*—lignocaine
- *Digitalis induced*—lignocaine potassium chloride
- *Ventricular premature beats*—beta blockers

Long QT syndrome
- *Congenital*—beta blockers
- *Acquired (acute attack)*—magnesium sulphate

Sick sinus syndrome (bradycardia phase)
- Theophylline

Perioperative arrhythmia
- Esmolol

Ventricular tachycardia
- Lignocaine and cardioversion

Torsade de pointes
- Pacing

Wolff-Parkinson-White syndrome
- Cardioversion/class I A/C antiarrhythmics

CHF
- *Congestive and low output symptoms*—enalapril and/or furosemide +/– digoxin/dobutamine
- *To reduce mortality*—spironolactone +/–ACE inhibitors
- *Acute ventricular filling pressure*—nesiritide
- *Ionotropic effects*—dobutamine
- *Digitalization of choice*—slow oral digoxin
- *Digoxin overdose*—digibind (Fc fragment IgG Ab)
- *Digoxin toxicity*—potassium
- *Digoxin induced arrhythmia*—lidocaine
- *First line drug*—ACE inhibitors
- *Rapid diuresis*—loop diuretics (most efficacious and fastest acting diuretics)

Hyperlipoproteinemia
- Statins (simvastatin)

Hypertension
- *Diabetes, CHF, unilateral renal artery stenosis, nephropathy, normal renin HTN*—ACE inhibitors
- *Renovascular disease*—ACE inhibitors/methyldopa
- *IHD, young and stressfull patients, high renin HTN*—beta blockers
- *Low renin HTN, isolated systolic HTN*—CCBs
- *Anxiety, migraine, tremors*—beta blockers
- *Bronchial asthma*—CCB/ACE inhibitors
- *Obesity, edema, old age*—thiazides
- *Pregnancy*—methyldopa
- *Emergency in pregnancy*—hydralazine
- *Pheochromocytoma, clonidine withdrawal and cheese reaction with MAO inhibitors*—phentolamine +/– beta blockers
- *Hypertensive emergency, controlled HTN*—sodium nitroprusside
- *Pre-eclampsia and eclampsia*—magnesium sulphate.

Male pattern baldness
- Minoxidil (topical) + finasteride (oral)

Diabetic dyslipidemia, postmenopausal dyslipidemia, hypertriglyceridemia, hyperlipoproteinemia
- Statins

Hepatic pruritis
- Colestipol/cholestyramine

Dysbetalipoproteinemia
- Fibrates (clofibrate, fenofibrate, gemfibrozil)

Familial hypercholesterolemia
- Nicotinic acid

Severe hypercholesterolemia
- Rosuvastatin (longest acting statin)

Lipid lowering in pregnancy, lactation and children
- Resins (cholestyramine, colestipol, cholesevelam)

LDL cholesterol reduction
- Atorvastatin

Reduction of TAG level
- Fibrates (clofibrate, fenofibrate, gemfibrozil)

Increasing HDL cholesterol, Hartnup disease
- Niacin (nicotinamide)

Thrombosis prevention in SLE positive antiphospholipid Ab
- Heparin

Aortic regurgitation
- *Initial*—diagoxin + diuretics + ACE inhibitors
- *Severe*—sodium nitroprusside
- *Long-term*—ACE inhibitor/valve replacement (end diastolic dimension >55% and EF <55%)

DOC IN ANS

Paralytic ileus, postoperative urinary retention, congenital megacolon
- Bethanechol

Sjögren syndrome (sicca manifestations)
- Cevemeline

Dry eyes
- Methylcellulose

Reversal of neuromuscular blockade, Cobra bites
- Neostigmine

Myasthenia gravis
- *Initial stage*—neostigmine
- *Maintenance*—pyridostigmine
- *Diagnosis*—edrophonium

Glaucoma
- *Refractory*—echothiophate
- *Low tension*—latanoprost
- *Primary open angle*—timolol
- *Glaucoma with asthma*—betaxolol

Priapism due to papaverine, trazodone and sildenafil, anaphylactic shock, prolonging the duration of LA, angioedema, cardiac arrest
- Epinephrine

Weight reduction
- Sibutramine

Postural hypotension
- Midodrine/proamitine

Hypotension during spinal anaesthesia
- Ephedrine

Narcolepsy
- Modafinil (sympathomimetic)

Suppression of premature labour
- Isoxsuprine/atosiban (oxytocin receptor antagonist)

Heart block
- Isoproterenol

Localised bleeding in GIT/ulcer
- Norepinephrine

Pupillary dilation without cycloplegia
- Phenylephrine

Short-term increase in BP
- Mephentermine

Nasal and eustachian tube congestion
- Pseudoephedrine

Pump failure due to MI, refractory CHF and cardiac surgery
- Dobutamine

Vagal mediated/sinus bradycardia, sick sinus syndrome, prevention of reflex laryngospasm, hyperhidrosis (excessive sweating), mashroom poisoning, carbamate poisoning, organophosphate poisoning, drying of respiratory secretion, iridocyclitis, corneal ulcer, mydriasis in children
- Atropine

Initial colic
- Pipenzolate

Motion sickness
- Scopolamine

Morning sickness
- Prochlorperazine

Motion sickness prevention
- Acetazolamide

Spasmodic abdominal pain with vomiting
- Dicyclomine

Spasmodic pain (renal/intestinal colic)
- Drotaverine

Ureteric pain
- Diclofenac

Chronic vertigo
- Cinnarizine

Essential tremors, lithium induced tremors, prevention of migraine, hypertrophic cardiomyopathy, somatic anxiety in social phobia, toxic multinodular goiter/hyperthyroidism, catecholamines dependent cardiac arrhythmia, akathesia (MC acute EPS of adults), cardiac instability during ET intubation, delaying aortic dilation in Marfan syndrome, intraoperative tachycardia
- Propranolol

Congenital torsade de pointes
- Metoprolol

Beta blockers for CHF
- Bisoprolol (mainly), Carvedilol, Metoprolol   **BCM**

Beta blockers with LA like actions
- Propranolol, pindolol   **PALM**
- Acebutolol   **ANS CCC**
- Labetalol
- Metoprolol
- Atenolol
- Nadolol
- Sotalol
- Carteolol
- Carvedilol
- Celiprolol

Aortic dissection
- Labetalol

Perioperative cardiac arrhythmia, fast cardiac arrhythmia, perioperative HTN
- Esmolol

Hypertension: Cheese reaction, opioid withdrawal, clonidine withdrawal, pheochromocytoma surgery
- Phentolamine

Malignant and inoperable pheochromocytoma
- Phenoxybenzamine

Drug induced necrosis and gangrene by thiopentone
- Phentolamine

Functional impotance
- Yohimbine

Erectile dysfunction
- Sildenafil citrate

Pulmonary HTN in newborn
- Tolazoline

DOC IN BLEEDING DISORDERS

Anticardiolipin antiphospholipid Ab/ lupus anticoagulant syndrome, pregnancy
- Heparin

Autoimmune hemolytic anemia
- Prednisolone

AMI
- Streptokinase with EACA to control bleeding

Hemophilia A
- Factor 8

Christmas factor
- Factor 9

Massive bleeding
- EACA/tranhexanemic acid

Bleeding due to aspirin, warfarin overdose
- Vitamin K

Heparin overdose
- Protamine sulphate

Capillary bleeding, bleeding in pulmonary TB
- Adrenochrome/ethamsylate

Local haemostasis in GIT
- Noradrenaline

Atrial fibrillation induced clotting
- Warfarin

Prevention of stroke, TIA
- Aspirin

Prevention of DVT
- Enoxaparin

Prevention of arterial thrombosis
- Aspirin/clopidogrel

Hypofibrigenaemia in DIC, Factor 8 deficiency, von Willebrand's disease
- Cryoprecipitates

Bleeding prevention due to thrombolytic therapy
- Epsilon

Subacute combined degeneration of spinal cord
- Vitamin B_{12}

Prevention of neural tube defects
- Folic acid

Anaemia in CRF
- Erythropoietin

DOC IN RESPIRATORY DISEASES

Asthma
- *Mild intermittent*—salbutamol, terbutaline
- *Mild persistent*—salbutamol/terbutaline + corticosteroids
- *Moderate to severe persistent*—salmeterol/formeterol + corticosteroids
- *Severe (air flow obstruction)*—inhaled corticosteroids (fluticasone, beclomethasone)
- *Initial treatment*—beta-2 agonist
- *Acute severe asthma*—oxygen 60% + nebulised beta-2 agonists + systemic corticosteroids
- *Acute severe*—nebulised salbutamol
- *Aspirin induced*—leukotriene antagonists (zafirlukast, montelukast)
- *Food allergy prophylaxis*—mast cell stabilizers
- *Poorly controlled*—theophylline
- *Relief of acute symptoms*—inhaled formeterol

Exercise induced asthma
- *Prophylaxis*—mast cell stabilizers/beta-2 agonists/leukotriene antagonists
- *Treatment*—mast cell stabilizers

COPD
- *Smoking cessation*—behaviour therapy, nicotine replacement, bupropion
- *Bronchodilators*—anticholinergics (ipratropium, tiotropium), beta-2 agonists, theophylline
- *Hypoxemia*—ambulatory oxygen, long-term oxygen therapy
- *Acute exacerbation*—glucocorticoids

Cough
- *Dry*—dextromethorphan + antihistaminics and decongestants
- *Productive*—expectorant (KI) and/or mucolytic (acetylcysteine)

- *Suppression* — dextromethorphan (non-opioid NMDA antagonist)
- *ACE inhibitor induced* — aspirin (acetyl salicylic acid)

For liquefying plaques of sputum in cystic fibrosis
- Acetylcysteine (opens disulfide bonds)

Test of bronchial hyperactivity
- Methacholine (pure muscarinic agonist)

Apnea in premature infants
- Theophylline

Temporal arteritis
- Prednisolone

Spinal cord injury induced sexual impotence
- Alprostadil (PGE_1 analogue)

Priming/ripening of cervix
- Dianoprost (PGE_2 analogue)

Early abortion
- Mifepristone (RU_{486}) + misoprostol

Second trimester abortion
- Dianoprost/carboprost tromethamine

Intermittent claudication
- Pentoxifylline/cilastazol (antiplatelets)

Beta blocker induced bronchospasm
- Ipratropium (selective M_3 blocker)

DOC IN GASTROINTESTINAL DISEASES

Bowel evacuation before X-ray, surgery and colonoscopy
- Saline purgatives, polyethylene glycol

Constipation
- *Functional* — fibres/bulk forming drugs (isaphagula, bran)
- *Chronic renal failure* — aluminium hydroxide
- *Bedridden* — phenolphthalein
- *Children* — castor oil
- *Stool and wax softening* — dioctyl sodium sulfosuccinate (acts like detergents)

Cleaning bowel for endoscopy
- Polyethylene glycol

Cleaning bowel before delivery
- Sodium phosphate enema

Diarrhoea due to carcinoid tumour, glucagonoma, VIPoma, HIV
- Octreotide

Functional/noninfectious diarrhea
- Loperamide

Secretory diarrhea
- Cholestyramine

Diabetic diarrhea
- Clonidine

Motion in morning
- Besacodyl

Emesis
- *Disease associated (migraine, uremia)* — metoclopramide, prochlorperazine
- *Drug induced (levodopa)* — domperidone
- *Morning sickness, migraine* — prochlorperazine
- *Motion sickness* — hyoscine
- *Postoperative, radiotherapy, cancer chemotherapy* — ondansetron

Chronic vertigo
- Cinnarizine (CCB with antihistaminic properties)

Gastroparesis due to diabetes and postvagotomy, increased motility
- Cisapride

Zollinger-Ellison syndrome, GERD (reflux esophagitis), dyspepsia, erosive esophagitis, gastric and duodenal ulcer
- Omeprazole (PPIs are most effective)

Hepatic encephalopathy, rapid relief
- Lactulose

Induction of emesis
- Apomorphine

Inflammatory bowel disease
- *Acute*—prednisolone
- *Maintenance*—Mesalazine

Irritable bowel syndrome
- Tegaserod

Ulcers
- *Acute stress ulcer*—pantoprazole, ranitidine
- *Stress ulcer*—misoprostol
- *Peptic*—omeprazole, ranitidine
- *NSAIDs induced (prevention and treament)*—omeprazole

Pain in ulcers
- Antacids (fastest action)

Reducing gastric emptying time before surgery
- Metoclopramide

Carcinoid syndrome, GH deficient and poor eater children, SSRIs induced sexual dysfunction, cold induced urticaria
- Cyproheptadine

Vomiting production
- *Oral route*—ipecacuanha
- *Parenteral route*—apomorphine

Spasmodic abdominal pain
- Drotaverine (PDE inhibitors)

D_2 blockers (haloperidol) induced EPS
- Promethazine

Nausea and vomiting: Reducing gastric emptying time, prevention of aspiration pneumonia (Mendelson's syndrome)
- Metoclopramide

DOC IN ENDOCRINOLOGICAL DISEASES

Acromegaly
- Octreotide

Acute and chronic adrenal insufficiency, adrenogenital syndrome, congenital adrenal hyperplasia
- Hydrocortisone

Diagnosis of Cushing's disease, tumour induced brain edema, to enhance lung maturation in developing baby
- Dexamethasone (longest acting glucocorticoid)

Mineralocorticoid deficiency
1. Idiopathic hypotension
2. Hypotension due to autonomic degeneration
3. Treatment refractory hypotension
4. Mineralocorticoid replacement
- Fludrocortisone

Addison's disease (chronic adrenal insufficiency)
- Hydrocortisone + fludrocortisone

Diabetes insipidus (central)
- Desmopressin

DM
- *Type I, severe weight loss, sugar >250 mg%, acute illness and lean type II*—insulin
- *Type II*—sulfonylureas
- *Elderly*—tolbutamide
- *Renal failure*—repaglinide
- *Prevention*—metformin
- *New onset*—insulin secretagogues (repaglinide)

Severe hypoglycemia in insulinoma
- Diazoxide (K^+ channel openers)

Beta blocker poisoning
- Glucagon

Diabetic ketoacidosis, sugar control in infection, DM in pregnancy, type I DM, surgery in DM, DM in renal and liver failure
- Regular insulin (only insulin given IV)

Obese diabetes
- Metformin

To reduce insulin resistance
- Pioglitazone

To reduce postprandial hyperglycemia
- Repaglinide (meglitinide derivatives)/acarbose

Hypoglycemia
- Dextrose 50%/glucagons/epinephrine

Dwarfism
- *Pituitary origin*—somatotropin
- *Laron type*—recombinant IGF-1

Hypoparathyroidism
- *Hypocalcemia and tetany*—calcium gluconate IV
- *Persistent*—alpha calcidiol/dihydrotachysterol

Hypothyroidism
- Levothyroxine

Hyperparathyroidism/hypercalcemia, osteoporosis, Paget's disease
- Bisphosphonates

Hyperprolactinemia
- Bromocriptine

Hyperthyroidism/Graves' disease
- *Mild/small goiter*—antithyroid drugs
- *Severe/large goiter*—radioactive iodine
- *Toxic nodular*—radioactive iodine

For suppressing somatic manifestation of
1. *Hyperthyroidism*
2. *Toxic multinodular (goitre and its prophylaxis)*
- Propranolol

For reducing thyroid gland vascularity, for making patient euthyroid before surgery
- KI

Thyroid storm
- Propranolol, propylthiouracil, sodium ipodate
- *In India*—KI/iodipate

Hypothyroidism/hypothyroidism during pregnancy
- Propylthiouracil

Myxoedema coma, cretinism, papillary CA
- Liothyronine IV/thyroxine

Pheochromocytoma
- Phenoxybenzamine, Phentolamine

Primary hyperaldosteronism
- Spironolactone

Rickets (metabolic) and osteomalacia
- *Vitamin D dependent*—calcitriol/alpha calcidiol
- *Vitamin D resistant*—phosphate + calcitriol/alpha calcidiol

Renal rickets
- Calcitriol/alpha calcidiol + dihydrotachysterol

Uterine fibroids, precocious puberty, CA prostate, endometriosis, prophylaxis of heavy DUB
- GnRH analogues (buserelin, goserelin)

Gynaecomastia, fibrocystic breast disease, hereditary angioneurotic edema
- Danazol (inhibits mid cycle surge)

DUB
- NSAIDs

Premenstrual syndrome
- SSRIs

Menorrhagia
- Ethamsylate/adrenochrome

Massive bleeding
- Tranhexemic acid/EACA (epsilon aminocaproic acid)

Emergency contraceptive (post-coital contraception), Cushing's syndrome, meningioma
- Mifepristone

Medical curettage in abnormal premenopausal bleeding
- Medroxyprogesterone acetate/norethindrone acetate

For medical curettage in abnormal premenopausal bleeding
- Medroxyprogesterone acetate/norethindrone acetate

To reduce bleeding before fibroid surgery
- Medroxyprogesterone acetate/danazole

Prevention of CA breast
- Tamoxifen

Anovular infertility, corpus luteum insufficiency, *in vitro* fertilization, polycystic ovarian disease, oligospermia
- Clomiphene citrate

Osteoporosis, postmenopausal osteoporosis
- Raloxifen/HRT

Prevention of postmenopausal osteoporosis
- Vitamin D and calcium

Glucocorticoid induced osteoporosis
- Alendronate

Vaginal atrophy
- Topical estrogen/HRT

To reduce itching in CA vulva
- Crotamiton

Induction of labour
- Oxytocin

If oxytocin is contraindicated
- Latanoprost (PGF$_2$ alpha)

Maitenance of PDA
- PGE$_2$/PGI$_2$

Primary pulmonary hypertension
- PGI$_2$ analogue

PID
- *Hospital*—cefoxitin/cefotetan + doxycycline
- *Outpatient*—fluoroquinolones + metronidazole or cefoxitin + probenecid or ceftriaxone + doxycycline +/− metronidazole

Hirsutism
- Cyproterone acetate

CA prostate
- GnRH analogue (buserelin, goserelin) +/− androgen antagonists (biclutamide/flutamide)

Large prostate and male pattern baldness
- Finasteride

BPH
- Tamsulosin (relaxes smooth muscles and inhibits reflexes)

Vasomotor symptoms in menopausal syndrome
- Estrogen + progesterone

Sarcoidosis
- Prednisolone

Pituitary edema
- Cabergoline

DOC IN INFECTIOUS DISEASES

Acinebacter (nosocomial infections)
- Imipenem/aminoglycosides + ciprofloxacin

Actinomyces israelii **(cervicofacial, abdominal and thoracic lesions)**
- Penicillin G, ampicillin

Bacteroides
- Clindamycin/metronidazole

Bacillus anthracis **(pneumonia, malignant pustule)**
- Penicillin G/ciprofloxacin/doxycycline
- *Systemic*—ciprofloxacin/doxycycline +/− imipenem/clindamycin

Borrelia burgdorferi/**Lyme disease**
- *Skin/erythema chronic migrans*—doxycycline
- *Nerve, heart and joints (stage 2)*—ceftriaxone

Borrelia recurrentis **(relapsing fever)**
- Doxycycline

Brucella
- Doxycycline + gentamicin/rifampicin and trimethoprim + rifampicin
- Aminoglycosides

Bartonella (cat scratch)
- Ciprofloxacin/macrolides

Bordetella pertussis
- Macrolides

Clammatobacterium granulomatosis (granuloma inguinale)
- Doxycycline

Campylobacter fetus
- *Bacteremia and endocarditis*—gentamicin and ampicillin
- *Meningitis*—ampicillin

Campylobacter jejuni **(enteritis)**
- Ciprofloxacin

Chlamydia psittaci
- Doxycycline

Chlamydia pneumoniae
- Doxycycline, azithromycin/clarithromycin

Chlamydia trachomatis
- *Lymphogranuloma venereum*—doxycycline
- *Trachoma*—azithromycin
- *Inclusion conjunctivitis*—azithromycin
- *Nonspecific urethritis and cervicitis*—azithromycin

Clostridium difficile
- *Antibiotic associated colitis*—metronidazole
- Metronidazole/vancomycin

Clostridium perfringens
- *Gas gangrene*—penicillin G + clindamycin

Clostridium tetani
- *Tetanus*—penicillin G, vancomycin
- Metronidazole +/– penicillin

Corynebacterium diphtheriae
- *RTI and carrier*—macrolide/clindamycin

Corynebacterium species (aerobic and anaerobic)
- Penicillin G and/or aminoglycoside and vancomycin

Cutaneous anthrax
- Doxycycline/ciprofloxacin

Entercoccus
- *Endocarditis (vancomycin sensitive)*—penicillin G/ampicillin + gentamicin
- *Endocarditis (vancomycin resistant)*—quinapristin + delfopristin, linezolid
- *UTI (vancomycin sensitive)*—penicillin/ampicillin/amoxicillin
- *UTI (vancomycin resistant)*—quinapristin + delfopristin and linezolid

Erysipelothrix rhusiopathiae
- Penicillin G

Enterobacter species
- Cotrimoxazole, ciprofloxacin, imipenem/meropenem
- Piperacillin + gentamycin

E. coli
- Ciprofloxacin/levofloxacin, first generation cephalosporin

E. coli, **Klebsiella, Proteus, Providencia, Serratia**
- Cephalosporin

Eikenella corrodens
- Penicillin

Flavobacterium meningosepticum **(meningitis)**
- Vancomycin

Francisella tularensis
- Streptomycin/gentamycin/tobramycin

Fusobacterium nucleatum
- Penicillin G, clindamycin

Gonococci
- Penicillin/ceftriaxone

Haemophilus ducreyi (chancroid)
- Ceftriaxone, cotrimoxazole, erythromycin

Haemophilus influenzae **(otitis media, sinusitis, pneumonia)**
- Cotrimoxazole, cefuroxime axetil, amoxicillin + clavulanate/cephalosporins

Klebsiella pneumoniae
- Cephalosporin

Legionella pneumophilla (**Legionnaires disease**)
- Azithromycin, fluoroquinolone

Leptospira (Weil's disease, meningitis)
- Penicillin G

Listeria monocytogenes
- Penicillin G/ampicillin and/or gentamycin

Moraxella catarrhalis
- Amoxycillin + clavulanate, ampicillin + sulbactam, gentamycin, cotrimoxazole

Mycobacterium avium intracellulare
- Ethambutol + clarithromycin

Mycobacterium leprae
- Dapsone + rifampicin

Mycobacterium tuberculosis   **PERI**
- **P**yrazinamide + **E**thambutol + **R**ifampicin + **I**soniazid

Mycoplasma pneumoniae
- *Atypical pneumonia*—doxycycline
- *Generally*—macrolides

Neisseria gonorrhoeae
- Ceftriaxone, cefixime, cefpodoxime, ciprofloxacin/levofloxacin

Neisseria meningitis
- *Meningitis*—penicillin G/ceftriaxone
- *Carrier state*—rifampicin

Nocardia asteroides (**pulmonary lesion, brain abscess**)
- Cotrimoxazole

Pasteurella multocida
- Ampicillin + clavulanate, penicillin G

Pneumocystis carinii
- Cotrimoxazole

Proteus mirabilis
- Ampicillin/amoxicillin, cotrimoxazole

Proteus (other species)
- Ciprofloxacin, 3rd generation cephalosporin

Pseudomonas aeruginosa
- *UTI*—penicillin, ceftazidime, cefepime, ciprofloxacin
- *Pneumonia, bacteremia*—penicillin + tobramycin, ceftazidime/cefepime + tobramycin

Pseudomonas mallei (**Glanders**)
- Streptomycin + tetracycline

Pseudomonas pseudomallei (**Melioodosii**)
- Ceftriaxone/ceftazidime, cotrimoxazole

Pneumococcus
- Penicillin

Peptostreptococcus
- Metronidazole + penicillin/clindamycin

Rickettsia
- Doxycycline

Salmonella
- Ciprofloxacin/levofloxacin/norfloxacin, ceftrixone

Serratia
- Imipenem, cefoxitin

Shigella
- Ciprofloxacin

Staphylococcus aureus
- *Generally*—nafcillin/oxacillin, dicloxacillin, cephalexin
- *MRSA*—vancomycin +/− rifampicin/linezolid
- *Vancomycin intermediate*—quinapristin + dalfopristin, linezolid, vancomycin + nafcillin/oxacillin

Staphylococcus epidermidis (**coagulase −ve**)
- Vancomycin +/− rifampicin

Streptococcus agalactiae
- Ampicillin/penicillin and/or gentamicin

Streptococcus bovis
- Penicillin G and/or gentamicin

Streptococcus pneumoniae
- *Generally*—penicillin, amoxicillin

- *Penicillin resistant*—ceftriaxone/cefotaxime, vancomycin
- *Penicillin G resistant*—vancomycin + rifampicin + cefotaxime/ceftriaxone

Streptococcus pyogenes
- Penicillin, amoxicillin, cephalosporin

Streptococcus viridans
- Penicillin G and/or amoxicillin

Streptococcus **(anaerobic)**
- Penicillin G

Streptococcus moniliformis
- Penicillin G

Spirochaetes and Borrelia burgdorferi
- Cephalosporin/amoxicillin/doxycycline

Treponema pallidum
- Penicillin G

Treponema pertenue
- Penicillin G, streptomycin

Generally, all cocci and bacilli
- Beta lactam especially penicillin

Ureaplasma urealyticum
- Doxycycline

Vibrio cholerae
- Doxycycline, ciprofloxacin

Yersinia enterocolitica
- *Yersinosis*—cotrimoxazole
- *Sepsis*—aminoglycoside, chloramphenicol

Yersinia pestis **(plague)**
- Streptomycin and/or tetracycline

Vibrio cholerae, balantidiasis, relapsing fever (undulant fever, malt fever), lymphogranuloma inguinale, donovanosis (granuloma inguinale), *Mycoplasma pneumoniae,* **Chlamydiae, tropical sprue, blind loop syndrome, prevention of plague, rickettsiae**
- Tetracycline mostly doxycycline

Tetanus, syphilis, diphtheria, actinomycetes, *P. multocida,* **erysipeloid, rat bite fever, oral and periodontal infections, meningococci, pneumococci, group A beta hemolytic and group B streptococci, Leptospira,** *B. anthrax,* **yaws, pinta**
- Penicillin (penicillin G)

Acne
- *Inflammed*—minocycline
- *Cystic*—isotretinoin

SIDAH
- Demeclocycline

Anaerobic brain abscess
- Metronidazole/chloramphenicol

Bowel sterilization before surgery
- Neomycin

UTI
- *Generally*—norfloxacin
- *E. faecalis*—amoxycillin

Dysuria
- Phenazopyridine

Acute attack of plague, rhinoscleroma, tularemia, brucella
- Streptomycin

Pseudomonas
- Tobramycin among aminoglycoside

Listeria monocytogenes, Enterococcus faecalis
- Ampicillin

Leptospirosis
- Penicillin, cotrimoxazole in allergy

Pneumocystis carinii/jiroveci, **uncomplicated UTI, URI in children, toxoplasmosis (DOC in pregnancy—spiramycin), nocardiosis, invasive dysentery, actinomycetes allergic to penicillin, severe Listeria meningitis, severe Listeria meningitis allergic to pencillin, cyclosporiosis, Whipple's syndrome**
- Cotrimoxazole

Community acquired pneumonia
- Clarithromycin

Surgical prophylaxis
- Cefazolin

MRSA
- Vancomycin

Vancomycin resistant enterococci
- Teicoplanin

MDR Staphylococcus
- Streptogramins

Ameobiasis (hepatic, intestinal), giardiasis, trench mouth, *H. pylori*, trichomoniasis, pseudomembranous enterocolitis, anaerobic infections
- Metronidazole

Leishmaniasis
- *Visceral and cutaneous*—sodium stibogluconate
- *Most effective drug*—miltefosine/liposomal amphoterecin B

Diphtheria carrier, Chlamydial urethritis in pregnancy, Campylobacter, cat scratch disease, whooping cough, bacillary angiomatosis
- Erythromycin

Non-gonococcal urethritis
- Doxycycline

***M. avium intracullulare*, community acquired pneumonia**
- Clarithromycin

Systemic *Bacteroides fragilis*, bacterial vaginosis
- Clindamycin

Diabetic foot
- Clindamycin + ciprofloxacin/cefuroxime

Chancroid, trachoma and gonococcal urethritis (single dose), short course chemotherapy, legionellosis
- Azithromycin (longest acting macrolide)

Norfloxacin in UTI, cartilage damaged by ciprofloxacin
- Prednisolone

Salmonella, *H. influenzae*, All meningitis except *L. monocytogenes*, Ophthalmia neonatorum, gonorrhea
- Ceftriaxone

Inflammatory bowel disease
- Sulphasalazine

Prophylaxis of newborn to mother with TB
- INH

Pyrazinamide induced hyperuricemia
- Aspirin

Dermatitis herpetiformis
- Dapsone

Acute attack of *P. vivax* in pregnancy
- Chloroquine

Severe falciparum and chloroquine resistant malaria except in pregnancy
- Quinine

Hepatic hypnozoites eradication and mosquito transmission reduction
- Primaquine (most effective gametocidal)

Cyst of amoebiasis
- Puromomycin/diloxanide furoate

Trypanosoma cruzi
- *Generally*—nifortimox
- *Hemolymphatic stage*—suramin
- *CNS stage*—milarsoprol

Systemic fungal infections
- Amphotericin B

Cryptococcal meningitis, vulvovaginal candidiasis (KTZ is DOC in recurrent), esophagitis in AIDS
- Fluconazole

Onychomycosis
- Terbinafine

Dermatophytes
- Griseofulvin

Aspergilloma, Sporothrix, blastomycosis, paracoccidioidomycosis
- Itraconazole

Herpes infections
- *Generally*—acyclovir
- *Resistant*—Foscarnet

HPV
- Interferon alpha

CMV retinitis
- Ganciclovir

HCV
- Ribavirin + interferon alpha

HBV
- Lamivudine

HIV
- *Accidental exposure*—AZT + lamivudine × 4 weeks
- *Vertical transmission*—AZT + nevirapine
- *Generally*—2 NRTIs / 2 NRTIs + 1 NNRTI / NRTI + NNRTI + PI

RSV
- Ribavirin

VZV
- Acyclovir

Condyloma accuminatum
- Podophylline

Podophylline resistant warts
- Imiquimod

On-off phenomena in PD
- Amantadine

Echinococcus granulosus, **neurocysticercosis**
- Albendazole

Guinea worm (*D. medinensis*)
- Niridazole / metronidazole (eradicated from India)

Tropical eosinophilia
- DEC

Loa loa, second DOC for cutaneous and visceral larva migrans, *O. volvulus, S. stercoralis*, Norwegian scabies
- Ivermectin (GABA agonist)

Mycobacteria
- *Renal failure*—rifampicin
- *HIV positive taking PI*—rifabutin
- *Sensitive patients*—INH
- *Prophylaxis of influenza B*—rifampicin
- *Staphylococcus*—rifampicin + anti-Staphylococcus penicillin
- *Penicillin resistant pneumococci*—rifampicin + ceftriaxone
- *Streptomycin resistant/MDR*—amikacin
- *Disseminated atypical mycobacteria in AIDS*—rifabutin
- *M. kanasasii*—INH + rifampicin + ethambutol
- *Latent TB*—INH
- *INH resistant latent TB*—rifampicin
- *Lepra reaction type I*—glucocorticoids
- *Lepra reaction type II*—thalidomide
- *Prophylaxis of M. kansasii (pyrazinamide resistant)*—azithromycin
- *Cutaneous TB due to atypical mycobacteria*—clarithromycin
- *M. murium TB*—clarithromycin + ethambutol
- *Leprosy*—rifampicin + dapsone (to reduce resistant)
- *Leprosy with extensive skin pigmentation*—dapsone + ethionamide
- *Paucibacillary leprosy*—rifampicin + dapsone (6 months)
- *Multibacillary leprosy*—rifampicin + dapsone + clofazimine
- *M. xenopi*—clarithromycin
- *Severe liver disease*—ethambutol + streptomycin

Sepsis
- *Gram-negative (Pseudomonas)*—piperacillin / tazobactam, ceftazidime + tobramycin
- *Gram-positive (staphylococci)*—vancomycin + gentamicin
- *Post-splenectomy*—ceftriaxone
- *Babesiosis (B. microti, B. divergenes)*—clindamycin + quinine / atovaquinone + azithromycin
- *Meningococcemia (N. meningitis, S. pneumoniae)*—penicillin / ceftriaxone
- *R. rickettsii (Rocky Mountain spotted fever)*—doxycycline
- *Toxic shock syndrome*—clindamycin + penicillin / oxacillin

- *Group A streptococci (necrotizing fascitis)*—penicillin +/– clindamycin
- *Brain abscess*—penicillin/oxacillin +/– metronidazole

Prophylaxis
- *Infective endocarditis*—amoxycillin
- *Endocarditis allergic to penicillin*—vancomycin
- *Dental prophylaxis in infective endocarditis*—clarithromycin
- *S. aureus*—mupirocin (intranasal)
- *Meningococcal meningitis*—rifampicin
- *Dirty wounds*—cefazolin
- *Otitis media/sinusitis in adults*—amoxycillin
- *Pneumococcal pneumonia in adults*—amoxycillin
- *Animal bites*—coamoxyclave (early case), amoxycillin/sulbactam (late case)
- *Cellulitis*—nafcillin/oxacillin
- *Enterobacter*—imipenem/meropenem
- *Serious infection in penicillin allergy*—vancomycin
- *Corynebacterium jeikeium*—vancomycin
- *Serious Gram-negative septicemia with neutropenia*—aminoglycosides
- *Serious upper UTI*—aminoglycosides
- *Upper RTI due to atypical pathogens*—doxycycline
- *E. faecum*—streptogramin
- *Children (typhus fever, Rickettsia—RMSF)*—chloramphenicol
- *Erythema gangrenosum*—carbenicillin
- *Microspora*—albendazole
- *Isospora belli*—cotrimoxazole

Toxocariasis, tropical eosinophilia, microfilarias, Norwegian scabies
- DEC

Trichuriasis (*Trichuris trichiura*/whipworm)
- Mebendazole

Intestinal cysticercosis
- Niclosamide

Mixed infestation
- Mebendazole (broadest spectrum antihelminth)

Infestation in pregnancy
- Piperazine/pyrantel

Sheep fluke (*Fasciola hepatica*)
- Biothionol

Trichinosis (*Trichinella spiralis*), Capillariasis (*Capillaria philippinensis*), Echinococcosis, Nematodes, Cestodes, Neurocysticerosis
- Albendazole

Ascariasis (*A. lumbricoides*), hookworms (*N. americanus, A. duodenale*)
- Mebendazole/albendazole

Cutaneous larva migrans
- Thiabendazole

Schistosomiasis (bilharziasis), Taeniasis (*T. saginata, T. solium*), lung fluke (Paragonimiasis), Schistosomiasis (*Schistosoma species*), Diphyllobothriasis, Hymenolepiasis (*H. nana*), intestinal fluke (*F. buski*, Heterophyes, Metagonimus), liver fluke (Clonorchis, Opisthorchis, *O. viverrini*)
- Praziquantel

Dracunculiasis (guinea worm)
- Metronidazole

Enterobiasis (hydatid disease)
- Pyrantel pamoate

Oncocerca volvulus, **Strongyloidiasis**
- Ivermectin

Aspergillus
- Voriconazole

Blastomyces dermatitidis
- AMB, itraconazole

Candida
- *Systemic*—AMB, fluconazole
- *Topical*—miconazole, clotrimazole, nystatin
- *Oral*—KTZ, fluconazole, itraconazole

Coccidioides immitis, Pseudallescheria boydii, **chromomycosis**
- Itraconazole

Cryptococcus neoformans, Histoplasmosis capsulatum, **Mucor**
- AMB

Paracoccidioides brasiliensis
- Itraconazole/KTZ

Sporothrix schenckii
- *Cutaneous*—KI
- *Systemic*—itraconazole

Amoebiasis
- Metronidazole +/− diloxanide furoate

Balantidiasis
- Tetracycline

Babesiosis
- Clindamycin + quinine

Giardiasis
- Metronidazole

Leishmaniasis
- Stibogluconate sodium/AMB

Malaria
1. *P. falciparum*
   - *Prophylaxis and treatment of P. falciparum*—chloroquine
   - *MDR (prophylaxis)*—mefloquine
   - *MDR treatment*—quinidine + antifolates/antibiotics such as quinidine/quinine + (pyrimethamine + sulfadoxine/sulfadiazine)/ (tetracycline/clindamycin); or mefloquine +/− artesunate; or atovaquone + proguanil
2. *P. ovale* and *vivax* (prophylaxis and treatment)
   - Chloroquine + primaquine
3. *P. malariae* (prophylaxis and treatment)
   - Chloroquine

Filariasis
- *W. bancrofti* and *B. malayi*—DEC + albendazole
- *Dipetalonema*—ivermectin + albendazole
- *Loa loa*—DEC
- *O. volvulus*—ivermectin

Toxoplasma gondii
- Pyrimethamine + sulfadiazine

Trichomonas vaginalis
- Metronidazole

Trypanosoma cruzi
- Nifurtimox

Trypanosoma brucei
- *Early CNS stage*—suramin + pentamidine/eflornithine
- *Late CNS stage*—melarsoprol +/− suramin

DOC IN SKIN DISEASES

Pediculosis (head—*P. capitis*, body—*P. corporis*, pubic—*P. pubis*) and *Sarcoptes scabiei* (scabies)
- Permethrin (disrupts Na channel of nerves)

Solar lentigenes
- Tretinoin

Recurrence of melanoma
- Alpha interferon + vaccine therapy

Atopic dermatitis
- *Topical*—corticosteroids
- *Severe systemic*—corticosteroids
- *Pruritis*—doxepin/hydroxyzine
- *Recalcitrant*—oral cyclosporin

For sparing steroids in atopic dermatitis
- Tacrolimus

Lichen simplex chronicus
- Highly potent corticosteroids

Psoriasis
- *Initial choice*—highly potent corticosteroids
- *Plaque type*—calcipotriene/tazoretene
- *Scalp*—tar
- *Advanced on scalp*—corticosteroids + keratinolytics
- *Extensive (>30% body surface)*—Goeckerman's regimen UVB
- *Non-responsive to Goeckerman's regimen*—PUVA therapy (psoralen + ultraviolet A)
- *Severe*—methotrexate/cyclosporin
- *Postular*—acitretin (teratogenic—not for pregnancy)

Psoriatic arthropathy
- *Initial stage*—NSAIDs
- *Later stage*—methotrexate

Gardnerella vaginalis
- Metronidazole

Ovulation induction
- Clomiphene citrate

Clomiphene resistant patients
- Chorionic gonadotropin with menotropins/urofollitropins

Porphyria cutanea tarda
- Hydroxychloroquine

Acne rosacea
- Oral tetracycline

Seborrheic dermatitis
- *Scalp*—zinc/selenium shampoo
- *Face*—weak corticosteroids (fluorinated)
- *Non-hairy and intertriginous areas*—weak corticosteroids

Taenia (body ringworms)
- Topical clotrimazole

Systemic dermatophytosis, recalcitrant dermatophytosis
- Griseofulvin

Stevens-Johnson syndrome
- Ig IV

Erythropoietic protoporphyria
- Beta carotene

Tinea cruris (Jock itch)
- Terbinafine

Long-term contraception
- Norplant (levonorgestrel)

Tinea pedis (athlete foot—MC cause of leg cellulitis)
- *Maceration stage*—aluminium subacetate
- *Dry and scaly stage*—azole antifungal

Tinea versicolor
- Selenium sulphide/ketoconazole

Discoid lupus erythematous (DLE)
- *Initial choice*—topical corticosteroids
- *Long-term*—hydroxychloroquine
- *Refractory*—thalidomide

DOC IN OPHTHALMOLOGY
Inclusion conjunctivitis
- Ceftriaxone

Keratitis
- *Herpetic*—idoxuridine
- *Acanthamoeba*—amphotericin B + pentamidine
- *Recalcitrant stromal/uveal herpetic*—acyclovir
- *Fusarium solani*—natamycin

Herpes zoster ophthalmicus
- Acyclovir

Secondary glaucoma
- Beta blockers

To reduce IOP
1. Before surgery
2. Severe rise
3. Diabetes
   - Mannitol

Glaucoma

PG analogues, **C**holinomimetics for increase **O**utflow   **PCO**

Beta blockers, **D**iuretics for reduced **S**ecretion   **BDS**

Scleritis, uveitis, allergic conjunctivitis (vernal catarrah), phlyctenular conjunctivitis, cystoid macular edema after intraocular edema, allergic keratitis
- Topical corticosteroids

Corneal graft rejection prevention, posterior uveitis, Vogt-Koyanagi-Harada syndrome, retrobulbar neuritis, malignant exophthalmos, orbital lymphangioma and pseudotumors, anterior ischaemic optic neuritis, papillitis
- Systemic corticosteroids

Drugs of Choice (DOC)

Prevention of meiosis during cataract surgery, to reduce postoperative cystoid macular edema after ECC extraction
- Flurbiprofen

Recurrent anterior uveitis
- NSAIDs

Mild allergic conjunctivitis
- Topical antihistaminics

Iridocyclitis
- Atropine

Mydriasis
- *Adults*—tropicamide/phenylephrine
- *Children*—atropine

Glaucoma
- *Primary open angle*—timolol
- *Angle closure*—acetazolamide/mannitol
- *Low tension*—latanoprost
- *Hypertension*—timolol

Corneal ulcers
- Cyclopentolate

DOC IN ENT DISEASES

Acute otitis media
- Coamoxyclave

Acute otitis externa, otomycosis

Necrotising otitis externa
- Ciprofloxacin/meropenem/gentamycin

Chronic suppurative otitis media
- Ciprofloxacin

Acute mastoiditis
- Vancomycin + ceftriaxone

Acute rhinosinusitis
- Coamoxyclave/ceftriaxone/clindamycin

Chronic rhinosinusitis
- *Pseudomonal*—ciprofloxacin
- *Fungal*—voriconazole

Tonsilloadenoiditis
- Cephalosporin +/– metronidazole

Acute pharyngitis
- Erythromycin/clarithromycin

Diphtheria
- Erythromycin/clindamycin/penicillin + antitoxin

Sialadenitis
- Penicillin/cephalosporin/clindamycin

Tonsillitis
- Penicillin

Severe peripheral vestibular dysfunction
- Gentamicin

Facial pain
- TCA/gabapentin

Glossopharyngeal neuralgia
- Carbamazepine

Otosclerosis
- Sodium fluoride

CSOM
- Ciprofloxacin

DOC IN CANCERS

ALL
- *Induction*—**DVPLasp** (**D**aunorubicin + **V**incristine + **P**rednisolone + **L**-asparaginase
- *Maintenance*—methotrexate + mercaptopurine + cyclophosphamide

AML
- Cytarabine + mitoxantrone/anthracycline

CML
- Imatinib/busulphan/hydroxyureas/alpha interferon

CLL
- Chlorambucil, fludarabine, prednisolone

Hodgkin's disease (stages III and IV)
- **ABVD** (**A**driamycin, **B**leomycin, **V**inblastine, **D**acarbazine)

Non-Hodgkin's lymphoma (intermediate and high grade)
- CHOP (**C**yclophosphamide, **V**incristine, **D**oxorubicin, **P**rednisolone) +/− rituximab

Cutaneous T cell lymphoma (mycosis fungoides)
- Topical carmustine, targretin, denileukin diftitox, radiotherapy

Microglobulinemia
- Fludarabine/chlorambucil

Essential thrombocytosis
- Anagrelide

Polycythemia vera
- Chlorambucil/busulphan

Adrenal glands
- Mitotane

Thyroid glands
- Cisplatin + ^{131}I + doxorubicin

Wilms' tumor
- Vincristine + dactinomycin

Carcinoid
- 5-FU + streptozocin +/− alpha interferon

Osteogenic sarcoma
- Methotrexate, doxorubicin, vincristine

Melanoma
- Dacarbazine, alpha interferon, IL-2

Neuroblastoma
- Cyclophosphamide + cisplatin + vincristine + doxorubicin + dacarbazine

Endometrium
- Progestin

Stomach
- Cisplatin + 5-fluorouracil

Colon
- Cisplatin + irinotecan/oxaliplatin

Rectum
- 5-fluorouracil + RT

Kidney
- Floxuridine, vinblastine, alpha interferon, IL-2

Insulinoma
- Streptozocin

Acute promyelocytic leukemia
- Retinoic acid + idarubicin

Pancreas
- Gemcitabine

Hairy cell leukemia
- Cladarabine

Kaposi sarcoma
- IF$_2$ alpha, doxorubicin, vincristine

Liver CA with secondaries, colorectal cancer
- 5-fluorouracil

Pustular psoriasis, psoriatic arthropathy, ectopic pregnancy, malignant meningitis due to leukemia, prophylaxis of CNS due to leukemia
- Methotrexate

Choriocarcinoma
- Methotrexate + dactinomycin + chlorambucil

Multiple myeloma
- Melphalan + prednisolone/**VAD** (**V**incristine + **A**driamycin + **D**examethasone)
- Melphalan + cyclophosphamide + carmustine + vincristine + doxorubicin + prednisolone
- Bortezomib for relapse

Waldenström's macroglobulinemia
- Fludarabine/chlorambucil/cyclophosphamide, vincristine + prednisolone

Brain cancers
- Nitrosoureas

Hemorrhagic cystitis due to cyclophosphamide/ifosfamide
- Mesna

Anticancers induced toxicity
- Amifostine (SH donating agent)

Anthracycline induced cardiotoxicity/myopathy
- Dextrozoxane

To increase neutrophils in immunocompromised
- Lithium

Severe pancytopenia due to anticancer
- Erythropoietin/GM-CSF

Small cell lung CA
- Etoposide + cisplatin

Non-small cell lung CA
- *Localised*—cisplatin/carboplatin, docetaxel
- *Advanced*—cisplatin/carboplatin, docetaxel, gemfitizib, etoposide, vinblastine, venorelbine

CA head and neck
- Cisplatin + 5-fluorouracil + paclitaxel

CA esophagus
- Mitomycin + cisplatin + 5-fluorouracil

Hypercalcemia in malignancy
- Glucocorticoids

Advanced ovarian and breast cancer
- Pacitaxel and docetaxel/paclitaxel + cisplatin/carboplatin
- *Node +ve*—doxorubicin/epirubicin + 5-FU/cyclophosphamide/docetaxel/paclitaxel
- *Node –ve*—drugs listed above/CMV (cyclophosphamide + methotrexate + 5-FU)
- *Estrogen/progesterone +ve*—tamoxifen

Breast cancer expressing HER 2 receptors
- Trastuzumab

Superficial cancer of urinary bladder
- BCG (intravesical)
- **CMV/MVAC** (**M**ethotrexate + **V**inblastine + **A**driamycin + **C**isplatin)

Testes
- Etoposide + cisplatin

Prostate
- Estrogen/GnRH analogues/flutamide

Uterus
- Progestin/tamoxifen

Ovary
- Paclitaxel + cisplatin/carboplatin

Cervix
- Methotrexate, doxorubicin, cisplatin, vinblastine
- Mitomycin, bleomycin, vincristine, cisplatin

DOC FOR POISONING

Acute arsenic and mercury
- Dimercaprol

Chronic mercury
- N-acetyl penicillamine

Iron
- Deferoxamine

Copper and Wilson's disease
- Zinc acetate/D-penicillamine

Lead
- DMSA (succimer)

Acute lead toxicity
- EDTA + BAL

Asymptomatic child of lead
- Vitamin C

Alpha-1 agonist
- Phentolamine

Beta-2 agonist
- Propranolol

Ergot alkaloid
- Sodium nitroprusside

Methylxanthines
- Propranolol

Carbon dioxide
- Hyperbaric oxygen

Warfarin
- Vitamin K

Heparin
- Protamin sulphate

Iodine
- Starch

MAO inhibitors
- *HTN phase*—Na nitroprusside
- *Hypotension phase*—NE

Anticholinergics
- Physostigmine

Carbamate
- Atropine

BZD
- Flumazenil

Cyanide
- Amylnitrite, EDTA, oxygen, Na thiosulphate, hydroxycobalamin

Ethylene glycol/methanol
- Ethanol/fomepizole (4-methylpyrrazole)

Cardiac glycosides
- Digoxin specific Ab fragments (Fab)

Aspirin
- Vitamin K + fresh frozen plasma

Paracetamol
- N-acetylcysteine

Opioid
- Naloxone

INH
- Vitamin B_6

CCBs
- Calcium + glucagon

Antipsychotics
- Lidocaine + Na bicarbonate

TCA
- Na bicarbonate

EDTA is commonly used in poisoning of
- Mn   MIC CPZ
- I*ron*
- C*u*
- C*d*
- P*b*
- Z*n*

CI of EDTA: Hg because it is firmly bound to tissue.

Penicillamine is commonly used in poisoning of
- Mercury
- Au
- Cu
- Cd
- Pb
- Zn   MAC CPZ

CI of penicillamine: As

Dimercaprol (BAL) is commonly used in poisoning of
- Bi   BAL HANGC
- As
- Lead
- Hg
- Antimony
- Ni
- Gold
- Cu

CI of BAL: Fe and Cd because of Fe-BAL and Cd-BAL complex are toxic.

DOC FOR MISCELLANEOUS DISEASES

Midline shift on CT scan due to severe brain edema
- Dexamethasone

Post-traumatic/surgical brain abscess
- Ceftriaxone + metronidazole + nafcillin/vancomycin

Lactation abscess
- Nafcillin/oxacillin

Metastatic bone pain, vitamin D intoxication, idiopathic hypercalcemia
- Calcitonin

Right ventricular infarction
- Vasodilators

Breast cancer
- Cyclophosphamide

TSH producing edema, VIPoma, GIPoma
- Octreotide

Darrier disease
- Retinoic acid

Raised ICT due to tumors
- Glucocorticoids

Pleuropulmonary anaerobic infections
- Penicillin

Initial treatment liver abscess triple therapy
- **P**enicillin + **A**minoglycosides + **M**etronidazole   **PAM**
- *Percutaneous abscess drainage under CT guidance (TOC)*

Pelvic infection triple therapy
- Gentamicin + metronidazole + clindamycin

Perirectal abscess
- *Outpatients*—metronidazole + augmentin/ciprofloxacin
- *Inpatients*—cefotetan + piperacillin/tazobactam + imipenem

Pustular acne
- *Topical*—tretinoin/benzoyl peroxide
- *Oral*—minocycline/doxycycline

Antibiotic resistant acne: Isotretinoin

Acromegaly
- *Initial*—bromocriptine
- *Non-responsive*—octreotide/pegvisoment

Actinomycosis
- Penicillin

Alpha-antitrypsin deficiency
- Pooled human alpha-1 antitrypsin

High altitude pulmonary edema, peripheral vascular disease
- Nifedipine

Renal amyloidosis
- Colchicine

Amurosis fugas (Holenhost plaque in retinal artery)
- Heparin

Hereditary sideroblastic anemia
- Vitamin B_6

Still's disease
- Aspirin

Lupus nephritis
- Cyclophosphamide

Acute rheumatic fever
- Penicillin

Vertical transmission of HBV
- Ig at 1 and 6 month

Radiation induced diarrhea
- Aspirin

Reactive arthritis
- Indomethacin

Familial mediterranean fever, prevention of acute attack of amyloidosis
- Colchicine

Cogan's syndrome, idiopathic cutaneous vasculitis, Henoch-Schönlein purpura
- Prednisolone

Lyme disease
- Doxycycline

Fibromyalgia
- TCAs

Urate nephropathy, overproduction of uric acid, advanced renal failure
- Allopurinol

Kawasaki disease
- Aspirin + Ig IV

Painful gynaecomastia
- Tamoxifen

To dissolve gallstones
- Chenodeoxycholic acid/urodeoxycholic acid

Stone prevention in cystinuria
- Penicillamine

Acute gout
- Indomethacin

Acute intermittent porphyria
- Hematin

Photodermatitis
- Chloroquine/aspirin

Phantom limb
- Mexiletine

Thiazide induced hyperuricemia
- Probenecid

AUTOIMMUNE

Idiopathic thrombocytopenic purpura
- Prednisolone
- Vincristine
- Azathioprine

Autoimmune haemolytic anaemia
- Prednisone
- Cyclophosphamide
- Mercaptopurine

Acute glomerulonephritis
- Prednisone
- Mercaptopurine
- Cyclophosphamide

Systemic lupus erythematosus, rheumatoid arthritis, chronic active hepatitis, inflammatory bowel disease
- Prednisone
- Cyclophosphamide
- Azathioprine
- Cyclosporin

Acquired factor XIII Ab
- Cyclophosphamide + factor XIII

ISOIMMUNE

Hemolytic anaemia of the newborn
- Rho (D) immunoglobulins

Organ transplantation
- *Heart*—azathioprine, cyclosporin
- *Kidney*—prednisone, Ab
- *Liver*—cyclosporin and prednisone
- *Bone marrow*—cyclosporin, cyclophosphamide, methotrexate, prednisone

DOC IN RENAL DISEASES

Allergy to thiazides/loop diuretics
- Ethacrynic acid (due to different chemical structure)

Idiopathic hypercalciuria, calciuria in hyperparathyroidism, calcium oxalate type renal stone, Liddle's syndrome, hypertension and nephrogenic DI
- Thiazides

Hypercalcaemia, hypertensive encephalopathy, edema in CHF, renal and liver disease
- Furosemide

Cerebral edema
- Mannitol

Alkalization of urine, acute mountain sickness, familial periodic paralysis and acute narrow angle glaucoma
- Acetazolamide

Primary hyperaldosteronism (Conn syndrome), secondary aldosteronism, thiazide induced hypokalemia, refractory ascites and reducing mortality in CHF
- Spironolactone

Lithium induced nephropathy
- Amiloride

Urate nephropathy, gout with renal failure, hyperuricemia in renal failure, hyperuricemia during anticancer chemotherapy and Lesch-Nyhan syndrome
- Allopurinol

ANAESTHETICS OF CHOICE (AOC)

LA of choice, regional block (Bier's block), spinal anaesthesia
- Lidocaine

Lidocaine allergy
- Prilocaine

Prilocaine-induced Methaemoglobinemia (due to O-toluidine)
- Methylene blue

LA in obstetrics
- Bupivacaine (levobupivacaine is non-cardiotoxic)

Epidural block
- Bupivacaine

LA-induced cardiac arrhythmia
- Bretylium

ENT, dental, maxilofacial, head, neck and obstetrical surgeries
- Nitrous oxide

AOC without monitoring
- Ether

Neurosurgery, cardiothoracic surgery, cardiac, hepatic and renal surgery, day care surgery and hypotensive AOC.
- **Isoflurane surgery in children**
- Ketamine (NMDA antagonist. Sevoflurane is alternative)

Induction, Lie detection in criminals and facilitating communication in psychiatric patients
- Thiopentone (scopolamine is alternative)

Fast induction
- Sevoflurane (desflurane—fastest action, most irritant, highest vapour pressure)

Day care surgery
- Propofol

Manual removal of placenta, external obstetrical version
- Halothane

Shock, sepsis and hypotensive patients
- Ketamine (cyclopropane is alternative)

Porphyrias
- Ketamine

Thiopentone induced shivering
- Pethidine

GA induced cardiac arrhythmia (halothane is MC)
- Lidocaine

Malignant hyperthermia, Stiffman syndrome
- Dantrolene

LA in malignant hyperthermia
- Procaine

Short procedures
- Succinylcholine (MC ADR—muscle pain)

Hepatic and renal failure, hepatobiliary atresia, myasthenia gravis (10% of normal dose)
- Atracurium

Bronchial asthma
- Pancuronium

Day care surgery
- Mivacurium (shortest acting MR)

Motor neurone disease
- Riluzole (glutamate antagonist)

Spasm in multiple sclerosis, spinal spasticity
- Baclofen

Stereotectic brain surgery
- Neurolept anaesthesia

Laparoscopic surgery
- Carbon dioxide

Histotoxic hypoxia, acute hypoxic respiratory failure, pure vetilatory failure and carbon monoxide poisoning
- Oxygen

Index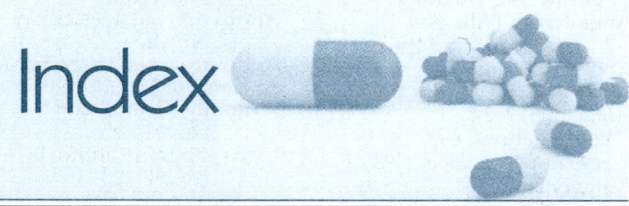

A

Abacavir *See* Antiviral
Abciximab 495
Abortion *See* Oxytocin
Acarbose 350
Acebutolol *See* Ppl
Acenocoumarol *See* Warfarin
Acetaminophen *See* Paracetamol
Acetazolamide 302, 384
Acetomenaphthone 720
Acetylation *See* MFO
Acetylcholine (ACh) 56
Acetylcholinesterase (AChE) 59
Acetylcysteine 520
Acetyldigoxin *See* Digoxin
Acetylsalicylic acid *See* Aspirin
Acid neutralizing capacity (ANC) 490
Acne vulgaris, drugs for 701
Acromegaly *See* GH
ACTH (Adrenocorticotropic hormone) *See* Adrenal cortex 279
Actinomycin D 674
Action potential (AP) 360
  in heart effect of digit on fast channel 361
  slow channel in nerve 42, 361
Activation of drugs 22
Active transport of drugs 8
Acyclovir 649
Addiction to drugs *See* ADR
Addison's disease *See* ACTH
Adenosine 390
Adenylyl cyclase, cAMP pathway 27
Adrenaline (Adr) 67
Adrenergic 64–74
  blockers 75
  drugs 69
  neuron blockers 83
  receptors 73
  transmission 46

Adrenochrome monosemicarbazone 445
Adrenocorticosteroids 227
Adroamycin *See* Doxorubicin
Adverse drug effects 33, 770–83
Affinity 29
Agonist 29
Albendazole 638
Alcohol 179, 221
  drinking: safe guidelines 180
  drinking: motivation for 181
  ethyl, methyl 183
Alcoholic beverages *See* Ethanol
Alcoholism *See* Ethanol
Aldehyde dehydrogenase inhibitors *See* Disulfiram
Aldosterone 281
Aldosterone induced protein (AIP) *See* Aldosterone
Alendronate *See* Bisphosphonate
Alfa adrenergic blockers 75–79
Alfacalcidol *See* Vit D
Alkylating agents 655
Allergy to drugs *See* ADR
Allopurinol 258
Alopecia *See* Finasteride
Alprazolam *See* BZD
Alprostadil *See* PGE
Alteplase (rt-PA) 492
Aluminium hydroxide 232, 491
Alzheimer's disease *See* Taecrine
Amantadine 654
Ambroxol 544
Ambemonium 56
Amdinocillin *See* Pn
Amethocaine *See* Tetracaine
Amifostine 675
Amikacin (Am) 584
Amylobarbitone 126
Amiloride 426

Amineptine *See* SSRI
Aminoglycoside antibiotics 582
  common properties 582
  mechanism of action 583
  shared toxicities 584
Aminoglutethimide 290
Aminopenicillins *See* Pn
Aminophylline *See* Theophylline
5-Aminosalicylic acid (5-ASA) *See* Mesalazine *See* Sulfasalazine
Amineptine 160
Amiodarone 381
Amithiozone *See* Thiacetazone
Amitriptyline 160
Amlodipine 388
Ammonium chloride 430
Amodiaquine *See* Mefloquine
Amoebiasis, treatment of 609
Amoxapine 160
Amoxicillin *See* Penicillin
Amphenone 290
Amphetamine 70, 211
Amphotericin B (AMB) 630
Ampicillin 547
Amprenavir 658
Amrinone 373
Anabolic steroids 292
Analgesic: definition *See* NSAIDs
  nonopioid *See* NSAIDs
  opioid *See* Morphine
Analgin *See* Chap 70
Anaemia 687–93
Anaesthesia *See* Chap 10
Analeptic 171
Anaphylactic reaction *See* ADR
Anaphylactic shock, treatment of *See* ADR
Anastrozole 675
Ancrod 482
Androgens 290
  transdermal 5

Androsterone *See* Androgen
Aneurine *See* Thiamine
Angiotensin (All) *See*
    Captopril 438–47
Anorectic drugs 73
Antabuse *See* Disulfiram
Antacid 519–24
  combinations 493
  role in peptic ulcer 493
Antagonism 29
Antagonist, competitive 29
Antazoline 414
Anterior pituitary
    hormones *See*
    Hormones
Anthelmintics *See*
    Albendazole
Anthraquinone purgatives 510
Antibiotic 531
Anticancer drugs 663–86
Anticholinergic drugs *See*
    Atropine 57
Anticholinesterases *See*
    Physostigmine 52
Anticoagulants 479
Anticonvulsants *See* Diazepam
Antidepressants *See* TCA 207
Antidiuretics 432
Antidiuretic hormone
    (ADH) 433
Antiemetics 449
Antifungal 629–36
Antiepileptics *See* CBZ
Antiestrogens 248
Antifolate 578
Antifungal drugs *See* KTZ
Antihaemophilic factor 445
Antihistamines *See* Citrizine
  H_1 blockers 448–56
  H_2 blockers 448–56
  H_3 antagonist 448
  second generation 448–56
Anti *H. pylori* drugs 523
Antihypertensive drugs *See*
    Chap 32
  combination of *See* Chap 31
Antileprotic drugs 591
Antimalarial drugs 614
  causal prophylaxis 615
  clinical cure 615
  for chloroquine resistant
    falciparum malaria 616, 617
  gametocidal 615
  radical cure 615
  suppressive prophylaxis 617
Antimicrobial 531
Antimonials, antineoplastic *See*
    Anticancer drugs
Antioxidant vitamina *See* Vit A
Antiparkinsonian drugs 68
Antiplatelet drugs *See*
    Ticlopidin

Antipsychotic drugs *See*
    Fluoxetine
Antipyretic-analgesics *See*
    NSAIDs
Anti-retrovirus drugs *See* AZT
Antisera 693
  diphtheria antitoxin
    (ADS) 693
  gas gangrene antitoxin
    (AGS) 693
  rabies (ARS) 693
  snake venom polyvalent 696
  tetanus antitoxin (ATS) 693
Antithrombotic *See* Atiplatelet
    drugs 462
Antithymocyte globulin
    (ATG) 671
Antithyroid drugs *See* TH
Antitubercular drugs *See*
    INH 604–13
Antitussive 543
Antivirial drugs 647–62
Apomorphine 525
Aprotinin 497
Arecoline 52
Arteether 621
Artemisinin 621
Artesunate 622
Ascorbic acid *See* Vit C
Aspirin 263
Astemizole 454
Asthma 527
  bronchial 527
Astringents 707
Atenolol *See* β blocker
ATG 684
Atovaquone 605
Atracurium 91
Atrial fibrillation *See* Chap 31
Atrial flutter (Afl) *See* Chap 31
Atropine 58
Atypical antidepressants *See*
    TCA
Atypical neuroleptics *See* SSRI
Auranofin *See* Gold
Aurothiomalate sod *See* Gold
Autacoids, definition 397
Autonomic influences on
    heart *See* ANS
Autoreceptors *See* Receptors
Azathioprine 671
Azelastine 456
Azithromycin 587
AZT (Azidothymidine) *See*
    Zidovudine
Aztreonam 553

B

Bacampicillin 547
Bacitracin 590
Baclofen 101
BAL *See* Dimercaprol
Bambuterol 545
Barbiturates *See*
    Phenobarbitone 158, 209

BCNU *See* Carmustine
Belladonna poisoning *See* Anti
    Ch E
Benazepril 403
Benidipine *See* Chap 70
Benzathine penicillin *See*
    Pn 565
Benzhexol *See*
    Trihexyphenidyl
Benzocaine *See* LA
Benzodiazepines (BZDs)
    164–70
Benzoic acid 636
Benzthiadiazines *See*
    Thiazides
Benzoyl peroxide 705
Benzyl benzoate 712
Beta adrenergic blockers 80–86
Beta-lactam antibiotics 543
Beta-lactamase 564–74
  inhibitors 569
Betamethasone, also *See*
    Corticosteroids 282
Betaxolol *See* Beta blockers:
    ocular
Bethanechol 52
Bezafibrate 477
Bhang See CNS stimulant
Bicuculline 171
Biguanides 349
Bile acid sequestrants
    (resins) *See* Lovastatin
Bioavailability 9
Bioequivalence 10
Biotin *See* Vit B
Biotransformation 13
Bisacodyl 536
Bisoprolol *See* β blocker
Bisphosphonates 326–28
Beta stimulant 72
Bitters 531
Black wilder spider toxin *See*
    Chap 5
Bleomycin 674
Blood–brain barrier 12
Bradykinin 398
  antagonists 403
Bran 534
Bretylium 383
Bromhexine 544
Bromocriptine 193
Bronchodilators *See*
    Salbutamol 545
Buclizine 414–19
Bulaquine 605
Bupivacaine *See* LA
Buprenorphine 185
Bupropion 160
Buserelin *See* Hormone
Buspirone 191
Busulfan 668
Butobarbitone 126
Butorphanol 185

Index

C

Butyrocholinesterase (BuChE) *See* Pseudocholinesterase

Caffeine 522
Calciferol 720
Calcipotriol 720
Calcitonin 278
Calcitriol 720
Calcium 324–28
  channels 384–88
  channel blockers (CCBs) 341
  edetate (calcium EDTA) 696
Camphor 708
Cancer chemotherapy *See* Anticancer drugs
Candesartan 446
Cannabinoids 170
Cannabis 215
Canthridin 708
Capecitabine 678
Capreomycin (Cpt) *See* Fusidic acid
Capsicum 708
Captopril 442
Captopril test 408
Carbachol 52
Carbamazepine 174
Carbapenems 554
Carbenicillin 547
  indanyl 547
  phenyl 547
Carbenoxolone 523
Carbetapentane 521
Carbidopa 246
Carbimazole 319–23
Carbocisteine 520
Carbolic acid *See* Phenol
Carbonic anhydrase inhibitors 423–25
Carboplatin 677
Carboprost (15-methyl PGF$_{2\alpha}$) *See* PGF
Cardiac glycosides *See* Digitalis 365–73
Cardiotonic drugs also *See* Digitalis
Carisoprodol 101
Carminatives 531
Cartiolol *See* β blocker
Carvedilol *See* β blocker
Castor oil 510
Catecholamines (CAs) *See* DA
CCNU *See* Lomustine
Cefaclor 550
Cefadroxil 550
Cefazolin 550
Cefdinir 550
Cefepime 551
Cefixime 551
Cefoperazone 550
Cefotaxime 550

Cefoxitin 550
Cefpirome 551
Cefpodoxime proxetil 551
Ceftazudume 550
Ceftibuten 551
Ceftizoxime 550
Ceftriaxone 550
Cefuroxime 550
Cefuroxime axetil 550
Celecoxib 274
Celiprolol *See* β blocker
Cell cycle *See* Vit A
Centchroman *See* OC
Cephalexin 550
Cephalosporins 570
Cephalothin 572
Cephradine 573
Cerebral malaria *See* Chloroquine
Cetirizine 414–19, 424
Charas See CNS stimulants
Cheese reaction *See* MAOI
Chelating agents *See* EDTA
Chemotherapy *See* Antimicrobial 553–63
Chenodeoxycholic acid (chenodiol) 505
Child dose calculation 31
Chlophedianol 521
Chloral hydrate 170, 213
Chlorambucil 668
Chloramphenicol 579
Chlordiazepoxide *See* BZD
Chlorhexidine *See* Chap 70
Chlormezanone 101
Chloroform 147
Chloroguanide *See* Proguanil 619
Chloroquine 616
Chlorothiazide *See* Thiazides
Chlorpheniramine 414–19
Chlorpromazine (CPZ) 186
Chlorpropamide 302
Chlorprothixene 153
Chlortetracycline 555
Cholecalciferol 720
Cholestyramine 501–03
Choline esters *See* ACh
Cholinergic 49
  crisis/weakness 58
  drugs 44–56
  transmission 51
Cholinesterases 51
Cholinesterase reactivators *See* Pralidoxime
Cholinoceptors 45
Cholinomimetic alkaloides *See* ACh
Cidofovir 657
Cilazapril 403
Cilostazol *See* Chap 70
Cimetidine *See* H$_2$ antagonists 514
Cinalukast 526

Cinchocaine *See* Dibucaine
Cinchonism 601
Cinnarizine 455
Ciprofloxacin 599
Cisapride 529
Cisatracurium 101
Cisplatin 676
Citalopram 160
Citrovorum factor *See* Folinic acid rescue
Clarithromycin 587
Classification of drugs 737–69
Clavulanic acid 569
Clearance (CL) of drugs 18
Clemastine 414–19
Clindamycin 588
Clioquinol *See* Quiniodochlor
Clobetasol butyrate 704
Clobetasol propionate 704
Clofazimine (Clo) 610
Clofibrate 506
Clomiphene citrate 248
Clomipramine 160
Clonazepam *See* BZD
Clonidine 405
Clopidogrel 495
Clorgiline 160
Cloffing factors 441
Clotrimazole 635
Clotting factors 474
Cloxacillin 547
Clozapine 424, 425, 461
CNS stimulants *See* Bhang
Coagulants 444–45
Coal tar 705
Cocaine 202, 215
Codeine 179, 521
Codergocrine *See* Dihydroergotoxine
Cognition-enhancers *See* Tacrine
Colchicine 255 *See* Gout
Colestipol 472
Colistin 589
Colloidal bismuth subcitrate (CBS) 522
Coma 691
Congestive heart failure (CHF) 313
Conjugation reactions 535
Contraceptives *See* OC
Converting enzyme inhibitors *See* Angiotensin
Convulsants *See* BZD
Corticosteroids 329–37
Corticotropin *See* ACTH 329–37
Cortisol *See* Hydrocortisone 329–37
Cosyntropin *See* Steroid
Co-transmission 48
Cortimazine 577
Cotrimoxazole 577

Cough *See* Respiratory drug
Counter-irritants 708
COX-1/COX-2 (cyclo-
    oxygenase)
    isoenzymes *See*
    NSAIDs
Cromoglycate sod (cromolyn
    sod) *See* Asthma
Cross resistance 536
Crotamiton 703
Cumulation *See* ADR
Curare, also *See*
    Tubocurarine 97
Cyanocobalamin 726
Cyclic GMP (cGMP) 27
Cyclizine 414–19
Cyclophosphamide 666
Cycloserine (Cys) 588
Cyclosporine 683
Cyproheptadine 414–19, 461
Cyproterone acetate 293
Cytarabine 672
Cytochrome P450 (CYP)
    isoenzymes 21
Cytotoxic drugs *See* 5-FU

D

Dacarbazine (DTIC) 668
Dactinomycin *See*
    Actinomycin D
Dalfopristin/Quinupristin *See*
    Fusidic acid
Danaparoid 464
Danazol 294
Danthron *See* Chap 70
Dantrolene 92
Dapsone (DDS) 610
Daunorubicin
    (Rubidomycin) 675
Dazoxiben 494
DDS *See* Dapsone
DDT *See* Dicophane
Decamethonium (C-10) *See*
    SCh
Deglycyrrhizinized 495
Dehydroemetine *See* DHE
Delavirdine 658
Demecarium 56
Demeclocycline 555
Demecarium 56
Demelanizing agents 707
Demulsants 520, 707
Deprenyl *See* Selegiline 160
Depression (of function)
    mental *See* TCA
Desamino oxytocin *See*
    Oxytocin
Desferrioxamine 692
Desflurane *See* GA 138
Desipramine *See* SSRI
Desloratadine 454
Desmopressin 435
Desogestrel *See* OC

Dexamethasone, also *See*
    Corticoster 282, 704
Dexamphetamine 76
Dexfenfluramine 76
Dextran 510
Dextromethorphan 545
DFP *See* Dyflos
DHE (Dihydroergotamine) *See*
    Ergotamine
Dibenamine 83
Dibetes
    insipidus *See* ADH
    mellitus 338–53
Diabetic hyperosmolar
    (nonketotic) coma 302
Diabetic ketoacidosis (diabetic
    coma) 301
Diacetylmorphine (heroin) *See*
    Opium
Diarrhoea 512
Diazepam 126
Diazinon (TIK-20) *See*
    Organophosphates
Diazoxide 402
Dibucaine *See* LA
Diclofenac sod 218
Dicloxacillin 547
Dicumarol *See* Bishydroxycou-
    marin
Dicyclomine 69
Didanosine *See* AZT
Diebestrol *See* OC
Diethyl carbamazine
    (DEC) 640
Diethylstilbestrol
    (stilbestrol) *See* OC
Diffusion hypoxia *See* GA (gas)
Diflorasone 704
Diflunisal 269
Degestants 531
Digitalis 365–73
Digitalization 365–73
Digitoxin 365–73
Digoxin (also *See* Digitalis)
Dihydralazine *See*
    Hydralazine 358
Dihydroergotoxine 428
Dihydrofolate reductase
    (DHFRase)
    inhibitors *See*
    sulfonamide
Dihydrotestosterone *See*
    Androgen
Dilazep *See* Chap 70
Diloxanide furoate 625
Diltiazem 338
Dimenhydrinate 414
Dimercaprol (BAL) 695
Dimercaptosuccinic acid *See*
    Succimer
Dimethicone *See* Skin drugs
Dimethindene 414
Dimethylpolysiloxane *See*
    Dimethicone

Dinoprost (PGF$_{2\alpha}$) *See* PG
Dioctyl sulfosuccinate
    (DOSS) 509
Diosmins *See* Chap 71
Diphenhydramine 414
Diphenylhydantoin *See*
    Phenytoin
Dipivefrine 149
Dipyridamole 493
Dipyrone *See* Metamizol
Disopyramide 379
Dissociative anaesthesia *See*
    Ketamine
Disulfiram 182
Diuretics 416
Divalproex *See* Chap 70
DMPA (depot
    medroxyprogesterone
    acetate) *See* OC
DMPP (dimethyl phenyl
    piperazinium)
Dobutamine *See* DA
DOCA (desocycorticosterone
    acetate) also *See*
    Mineralocorticoid
Docetaxel 674
Dofetilide 362
Domperidone 530
Donepezil 56
Donovanosis *See* Granuloma
    inguinale
DOPA 76
Dopamine (DA) 69
Dorzolamide *See* CAse I
Dose-response relationship 25
Dothiepin 160
Doxazosin 83
Doxepin 160
Doxycycline 555
Doxylamine 414
Droperidol 153
Drotaverine *See* Chap 70
Drug
    absorption 7, 9
    abuse *See* ADR
    action 22
    activation 23
    addiction *See* ADR
    adverse effects 38
    allergy 40
    combined effect of 29
    definition 1
    diffusion 7
    distribution 10
    development and testing 2
    dosage 19
    effect 28, 29
    efficacy 29
    essential 4
    factors modifying action
        of 30
    habituation *See* ADR
    induced diseases *See* ADR

interactions: mechanisms
of 12
nomenclature 3
orphan 4
routes of administration 4
Drugs of choice 790–819
DTIC *See* Dacarbazine
Dyflos *See*
Organophosphates
428–32

E

Ebastine 414
Echothiophate 56
Econazole 619
Edetate *See* EDTA
Edrophonium 56
EDRF (endothelium dependent
relaxing factor) *See*
Chap 7
Efavirenz 653
Eicosanoids *See* PG
Emesis 497
Emetine 625
Emetics 499
Emollients 707
Enalapril, also *See* Angiotensin
converting
enzyme inhibitors 443
Endogenous opioid 187
Endorphins 187
Enfenamic acid 217
Enflurane *See* GA
Enkephalins *See* Opioid
Enoxaparin *See* Heparin
Entacapone 194
Enteric fever *See* Typhoid fever
Enzyme
induction 29
inhibition 29
stimulation 29
Ephedrine 71
Epidural anaesthesia *See* LA
Epilepsies *See* Phenytoin
experimental models of
treatment 143
Epinephrine *See* Adrenaline
Epirubicin 675
Epoetin *See* Erythropoietin
Eprosartan 403
Epsilon amino caproic acid
(EACA) 466
EPSP (excitatory postsynaptic
potential) *See* Chap 5
Eptifibatide 465
Erogometrine
(ergonovine) 462
Ergot alkaloids 462–67
Ergotamine 462–67
Ergotoxine 462–67
Erythromycin 586
Esmolol *See* β blocker
Esomeprazole 489

Esophagitis *See*
Gastroesophageal
reflux
Essential drugs 4
Estradiol also *See* Estrogens
Estrogens, also *See* Oral
contraceptives 246, 295
Estrone *See* OC
Etanercept 253
Ethacrynic acid *See* Diuretics
Ethambutol (E) 606
Ethamsylate 445
Ethanol *See* Alcohol ethyl 148
Ether 134
Ethinyl estradiol, also *See* Oral
contraceptives
Ethinyl estranol *See*
Lynestrenol
Ethionamide (Etm) 588
Ethoheptazine 184
Ethosuccimide 175
Ethyl alcohol *See* Alcohol ethyl
Ethylene glycol poisoning *See*
Ethanol
Ethyl morphine 521
Etomidate 141
Etoposide 674
Eutectic lidocaine/
prilocaine *See* LA
Excretion of drugs 16

F

Facilitated diffusion *See*
Diffusion
Factors modifying drug
action 30
Famciclovir 658
Famotidine, *See* H_2
antagonists 487
Febrile convulsions *See*
Epilepsy
Felodipine 345
Fenofibrate 506
Fenfluramine 76
Fentanyl *See* GA 144
Feracrylum *See* Chap 70
Ferric *See* Anemia
Fexofenadine *See* Terfenadine
Fibric acid derivatives 505
Fibrin 457
Fibrinogen 477
Fibrinolytic drugs 488–97
Finasteride 293
First pass metabolism 16
Flavonoids *See* Chap 70
Flecanide 381
Flucloxacillin 547
Fluconazole 634
Flucytosine (5-FC) 633
Fludrocortisone 282
Flumazenil 135
Flunarizine 430
Flunitrazepam *See* BZD

Fluocinolone acetonide 704
Fluoroquinolones (FQs) 598
5-Fluorouracil (5-FU) 671
Fluoxetine 160
Flupenthixol 153
Fluphenazine 153
Flurazepam *See* BZD
Flurbiprofen *See* NSAIDs
Flutamide 295
Fluticasone propionate 704
Fluvoxamine 160
Folic acid 733
antagonists *See*
Dihydrofolate reductase
inhibitor
Folinic acid (THFA) 730
Fomepizole 183
Formoterol *See*
Salbutamol 545
Foscarnet 651
Fosinopril 403
Framycetin 564
Frusemide *See* Furosemide
FSH (follicle stimulating
hormone) *See* GnRH
Ftorafur 672
Furazolidone 610, 612
Furosemide 417
See High ceiling diuretics
Fusidic acid (fusidate sod) 568

G

$GABA_A$-benzodiazepine
receptor *See* BZD
$GABA_A$-receptor *See* BZD
Gabapentin *See* BZD
Gallamine 99
Gall stone dissolving
agents 532
Y-Vinyl GABA *See* Vigabatrin
Ganciclovir 651
Ganglionic blocking agents *See*
Lobeline 62
Gatifloxacin 600
Gemcitabine 678
Gemfibrozil 505
General anaesthetics
(GA) 121–54
Gene therapy 672
application of 672
Gentamicin 583
Gentamicin-PMMA
chains 563, 564
Gepirone 159
Giardiasis 610
Ginkgo biloba
(ginkgolide) 173, 438
Glaucoma *See* Mydriatics
Glibenclamide 348
Gliclazide 348
Glimepiride 348
Glipizide 348
Glucagon *See* Insulin

Glucocorticoids, 331–35
Glyburide See Glibenclamide
Glyceryl trinitrate (GTN) 353
Glycopeptide antibiotics 568
Glycoprotein (GP) II$_b$/III$_a$ antagonists See Ticlopidine
GnRH agonists See Chap 23
GnRH antagonists See Chap 23
Goiter See Chap 26
Gold 251
Gonadotropins (Gns) 235
Gonadotropin releasing hormone (GnRH, gonadorelin) 238
Gossypol 306
Gout See Allopurinol
G-proteins See CAMP
Granisetron 530
Grepafloxacin 583
Griseofulvin 632
Growth hormone (GH) 282–85
Guanethidine 404
Guar gum 351
Gugulipid 507

H

H$_1$ antagonists 453
H$_2$ antagonists 454
H$_3$ antagonists 454
Habituation See ADR
Haematinics 677
Haemostatic See Anaemia
Half life (t½) 18
Hallucinogens 170
Halofantrine 604
Haloperidol 153
Haloprogin 701
Halothane 135
Hamycin 61
Heavy metal antagonists See Chelating agents
Hemicholinium See Nicotine
Heparan sulfate 446–49
Heparin 479, 494
Heroin See Opium
Hetastarch (See Hydroxyethyl starch) 481
Hexamethonium 69
Hexamine See Methenamine
Hexobarbitone 126
High-ceiling diuretics See Furosemide
Histamine 411–13
'Hit and run' drugs See Tyramine
HMG-CoA Reductase inhibitors (statins) See Lovastatin
Homatropine See Atropine
Hormone, definition of 276–81
Hormone replacement therapy (HRT) 287
Hydralazine 400
Hydrochlorothiazide, also See Thiazide diuretics
Hydrocortisone 281 See Coritcosteroids
Hydrogen peroxide See Skin drugs
Hydroquinone 707
Hydroxocobalamin 726
Hydroxychloroquine See Chloroquine
Hydroxyethyl starch (HES) See Drugs for gut
Hydroxyprogesterone caproate See OC 303
8-Hydroxyquiniline 625
5-Hydroxytryptamine (5-HT) receptor subtypes See Serotonin
Hydroxyurea 666
Hydroxyzine 159, 414
Hyoscine 68
Hyperkinetic children See Attention deficit disorder
Hypersensitivity (allergic) reactions See ADR
Hypertension 411
Hypertensive emergencies/urgencies See Chap 32
Hyperthyroidism See Thyrotoxicosis
Hyperthyroidism See Thyrotoxicosis
Hypervitaminosis A See Vitamin A
Hypervitaminosis D See Vit D
Hypnotics See BZD
Hypoglycaemia See Insulin
Hypolipidemic drugs See Lovastatin
Hypothalamic hormones/factors 225
Hypsarrhythmia See Siezures

I

Ibuprofen See NSAIDs
Idarubicin 680
Idiosyncrasy See ADR
Idoxuridine 650
Ifosphamide 667
Imidazole antifungals 617
Imipenem 554
Imipramine See SSRI
Immunoglobulins (IGs) 671
Immunosuppressants 669
Impeded androgens See Danazol
Inamrinone See Amrinone
Indapamide See Diuretics
Indinavir See Acyclovir
Indomethacin See NSAID
Infliximab 254
INH See Isoniazid
Inhaled steroids See Skin drugs
Inhibin 236
Insulin 339–53
Insulin like growth factors (IGFs) 339
Interferon See Amantadine 655
Intolerance See ADR
Intra-arterial injection See Chap 1
Intradermal injection See Chap 1
Intramuscular injection (IM) See Chap 1
Intravenous anaesthetics See LA
Intravenous injection (IV) See Chap 1
Intravenous regional anaesthesia See LA
Intrinsic activity 24
Inverse agonists 24
Iodide, sod/pot 273
Iodine, radioactive (^{131}I) 322
Iodochlorohydroxyquin See Quiniodochlor
Iodoquinol See Diiodohydroxyquin
Ion trapping 265
IP$_3$ (Inositol trisphosphate) See G protein
Ipecauanha (Ipecac) 499
Ipratropium bormide See Atropine
Ipsapirone 159
IPSP (inhibitory postsynaptic potential) See Chap 5
Irbesartan 403
Irinotecan 679
Iron 689
Iritants 708
Isocarboxazide 160
Isoflurane See GA 137
Isoniazid (INH) 604
Isoprenaline (Iso) 76
Isopropanol See β blocker
Isosorbide 355
Isosorbide dinitrate 355
Isosorbide mononitrate 355
Isotretinoin See Vit A
Isoxsuprine 76
Ispaghula 509
Itraconazole (ITR) 635
Ivermectin 643

J

Jarisch-Herxheimer reaction See Pn

K

Kala-azar See Leishmaniasis
Kanamycin (Kmc) 562
Keratolytics 704

Index

Ketamine *See* GA 142
Ketanserin 83, 461
Ketoconazole (KTZ) 633
Ketoprofen *See* NSAIDs
Ketorolac 219
Kidney disease and drugs 371
Kinetics of drugs
    elimination 17
Kinins: plasma 398
  receptors 409
Kinin antagonists 403

L

Labetalol *See* α + β blocker 85
Labour: induction/
    augmentation *See*
    Oxytocin
Lacidipine *See* CCB
Lactulose 511
Lamivudine 648
Lamotrigine 176
Laxatives 533, 537
Levamisole 637
Linezolid 568
Lansoprazole 518
Laplace equation *See* Chap 30
L-Asparaginase 676
Latanoprost *See* Chap 70
L-Dopa *See* Levodopa
Lead poisoning 690
Leavulose *See* Chap 70
Leflunomide 252
Leishmaniasis 610
Lepirudin 496
Lepra reaction 594
Leprosy, drugs for 591
  alternative regiments 594
  multidrug therapy
    (MDT) 594
Leracanidipine *See* Chap 70
Letrozole 675
Leucovorin *See* Folinic acid
Leukotrienes (LTs) 467–73
  antagonists *See* NSAIDs
Leuprolide 293
Levallorphan 185
Levarterenol *See* Noradrenaline
Levetiracetam 178
Levobunolol *See* Chap 70
Levobupivacaine *See* LA
Levodopa 246
Levofloxacin 583
Levonorgestrel *See* OC
LH (luteinizing hormone) *See*
    GnRH
Lidocaine *See* Lignocaine
Lie detector *See*
    Amphetamine
Lidoflazine *See* Chap 70
Ligand *See* EDTA
Lignocaine *See* GA
Lincomycin 591
Linezolid *See* Clindamycin

Liothyronine *See*
    Triiodothyronine
Lipid transport *See* Chap 2
Liquid paraffin 535
Lisinopril *See* Angiotensin
    converting enzyme
    inhibitors 403
Lethidrone 184
Lithium 160, 199
Lobeline 56
Local anaesthetics (LAs) 99–121
Lomefloxacin *See* Ganfloxacin
Lomustine (CCNU) *See*
    Anticancer
Loperamide 542
Lopinavir *See* Antiviral
Loratadine 414–19
Lorazepam *See* BZD
Losartan also *See* Angiotensin
    antagonist
Lovastatin 403
Loxapine *See* Reserpine
Loxatidine 153
Lugol's solution,
Lymecycline 575
Lypressin *See* ADH
Lynesternol *See* OC
Lysergic acid amide *See*
    LSD 211
Lysergic acid diethylamide
    (LSD) 211

M

MAC (Minimal alveolar
    concentration) *See* N_2O
MAC (*Mycobacterium avium*
    complex) drugs for *See*
    INH
Macrolides antibotics 586–92
Magaldrate 492
Magnesium 310, 491, 492
Male contraceptive 257
Malignant hyperthermia *See*
    Dautrolene
Malignant neuroleptic
    syndrome *See* Fentanyl
Mannitol 388
Mania 153
Manic depressive illness (MDI,
    bipolar disorder) *See* Li
Mannitol 388
Maprotiline 160
Marijuana *See* Bhang
Masking of infection 536
Mast cell stabilizers *See*
    Asthma
Mebendazole 637
Mebeverine *See* Chap 70
Mebhydroline 414
Mecamylamine 69
Mechlorethamine (mustine
    HCI) *See* Anticancer
Meclizine (meclozine) 414–19

Medroxyprogesterone
    acetate *See* OC
Mefloquine 617
Meglitinide 302
Melanizing agents 715
Meloxicam 220
Melphalan 656
Menadione 720
Mepacrine 600, 610
Meperidine *See* Pethidine
Mephenamic acid *See* NSAIDs
Mephenesin 91
Mephentermine 76
Mephobarbitone 126
Mepyramine 414
Mercaptopurine (6-MP) 670
Mercurial diuretics *See*
    Furosemide
Mersalyl *See* Diuretics
Mesalazine (5-ASA,
    mesalamine) 541
Mesterolone *See* Chap 70
Metabolism *See*
    Biotransformation 530
Metabolism *See* Presystemic
    (first pass)
Metamizol 220
Metaraminol 76
Metformin 302
Methacholine *See* ACh
Methacycline 575
Methadone 238
Methamphetamine 76
Methanol 183
Methaquolone 170
Methdilazine 414
Methenamine 590
Methicillin 547
Methicillin resistant *Staphylococcus aureus* (MRSA) *See*
    Pn
Methimazole 319
Methohexitone 126
Methotrexate (Mtx) 669
Methoxamine 76
Methoxsalen 707
Methyl alcohol *See* Ethanol
Methyldopa 407
Methylergometrine *See* DHE
Methyl polysiloxane 504
Methyl prednisolone 281
α-Methyl-p-tyrosine *See*
    Chap 5
4-Methyl pyrazole
    (fomepizole) *See*
    Chap 13
Methyl xanthines 546
Methysergide 464
Metipranolol *See* β blocker
Metoclopramide 528
Metoprolol *See* β blocker
Metronidazole 623
Metyrapone 209
Mezlocillin *See* Pn

Miconazole 619
Microsomal enzymes 15
Midazolam See BZD
Mifepristone 302
Miglitol 302
Migraine See Sumatriptan 465, 466
Milrinone 372
Mineralocorticoid See Steroid
Minimum bactericidal concentration (MBC) 537
Minimum inhibitiory cincentration (MIC) 537
Minocycline 575
Minoxidil 401
Mirtazapine See SSRI
Misoprostol See PG
Mitomycin C 675
Mitotane 290
Mitoxantrone 676
Mivacurium See SCh
MMF 683
Moclobemide 160
Molindone 153
Monoamine oxidase (MAO), inhibitors (MAOI) 160, 192–94
Monobactams 553
Montelukast 549
Mood stabilizer See Li
MOPP regimen See Anticancer
Moricizine See Cetrizine 379
Morphine 233–37
  dependence 179
  epidural/intrathecal See LA
  poisoning 181
Mosaprode 530
Motion sickness 506
Moxifloxacin See Ciprofloxacin
Mucokinetics See Expectorants 543
Mucolytics 520
Muromonab CD3 683
Muscarine 56
Muscarinic 51
  actions 56
  receptor 57
Muscle relaxants See SCh
Mushroom poisoning See ACh
Mustard Seeds 708
Mutagenicity of drugs See ADR
Mustine See Mechlorethamine 667
Myasthenia graivs See Anti-Ch E
Mycobacterium avium complex (MAC) infection See INH
Mycophenolate mofetil (MMF) 670
Mydriatics 69

Myocardial infarction (MI), drugs for 310
Myxoedema, also See Hypothyroidism

N

N-acetyl cysteine 222
Nafcillin 547
Nafazodone 160
Nalbuphine 241
Nalidixic acid 570
Nalorphine 240
Naloxone 241
Naltrexone 241
Naphazoline 76
Naproxen See NSAID
Narcotine See Noscapine 521
Nasal decongestants See Ephedrine 73
Natamycin 615
Nateglinide 302
Natural progesterone 250
Nefazodone 160
Nefopam 272
Nelfinavir See Acyclovir
Neomycin 584
Neostigmine 56
Netilmicin 564
Neurohumoral transmission 47
Neurolept analgesia See Fentanyl
Neuroleptic drugs See Antipsychotic drugs 190, 500
Neuromuscular blocking agents 97
Nevirapine 658
Newer drugs 784–89
Niacin (Vit B_3) 734
Nicardipine 345
Niclosamide 642
Nicorandil 356
Nicotinamide See Niacin
Nicotine See ACh
Nicotinic acid (Vit B_3)
Nicotinic actions See ACh
Nicotinic receptors See ACh
Nicoumalone See Acenocoumarol
Nidocromil 550
Nifedipine 387
Nimesulide 270
Nimodipine 346 See Chap 70
Nimorazole 610
Niridazole 629
Nitrates 392–97
Nitrate dependence/tolerance 353
Nitrazepam See BZD
Nitrendipine 388
Nitric oxide (NO) See Chap 7 132–34

Nitrofurantoin 570
Nitroglycerine See Glyceryl trinitrate
Nitroprusside sod 361
Nitrosoureas 668
Nitrous oxide (N_2O) See GA
Noncompetitive antagonism 29
Nonmicrosomal metabolism See Chap 2
Non-nucleoside reverse transcriptase inhibitors (NNRTIs) See AZT
Nonsedating anti-inflammatory drugs (NSAIDs) 206–23
Noradrenaline (NA) See Chaps 5 and 7
Norepinephrine See Noradrenaline
Norethisterone See Norethindrone
Northindrone enanthate (NEE) See OC
Norethynodrel See OC
Norfloxacin See Ciprofloxacin
Nortriptyline 160
Nortriptyline See SSRI
Nucleoside reverse transcriptase inhibitors (NRTIs) See AZT
Nylidrin See Chap 70
Nystatin 615

O

Obidoxime 56
Octreotide See Androgen
Ofloxacin See Ciprofloxacin 600
Oil of wintergreen See Methyl salicylate
Olanzapine 153
Olmesartan 403
Olsalazine 541
Omega-3 FA See Chap 70
Omerprazole 517
Oncovin See Vincristine
Ondansetron 530
On-off effect See Levodopa
Opioid See Morphine 217
Opium See Morphine
Oral
  absorption of drugs See Chap 1
  anticoagulants See Warfarin
  contraceptives (OCs) 254
  hypoglycaemics 302
  ion preparations See Anaemia
  oral rehydration salt/solution (ORS) 539
  route of administration See Chap 1

Organophosphates 229 *See* Chap 6
Organophosphate poisoning *See* Chap 6
Ormeloxifene 300
Ornidazole 626
Osmotic diuretics *See* Diuretics 429
Osmotic (saline) purgatives 536
Ouabain *See* Digitalis
Oxacillin 547
Oxazepam *See* BZD
Oxazolidinone antimicrobial 571
Oxeladin 521
Oxiconazole 701
Oxidation *See* Chap 2
Oximes *See* Chap 6
Oxotremorine 56
Oxpentifylline *See* Pentoxiphylline
Oxymetazoline 76
Oxyphedrine 398 *See* Chap 70
Oxyphenbutazone 214
Oxyphenonium *See* Chap 6
Oxytetracycline *See* Tetracycline
Oxytocics 308
Oxytocin 308
Oxytocin challenge test 261
Oxyuresis *See* Enterobiasis

P

PABA (Para-aminobenzoic acid) 705
Paclitaxel 673
2-PAM *See* Pralidoxime
Pancreatin 431
Pancuronium *See* SCh
Pantoprazole 489
Para-amino salicylic acid (PAS) 588
Paracetamol 221
Paraldehyde 135
Paramethasone 282
parasympathomimetic drugs *See* Cholinergic drugs
Parathion *See* Organophosphates
parathyroid hormone (PTH) 325–28
Parkinsonism *See* Levodopa
Paroxetine 160
Paroxysmal supraventricular tachycardia (PSVT) *See* Chap 32
Partial agonist *See* Chap 3
Pectin *See* Chap 70
Pefloxacin *See* Ciprofloxacin
Pempidine 69
Penciclovir 657

Penfluridol 153
Penicillamine 697
Penicillinase 543
Penicillins 564–74
 acid resistant 566
 benzathine 566
 benzyl (G) 566
 extended spectrum 567
 penicillinase resistant 568
 phenoxymethyl (V) 569
 procaine 569
 semisynthetic 568
Pentamidine 628
Pentazocine 185
Pentobarbitone 127
Pentolinium 69
Pentoxiphylline 398
Pentylene tetrazole (PTZ) 171
Pepsin 483
Peptic ulcer 483
Pergolide 193
Perindopril 444
Peripheral decarboxylase inhibitors *See* Levodopa
Permethrin 703
Pernicious anaemia *See* Iron
Pethidine 238
Pharmaceutics 2
Pharmacodynamics *See* Chap 3
Pharmacokinetics 7
Pharmacology, definition 1
Pharmacotherapeutics 2
Pharmacy, definition 3
Phenazopyridine 571
Phenformin 302
Pheniramine 414–19
Phenobarbitone 127
Phenolphthalein 535
Phenothiazines *See* SSRI 188
Phenoxybenzamine 83
Phentolamine 83
Phenylbutazone 266
Phenylephrine 76
Phencyclidine 170
Phenyl propanolamine *See* Chap 5
Phenytoin 172
Pholcodeine 182
Phospholipase C-IP$_3$-DAG pathway *See* Chap 3
Photochemotherapy (PUVA) 706, 707
Photosensitivity 706
Phylloquinone *See* Vitamin K
Physostigmine 56
Phytonadione *See* Vitamin K$_1$
Picrotoxin 202
Pilocarpine 56
Pimozide 153
Pindolol *See* β blocker
Pinocytosis *See* Chap 2
Pioglitazone 352

Pipecuronium *See* SCh
Piperacillin 547
Piperazine 641
Piracetam 203
Piribedil 193
Piroxicam 271
Pizotifen 461
pKa *See* Chap 2
Plantago 535
Plasma expanders 509–12
Plasma half life (t½) *See* Chap 2
Plasma protein binding 12
Platelet activating factor (PAF) 472, 473
 anatagonists 438
Plicamycin 675
Polydocanol *See* Chap 70
Polygeline 510
Polymyxin B, E 569
Polypeptide antibiotics *See* Clindamycin 589
Polyvinyl pyrrolidone (PVP) 481
Post antibiotic effect (PAE) 537
Potassium 390
 channel openers 397–99
 sparing diuretics 425, 426
Povidone iodine *See* Chap 70
Pralidoxime (2-PAM) 56
Pramipexole 196
Pravastatin *See* Lovastatin
Praziquantel 629
Prazosin 83
Preanaesthetic medication *See* GA
Prednisolone also *See* Corticosteroids 333
Presystemic (first pass) metabolism *See* Chap 2
Prilocaine *See* LA
Primaquine 620
Primidone 138
Prinzmetal's angina *See* Variant angina
Probenecid 256
Probucol 507
Procainamide 378
Procaine *See* LA
Procarbazine 677
Progabide 102
Progesterone 300
Progestins also *See* Oral contraceptives 250, 254
Prolactin (Prl) 284
Promethazine 414–19
Propafenone 338
Propionic acid derivatives 268
Propofol *See* GA 140
Propoxur 81 (also *See* Anticholinesterase poisoning)
Proptriptyline 160
Propranolol (Ppnl) 89
Propyl thiouracil 319

Prostacycline (PGI$_2$) 432
Prostaglandins (PGs) 432, 467–73, 489
  synthesis inhibitors See NSAIDs
Prostanoid receptors See PG
Protamine sulfate 482
Protamine zinc insulin (PZI) See Insulin
Protease inhibitors (PIs) See Antiretroviral
Proton pump inhibitors (PPIs) See Ranitidine
Pseudocholinesterase (BuChE) 53
Pseudoephedrine 76
Psoralen 707
Psychopharmacological agent (psychotropic drugs) See LSD
Psychostimulants 170
Psychotogens See Hallucinogens
Psychotomimetics See Hallucinogens
Putgatives 534
Purinethol See Mercaptopurine
Pyracetam 172
Pyrantel pamoate 641
Pyrazinamdie (Z) 608
Pyridostigmine 56
Pyridoxine See Vit B$_6$ 247
Pyrimethamine See Antimalarial 620
Pyritinol (pyrithioxine) 173 See Chap 70
Pyroxylon See Collodion

Q

Quinacillin 547
Quinacrine See Mepacrine 600
Quinapril 403
Quinidine 376
Quinine 618
Quiniodochlor 610
Quinolones 598
Quinupristin/Dalfopristin See Chindamycin

R

Rabeprazole 489
Raloxifene See Tamoxifen 299
Ramipril 403
Ranitidine, also See H$_2$ antagonists 517
Rapacuronium See SCh
Rauwolfia alkaloid See Reserpine
Receptors 23, 49
  enzymatic 23
  G protein coupled 26, 44

transducer mechanisms 26
  with intrinsic ion channel 22, 27
Rectal administration See Routes
Reflux esophagitis See Gastroesophageal reflux
Rehydration See ORS
Renal excretion of drugs See Excretion
Renin-angiotensin system (RAS) 439
Repaglinide 351
Replacement therapy See ORS
Reserpine 153, 362
Resistance: to AMAs 536
Resperidone 153, 425
Retinoic acid 705, 712
Retroviral protease inhibitors (PIs) 654–62
Reversal reaction See Leprosy
Reverse transcriptase inhibitors 656
Reversible inhibitors of MAO-A (RIMAs) See Selegiline
Ribavirin See Interferon 656
Riboflavin (Vit B$_2$) 722
Rickets See Vit D
Rifabutin See INH
Rifampin (Rifampicin R) 605
Rimantadine 655
rINN (recommended international nonproprietary name) See Chap 1
Reserpine 404
Risperidone See SSRI
Ritanserin 425
Ritodrine 76, 310
Ritonavir See Acyclovir
Rivastigmine 56
Rocuronium 70 See SCh
Rofecoxib 222
Ropinirole 194 See Chap 70
Ropivacaine See LA
Rosiglitazone 352
Routes of administration See Chap 1
Roxatidine, also See H$_2$ antagonists 517
Roxithromycin 507
Rubefacients 708
Rubidomucin See Daunorubicin
Rutin 445

S

Salbutamol 76
Salicylates See NSAID
Salicylazosulfapyridine See Sulfasalazine

Salicylic acid 705
Saline purgatives See Osmotic purgatives
Salmeterol 76
Saquinavir See Acyclovir
Satranidazole 612
Scabies, drugs for 703
Schizophrenia 152
  drugs for See Antipsychotic drugs
Sclerosing agents 446
Scopolamine See Hyoscine
Secobarbitone 126
Secnidazole 626
Secondary effects See GA (gas)
Second gas effect See GA (gas)
Sedative See BZD
Selective estrogen receptor modulators (SERMs) See Tamroxifen
Selegiline See MAOI
Selenium sulfide 705
Serotonergic receptors 420
Serotonin, See 5-hydroxy-tryptamine 457
Serotonin and noradrenaline reuptake inhibitor (SNRI) 160
Sertraline 160
Sevoflurane See GA
Sexually transmitted diseases, treatment of See Sulfonamide
Sibutramine See Anorectics
Side effects 731–51
Sildenafil 78
Simethicone See Dimethicone
Simvastatin See Hypolipidemics
Sisomicin 562
Skeletal muscle relaxants See SCh
Sleep 125
Smoking cessation: aid to 173
Sodium
  bicarbonate 490
  citrate 491
  cromoglycate 549
  nitroprusside See HTN 403
  stibogluconate 628
  valproate See Valproic acid
Soman See Physostigmine
Somatomedins See GH
Somatostatin 284
Sotalol See β blocker
Sparfloxacin See Ciprofloxacin
Spectinomycin 589
Spinal anaesthesia See LA
Spiramycin 587
Spironolactone 385
Spirulina See Chap 70
SRS-A See Leucotrienes
Stanozolol See Danazol

Statins (HMG-CoA reductase inhibtors) 500–508
Stavudine *See* AZT
Steroid receptor 225
Stilbestrol *See* Diethylstilbestrol
Streptogramin 591
Streptokinase 491
Streptomycin (S) 563
Streptozocin 668
Styptics 478
Subcutaneous injection (SC) *See* Route
Sublingual administration *See* Route
Succinylcholine (SCh) 88–90
Sucralfate 522
Sufentanil *See* Opium
Sulbactam 547
Sulbutamol 76
Sulbutiamine *See* Chap 70
Sulconazole 701
Sulfacetamide sod 575
Sulfadiazine 594
Sulfadoxine 595
Sulfamethoxazole 594
Sulfamethopyrazine 595
Sulfamoxole 575
Sulfanilamide 575
Sulfasalazine 541
Sulfinpyrazone 257
Sulfonamides 594
Sulfonylureas 348
Sulindac 221
Sulpiride 153
Sumatriptan 430
Sun screens 705
Superinfection (suprainfection) 536
Super ORS *See* ORT
Suramin 644
Surface anaesthesia *See* LA
Suxamethonium *See* Succinylcholine
Sympathetic nervous system *See* Chap 5
Sympathomimetics *See* Chap 7
Synthesis ACh, NA 46, 47

T

Tabun *See* Physostigmine
Tacrine *See* CNS stimulant
Tacrolimus 683
Tamoxifen citrate 299
Tamsulosin *See* Chap 70
Tannic acid/Tannins 707
Tarfenadine 414
Taxanes *See* Anticancers
Tazobactam *See* Pn
Tegoserod *See* Chap 70
Teicoplanin 568
Temazepam *See* BZD
Temoxicam *See* NSAIDs

Teratogenicity *See* ADR
Terazosin *See* α agonist
Terbinafine 635
Terfenadine *See* Cyproheptadine
Terlipressin 396
Testosterone *See* Androgen
Tetmosol 703
Tetracaine *See* LA
Tetracyclines 575–78
D^9-Tetrahydrocannabinol (D^9-THC) *See* CNS stimulant
Tetramisole 642
Tetrodotoxin *See* Chap 5
Theobromine 548
 theophylline 548
 Aminophylline 549
Therapeutic index 19
Therapeutic window phenomenon 19
Thiabendazole 639
Thiacetazone (Tzn) 607
Thiamine *See* Vit B_1
Thiazide diuretics 420–23
Thiazolidinediones *See* Oral hypoglycaemic
6-Thioguanine (6-TG) *See* Anticancer
Thiopentone 160
Thioproperazine 153
Thioridazirie 153
Thio-TEPA *See* Anticancer
Thioxthixene 153
Thread worm *See* Enterobiasis
Thrombolytics *See* Fibrinolytic drugs 459
Thromboxane A_2 (TXA_2) *See* PG
Thyroid disease and drugs 311
Thyroid hormones 311
Thyroid inhibitors 311–23
Thyrotoxicosis 264
 drugs for 270
Thyrotropin *See* TSH 311
Thyroxine (T_4) 262
Tiagabine 177
Tianeptine 160
Tibolone 298
Ticarcillin 547
Ticlopidine *See* Platelet inhibitor
TIK-20 *See* Diazion
Timolol *See* β blocker
Tinidazole 624
Tirofiban 495
Tissue type plasminogen activator (rt-PA, alteplase) *See* Fibrinolytics
Tizanidine 103
Tobacco *See* CNS stimulant 204–07
Tobramycin *See* Amikacin

Tocainide 380
Tocolytics *See* Uterine relaxants
Tolazamide 302
Tolbutamide 302
Tolcapone 194
Tolerance *See* ADR
Tolnaftate 701
Topical application of drugs 703–08
Topical NSAIDs 703
Topical steroids 703
 adverse effects of *See* ADR
Topiramate 177
Topotecan 679
Tramadol *See* Opium
Toxic effects 731–51
Toxicology, definition of 685
Toxoids *See* Vaccines
Tramadol *See* Opium
Tranexaemic acid 496
Transdermal therapeutic systems (TTS) 5
Transducer mechanisms *See* G protein
Transduction 557
Transmission 39
Transformation 557
Tranylcypromine 160
Traveller's diarrhoea *See* Doxycycline
Trazodone 160
Tretinoin *See* Vit A
Triamcinolone 281
Triamterene 426
Triazolam *See* BZD
Triazole antifungals 617
Trichlophos 170
Tichomoniasis, drugs for 610
Tricyclic antidepressants 164, 198
Trifluoperazine 186
Trifluperidol 186
Triflupromazine 186
Trihexyphenidyl *See* Atropine
Triiodothyronine (T_3) *See* TH
Trimazocin *See* β blocker
Trimetazidine *See* Chap 70
Trimethadione 141
Trimethaphan camforsulfonate 69, 361
Trimethoprim + sulfamethoxazole *See* Cotrimoxazole 596
Trimipramine 414
Trioxasalen 707
Tripotassium dicitrato-bismuthate (CBS) *See* Antacid
Troglitazone 302
Troprolidine 414
Trovafloxacin 703–08
Tuberculosis 585
 biology of infection 589
 chemoprophylaxis 589

conventional regimens 590
corticosteroids in 589
in AIDS patients 589
in breast feeding
    women 590
in pregnancy 590
multidrug resistant
    (MDR) 590
short course chemotherapy
    (SCC) 590
treatment of 589
Tunocurarine (d-TC) 97
Tyramine See MAOI
Tyrothricin 569

U

Ulcer healing drugs See
    Omeprazole
Ulcer protectives See Antacid
Universal antidote See
    Poisoning
Ureido penicillins See Pn
Uricosuric drugs See
    Allopurinol
Urokinase 491
Ursodeoxycholic acid
    (ursodiol) 505
Uterine
    relaxants 259–61
    stimulants 259–61

V

Vaccines 701
    bacterial 701–08
    BCG 701–08
    cholera, inactivated 701–08
    cholera, oral 701–08
    double antigen (DT-
        DA) 701–08
    Haemophilus influenzae type b
        (Hib) 701–08
    hepatitis A 701–08
    hepatitis B 701–08
    influenza 701–08
    killed (inactivated) 701–08
    live attenuated 701–08
    measles: live
        attenuated 701–08
    meningococcal 701–08

MMr (measles, mumps,
    rubella) 701–08
plague 701–08
polio: inactivated (IPV,
    Salk) 701–08
polio: oral (OPV,
    Sabin) 701–08
rabies: carbolized (Semple
    vaccine) 701–08
rabies : purified chick embryo
    cell vaccine
    (PCEV) 701–08
rabies: human diploid cell
    (HDCV) 701–08
rabies: purified vero cell
    (PVRV) 701–08
rubella 701–08
TAB 701–08
TABC 701–08
triple antigen (DPT) 701–08
typhoid-Ty21a (oral) 701–08
typhoid: Vi
    polysaccharide 701–08
varicella (live
    attenuated) 701–08
viral 701–08
whooping cough
    (pertussis) 701–08
Valacyclovir 657
Valdecoxib 223
Valethamate See Chap 70
Valproic acid 175
Valsartan 403
VAMP regimen See Anticancer
Vancomycin 588
Vasicant 708
Vasomotor reversal 83
Vasopressin See Antidiuretic
    hormone
Vecuronium 100
Venereal diseases: treatment of
    See Sexually transmitted
    diseases
Venlafaxine 160
Verapamil 341, 389
VIAGRA See Sildenafil
Vidarabine 651
Vinblastine 662
Vinca alkaloids 673
Vincristine 673
Vinorelbine 675
Visual cycle, Vit A 712

Vitamins 717–36
    definition 717
    fat soluble 717
Vit A 717
Vit B complex 729
Vit B_{12} 723
Vit C 727
Vit D 722
Vit E 729
Vit K 4 77, 728
Volume of distribution (V) 11

W

Warfarin sod 483
Wines See Ethanol
Withdrawal reactions See ADR
Wood alcohol See Ethanol

X

Xanthines See
    Methylxanthines
Xanthinol nicotuate See
    Chap 70
Xipamide See Diuretics
Xylometazoline 76

Y

Yohimbine 83
Young's formula 29

Z

Zafirlukast 549
Zalcitabine 653
Zaleplon See Chap 70
Zephiran, See Benzalkonium
Zidovudine (AZT) 652
Zileuton 526
Zinc See Skin drugs
    pyrithione 705
Zofenopril 403
Zolasartan 403
Zollinger-Ellison
    syndrome See
    Ranitidine
Zolpidem 127
Zopiclone 127